Social Paediatrics

Social Paediatrics

Edited by

Bengt Lindström
*The Nordic School of Public Health,
Gothenburg, Sweden*

and

Nick Spencer
*School of Postgraduate Medical Education
and Department of Applied Social Studies,
University of Warwick, Coventry, UK*

Oxford   New York   Tokyo
OXFORD UNIVERSITY PRESS
1995

Oxford University Press, Walton Street, Oxford OX2 6DP
Oxford   New York
Athens   Auckland   Bangkok   Bombay
Calcutta   Cape Town   Dar es Salaam   Delhi
Florence   Hong Kong   Istanbul   Karachi
Kuala Lumpur   Madras   Madrid   Melbourne
Mexico City   Nairobi   Paris   Singapore
Taipei   Tokyo   Toronto
and associated companies in
Berlin   Ibadan

Oxford is a trade mark of Oxford University Press

Published in the United States
by Oxford University Press Inc., New York

Bengt Lindström, Nick Spencer, and the contributors list on pp. xiii–xiv, 1995

All rights reserved. No part of this publication may be
reproduced, stored in a retrieval system, or transmitted, in any
form or by any means, without the prior permission in writing of Oxford
University Press. Within the UK, exceptions are allowed in respect of any
fair dealing for the purpose of research of private study, or criticism or
review, as permitted under the Copyright, Designs and Patents Act, 1988, or
in the case of reprographic reproduction in accordance with the terms of
licences issued by the Copyright Licensing Agency. Enquiries concerning
reproduction outside those terms and in other countries should be sent to
the Rights Department, Oxford University Press, at the address above.

This book is sold subject to the condition that it shall not,
by way of trade or otherwise, be lent, re-sold, hired out, or otherwise
circulated without the publisher's prior consent in any form of binding
or cover other than that in which it is published and without a similar
condition inducing this condition being imposed
on the subsequent purchaser.

A catalogue record for this book is available for the British Library

Library of Congress Cataloging in Publication Data
(Data available)

ISBN 0 19 262179 3

Typeset by EXPO Holdings, Malaysia
Printed in Great Britain by Biddles Ltd, Guildford and King's Lynn

Preface

Childhood is the anvil of adulthood—it shapes future generations. Childhood also has a value of its own, not merely as a passage to adult life. Recognition of the importance and vulnerability of childhood is relatively recent and has reached its peak in the *United Nations Convention on the rights of the child*, a document prepared 'for the best interests of the child'. The *Convention* and the child health targets of the WHO *Health for all by the year 2000* (*HFA* 2000) initiative constitute both a goal for governments and professional and voluntary agencies and a guide and incentive to multi-agency, intersectoral working.

Individual child health professionals have made significant contributions to the realization and philosophy of the UN Convention and the *HFA* child health targets. However, traditional paediatrics has been concerned primarily with the disease process in the individual child, an orientation reflected in the main paediatric textbooks and research literature. A different approach is required to respond to the challenge of the Convention and the HFA child health targets.

Social paediatrics is concerned with social, political, environmental, and family influences on child health at population and individual levels. It is not divorced from traditional paediatrics but sets it in its social and family context. It builds on the work of Robert Debre, John Apley, Ronnie McKeith, Michel Manciaux, Lennart Köhler, and many other far-sighted child health professionals. It enables child health professionals to look beyond the disease process in the individual child and address the major social determinants of childhood ill-health.

This book, the first comprehensive English language textbook of social paediatrics, joins the French text, Mande *et al.* (1977) *Pédiatrie sociale*, Flammarion, Paris, in providing the theoretical framework for child health professionals, both in training and in established practice, striving to adopt new approaches and meet new challenges. The book has a European orientation reflecting the disintegration of post-war barriers within Europe and the cooperation between states with different traditions implicit in the development and proposed expansion of the European Community. At the same time, it addresses some of the adverse consequences for child health of the resurgence of dormant conflicts and the breakdown of social structures which have followed the collapse of communism in Eastern and Central Europe.

The rapidity of change in Europe has overtaken the preparation of this book. Throughout the text where reference is made to countries such as Yugoslavia, the USSR, and the German Democratic Republic, they are referred to as 'former'.

As members of the executive committee of the European Society for Social Paediatrics (ESSOP), we have been privileged to organize and teach on a series of training courses held across Europe since 1985. This experience has helped us formulate the structure and philosophy of the book and provided us with invaluable insights and contacts. The authors are drawn from all over Europe, as well as a few from the United States, giving a broad perspective on child health themes and problems. The important lessons of the struggle for health in the developing world are summarized in a chapter in the opening section in order to set the largely European experience in a wider context.

The book has a common theme—a positive approach to the promotion of the health of children, individually and collectively, by recognizing and seeking to change adverse social, political, environmental, and family influences and enhancing the quality of life for all children. The important aspects of social paediatrics are covered but no attempt is made to describe in detail the clinical features of specific problems such as child abuse and neglect. These are dealt with in much greater detail in many other texts; here they are viewed in a broader context with emphasis on European comparisons and a positive approach to prevention and management.

In the first part, an introduction to social paediatrics, Michel Manciaux, a leading European social paediatrician, considers the history of social paediatrics and the public health approach to child health. The historical development of the approach to child health, which forms the basis of social paediatrics, is traced. Lennart Köhler and Keith Barnard focus on child populations and argue for a 'child public health' approach. They consider the development of a distinctive child public health approach through the WHO *HFA 2000* targets and the *Healthy cities* initiative. The editors, with Concha Colomer, survey the current state of social paediatrics in Europe and the research interests of the members of ESSOP. The development of the social paediatric approach to child health is recorded in the survey, as are the limitations and barriers to future progress. The continuing philosophical and organizational bias towards curative paediatrics across most of Europe is highlighted and the tasks facing social paediatricians outlined.

The crucial importance of the UN Convention and the *HFA 2000* initiative in reorientating child health practice is reflected in the introductory section and, in the reminder of the book, constant reference is made to these key initiatives. Their philosophy and aims are essentially those of this textbook. The final chapter of the first part serves to illustrate the enormous tasks facing those who wish to see the realization of the aims of the Convention and *HFA 2000*; children in developing countries suffer deprivations long forgotten in parts of Europe and it is important to keep their plight in focus and learn from the important gains that have been made in primary child health care against huge odds. These lessons are of particular importance to child health professionals working in areas of Europe affected by industrial decline, poverty, and war.

The second part examines socio-demographic trends in Europe which have particular relevance to child health. Jitka Rychtaříková outlines the changes in pregnancy and birth-weight since the Second World War and Aldona Sito looks at family structure changes with particular reference to Poland. The changing patterns of childhood mortality and morbidity are addressed by Roy Carr-Hill. The trends outlined in this section form an essential background to subsequent chapters as they exert a profound influence on all aspects of child health.

The next part considers two major global threats to child health: the first is an ancient threat which has reared its head again in Europe and the other is a new threat which offers a major challenge to health promotion and carries with it many moral and ethical dilemmas. Tytti Solantaus details the effects of war on children directly and in the form of the psychological damage associated with the fear of war. Catherine Peckham and Marie-Louise Newell examine HIV and its implications for child health.

The fourth part considers major environmental influences on child health, the importance of which are increasingly being recognized. Sheena Nakou examines in detail the evidence for the effects of pollution on child health and Bjarne Jansson and Leif Svanström, based on the extensive Swedish experience of child accident prevention, consider community-based responses to the mortality and morbidity associated with childhood accidents.

Part V is concerned with concepts of normality. Knowledge of the normal range of child development and growth are essential to the identification of variations from normal. However, concepts of normality and childhood itself are changing constantly. Chris Jenks explores the historical basis of the modern concept of childhood and the conflicting trends within its development. Jean-Claude Vuille and Clas Sundelin consider differing perspectives on growth and development and the concept of critical periods in child development illustrated by specific examples. Risk and risk-taking as a 'normal' part of growing up is addressed in detail by Vivien Igra and Charles Irwin; the correlations and associations of particular forms of risk-taking are considered.

In Part VI the focus shifts to more specific child health problems. Ulla Fasting looks at the problems, clinical and ethical, associated with new treatments and treatment opportunities. A range of problems which can be grouped under the 'new' morbidity—behaviour disorders, suboptimal nutrition, unexpected infant death, child abuse, and special needs—are considered in their European context. The authors do not deal with clinical presentations but review these problems in their social and family contexts.

The next part considers those children who are especially vulnerable within modern societies and who are disadvantaged either by poverty, low birthweight, ethnic origin, or family breakdown. The chapters consider each of these groups whilst recognizing that there are frequently a multiplicity of deprivations which affect children. In the final chapter of the section, Ian Goodyer presents a detailed account of protective factors which seem to ensure that some vulnerable children survive adversity more effectively than others. Positive approaches arising from this detailed review should assist child health services in formulating appropriate interventions to counteract the adverse effects of disadvantage.

The final two parts consider issues for the child health services and some important innovations which positively enhance child health and quality of life. Traditional divisions between agencies have acted as barriers to the achievement of improved child health. The intersectoral strategies considered in Part VIII indicate some of the ways of working to break down these barriers. Immunization has been one of the most effective preventive strategies; Stuart Logan and Helen Bedford discuss the problems and possible solutions in implementing immunization programmes. They point out that the information systems required are more complex than might first appear and that immunization programmes need a higher priority; they cannot be left to run themselves.

Aidan Macfarlane, in considering the difficult issue of outcome measures in child health, argues that health services cannot avoid scrutiny of the effectiveness of the services they offer. His chapter explores 'best practice' in evaluating services for children whilst warning against the inappropriate use of outcome measures to answer questions they are unable to address.

Child health promotion is considered separately though its philosophy underpins much of the content of this book. Concha Colomer stresses the distinction between promotion and health education; promotion is concerned with creating healthy environments within and outside the home rather than simply educating parents and placing the onus on them to ensure the health of their child. Berlith Persson give an account of a the creation of a nourishing and positive environment in the heart of technological paediatrics—the neonatal intensive care unit. Her chapter illustrates that strategies designed to enhance health and life quality can be introduced even in the most adverse circumstances. The parents to whom her chapter gives voice speak eloquently of the value and importance of these strategies.

Partnership with parents, which remains a dream in current child health services, is considered along with community diagnosis and participation strategies. The increasing experience in these innovative approaches is considered as well as their far-reaching implications for all professional agencies. The final chapter explores the new frontier of health—the measurement and enhancement of quality of life for all children. The success of future child health services could be decided not on the number of new medical treatments devised but on their contribution to quality of life for all children.

This textbook has neither the form nor the content of a traditional paediatric text. We make no apologies for this difference; this book sets out to address issues beyond the disease process in individual children. We have attempted to provide a theoretical and philosophical framework for those wishing to face the challenge of enhancing life quality for all children and to indicate practical approaches for whole services and individual child health professionals.

1994

B.L.
N.S.

Contents

List of contributors   xiii

PART I INTRODUCTION TO SOCIAL PAEDIATRICS

1. What is social paediatrics and where does it come from?   3
   Michel Manciaux

2. Child health as a public health issue   12
   Lennart Köhler and Keith Barnard

3. Social paediatrics in Europe   22
   Nick Spencer, Bengt Lindström, and Concha Colomer

4. For the best interests of the child—the *UN Convention on the rights of the child*   36
   Bengt Lindström

5. The situation of children in developing countries   45
   Oriol Vall and Oscar Garcia

PART II SOCIAL AND DEMOGRAPHIC TRENDS IN EUROPE

6. Demographic trends in pregnancy and birth-weight   71
   Jitka Rychtaříková

7. Demographic trends in families in Europe—with particular reference to Poland   81
   Aldona Sito

8. Trends in childhood mortality and morbidity   95
   Roy A. Carr-Hill

Part III GLOBAL THREATS TO CHILD HEALTH

9. Children and war   111
   Tytti Solantaus

10. Children and HIV infection   128
    Marie-Louise Newell and Catherine Peckham

PART IV CHILDREN AND THE ENVIRONMENT

11. Pollution and child health   153
    Sheena Nakou

12	National inequalities in accident mortality among children and adolescents in the European countries *Bjarne Jansson and Leif Svanström*	174

PART V CONCEPTS OF NORMALITY

13	Historical perspectives on childhood *Chris Jenks*	195
14	Growth and development *Jean-Claude Vuille and Claes Sundelin*	210
15	Risk and risk-taking in adolescents *Vivien Igra and Charles E. Irwin Jr*	225

PART VI THE NEW MORBIDITY

16	The new iatrogenesis *Ulla Fasting*	259
17	Suboptimal nutrition *Ann Aukett and Brian Wharton*	270
18	Unexpected death in infancy *Elizabeth Taylor*	297
19	Child abuse and neglect *Stella Tsitoura*	310
20	Young children with special needs *Agnes Lànyi Engelmayer*	331
21	Adolescents and young people with special needs *Robert Wm Blum, Joan-Carles Suris, and Joan Patterson*	341

PART VII VULNERABLE CHILDREN

22	Children in poverty *Nick Spencer and Hilary Graham*	361
23	Low birth-weight infants *Pauline Verloove-Vanhorick*	380
24	Children and families in distress: the case of family breakdown *Bengt Lindström and Lennart Köhler*	397
25	Immigrant and ethnic minority children *John Black*	412
26	Risk and resilience processes in childhood and adolescence *Ian M. Goodyer*	433

PART VIII SERVICE AND INTERSECTORAL ISSUES

27	Planning and managing child health services *Louis Martín Alvárez and Joaquín Uris Sellés*	459
28	Intersectoral approaches to promoting health and children *Bob Chamberlin and Barbara Wallace*	469
29	Outcome and performance measures in child health *Aidan Macfarlane*	477
30	Implementing immunization programmes *Stuart Logan and Helen Bedford*	498
31	Child health promotion *Concha Colomer*	512

PART IX EXPLORING SOLUTIONS AND PRACTICAL POSITIVE CHANGE

32	Can we create a more optimal hospital environment? *Berlith Persson*	527
33	Partnership with parents *Nick Spencer*	540
34	Community diagnosis and participation *Jon Cook, Michel Pechevis, and Tony Waterston*	550
35	Measuring and improving quality of life for children *Bengt Lindström*	570
Index		587

Contributors

Dr Ann Aukett   Consultant Community Paediatrician, Dudley Road Hospital, Birmingham, UK.
Keith Barnard   WHO Consultant, Nordic School of Public Health, Gothenburg, Sweden.
Helen Bedford   Institute of Child Health, University of London, 30 Guilford Street, London, UK
Dr John Black   Paediatrician, Denmark Hill, London, UK.
Professor Robert Wm Blum   Division of General Pediatrics and Adolescent Health, National Center for Youth with Disabilities and the Center for Children with Chronic Illness and Disability, University of Minnesota, Minneapolis, USA.
Dr Roy A. Carr-Hill   Institute of Education, University of London, 20 Bedford Way, London, UK.
Dr Bob Chamberlin   Paediatrician, Maternal and Child Health, Canterbury, New Hampshire, USA.
Dr Concha Colomer   School of Public Health (IVESP), Valencia, Spain.
Jon Cook   Anthropologist, Centre International de l'Enfance, Paris, France.
Agnes Lànyi Engelmayer, Educationalist, Institute of Psychology, Budapest, Hungary.
Ulla Fasting   Nurse Specialist, Aarhus, Denmark.
Oscar Garcia   Paediatric Registrar, Barcelona, Spain.
Professor Ian M. Goodyer   Section of Developmental Psychiatry, University of Cambridge, UK.
Professor Hilary Graham   Department of Applied Social Studies, University of Warwick, Coventry, UK.
Dr Vivien Igra   Senior Fellow, Division of Adolescent Medicine, University of California, San Francisco, California, USA.
Charles E. Irwin Jr
Dr Bjarne Jansson   Associate Professor, Karolinska Institute, Department of International Health and Social Medicine, Kronan Health Centre, Sundbyberg, Sweden.
Chris Jenks   Department of Sociology, Goldsmith's College, University of London, UK.
Professor Lennart Köhler, Director   The Nordic School of Public Health, Gothenburg, Sweden.
Dr Bengt Lindström   The Nordic School of Public Health, Gothenburg, Sweden.
Dr Stuart Logan   Senior Lecturer in Paediatric Epidemiology, Institute of Child Health, University of London, 30 Guilford Street, London, UK.
Dr Aidan Macfarlane   Consultant in Public Health Medicine, Oxfordshire Health Authority, Oxford, UK.
Professor Michel Manciaux   School of Public Health, University of Nancy, Nancy, France.
Dr Louis Martin Alvárez   Pediatra, Centro de Salud Barrio del Pilar, Asesor Salud Pública Consejería de Sanidad, Communidad Autónoma de, Madrid, Spain.

Dr Sheena Nakou   Institute of Clinical Health, Athens, Greece.
Dr Marie-Louise Newell   Institute of Child Health, University of London, 30 Guilford Street, London, UK.
Dr Joan Patterson   Assistant Professor, School of Public Health; Director of Research, The Center for Children with Chronic Illness and Disability, University of Minnesota, Minneapolis, USA.
Dr Michel Pechevis   Paediatrician, Centre International de l'Enfance, Paris, France.
Professor Catherine Peckham   Institute of Child Health, University of London, 30 Guilford Street, London, UK.
Berlith Persson   Nursing Director, Department of Paediatrics, Helsingborg Hospital, Helsingborg, Sweden.
Dr Jitka Rychtaříková   Department of Demography & Geodemography, Charles University, Prague, Czech Republic.
Dr Joaquín Uris Sellés   Paediatrician, Centro de Salud Cuidad Jardín, Alicante; Associate Professor, Department of Public Health, Faculty of Medicine, University of Alicante, Spain.
Dr Aldona Sito   Paediatrician, Associate Professor, Head, Department of Family Health, Institute of Mother and Child, Warsaw, Poland.
Dr Tytti Solantaus   Child Psychiatric Clinic, Helsinki University, Lastenlinnantie, Helsinki, Finland.
Professor Nick Spencer   School Postgraduate Medical Education and Department of Applied Social Studies, University of Warwick, Coventry, UK.
Dr Claes Sundelin   Associate Professor, Department of Paediatrics, Uppsala University, Uppsala, Sweden.
Dr Joan-Carles Suris   Fellow, Adolescent Health Program, University of Minnesota, Minneapolis, USA.
Professor Leif Svanström   Karolinska Institute, Department of International Health and Social Medicine, Kronan Health Centre, Sundbyberg, Sweden.
Dr Elizabeth Taylor   Senior lecturer in Community Paediatrics, Department of Paediatrics, Sheffield Children's Hospital, Sheffield, UK.
Dr Stella Tsitoura   Paediatrician, Agra Sophia Children's Hospital Athens, Greece.
Dr Oriol Vall   Head of Department of Paediatrics, Barcelona, Spain.
Professor S. Pauline Verloove-Vanhorick   Head, Department of Child Health, TNO Prevention and Health, The Netherlands.
Professor Jean-Claude Vuille   School Health Service, Bern, Switzerland.
Barbara Wallace   South of Tyne Health Commission, Newcastle, UK.
Dr Tony Waterston   Consultant Community Paediatrician, Newcastle General Hospital, Newcastle, UK.
Professor Brian Wharton   Professor Emeritus, Department of Child Health, Glasgow, UK.

PART I

Introduction to social paediatrics

This part introduces social paediatrics. The historical development of paediatrics and the place of social paediatrics within this development are considered. The relationship of child health to public health is discussed as part of the WHO *Health for all by the year 2000* and the *Healthy cities* initiatives. A survey of social paediatric practice and research presents the current activity of European social paediatrician and indicates the key areas for future development. In view of its seminal importance, the *UN Convention on the rights of the child* is considered in a separate chapter and the enormity of the task facing those wishing to see the Convention enacted for all children throughout the world is highlighted by the final chapter in the part which deals with children in developing countries.

1 What is social paediatrics and where does it come from?

Michel Manciaux

Trying to define social paediatrics at the outset of a textbook devoted to this topic is not easy. If paediatrics is, according to the Court report (Court 1976), 'the care of the developing and depending human being in health and disease', is it right to consider social paediatrics as only a branch of general paediatrics, like, for instance, neuro- or cardio-paediatrics? Certainly not. Is it then the part of public health concerning children? Yes it is, since it deals with the health of a given subgroup (or rather several subgroups, if only by age: infants, children, youngsters ...) of the global population, and represents a meeting point of several disciplines contributing interactively to the global health of these groups. However, it is more than that: social paediatrics is also concerned with the psychosocial aspects of health and disease of individual children.

Social paediatrics existed in fact before it was clearly defined, which was done in Lisbon, during the International Congress of Paediatrics in 1962. Two definitions were given in the course of a round table discussion on the subject. The first, by Robert Debré, ran thus: 'Since a collective—either local, national or international—action is in process, paediatrics becomes social' (Debré 1963). The second, by Nathalie Masse, seems more comprehensive: 'Social paediatrics considers the child—either healthy or ill—in the context of the human groups which he/she belongs to and of the circles in which he/she develops' (Masse 1962). Indeed, a combination of these two definitions would encompass both aspects of social paediatrics: its population dimension and its global approach.

As for public health, no definition is fully comprehensive and generally accepted. A more appropriate approach would be to concentrate on the field of activities pertaining to the health, care and welfare of children. This forms the basis of the rest of this chapter.

History

When did paediatrics as such appear for the first time? It is difficult to say, but the philosophy of the Enlightenment in the eighteenth century is a likely starting point: it was during this period that, in Europe, a great number of physicians began to show some concern about children's health and diseases. For example, Rosen von Rosenstein, a Swede, published in 1753 *The diseases of children and their remedies* which was issued five times, translated into eight languages, and circulated throughout the whole of Europe. In 1760, the physician Des Essarts, from Paris, wrote *Traité de l'éducation médicinale des enfants en bas âge*, while, in 1767, George Armstrong, a Scotsman who lived in London, published his *Essay on the diseases most fatal to infants*. These are only three of the great number of authors renowned at this period. Though oriented towards children's disease, these books also contain chapters that could belong to social paediatrics: on breastfeeding; on mother and child's education; and on inoculation of vaccine, the forerunner of immunization. In 1767, George Armstrong opened the first clinic for children of poor families. It was the launching of the movement.

The expression 'médecine sociale' was coined by Jules Guérin, a French physician, who was the first, in 1848, to create a heading on this subject in *La Gazette Médicale de Paris*. But the most famous physician in French social medicine was Villermé, who published some observations that were really epidemiological, even before this word was ever used. Two of them are worth mentioning. Measuring young men living in Paris and called for their military service, Villermé noticed marked differences between the height of these young recruits according to the part of Paris they came from. He deduced that the influence of poverty on growth is greater than that of climate. In 1840, Villermé wrote, in an essay entitled 'La misère des ouvriers de l'industrie du coton', 'While in the families of manufacturers, merchants, drapers, directors of factories half the children reach the age of 29, this same half disappears before the age of two in the families of weavers and workers in cotton mills'. Thus he brings in both the notions of differential growth according to socio-economic classes and of differential mortality according to the socio-professional status of the parents (Villermé 1979).

While the German school, following Czerny's ideas, was more concerned with hygiene and the feeding of children and, in Vienna, Semmelweis was fighting against puerperal fever, the great killer of mothers and newborn babies, Pasteur was developing Jenner's work towards the theory and practice of immunization. At the turn of the century, the Society for the Prevention of Cruelty to Children was created, in London.

This is how, little by little, the different components of social paediatrics were assembled, even before paediatrics existed in its own right.

It is during critical periods that humanity achieves the greatest progress. Indeed, social paediatrics has gained from the tragic situations created in Europe by industrialization in the second half of the nineteenth century and beginning of the twentieth century, and by the two world wars. The industrial revolution brought about a wild exploitation of children's labour. Villermé described in his report the condition of working children: 'The working hours are the same for all ages: 13 hours and a half a day. Night work and work on Sundays are not spared to them; in factories or in mines, from the age of six, they work in such conditions that their physical and mental health is rapidly ruined'. No wonder that in France the first legal text on the protection of the child was a bill prohibiting work in a factory under the age of eight and limiting the number of working hours in a day to 12 for children under the age of 12. However, not until 1894 was children's working in the mines definitively prohibited. The situation was the same in England where Engels and Owen, even before Marx, give a description of the industrial slavery of children (Engels 1960). We must not forget this relatively recent shameful history when we pass judgement on the labour of children in the Third World.

As a counterpoint, interesting initiatives appeared occasionally in Europe in favour of children of poor families: free clinics, centres for the distribution of free milk, where it is notable that generosity was accompanied by a concern for hygiene which was based on the Pasteur discoveries. Here, the protestant tradition of health education of the people played an important role. As paediatricians did not yet exist as such, these achievements were often initiated by obstetricians—Budin, for example, in Paris in 1901.

The consequences of the two world wars were such a disaster for children's health that the rise of infant mortality suppressed for a while the progress that had been made. But they were also, because of this situation, the origin of new initiatives, on local, regional, national, and international levels, which heralded better days.

After the First World War, activities that were in the interest of children became more and more numerous. The Red Cross, voluntary organizations, charities, and institutions took into care orphans and sick children suffering from undernourishment, tuberculosis, handicaps, and so on ... In Belgium in 1919, the Oeuvre National de l'Enfance was created, with ambitious objectives: medico-social and educational activities directed at families and young children; assistance for children with handicaps; information, documentation, and health education for the general public; research work. Similar organizations were set up in other places at that time and developed between the wars.

However, it was only after the Second World War that concern about mother and child health really developed; in France, a bill was passed which inspired legislation in many other developed countries and, later on but with less success, in countries of the Third World when they became independent. At the same time, a number of paediatricians interested in the preventive and social aspects of their discipline initiated the activities of social paediatrics.

Chairs of child health were created in Universities in Great Britain, along with the National Children's Bureau. An international study on growth and development of the child, coordinated by the International Children's Centre, brought together teams of researchers: Graffar and Sand in Belgium; Tanner and Hindley in Great Britain; Masse, Sempé, and Roy in France; Karlberg and Duchateau in Sweden; Andrea Prader in Switzerland; not to mention countries outside Europe (Centre International de l'Enfance 1980).

Evidence of the dynamic development which has enabled the purely clinical aspects of paediatrics to evolve into real social paediatrics include nutrition and immunization; the work of the Newcastle team (Miller *et al.* 1974) with '*One thousand families*'; perinatal problems studied in the well known 'British perinatal survey' initiated in March 1946 by Douglas and followed up through the years by Alberman, Butler, Illsley, and others (Butler and Alberman 1969); prevention of accidents with the pioneer work of Berfenstam in Uppsala; the rapid expansion of child psychiatry; the teaching of paediatrics and the creation, under the aegis of the World Health Organization Regional Office for Europe, of the 'Association for paediatric education in Europe' with Doxiadis, Jackson, Sjölin, and Veneklaas. Together with Raymond Mande and Nathalie Masse we tried to achieve a synthesis of all these activities in the first French textbook on social paediatrics, published in 1972, re-edited in 1976, and subsequently translated into Spanish (Mande et al. 1977)

This interest in the child took an international turn with the creation of UNICEF in 1946. Two of its promoters were Robert Debré and Ludwik Rajchmann. Before talking about the latter, let us recall the memory of Janusz Korczak, a Polish Jew—a physician, teacher, and health educator, he was entirely devoted to the orphans of Warsaw and accompanied them to their death in the gas chambers of the camp at Treblinka. Of his literary work one book especially must be mentioned: *Le droit de l'enfant au respect* (Korczak 1979), which was half a century in advance of the *UN Convention on the rights of the child*.

Ludwik Rajchmann, Director of the Institute of Hygiene in Warsaw was, between the two world wars, founder and driving force of the Committee of Hygiene of the League of Nations before he created UNICEF in December 1946, of which he was the first Executive director (Balinksa 1991). UNICEF (United Nations International Children's Emergency Fund) was created in order to help children in Europe who were victims of the war—those who were orphans, sick, handicapped, displaced, under-nourished, and so on. But the situation evolved very quickly. With the help of the Marshall Plan and their own efforts, many of the countries of Western Europe were soon able to meet the needs of their children. The Iron Curtain became a limit to the field of action of UNICEF; there was a risk of its being disbanded, its task at times being made impossible. Rajchmann and Debré pooled their efforts to convince the United Nations and their State Members that the fate of the world's children was at stake and that UNICEF should develop and spread its mandate. Their clear-sightedness gave UNICEF a new direction towards a multidisciplinary action in which health, education, nutrition, and social promotion were closely linked.

A little later, the International Children's Centre (ICC) was created in Paris. At that time UNICEF had laid stress, quite rightly, on the training of personnel having to deal, in different disciplines, with children of pre-school age, and this is how the idea of International Children's Centres arose in some countries, such as Great Britain, Poland, India, and France, on the basis of a financial agreement between UNICEF and the governments of these countries. It was only in France that this project fully achieved its aims, owing to Debré's persistence and also to his political connections. Great Britain created the Institute of Child Health; Poland the 'International advanced MCH course' which lasted for more than 25 years; and India, in Bombay, a Child's Bureau which has been particularly effective.

The outstanding action of the World Health Organization in promoting maternal and child health throughout the world should also be emphasized, and deserves tribute. Whereas most of the MCH (maternal and child health) national programmes are unbalanced—with their maternal component underdeveloped—WHO has always promoted maternal and child welfare together, in an integrated approach which, quite logically, led to the concept of family health and its practical applications (WHO 1973).

Development of concepts

Is it really true that events, often harmful, could have inspired the creation, by a few clever individuals, of a new concept in medical practice? First of all, it is true that a handful of 'great names' have, in most countries, played a crucial role in launching social paediatric activities. However, they were at the same time stimulated by challenges originating from very poor situations and international comparisons which engendered emulation, and supported by colleagues, teams, officials, and to some extent the general public—progress occurred as a result of the right person being in the right place at the right time. For instance, the *One thousand families* report mentioned above created a shock which activated the need to work to improve a critical situation. In the UK, the Court report (Court 1976) arose from a perceived poor 'national performance' in terms of infant mortality. The same kind of stimulation has arisen from increasing consciousness of the great effect of social class on children's health (remember the report *Born to fail?* published by the Children's Bureau (Wedge 1974)), of persistent abuse of young children and of excess perinatal loss. And, in spite of a lot of progress, a great deal remains to be done, as is well expressed in this quotation which is still unfortunately true for millions of children in the world, and not only in developing countries:

> If I were asked to compose an epitaph on the twentieth century, it would read 'Brilliant in its scientific discoveries, superb in its technical breakthrough, but woefully inept in its application of knowledge to those most in need …' We are now experienced; and all that remains is the problem of translating what is current common knowledge and routine medical and health practice to the other two thirds of the world: the implementation gap must be closed. (Fendall 1972.)

Beside this, it must be realized that social paediatrics is still largely split into many thematic topics and approaches. Can we content ourselves with this statement by Robert Debré, '*Social paediatrics is not a discipline, it is a state of mind*'? It is, in fact, a meeting point and cross-fertilization of various disciplines.

In a great number of European countries as well as on an international level, social paediatrics has brought about crucial contributions to the development of our knowledge of the child and of our activities directed towards children's welfare. At the same time it has benefited from the remarkable scientific and technical progress of the past 50 years. As mentioned above, social paediatrics is at the crossroads of many disciplines. It is obviously linked with clinical paediatrics, but it also has links with social obstetrics through the progress and programmes of perinatology and genetics. It is becoming increasingly connected with the human sciences: not only psychology and sociology but also ethnology and anthropology, especially so in multi-racial societies; and with pedagogy: teachers can tell us a great deal about the children, who may or may not be in difficulty, with whom they associate throughout the year. Social paediatrics has also established successful bonds with the basic sciences, i.e. developmental biology, and with public health, law, and economics. Epidemiology perhaps deserves a special mention, with its approach to children's problems being complementary to the clinical approach.

It is clear that social paediatrics pertains to many disciplines while keeping its own identity. The links between social paediatrics and family health, community health, public health, and developmental paediatrics are subtle and the concept of 'child global health' is probably an appropriate way to reconcile these disciplines with social paediatrics and give us a clearer view on the subject. 'Child global health' means taking into account health and development as a whole, as a continuity, as well as interactions between various environments (physical and social) and healthy children (the majority of them) or physically or socially handicapped ones. All these aspects we have tried to describe and develop in *L'enfant et sa santé* (Manciaux *et al.* 1987). Other books take a similar direction, such as *Children's health and well-being in the Nordic countries* edited by Lennart Köhler (Köhler and Jakobsson 1987) and *Child health in changing society* by Forfar (1988).

From this expanded conception ensue various programmes of activity and training, which, in 1972, the Council of Europe formulated as microsocial, mesosocial, macrosocial, and megasocial paediatrics (Conseil de l'Europe 1986). The programme it suggests may appear ambitious but is perhaps well adapted in today's societies.

Microsocial paediatrics:
   the child: mutual influences of genetics and the environment;
   the child in his family.
Mesosocial paediatrics:
   relationships between the child, other children, and social groups.
Macrosocial paediatrics:
   socio-economic context;
   health policy and programmes.
Megasocial paediatrics:
   population dynamics;
   ecology: pollution, waste of natural resources.

From this broad field, one could conclude that social paediatrics is at the cross-roads of epidemiology and statistics, clinical sciences, and human sciences relevant to psychosocial development, and that social paediatrics should enlarge its concern and involvement to become known as 'pedontology' just as social geriatrics has evolved towards gerontology.

Challenges for the future

'The longer you can look back, the further you can look forward.'
Sir Winston Churchill, 1944.

We are confronted with the necessary rebalancing between sciences such as epidemiology and statistics on the one hand and the social sciences on the other, the data from which, often difficult to quantify, are nevertheless extremely useful to social and preventive medicine. The weight of social factors in a number of morbid syndromes, as pointed out by Villermé 150 years ago, must be underlined in the fields of perinatology, accidents, handicaps, and communicable diseases, and also in the way health-care services are available and used and prevention accepted. It is impossible for the physician to be responsible for all the abnormal situations that favour diseases and handicaps, but a true paediatrician must consider the social factors whose impact is important in family health and cooperate with those professionals dealing with social problems.

The health of adolescents, too, deserves our concern: this subject was the theme of technical discussion at the WHO General Assembly in 1989 (WHO 1989). Youth health is often not good, though they are poor health care consumers. Paediatricians who, in the past, have favoured the other end of childhood, i.e. the perinatal period, should, from now on, show more interest in adolescents and their problems, since many of the health problems of young people have a psychosocial origin, and are rooted in childhood. Many of them have already done so, in North America and in Australia for instance, but less so in Europe.

Activities in university hospitals and in the field should also be rebalanced. Social paediatrics should first and foremost be developed in the community; but most of the teachers in social paediatrics are academics and work in hospitals. It is interesting to note that research in ambulatory paediatrics is developing in many places in Europe, the first example being in GREPA (Groupe romand d'études en pédiatrie ambulatorie) initiated by Girardet in Neufchâtel, Switzerland, 15 years ago. Social paediatrics, whose research and studies are carried out in the community, by community workers, fits in very well in such experiences and should play a crucial role in promoting a 'combined child health service' (British Paediatric Association 1991).

Last but not least, prevention does not have an adequate position in today's medical practice. For instance, there is no country in Europe where the budget for prevention reaches more than five per cent of the total health expenditure. This situation is untenable and must be remedied. The renowned French paediatrician, Jean Bernard, expressed it very clearly: '*It is not in treatment, but in prevention and its progress that lies the solution of the harrowing and paradoxical problem of tomorrow's medicine'.*

To meet these challenges, training in social paediatrics has to be improved. Apart from a few notable exceptions, it is globally inadequate. A survey (IPA 1989) on the teaching of social paediatrics in various countries was conducted recently by the International Paediatric Association. Of the 12 countries in Europe which participated, only three of them mentioned a connection with a public health department, two of which plus another use the community as a training field for students. Two others mention explicitly the psychosocial aspects of health and disease. It is therefore urgent to find a remedy to this very serious deficiency, and this problem will be dealt with in later chapters.

Finally, the importance of ethical issues in modern paediatrics must be emphasized (Campbell 1988). The position which considers the child as incapable, in the juridical sense of the word, just as mentally ill patients, is to us unacceptable. But to consider a child as a miniature adult in respect of the law is equally unbearable. Paediatrics shows us quite a number of specific situations which do not exist in adults' health and disease, and the problems of the child—a being in development—need a special approach. Social paediatrics has an active role to play in the working out of a modern ethics which is necessary due to the rapid progress of science and technology. One thinks first of medically assisted procreation, with its twofold dimensions: the right to have a child, and the rights of the child born under such conditions. But there are other fields in paediatrics where ethical problems appear and we have to try to consider the rights of the child from an ethical viewpoint. The *International Convention on the Rights of the Child* adopted in 1989 by the General Assembly of the United Nations has been ratified by many countries in the world (Manciaux 1991). Paediatricians, as advocates of the child, have an important role to play in the enforcement and implementation of the Convention (Manciaux 1991, 1989) and the Children Act enforced in the UK (Cretney 1991).

In spite of some brilliant breakthroughs, there is still a lot to do to improve the health, welfare, and fate of millions of children in Europe and the rest of the world. Preventive and social paediatrics, whatever the name it will take in the future, has a prominent role to play if it is to succeed in adapting itself to these new challenges in the integrated approach of global health applied not only to children but also to mothers, parents, families, and society as a whole.

References

Balinska, M.A. (1991). Ludwik Rajchmann, un militant de l'action sanitaire internationale. Forum mondiale la santé: Organisation Mondiale de la Santé. (OMS). **12**, 503–13.

British Paediatric Association (1991). *Towards a combined child health service*. BPA, London.

Butler, N.R. and Alberman, E.D. (1969). *Perinatal problems. The second report of the 1958 British perinatal survey.* Livingstone, Edinburgh.
Campbell, A.G.M. (1988). Ethical issues in child health and disease. In *Child health in a changing society* (ed. John O. Forfar). Oxford University Press.
Centre International de l'Enfance (1980). Croissance et développement de l'enfant. *Courrier du CIE*, **30**, n° spécial.
Conseil de l'Europe (1986). *Pédiatrie préventive et formation des pédiatres à la prévention et à l'éducation pour la santé.* Comité européen de la santé, Strasbourg.
Court, S.D.M. (1976). *Fit for the future.* Report of the Committee on Child Health Services. Her Majesty's Stationery Office, London.
Cretney, S.M. (1991). The implications of the Children Act 1989 for paediatric practice. *Arch. Dis. Child.* **66**, 536–45.
Debré, R. (1963). Définition de la pédiatrie sociale. Paris. *Courrier du CIE*, **13**, 621–6.
Engels, F. (1960). *La situation de la classe laborieuse en Angleterre.* Editions sociales, Paris.
Fendall, N.R. (1972). Auxiliaries and primary health care. *Bull. N.Y. Acad. Med.*, **43**, 1291–303.
Forfar, J.O. (1988). *Child health in a changing society.* Oxford University Press.
Köhler, L. and Jakobsson, G. (1987). *Children's health and well-being in the Nordic countries.* Blackwell Scientific, Oxford.
Korczak, J. (1979). *Le droit de l'enfant au respect.* Laffont, Paris.
Manciaux, M. (ed.) (1989). *Le pédiatre et les droits l'enfant.* Paris. UNESCO, Paris.
Manciaux, M. (1991). The UN Convention on the rights of the child: will it make a difference? *International Digest of Health Legislation*, **42**, 165–9.
Manciaux, M. (1992). Les droits des enfants dans les systémes de soins européens. *Le pédatre*, **28**, 103–9.
Manciaux M., Lebovici, S., Jeanneret , O., Sand, A.E., and Tomkiewicz, S. (1987). *L'enfant et sa santé.* Doin, Paris.
Mande, R., Masse, N.P. and Manciaux, M. (1977). *Pédiatrie sociale.* Flammarion, Paris.
Masse, N.P. (1977). Introduction à la pédiatrie sociale. In *Pédiatrie sociale* (ed. R. Mande, N.P. Masse, M. Manciaux). Flammarion, Paris.
Miller, F.J.W., Coori, S.D.M., Knox, E.G. and Brandon, S. (1974). *The school years in Newcastle upon Tyne.* Oxford University Press, London.
Paediatric education: IPA survey. *Bull. Intern. Pediat. Assoc.* **10**, 105–64.
Villermé, C. (1979). *Tableau de l'état physique et moral des employés dans les manufactures de coton.* Edhis, Paris.
Wedge, P. (1974). Born to fail? Social disadvantage. The facts and the practitioner. *Concern*, **13**, 6–14.
World Health Organization (1973). *Family health. Report of a consultation.* FHE 75, 4. WHO, Geneva.
World Health Organization (1989). *Youth health. WHA Technical Discussions.* Report, A42/13. WHO, Geneva.

2 Child health as a public health issue
Lennart Köhler and Keith Barnard

Paediatrics deals with children's diseases. Children's health is a much wider concept, including aspects of their well-being other than the purely medical ones. Many attempts have been made to define health, and however different the definitions there is general agreement that it is not only freedom from disease that is important, but there should also be positive elements in its physical, mental, and social aspects. Most well known and still most used is the original **WHO** definition: *'Health is not only the absence of disease but a complete physical, mental, and social well-being'*. This definition has been heavily criticized on the grounds that it is imprecise, utopian, and impractical. Today, many prefer a concept of health that is connected to the individual's situation and allows her or him to cope with the demands of life. Therefore, health is the ability to withstand strains of a physical, mental, and social nature, so that they do not lead to a reduced life span, function, or well-being.

The ultimate goal of WHO's later strategy *Health for all by the year 2000* is to make it easier for people to achieve a socially and economically productive life. This strategy, accepted by all governments in Europe, was then developed into 38 targets, which represent a common European view of what could and should be done to achieve health for all.

Central to the strategy is equity; both within and among European countries and between Europe and the rest of the world. Emphasis is placed on promotion of healthier lifestyles and a healthy environment and on the reorientation of health care systems, based on primary health care.

The study of these broad and complex issues of population health, which emphasize the cultural, social, economic, and political dimensions, is usually labelled *public health*. According to Sir Donald Achesons's influential report on public health in England, public health is defined as *'the science and art of preventing disease, prolonging life, and promoting health through organized efforts of society'*. Naturally, this also includes children as part of the population, and there are several major reasons why children's health and well-being is of special importance in public health.

1. Children make up a substantial part of the country's population, in Europe generally around 20 per cent.

2. Children have no political power and are not represented in formal or informal pressure groups able to influence health and related policies.

3. Children represent a vulnerable group in society, whose health and well-being thus reflect the will and ability of the society to care for its citizen.

4. Adult knowledge, attitudes, and behaviour in health matters are learned and commented in the formative years of childhood and youth.

5. The United Nations has proposed special protection for children through its *Convention on the rights of the child*, adopted in 1990.

Now that it is possible to articulate such a powerful argument for child public health it is instructive to trace its evolution over the past century and a half during which time the explicit and specific relevance of public health has emerged. The nineteenth century was the 'sanitary era' of public health with its focus on water and sewerage, nuisances and other matters relating to the physical environment, and epidemic control. By the Second World War, while the old issues remained important and others such as occupational hygiene had been taken up, most significantly there was a growing emphasis on families: maternal care, infant welfare and the reduction of infant mortality, the health and development of the school child and the adolescent, and family living conditions.

In 1946, the WHO Constitution citing the importance of the healthy development of the child amongst its basic principles proposed, as one of the specific functions of the organization, to promote maternal and child health and welfare and to foster the ability to live harmoniously in a changing total environment. It is interesting to note that this formulation, in retrospect, appears to anticipate the socio-ecological concept of public health which now sets the agenda for policy and action, i.e. the interplay of individuals and groups with all aspects of their natural and man-made environments.

This socio-ecological concept is reflected particularly in the current emphasis on health protection and promotion. Health protection and promotion can be characterized as the sum of policies and actions which together secure the conditions for healthy living, i.e. the prerequisites to be met, the various criteria for a healthy environment to be satisfied, the necessary social support, community organization, and other measures to assist groups and individuals in their health needs, including the prevention of disabilities and handicaps, the provision of such education and information as will enable people to make their own choice and decisions relating to their way of life and help sustain their knowledge and motivation for their own health maintenance. This broad concept is a response with the needs of children very much in mind, to the many manifestations of psychological and social as well as physical ill-health which are, in modern societies, undergoing profound rapid change. At the individual level social ill-health is seen, for example, in domestic violence, family breakdown, and child abuse. At the community level disaffected youths express their alienation through acts of vandalism to public and private property. At the societal level there is inter-ethnic violence and xenophobia expressed as hostility to migrants and would-be refugees. There are real risks of psychological ill-health in the loneliness which comes with the geographical and other forms of dispersal of families, the sense of isolation of the nuclear family in the absence of a supportive network of friends, and even in the cultural gap between the individual and family and seemingly impersonal providers of social services including medical care.

In these circumstances it is imperative to reinforce the notion of health protection as an essential dimension of public health. The whole concept of a welfare society providing a safety network of income and other form of support to protect its weaker or disadvantaged members should be seen as a set of health protection measures no less than traditional environmental health protection or, say, classic accident prevention measures. A further role of the welfare society is ensure that people do not, through force of circumstances become disadvantaged, but that they retain their personal resources of resilience and self-reliance which help maintain health.

Safety promotion for children is an integral part of protection. Even if it were desirable, it is difficult to conceive of an environment, at the neighbourhood or at the national and global levels, which is totally without danger (whether man-made or natural). Confronting hazards and taking risks of various kinds is natural behaviour. It is seen daily, for example, in the exploratory behaviour of children as they learn about the world around them and of young persons as they make the transition to adulthood. The expectation is that they will learn the importance of safety from their experiences. Safety promotion means the creation of a rational safety culture in the community and in particular settings will secure real compliance with legislation and regulations and the adoption and adherence to reasonable safety practices and systems.

Health promotion, a complimentary component to protection, covers measures which are intended to support and sustain people's healthy patterns of living and to facilitate health-improving behavioural change (reducing health-risky behaviour, adopting health-enhancing behaviour), and to secure needed environmental changes which would reduce or better eliminate social and other environmental causes of ill-health.

The Ottawa Conference on health promotion in 1986, co-sponsored by WHO, was the first formal occasion at which the potential of promotion was fully articulated. The charter formulated at this conference identified the requirements of a concerted effort from different professions and others in many sectors. In terms of action areas to which that concerted effort should be directed, the Ottawa Charter identified the following as the field of concern.

- Building health promotive public policy, in all sectors and levels of society, aimed at influencing public and private decision makers, and spanning the physical, economic, social, and cultural environment.

- Creating supportive environments, in both physical and social dimensions, in settings of everyday life (work, leisure, family, etc.), strengthening the community's social support systems.

- Strengthening community action, so that whether community is defined by locality or as a group of people with shared interests and objectives, these people are involved in debate, decision, and action for promoting health, drawing on people's own resources and giving them a greater sense of self-worth.

- Developing personal skills to increase self-esteem and to strengthen people's capacities to make their own choices and cope with the pressures they face.
- Reorienting health services to give greater emphasis on promotion in the remit of these services and their staffs and to stress the potential of health care institutions as health promotion settings.

It should also be noted that effective health education is a necessary condition for purposeful action in health protection and promotion: both to enhance health knowledge and awareness in the population and to help create the conditions which make health-supportive change possible. Health education, as now understood, seeks to empower people so that individually, by making informed choices, they may adopt healthy patterns of living, and collectively, as responsible and aware citizens, they intensify political and social action for policy and structural changes as envisaged in the Ottawa Charter. It is therefore essential that the concept of health education finds a place in the mainstream of the school curriculum, rather than at the margins.

The range of actions taken within a public health strategy which have the needs of children in mind and adhering to the goals and aims of health for all would need to cover

- the provision of education and later work in conformity with a person's physical and mental capacity;
- availability of suitable housing and safe water and sanitary facilities; and ensuring a safe and adequately nutritious food supply;
- improvement of the physical, economic, cultural, psychological, and social environment; and developing and maintaining community organization and various forms of social support;
- the raising of people's awareness about health matters; enabling them to cope with health problems by helping them develop personal skills; providing them with valid information on such basic matters of lifestyle as appropriate through diet, physical activity, relaxation, and sleep;
- the strengthening of support to community efforts of self-care and self-reliance through the steady availability of professional advice and services where needed, to ensure that community action develops and is sustained in a way which most effectively protects and promotes the community's health.

Evidence of effective action would be seen in the relevant environmental changes, in the provision of reasonable protection, in the adoption of healthy patterns of living, in the reduced prevalence of risky behaviour, in improved levels of population health, and in both observable and self-perceived improvements in peoples' quality of life.

We may go further and say that the fundamental task in health protection and promotion is to operationalize the concept of health and the goal of improved health status. Within the broad framework of health for all, this means a focus for action typified by the objectives of a functioning healthy city or neighbourhood which, having in mind child and family needs, might be generalized in such terms as

- to create and sustain a quality of life for its residents such that there is a positive rewarding experience, creating a sense of identification and belonging;
- to ensure that residents are aware and conscious that they have access to whatever resources of the locality can enhance their well-being;
- to manage the locality so that it 'works'; public and commercial services of all kinds are efficient, effective, reliable, and customer-sensitive;
- to promote at the policy level a prevailing climate of collaboration: both public bodies and private, commercial, and other organizations take decisions and make investments with proper regard for health criteria;
- to demonstrate ecological awareness and a commitment to preserving the natural environment and improving, where warranted, the man-made environment;
- to create (as a dimension of equity) as many opportunities as possible for choice in work, leisure, dwelling, and social participation/communal activity.

In particular, social participation or community involvement means taking all steps to ensure, through education, personal skills development, and other supportive means, that people can enhance their own health through their own personal efforts, individually and collectively, rather than be merely passive recipients of professional services.

Most recently the Regional Committee of the WHO European Region (1993) has adopted an updated set of 'health for all' targets which, for the first time, includes a target dedicated to promoting the health of children and young people, replacing the earlier narrow target of reducing infant mortality. The new target takes full account of the new objectives which typify health protection and promotion, including the promotion of children's rights, and also retains a proper concern for the well established activities of child health.

Target 7: Health of children and young people

By the year 2000, the health of all children and young people should be improved, giving them the opportunity to grow and develop to their full physical, mental, and social potential. This target aims at achieving

- comprehensive support of children and their families, according to their health needs and socio-economic circumstances;
- a reduction of infant mortality rates in countries with rates currently between 10 and 20 per 1000 live births to below 10, and in countries with rates currently above 20 per 1000 live births to below 15;
- a reduction of the differences in infant mortality rate between different geographical areas and socio-economic groups by 25 per cent;
- a reduction in mortality and serious injury in children and young people, notably due to accidents, by 25 per cent;

The target can be achieved by implementing strategies that

- protect children as vulnerable members of society, with all appropriate measures in accordance with the *UN Convention on the rights of the child*;
- organize disease prevention and health surveillance for all children including good antenatal, postnatal, pre-school, and school health services;
- promote breast-feeding of infants by the greatest possible proportion of mothers, including working mothers;
- promote healthy patterns of living among children and young people;
- ensure social, economic, and psychological support for disadvantaged children, including those with long-term illness and disability, and for their families;
- ensure that all young people are informed about, and have easy access to, facilities and support to avoid unplanned parenthood.

Thus the ideology of health for all, the fundamentals of public health, and the societal importance of children's health merge into *social paediatrics* or, as we may call it, *child public health*, the task of which is to place the health of children and their families in their full social, economic, and political context. In our times of superspecialization and fragmentation of medical sciences and medical professions, so obvious in clinical paediatrics, social paediatrics is the counterbalance, with its intersectoral and multidisciplinary approach to the fullness of health. Definitions of social paediatrics are many, and usually rather complex, but for the purpose of clarity three main areas could be identified as the principal targets for socio-paediatric activities:

1. child health problems with significant social determinants;
2. child health problems with social consequences; and
3. child health care in the society.

These are the areas defined for teaching and practical work, as well as for research.

Social paediatrics thus implies a very broad concept, taking professionals away from the narrow experience of specialized institutions into the community, making them aware of the social context in which children live in order to better understand their health problems, and also the need to promote genuine interdisciplinary and interprofessional team working.

More than ever before, there now seems to be unity and cohesion in this kind of thinking throughout the health sector. These developments do suggest a strong move towards the community and 'health for all' orientation which social paediatrics has always stood for. If the present sense of direction can be maintained it could mean that the clinical practice of physicians, the caring tasks of nurses and others, and the work of social paediatrics will be seen as complementary and not as entities competing for professional esteem, public recognition, and political and financial support.

Social paediatrics as a field of study has three principal concerns. Firstly it is concerned with the education and training and career developments of child health workers. Secondly, there is research in its various forms, conducted on multi- and interdisciplinary bases, designed to increase the understanding of different child health phenomena and to clarify the desirability and feasibility and policy measures and programmes to improve children's health. Thirdly, there is service-giving, working with practitioners, and policies and problems; and the acceptance of responsibility for ensuring that a participating community is an informed community, whether it be political representatives, community action groups, voluntary health workers of various kinds, or the professional workers of others sectors where actions have a potential impact on children's health.

In *education* it is important to instil socio-paediatric values and perspectives in a consistent way to practitioners and academics, from undergraduate through postgraduate to post-experience in continuing education.

The second task is that of *research*. A conventional argument has it that research work keeps the educator intellectually sharp and enriches teaching. The teacher who is active in research is a better teacher. This is probably true, but the duty of research is also to reveal how matters are interconnected. It is vital that socio-paediatric research relates to the world, is practical, and is relevant. It might be that this kind of research will take a somewhat different set of underpinning values than those of the classical elitist academic world. Of course this does not mean abandoning a certain sense of detachment in analysing problems, the ability to see more than one side to a problem, the ability to think through the implications and consequences of alternative courses of action or the search for truth. But social paediatrics cannot confine itself to activities that are only those which would follow the rules of academic science. In the real world, actions have sometimes to be taken on assumptions and judgement, showing empathy with the fellow health workers doing a practical job, and indeed colleagues in all other sectors working for children's health.

Thirdly, there is the task of *service*. The same considerations apply as for research; that social paediatrics become involved in ways that are seen by others to be relevant. Indeed, active involvement in service, including consulting, is arguably the best way to strengthen one's credibility as an educator with students. It can show them that academics do know the world the students are entering, that their understanding and messages to them are relevant, and that academics will be a continuing support to them in their working career.

The key word, again, is relevance. The goal of a unit of social paediatrics, whether in a university, school of public health, or in a community, should be a centre of relevance rather than a centre of excellence in the traditional academic sense. Only by leaving the ivory tower is it possible to understand the problems, to be visible and credible, and to obtain recognition from the public and from politicians. If we insist on equating social paediatrics with medicine we will always remain on the periphery of medicine when we could instead be at the centre of child health.

From recent research programmes on children's health in general and on handicapped children in particular, some interesting observations have been made. Although the studies were performed in countries that belong to the richest in the world, and, consequently, with children that are among the most healthy in the world, there are some lessons and experiences that are universal and could lead to conclusions that, perhaps, are generally applicable in research and education as well as in practice.

- Children are very seldom in focus in population-based studies on health, well-being, and quality of life. Consequently, the otherwise overwhelming collection of health data does not offer a child's perspective.

- Even when children's health is seen from a public health perspective, children are regarded as a group whose importance lies mainly in the fact that they will eventually grown up to adulthood.

- There is very little discussion as to whether the traditional health indicators used for adults, e.g. life expectancy and use of health services, are also the most suitable for children.

- Studies of children's health are usually limited to small areas or age groups, and are only by exception representative for major areas or a country.

- Definitions of diseases and their seriousness, traditions of care and services are seldom uniform and unambiguous, which is the case for age limits, social class, and geographical areas, etc. This makes the results difficult to interpret and comparisons more or less impossible.

- Too few data on children's health are based on repeated studies or follow-ups.

- Data on children's social background and living conditions are seldom encountered, neither in official statistics nor in research reports.

The overall conclusion, from a methodological point of view, is that there is no systematic, continuous, and thorough reporting of children's health, seen from a child's perspective and put into a social context.

One recommendation, therefore, in this study was the creation of a national system to coordinate the documentation of children's health and well-being and to develop theories and methodologies. This should lead to strong sociopaediatric research activity, which should be interdisciplinary and interprofessional, and relevant to the needs of children, families, and society.

Implications: an element of a strategy

Social paediatrics—research as well as training and practical work—should be based on the *Health for all* strategy, and place the health of children in their full social, economic, and political context. It means that the activities should be practical and relevant and carried out by interdisciplinary and multiprofessional teams, absorbing the insight that we have from different social sciences such as sociology, psychology, economics, organizational behaviour, and political science, and what can be offered by management sciences such as operational research, systems analysis and computer science.

With such a broad competence, social paediatrics is fit to attack a wide range of child health issues, be it a healthy public policy for children, social support for vulnerable groups, product safety, traffic planning, or immunization take-up. One important area to be covered by social paediatrics is the development of health indicators appropriate for use among children. Vulnerable groups should be more closely observed and followed, e.g. children with chronic disease, abused children, refugees, immigrants, and other underprivileged groups.

An ideal, although seemingly idealistic and utopian outcome of sociopaediatric research, would be the development of a complete, systematic, and continuous surveillance of children's health and well-being, seen from a child's perspective and placed in a social context. This would create an instrument to judge children's health, to compare it within and between countries and between periods of time, and allow the evaluation of health-promoting and disease-preventing activities in the child population.

To take social paediatrics to the centre of child health and keep it there, a strategy is needed. This strategy, with elements of ideology and vision as well as something still of orthodox planning, must take into account that the public sector, throughout Europe, will be more deregulated, consumer- and goal-oriented, and outcome-responsible than has traditionally been expected of it. This implies that some methods and means, more known and used in business life than in the public sector, might need to be used to attain the goals. Key elements indicated in the strategy, however, should not be very different from those traditionally followed in the best public health sector practice.

It seems evident that the first task of each socio-paediatric team or unit must be to establish, or perhaps in some cases to renew, its own sense of coherence, affirming its commitment to interprofessional and interdisciplinary working and finding a focus for its efforts which harnesses the energies and interest of all the staff; i.e. the development of a strong 'corporate image'. Secondly, there must be a conscious attempt to find allies and partners for action at all levels—local, national, and international in the professional and political spheres, paying particular attention to establishing a good relationship with the media, and finding ways of making contacts with the public at large, especially not forgetting the children themselves. Lastly, it should not be forgotten that in bodies such as ESSOP, the European Society for Social Paediatrics, there are means for collective action and for mutual aid and support. We must of course be realistic about all this. It is a slow process to make active and powerful international forces out of professional associations, especially if most of the work has to be done by voluntary and unpaid staff.

It will be evident from what has been said so far that the issues of concern for social paediatrics distinguish it clearly from the biomedical interests that dominate clinical paediatrics. Social paediatrics is an open multiprofessional field whose concerns relate to child *health*. Clinical paediatrics, as a closed medical speciality, has a no less necessary but equally very different orientation to child *morbidity*. Most paediatricians still identify themselves more easily with clinical paediatrics, which is a well established and respected discipline in medicine, rather than with the emergent and still fluid territory of social paediatrics. It is important for those working in social paediatrics, especially physicians, to accept that they will most often be seen by fellow physicians as being on the periphery of medicine. Social paediatricians must therefore see themselves quite clearly and unequivocally as at the centre of child health and to vigorously pursue their tasks in that spirit.

References

Acheson, Donald (1988). *Public health in England. The report of the committee of inquiry into the future development of public health function*. HMSO, London.
World Health Organization (1985). *Target for health for all*. WHO, Copenhagen.
Köhler, L. and Jakobsson, G. (1991). *Children's health in Sweden*. The National Swedish Board of Health and Welfare, Stockholm.
Ottawa Conference on Health Promotion (1986). *Health Promotion—An International Journal*, Vol. 1., No. 4.
Regional Committtee, WHO European Region (1933). *Health for all targets: health policy for Europe*. European Health for All Series, No. 4, WHO Regional Office for Europe, Copenhagen.

3 Social paediatrics in Europe

Nick Spencer, Bengt Lindström, and Concha Colomer

Introduction

This chapter sets the scene of social paediatrics in Europe and provides an overview of the current state of social paediatric practice, training, and research. It is based the results of two questionnaires (Tables 3.1 and 3.2) circulated to members of the European Society of Social Paediatrics (ESSOP). The questionnaires were circulated just before the major political changes occurred in eastern and central Europe; the responses from East Germany have been included though they will be of historic interest only by the time of publication. Political changes may affect the organization of health services for children rendering some of the information presented out of date. Replies to the practice and training questionnaire (Appendix I) were received from 19 countries (see Table 1). Albania, Austria, Bulgaria, and Luxembourg were not approached. Forty-eight individual members of ESSOP responded to the research questionnaire which forms the basis of a European social paediatric research register.

Questionnaire 1 was designed to obtain information on the following: the range of definitions of social paediatrics in different countries; the extent of recognition of social paediatrics as a sub-specialty; the variation of social paediatric practice and training; progress and obstacles to progress over the proceeding 10 years and prospects for the future. The design aimed to obtain the maximum information for the minimum effort on the part of the respondent with the inevitable result that the

Table 3.1 *Countries responding (Questionnaire 1)*

Northern Europe	Central/Eastern Europe	Southern Europe
France	Germany (West and East)*	Spain
Sweden	Poland	Greece
Denmark	Hungary	Portugal
Norway	Switzerland	Roumania
Finland	Czechoslovakia	
United Kingdom	USSR*	
Belgium	Croatia**	

* Questionnaires completed prior to recent changes in Eastern Europe.
** Questionnaire completed by a colleague from Zagreb partly represents situation in former Yugoslavia.

answer categories were inappropriate for some countries. Nevertheless, valuable data were collected. Questionnaire 2 was designed to obtain information on the research interests of social paediatricians in Europe and areas of current research. The research register is intended as a European resource for social paediatric researchers which will be updated on a regular basis.

The results of both questionnaires have been analysed for the whole European area; our expectation of regional patterns failed to emerge. Data are presented numerically with qualification based on the comments of respondents.

Definition

The following definition of social paediatrics was presented for consideration in the questionnaire:

Social paediatrics is the study of children, in health, illness, and development, with particular reference to social and environmental influences on their well-being; it encompasses, amongst others, paediatric epidemiology, biostatistics relevant to childhood, the optimal care of disadvantaged children and their families, prevention and early detection of handicap.

This was broadly acceptable to respondents from seven of the 19 countries though a number felt that social paediatrics should be concerned with the socialization of disadvantaged children rather than merely ensuring optimal care. For the majority the definition was only partially applicable to their countries; the major critique was that the definition tended to present social paediatrics as a paediatric sub-specialty and not as an integral part of all child health care. One respondent advanced an alternative definition:

Social paediatrics views the child, both well and ill, and groups of children, in relation to the societies and human groups of which they form a part and the milieux in which they develop.

The definition of social paediatrics has prompted a long-running debate in Europe but, this debate apart, the results suggest broad similarity in the orientation of social paediatricians across Europe. The interesting concordance of areas of child health care work undertaken by social paediatric practitioners (see Table 3.2) is confirmation of this.

Table 3.2 *Practitioners involved in social paediatrics*

Practitioners actively involved in social paediatrics	Yes	No	Partly
Trained social/primary care paediatricians	12	6	1
General hospital paediatricians	12	3	4
Family medical practitioners	12	4	3
Trained child health nurses	17	1	1
General community-based nurses	8	10	1

Recognition of social paediatrics

Social paediatrics is recognized as a sub-specialty in only two countries, Hungary and West Germany. In three countries recognition is partial: in Portugal it has the status of a 'special interest' within paediatrics; in Czechoslovakia, partial recognition has been achieved without the full status of other paediatric sub-specialties; and in the UK, community paediatrics is the fastest growing sub-specialty but its orientation tends to be more towards developmental rather than social paediatrics. The lack of sub-specialty status is seen by a number of respondents as a barrier to the development of concepts of social paediatrics within their countries.

The divergence of opinion on the place of social paediatrics in child health care (see above) may explain, in part, the low level of recognition in Europe. The principal reason, however, is likely to be the persistence of a curative and pathological orientation amongst paediatricians identified as a significant barrier to progress in social paediatrics by most respondents.

Current practice and teaching

Practitioners

Despite the lack of recognition of social paediatrics as a sub-specialty, there were only six countries with no trained social paediatricians. General hospital paediatricians are involved in social paediatric practice in most countries though in four countries their involvement is limited. Family medical practitioners have a role in social paediatric practice in the majority of countries; in four countries family practitioners are not involved in child health care. In almost all countries responding, trained child health nurses actively participate in social paediatric practice; general community-based nurses, however, have a role in a minority of countries.

Eight respondents identify paediatricians and child health practitioners, other than trained social paediatricians, engaged in social paediatric work: private paediatricians in Switzerland and Greece; primary care paediatricians in Czechoslovakia, Spain, Hungary, and West Germany; in West Germany school health officers and in the UK clinical medical officers, who come out of the social medicine movement; in France the *medecins de protection maternelle et infantile*. Midwives in France, the personnel of Social Paediatric Centres in West Germany, and physiotherapists in Sweden are involved in social paediatric practice.

Setting of social paediatric practice

Most social paediatrics is practised outside hospital though in eight countries hospital paediatric units play a significant part and in three, a minor role.

Table 3.3 *Social paediatric practice settings and child health care aspects undertaken by social paediatricians*

	Yes	No	Partly
Settings:			
Hospital paediatric units	8	8	3
Community-based units	15	4	0
Aspects of child health care			
Child health promotion	14	5	0
Immunization programmes	16	3	0
Child health surveillance	14	3	2
Acute curative care	9	8	2
Chronic curative care	14	3	2
Developmental paediatrics	17	1	1
Educational medicine (school health)	17	2	0
Child abuse and neglect	13	5	1
Care of socially deprived children	13	6	0
Care of fostered/adopted/abandoned children	13	5	1

Social paediatrics is practised in hospitals exclusively in three countries (see Table 3.3)

Areas of child health care work undertaken by social paediatric practitioners

Care of children with special needs is the responsibility of social paediatric practitioners in 16 countries. In the same number of countries educational medicine is practised by social paediatricians. Only three countries report no involvement of social paediatric practitioners in immunization programmes.

Social paediatric practice includes child health promotion, child health surveillance, chronic curative care, child abuse and neglect, care of socially deprived children, and care of fostered and abandoned children in the majority of countries. Just under half the respondents report the involvement of social paediatric practitioners in acute curative care and a further two identify partial involvement. Overall the areas of work undertaken by social paediatric practitioners in European countries appear to be very similar suggesting less variation than expected (see Table 3.3).

Intersectoral work

In all the countries responding, social paediatric practitioners work with teachers and educational psychologists and the majority work with the police and lawyers and judges (see Table 3.4). Intersectoral work with local government

Table 3.4 *Intersectoral working*

Regular work with other sectors outside the health services	Yes	No	Partly
Social workers	16	3	0
Teachers and educationalists	19	0	0
Police	8	9	2
Judges	7	9	3
Local government officers	6	10	3

Table 3.5 *Training*

	Yes	No	Partly
Social paediatrics included in undergraduate medical curriculum	6	5	8
Specialist social paediatric training for postgraduate doctors	10	6	3
Academic departments of social paediatrics	10	8	1

representatives is reported in only six countries. Other sectors mentioned by respondents were voluntary organization, politicians and central government, and in former East Germany, social welfare institutions.

The sectors with which social paediatric practitioners work in the majority of European countries reflect the main areas of practice. However, the limited work with police and legal institutions suggest that social paediatricians, though involved in child abuse work, do not take part in related legal proceedings in many European countries.

Educating and training

Three countries have no social paediatric training in the undergraduate curriculum, eight have some partial undergraduate training, and in six social paediatrics is an integral part of the curriculum. Postgraduate training is available in eight countries and partly in two. Academic social paediatric departments are established in ten countries.

Research

Replies were received to Questionnaire 2 from 48 ESSOP members from 14 European countries detailing their research interests. This clearly does not represent a comprehensive picture of social paediatric research in Europe but is sufficient to give an idea of the general areas of research interest. Research areas have been broadly grouped under general headings and are presented in Table 3.6 with the number of individual researchers who specified each area. Child health promotion and prevention, including accident prevention, was the most commonly identified research area. Growth, development and nutrition was another area in which a significant number of researchers expressed an interest.

Table 3.6 *Areas of research interest*

Research area	Number of responses (individuals frequently identified > 1 area)
Child health promotion/prevention	
Promotion/prevention/evaluation	12
Accident prevention	7
Immunization	2
Health behaviour of schoolchildren	2
Preventive dental care	1
Screening procedures	3
Total	27
Growth/development/nutrition	
Growth and nutrition (including breast-feeding)	9
Child development	3
Psychosocial development	2
Obesity	1
Total	15
Paediatric epidemiology	
General	7
Longitudinal studies	3
Morbidity surveillance	3
Infant mortality (including SIDS)	2
Measurement of health	1
Total	16
Specific conditions (related social factors)	
Respiratory	5
Malignancy	2
Metabolic diseases	2
Cytomegalovirus/toxoplasmosis (congenital infection)	2
Chronic serous otitis media	1
Diabetes mellitus	1
Diarrhoeal diseases	1
Total	14
Children with special needs	
General	5
Epidemiology of special needs	1

Table 3.6 (cont.)

Research area	Number of responses (individuals frequently identified > 1 area)
Rehabilitation	1
Quality of life in children with special needs	1
Total	8
Health service use	
Evaluation	2
User views	1
Hospital admission (reasons for)	1
Patient held record cards (adolescents)	1
Operation consent	1
Total	7
Child rights/child protection	
Child abuse (including neglect/CSA)	4
Child rights	1
Total	5
Mental health/behaviour problems	
Behaviour problems	3
Mental health	2
Total	5
Neonatology	
General	2
Follow-up	1
Total	3
International child health	
Total	1
Other social paediatric problems	
General	7
Adolescent health	3
Material deprivation/inner city children	4
Day care and acquired illness	3
Homelessness	1
Ethnic minority children	1
Family health	2
Total	21

Surprisingly few researchers identified child rights and child protection and children with special needs as their areas of interest. It is also of concern that only one researcher expressed an interest in international child health. Further experience with the register should permit comment on neglected research areas as well as information for individual researchers seeking assistance or collaboration.

Progress and barriers

Twelve of the countries report recent progress in social paediatrics. In one country, the enormity of current child health problems had ensured that little progress had been made in social paediatrics. In seven countries a growing interest in the social aspects of health was identified with three specifying increased attention to child abuse and neglect. This interest is reflected in child health services and medical training; increased posts for paediatricians working outside hospital, improved links with primary care, comprehensive care for the handicapped, and the development of systematic child health surveillance were identified as positive system changes and enhanced undergraduate and postgraduate training. An increase in short courses in social paediatrics for general paediatricians were some of the signs of progress in training. A further sign of progress is the development in more than half the countries responding of national social paediatric associations, often as subsections of the national paediatric groups.

The barrier to further progress identified by most respondents was the curative orientation of paediatricians. This resulted in lack of recognition for social paediatric work, limited research funding, and inadequate numbers of trained social paediatricians. Financial restraints were specifically mentioned by five respondents as a barrier to progress and the lack of financial reward for preventive and social paediatric work was identified as important in four countries. The poor coordination of services for children and the lack of public health programme were mentioned, as were negative service changes in two countries.

Discussion

Practitioners committed to social paediatrics remain a small group but there are signs of increasing recognition in many European countries of the importance of social influences on health and the need for expertise in the social aspects of child health care. The dominance of a curative orientation in child health work constitutes the main barrier to the development of a social paediatric approach in most countries; a direct consequence of this orientation is the low status of preventive and socially orientated child health work in financial, academic, and professional terms. Promotion and prevention have tended to suffer first as a result of financial restraints imposed on the services.

Broad agreement exists across European countries on the definition of social paediatrics. Divergence, in definition and practice, arises in relation to the place of social paediatrics as a philosophy for all child health work or a sub-specialty within paediatrics. Those favouring an approach based on establishing the social paediatric philosophy as the basic philosophy of all child health work argue that sub-specialty status detracts from this overall aim by accepting social paediatrics as 'just another branch of paediatrics'. Those favouring sub-specialty status argue that recognition will come about only as a result of developing academic units and training social paediatric specialists.

At present, social paediatric work is undertaken by a broad group of health professionals. This is both inevitable and desirable but may have the negative consequence of diffusing interest and expertise unless the key issue of intersectoral/interdisciplinary work and training is addressed. The results of the questionnaire indicate the need for more training, both undergraduate and postgraduate, in social paediatrics; this could result in a better trained broad group of child health professionals or more social paediatric specialists.

Considerable experience has already been gained in interdisciplinary and intersectoral training in the Nordic School of Public Health and the School of Public Health in Valencia. The series of training courses organized by the European Society of Social Paediatrics (ESSOP) have been interdisciplinary and have provided valuable resource material for social paediatric teaching (Nordic School of Public Health, 1987–89).

Whichever approach is adopted, there is a clear need for a more established academic position for social paediatrics and increased research activity related to the social influences on child health. As would be expected in view of the curative orientation of paediatrics in most countries, there is some indication of lack of research funding for social paediatric research.

Despite these constraints, research activity in social paediatrics is considerable, with particular attention to areas of growing importance such as child health promotion. More information is needed on social paediatric research in areas such as child abuse and neglect and child rights and there is a need for more social paediatric research concerned with international child health issues. The ESSOP research register should act as both a resource and an instrument of change in the next few years.

Social paediatric practitioners have taken a lead in intersectoral child health work; they work with teachers, psychologists, and social workers in most European countries and, in some countries, with legal agencies. Work with local government remains limited and this is an area for future development. Despite the many barriers, progress has been considerable in most countries. For the future the major task remains the reorientation of child health work from a narrow curative perspective towards a broader vision of the promotion of health for all children within their family and social settings. Common to this task is the need for better training, though different paths may be taken to its achievement in different countries.

Reference

Nordic School of Public Health (in collaboration with ESSOP) (1987–89). *Reports of training courses in social paediatrics: parts 1, 2 and 3* (ed. B. Lindstrom and N.J. Spencer).

Appendix I

SOCIAL PAEDIATRICS IN EUROPE QUESTIONNAIRE

BACKGROUND & RATIONALE

Social paediatrics is a relatively new and small discipline within Child Health. The definition, teaching and practice of social paediatrics seem, on anecdotal evidence, to vary greatly between and within European countries. As far as we are aware there is no reliable information on social paediatrics based on a survey of the whole of Europe.

Bengt Lindstrom and I are editing a European textbook of social paediatrics; we plan an introductory chapter outlining the state of social paediatrics in Europe. This questionnaire will form the basis for the chapter. Further, the European Society for Social Paediatrics (ESSOP) is exploring the possibility of setting up a European Masters Degree in Child Health base on participating centres throughout Europe. A survey of Social Paediatrics in different European countries will assist in the planning of a Masters Degree.

SURVEY METHOD

Key ESSOP members in each region of Europe are being approached to complete the questionnaire for their own country and a small number of other countries by contacting established ESSOP members in each country and obtaining the information from them. The information requested is qualitative so the accuracy of figures will not be in question. In the absence of ESSOP members in some countries, information will be sought from national paediatric associations.

SECTION 1:   COUNTRY _____

SECTION 2:   INFORMATION OBTAINED FROM
             _____

             INFORMATION OBTAINED BY
             _____

SECTION 3:   DEFINITION OF SOCIAL PAEDIATRIC

The following definition of Social Paediatrics is accepted by ESSOP:

Social Paediatrics is the study of children, in health, illness and development, with particular reference to social and environmental influences on their well-being; it encompasses, amongst others, paediatric epidemiology, biostatistics relevant to childhood, the optimal care of disadvantaged children and their families, prevention and early detection of handicap.

Is this definition appropriate for Social Paediatrics as taught and practised in _____ ? YES
NO
PARTLY

If the answer to the above is NO or PARTLY, please give a definition of Social Paediatrics as it applies in _____
_____
_____
_____

Additional comments on Definition:
_____
_____
_____

SECTION 4: RECOGNITION OF SOCIAL PAEDIATRICS

Is social paediatrics recognized as a paediatric sub-speciality in _____ ?
YES
NO

SECTION 5: SOCIAL PAEDIATRIC PRACTICE

a. Which of the following practitioners are actively involved in Social Paediatrics in _____ ?

	YES	NO
Trained Social Paediatricians		
General Hospital Paediatricians		
Family Medical Practitioners		
Specially trained Child Health Nurses		
General Community-based Nurses		
Others (if yes, specify below)		

_____
_____

b. Where is social paediatric work mainly carried out?

	YES	NO
Hospital paediatric units		
Community based units		

c. In which of the following aspects of child health care are social paediatricians in _____ working?

	YES	NO
Child health promotion (primary prevention)		
Immunisation programmes		
Child health surveillance (secondary prevention)		
Acute curative care		
Chronic curative care		
Care of children with special needs (developmental paediatrics)		
Educational medicine (school health)		
Child abuse and neglect		
Care of socially deprived children		
Care of fostered, adopted, abandoned children		

d. Do social paediatric practitioners in _____ work regularly with other sectors (agencies) outside the health services?

	YES	NO
Social workers		
Teachers and Educational Psychologists		
Police		
Lawyers and Judges		
Local Government Officers (town planners, safety officers etc.)		
Others (if yes, specify below) _____ _____		

SECTION 6: EDUCATION AND TRAINING

a: Which of the following are true for _____ ?

	YES	NO
Social paediatrics is included in the undergraduate medical curriculum		

Specialist social paediatric training is available for postgraduate doctors	_____	
There are academic departments of social paediatrics carrying out teaching and research	_____	

SECTION 7: RECENT PROGRESS

Has there been any notable progress in Social Paediatrics in _____ in the last 10 years?

                                                                           YES
                                                                           NO

If yes, specify:
_____
_____
_____
_____

SECTION 8: OBSTACLES TO FURTHER PROGRESS

What are the main obstacles to further social paediatric progress in _____ ?
_____
_____
_____
_____
_____

SECTION 9: GENERAL COMMENTS

Please give further comments on any aspects of Social Paediatrics relevant to _____ in this section
_____
_____
_____
_____
_____

THANK YOU FOR COMPLETING THE QUESTIONNAIRE

                         Bengt Lindstrom   Nick Spencer

d/Spencer/SPEQ

4 For the best interests of the child—*UN Convention on the rights of the child*
Bengt Lindström

At the turn of the century one of the initiators of the 1924 *UN Declaration on the rights of the child* declared this century as 'the century of the child'. Looking back, we can only conclude that this objective has not been reached: we still live in a world where the child is treated inhumanely. The century of the child is yet to come.

When the *UN Convention on the rights of the child* was accepted in 1989 some people questioned the need for such an international law. A glance at the text gives an indication of what reality a child of today can face. The Convention is forced to make statements on sexual exploitation of children, sale or traffic in children, torture, imprisonment, and children and war in order to protect and secure at least a minimum set of rights for the child. There is a deliberate formulation in the text, using *the child* as the subject instead of *children* as a collective group. The intention is to focus on the responsibility for each individual child and make the relationship more intimate, making it more difficult to hide child issues under collective covers.

Another basis for this textbook, the HFA target document, raises the question of equity as one of the fundamental principles securing equal rights to health for all groups in society. Some of the most vulnerable population groups have been given special target formulations, such as 'target 7 for the children'. This target mentions in particular that the *UN Convention on the rights of the child* should guide all public health efforts for children. In this text some of the basic principles of the Convention will be discussed in the context of child health in Europe. The complete text of the Convention is not included because of limited space but it is recommended that every body who deals with children get acquainted with the text in detail and also use it in their everyday practice.

History

Historically this convention is not the first attempt to create an international agreement on the rights of the child. In the first decades of the twentieth century there was a period of international 'thaw' and an increasing awareness of questions regarding human rights. Issues of equity and non-discrimination were put on the political agenda. Women gained their political rights and this movement in many ways made way for the focus on the child. The First World War and its grim experience was a setback for the human rights movement, but after the war, the League of Nations was formed. This organization prepared the declaration of human rights and created the first declaration on child rights. This was accepted in Geneva in 1924. Although the declaration has now only historical importance, its simplicity and straightforwardness are relevant even today.

The full statement (author's translation from Swedish) runs as follows.

1. The child must be allowed to develop normally both physically and mentally.
2. The child who starves must have food, the child who is ill must have treatment, the child who is emotionally neglected must have support, the child who is bewildered must be restored, the parentless and lost child must be sheltered.
3. The child must be the first to be cared for in disasters.
4. The child must be nurtured and must be protected from all kinds of exploitation.
5. Children must be fostered to make their best capacities beneficial to mankind.

Today the last paragraph, formulated mainly by the founder of the Save the Children Foundation, Englatyne Jebb, may elicit ambiguous reactions—after centuries of misinterpretation of what children's needs really are, of fostering principles where children were considered to be the property of adults who believed they were right to mould and adapt children to the needs of the adult society. This is a grim passage in the history of the child. The word 'benefit' may give connotations of self-obliteration and unconditional obedience. Originally there was rather a different intention: a call for education for peace and to give priority to an issue which has not lost its importance today, i.e. letting the child develop his or her own resources and best capacities and strengths, not only for the protection of the individual child but to bring a sense of solidarity to fellow humans and the oppressed.

The spirit of this paragraph was completely lost in the *UN Declaration of children's rights* of 1959 which succeeded the declaration of 1924. There it is stated, in paragraph 10:

Children are to be protected from pressures which cause prejudice and they are to be brought up in an atmosphere of friendship and peace.

The exact statement of 1924 has become a diluted, common phrase in 1959— unfortunately this is rather the rule of the latter document.

The preparation of the Convention

In the UN 'International year of the child', 1979, there was a proposition from Poland to create a new international law or convention for the child. In spite of a general acceptance of the proposition there were ten years of hard negotiations before the Convention could be accepted in 1989 and finally ratified in 1990. The difference between a declaration and a convention lies in the fact that the countries who have sign a convention also have to harmonize their national laws in accordance with the convention and abide by an international control and reporting system.

A subcommittee of the UN Commission on human rights was formed and made responsible for formulating the Convention. While this work was proceeding there was an increasing international awareness and interest in the development of the convention as people realized that this work might move the legal frontiers and create a real and important change for the children of the world. Several voluntary organizations participated actively in this work and made a strong impact on the formulation of some central articles. There are some compromises which have been seen as drawbacks, such as the question of the child and war where it was impossible to reach an agreement to protect all children from participating in wars, and the age limit was drawn at 15 rather than 18 years.

An overview of the contents

There are 13 introductory paragraphs and 54 articles in the Convention. The text itself contains three sections:

- an introduction which concludes the basic principles of the text and gives guidance to its interpretation;
- the 54 articles';
- a section on the implementation, reporting, and control mechanisms.

The articles include all different human rights, economic, social, and cultural, plus the political and constitutional rights. This is considered to be very important because earlier UN documents have separated these two categories of human rights, which has been a constraint in many negotiations.

The Convention includes three categories of articles:

- The right to fulfil basic needs:
  the basic needs are the right to food, health care, and education, i.e. the most fundamental needs for survival and normal development.

- The right to be protected from exploitation and discrimination:
  this means that the child has to be protected from sexual and economical exploitation; to be protected from wars and other similar situations; and to be protected from military recruitment. Special protection is needed for the vulnerable child, such as the child refugee and the disabled, also protection against traditional customs that may injure the child (such as female circumcision).

- The right to influence your own conditions; expressing personal view and having them respected:
the child's personal views are to be heard in matters that concern personal life, according to maturity and development.

Some of the articles are more important to the small child (such as questions of survival and health care) while others are more important to the young person (freedom of organization and religious freedom).

The basic principles of the Convention

What is a child?

The articles of the Convention are to be applied to all individuals under the age of 18 unless majority is gained earlier by national law (article 1). Thereby the article give a chronological definition of the child which can be used to protect each individual under the age of 18.

Non-discrimination

A basic principle is that the child is protected from discrimination irrespective of the child's own or parent's race, colour, sex, language, religion, political or other opinion, national, ethnic or social origin, property, disability, birth, or other status. This principle is similar to what is stated in the *UN Convention on human rights*.

'For the best interest of the child'

One of the most fundamental principles is stated in the formulation 'for the best interest of the child'. At first glance it might seem insignificant but it has a tremendous importance. It is an effort always to take the child's perspective in matters concerning the child. This principle is first mentioned in the third article, which states

In all activities concerning the child, whether undertaken by public or private social welfare institutions, courts of law, administrative authorities, or legislative bodies, the best interest of the child shall be a primary consideration.

In article 9, which deals with the child who is separated from one or both of their parents, it is stated that the child has a right to maintain a regular contact with both parents unless such separation is necessary for 'the best interest of the child'. This article concerns such 'common' matters as the child and divorce and more specialized situations such as the child who is born through donor insemination.

Article 18, which gives both parents mutual responsibility for the upbringing and development of the child, states that 'the best interest of the child will be their basic concern'. This formulation was much discussed when the Convention was being prepared. A convention usually regulates the responsibility of the state in respect of its citizen; here the parents are made responsible for the child, meaning that the obligation of the State is to be supportive and to safeguard the rights of the child while the parents execute the direct responsibility. However, the parental rights are never unconditional, while the State is obliged to be supportive to them and the child.

Articles 20 and 21, which deal with foster placement and adoption, are also based on the above principle. In article 20 it is stated that a child temporarily or permanently deprived of his or her family environment, or in whose best interest cannot be allowed to remain in that environment, shall be entitled to special police protection. Article 21 starts off by stating that 'State parties that recognise and/or permit a system of adoption shall ensure that the best interest of the child shall be the paramount consideration'.

There are other formulations in other parts of the Convention having the same intention but the basic principle is clear: 'the best interest of the child' is a ruling principle. This means that if there are contradictions in a particular situation, between one of the norms of the Convention and 'the best interest of the child'—'the best interest' always becomes the overruling principle!

Although the principle is clear it is difficult to decide who is the best person or institution to interpret what is 'for the best interest of the child'. The possible parties concerned are the parents or various welfare institutions representing the State, such as the courts and health or social care.

The parents are given the main responsibility for the child, which means the right and obligation to decide what is best: 'parents have the primary responsibility—the best interest of the child will be their basic concern' (article 18). On the other hand article 9 declares that 'competent authorities subject to judicial review can separate the child and its parents if this is necessary for the best interest of the child'. The legal system is obliged to make such a decision when there is a conflict between the parents and what is seen as best for the child. In such situations the court can overrule the parents but the parents are guaranteed a right to take the case to a higher court.

The experts of the social system and child psychiatry are supposed to motivate and support the decisions of the legal system. In a sense, one could argue that they have the ultimate power of decision. According to article 19, the State parties must create a professional system for 'identification, reporting, referral investigation, treatment, and follow-up' of cases where the 'best interest of the child' has been neglected by the family. The core intention of this statement is not perfectly clear but it seems that the expert opinions are to serve as important factual bases for the legal decisions. On the other hand it is made particularly clear that social and health care authorities can never make such decisions on their own.

Ultimately there is an another party involved, the child. The Convention makes a great effort always to permit the views of the child to be heard. Article 12 considers this issue in extension 'the child who is capable of forming his or her own views shall be assured the right to express those views freely in all matters affecting the child ...'. This means that no decisions on the child can be taken without hearing the views of the child. Note that there is no lower age limit to this statement. However, the court (or parents) do not have to make their decision according to the opinion of the child, 'the views of the child being given due weight in accordance with the age and maturity of the child'.

To summarize the discussion, it could be stated that the following adhere to the principle 'the best interest of the child':

- The child must always be provided with the opportunity to state his or her views; they are important.
- Parents have a right to decide as long as they follow the principle 'for the best interest of the child'.
- Legal parties are the only institutions that can overrule parental views on the best interest of the child.
- Legal decisions must be based on existing laws and use all available sources of information as a basis for such decisions.
- There must always be a legal opportunity to review a decision on these matters.

The spirit of 'the best interest of the child' should become the ruling principle in health care. There is no need for much imagination to find areas where this can be considered; for instance, when the child is taken into hospital care, when the child is separated from the parents because of medical interventions, in research on the child, and when the integrity of the child is threatened. The necessity of every medical intervention has to be scrutinized in this respect to assure that the interventions really are necessary and performed in a manner which is for the best interest of the child.

Specific health issues mentioned in the Convention

Article 24 recognizes the right of the child to the enjoyment of the highest attainable standard of health and facilities for the treatment of illness and rehabilitation of health. Particular attention must be paid by State parties to take appropriate measures

- to diminish infant and child mortality;
- to combat disease and malnutrition within the framework of primary care using appropriate technology, providing adequate food and drinking water and considering the risks of environmental pollution;

- to ensure appropriate prenatal and postnatal health care for mothers;
- to ensure that basic knowledge of child health and nutrition is disseminated to all segments of society, particularly to parents and children;
- to develop preventive health care, family guidance and family planning, and education services;
- to take all effective and appropriate measures to abolish traditional practices prejudicial to the health of the child.

Most of these statements are self-evident to the initiated child health worker and have a rather traditional format. There is also a reservation in that these measures are dependent on the resources available in the particular country or situation, but the child should always be given first priority in questions of resource allocation. It is noteworthy that issues of health are given such a priority and consideration in the Convention.

Article 23 deals with disability.

The mentally or physically disabled child should enjoy a full and decent life, in conditions which ensure dignity, promote self-reliance, and facilitate the child's active part in the community.

Special care for the disabled child should be provided free of charge, whenever possible, and designed to ensure that the child has access to and receives education, training, health care services, rehabilitation services, preparation for employment, and recreation opportunities. The role of international cooperation in the field of preventive health care and of medical, psychological, and functional treatment of the disabled child is mentioned with particular reference to the needs of developing countries.

There are many countries, even in Europe, which need to review their services to the disabled child according to the contents of this article. The past few years in Europe have been quite shocking and have revealed that many disabled children, especially the mentally retarded, live under conditions that are far from the intention of this article.

The health of the child when employed is considered in article 32, stating that need to protect the child from economic exploitation and from performing work that is hazardous or can interfere with the child's health or physical, mental, spiritual, moral, or social development. Minimum ages of admission to employment and appropriate regulations of the hours of employment have to be considered, including appropriate penalties to ensure an effective enforcement of this article. It is well known that there are countries in Europe which still allow exploitation of the child through organized child labour under conditions that are harmful and hazardous to the child. Even in the most developed countries children are being killed while at work because of conditions that are not appropriate for the child.

Drug abuse, exploitation, imprisonment, war, and refugees

Issues of child abuse are considered in article 33 demanding State parties to take appropriate measures to protect the child from illicit use of narcotic drugs and psychotropic substances and involvement in the production and trafficking of such substances. The State is ultimately made responsible to make it impossible for the child to either use or deal with illicit drugs.

The child must be protected from sexual abuse, exploitation in prostitution or pornographic performances and materials (article 34), and from torture or any inhuman degrading treatment or punishment (article 37). This is an international law which has the intention, when fully implemented, of making it impossible to exploit the child no matter who or where. Neither capital punishment nor life imprisonment without possibilities of release shall be imposed on persons below 18 years of age. Imprisonment of children shall be used only as a means of last resort and should be for the shortest possible period of time and separate from adults, unless it is considered in the child's best interest to the contrary. The last reservation is made to enable, for example, an imprisoned mother to breast-feed her child.

As mentioned earlier war and the child was given special consideration, where the Convention sets an age limit of 15 for recruitment of the child as a soldier. This was one of the most difficult compromises made in the development of the Convention. This low age limit kept several countries from signing the Convention and it was generally a disappointment that developed Western countries such as the USA, insisted that the age limit should be kept at 15. Fortunately, negotiations between the UN, members states and Non-Governmental Organizations (NGOs) mean it is likely that the age limit will soon change to 18.

It is made imperative that the child should not be affected by armed conflicts. It is a disgrace to humanity that armed conflicts are intentionally affecting civilians and the child to an increasing extent. Especially in conflicts which have the nature of civil wars, cruelty to the child and other civilians has become an effective way to break morale. Closely connected to the question of war, the Convention makes special considerations for the protection and treatment of the child as a refugee, with emphasis on the rehabilitation of child victims to promote physical and psychological recovery and social reintegration.

Right of education, play, and recreation

The Convention secures the child a right to an adequate standard living and care takers are enforced to secure financial capacities to ensure these means, if necessary supported by the State. The child is guaranteed a right to primary education which must be compulsory, available to all, and free to charge. The objective of education is to ensure the development of the child's fullest potential, to respect human rights and cultural identity, and to instil a spirit of peace, tolerance, equality of the sexes, and friendship among all peoples. School discipline must be administered in a manner consistent with the child's human dignity. This must be interpreted as a protection of the child from physical punishment for educational proposes. Two articles (31, 32) recognize the right of the child to rest and leisure, to engage in play, and to participate freely in cultural life and arts. Thus the child is entitled to be engaged in one of the most important elements of natural development—play.

Conclusion

The *UN Convention on the rights of the child* is a document that secures the fundamental minimum needs of the child. It takes great consideration to support the perspective of the child in every respect. For those who are sceptical of its effectiveness it must be understood that the implementation of the Convention will not happen overnight but it has both an immediate effect for the child in need and a long term objective, to create a better world for the child of the future. It is a document that has legal implementations and contains reporting systems and built-in control mechanisms. The first national reports on its implementations will be available in 1993. Basically it is a document that regulates the rights of the child in relation to the state but it also contains principles that should guide everyday life and practice. Child health workers must read it and learn how to use it in practice. The spirit of the Convention is not that it should be used in a distant legal fight on an international level but that it is a document which, if used correctly, has the potential to influence and change the everyday life of every child. It only becomes effective when it is made known to the general public and to the child with the full intention of serving the 'best interest of the child' principle.

Acknowledgement

Dr Lars H. Gustavsson kindly made his analysis of the principle 'for the best interest of the child' available for the preparation of this chapter.

Bibliography

UN Convention on the rights of the child (1989). UN, New York. (Most countries have it available in their own national languages at their Foreign Offices or at the National UNICEF Organization. Commentaries have been made by various voluntary organizations such as the Save the Children Foundation.)
UN Declaration on the rights of the child (1959). UN, New York.
Geneva Declaration on the rights of the child (1924). UN, New York.
WHO HFA Target Document (revised) (1992). WHO, Copenhagen.

5 The situation of children in developing countries

Oriol Vall and Oscar Garcia

Introduction

It has been estimated that by the year 2000 there will be around 2500 million children worldwide under the age of 14. The majority of them will live with the risk of becoming ill from one of three causes: infectious diseases, polyparasitism, or nutritional problems. The risk will increase and its spread and establishment will be furthered by poverty and immigration.

If we can expect one doctor for each 800 or 1000 inhabitants in Europe, in poor countries there is only one for every 25 or 50 thousand inhabitants who are mainly concentrated within cities. The lack of health care is especially alarming when we consider that the majority of the infant population lives in rural or deprived areas on the outskirts of major cities.

Poor countries are known by many names. They may be called Third World countries, which implies the need to define the first and second worlds; developing countries, despite many of them being in a negative state of development; underprivileged countries, although this implies a need to define the extent to which they are underprivileged; or simply poor countries, in contrast to rich countries, a term which obviously an oversimplification. Even with so many different options, none of them is absolutely right. Faced with this lack of agreement, we will indiscriminately use any of the above terms.

The causes of the great differences which exist between developing and undeveloped countries are numerous. However, we can group them into the famous 'three Ds': demography, desertification, and debt.

Demography

In the last quarter of a century the world population has exceeded 5000 million inhabitants and by the year 2000 it is estimated that there will be some 6000 million.[1,2]

Mortality has fallen—reflected in the increase of life expectancy at birth—not only because of the increase in the standard of living but also because of improvements in nutrition, water, education, and advances in medicine, but life expectancy in industrialized countries is still a third greater.[1]

In developing countries birth rates (number of live births per 1000 inhabitants) are usually high (on average 40) due in part to the absence of family planning, whilst in industrialized countries they are usually less than 20.[1,3]

In countries of low income per capita, children make up a large part of the population, in many cases up to 50 per cent.[3] (Fig. 5.1). The average population growth rate of these countries is normally around 2.5 per cent per annum, in contrast with one per cent for industrialized countries. Whilst the population has doubled in poor countries in 28 years, in rich ones it has taken 70 years to double.[1,3]

If the present demographic trend were to persist, by the year 2025 the world population would be 14 000 million. Whilst stabilization is forecast, with a world growth rate of zero, it is not possible to predict exactly when this will take place. In any case, world population will still increase, albeit in an irregular fashion; that is to say 60 percent of the population will live in Asia and in 50 years this figure will triple, the population of South America will double in 24 years, and that of Africa will double in 28 years (Fig. 5.2). The gravity centre of the population will move from the Northern hemisphere to the Southern hemisphere, average age will fall and urban concentration will increase.[1]

Evidently, the increase in the over 60s population up until the year 2000 will be greater in advanced countries (75 per cent) than in developing countries (35 per cent).[1]

Desertification

Ecological studies on Africa show that each year the forest area will decrease by 0.5 per cent in this continent. For instance, the central area of Tanzania, now almost desert-like, was a great jungle 100 years ago. All the trees were felled in order to build railways and to export enormous quantities of wood, a great source of fuel in the last century. Cities absorbed and displaced rural communities, and the end result is now known to be the consequence of development policies in which only immediate benefits were taken into account with conservation of resources, useful for less privileged classes, disregarded.

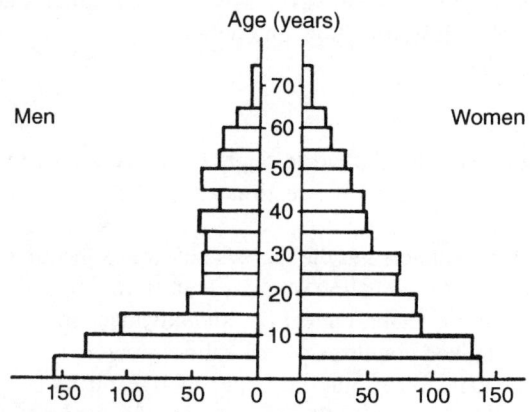

Fig. 5.1 Age pyramid of a rural African population. (Source: reference 1.)

The situation of children in developing countries

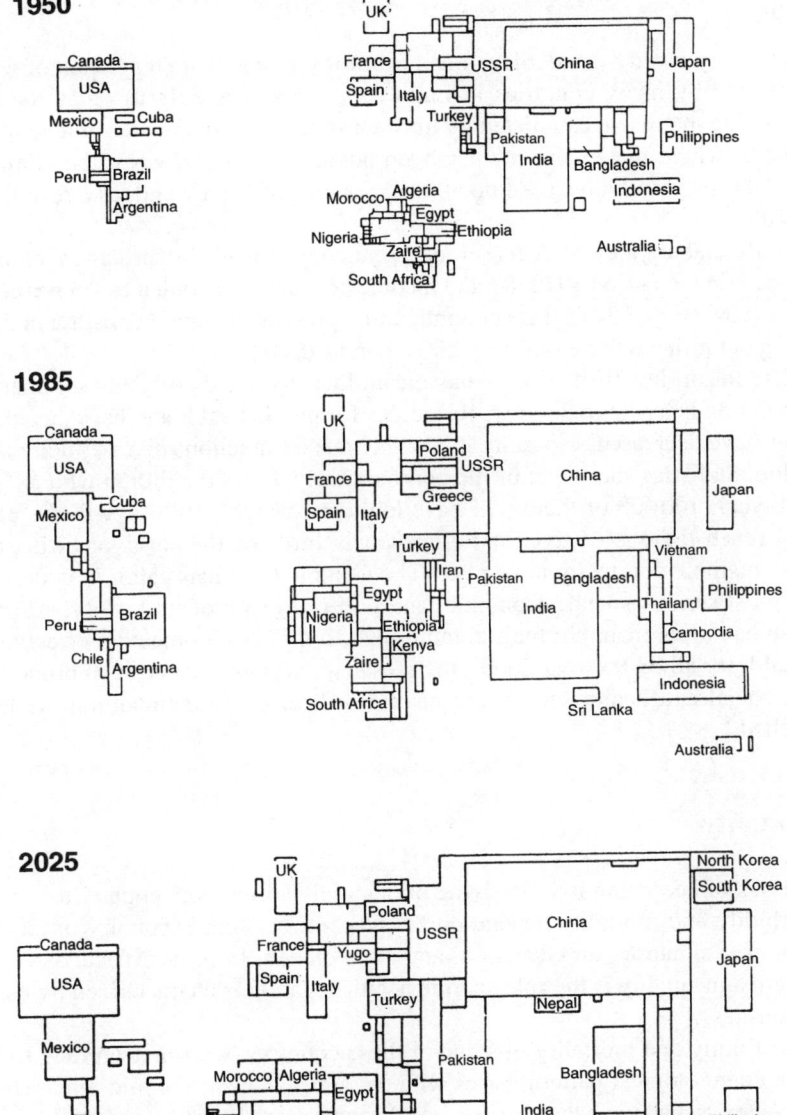

Fig. 5.2 Proportional representation of the world population. (Source: reference 1; reproduced from Vallin, J. (1986). *La population mondial*. Editions La Découverte, Paris.)

Debt

The money owed by underdeveloped countries is such that 80 per cent of wealth generated by many countries in Latin America serves only to repay the debt. Often, the interest accumulated by the debt is higher than they are able to afford, a factor which makes the country even poorer. Moreover, when they liquidate the debt, they will have used up all their sources of energy and, as a result, their wealth.

In the Sahara area of Africa, food production per inhabitant has fallen by 20 per cent in the period 1970–84 and income per capita has fallen by 15 per cent in the 1980s[4] (Fig. 5.3). If this economic trend persists, income per capita in developing countries will be lower by 2000 than in 1970.[4]

The fall in levels of income has meant that two-thirds of Central America's population is living in poverty. Resources for public health and basic health services have decreased. Mortality is growing due to infectious diseases and malnutrition. Statistics show that of the approximately 850 000 children who are born each year, 100 000 of them will have low birth weight, 100 000 will die before they reach the age of five, and almost two-thirds of the survivors will suffer from malnutrition to some degree.[5] The Central America region is undergoing the most serious social, economic, and political crisis of its history. Although these countries maintain their commitment to the social objective of achieving 'Health for all by the year 2000', the present crisis has reached such proportions that social and health sectors are having difficulties in maintaining the levels reached.[5]

Mortality

The risk of becoming ill or of dying prematurely varies from country to country. Morbidity and mortality depend on the place of residence (country or city), on economic situation, on education, and even on sex. In Asia, Africa, and South America inequality is the rule and the health situation is characterized by its precariousness.[1]

Morbidity and mortality in some of these countries worsen according to how the epidemiological pattern varies with the appearance of chronic diseases such as cancer, ischaemic heart disease, or tobacco-related illnesses and others resulting from a lack of hygiene.[1,6] Although life expectancy has increased—from 42 to 54 years—it could fall to 37 years in the poorest developing countries.[1]

Of the approximately 50 million deaths which occur in the world each year, 15 million are children under the age of five. The majority of these deaths are caused by infectious and parasitic diseases, although it is difficult to know specifically which disease is being dealt with since it is practically impossible to obtain reliable information. Morbidity and mortality data are scarce and often come from small sections of the population from which an estimation is taken.

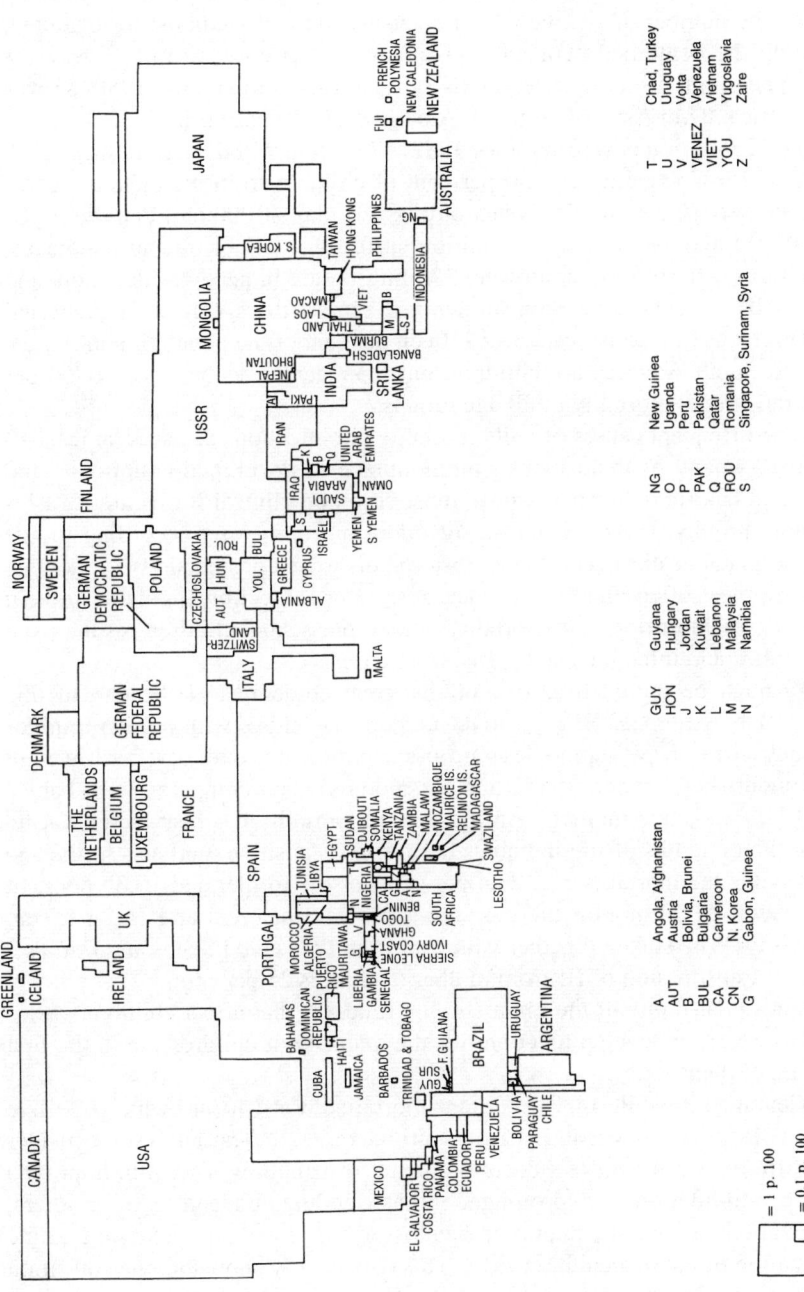

Fig. 5.3 Distribution of PNB amongst some countries (1982). (Source: reference 1; reproduced from *Informe sobre el desarrollo en el mundo* (1984). World Bank, Washington.)

In spite of this, WHO has been able to collect information obtained from different sources, above all that which concerns various important diseases, either by counting the number of sick people or by using indirect methods; for example, estimating the combined neonatal and infant mortality rates (up to five years old).[6,7] The infant mortality rate per 1000 live births in the period 1980–85 was 114 in Africa, 87 in Asia, 64 in South America, and 16 in Europe.[2]

Of the 125 million newborns since 1982, 17 million will die before they reach the age of 15. Comparatively, 50 per cent of children from the Sahara area of Africa die before they are five years old.[1] Every day 40 000 children die in the Third World and every year 100 million suffer physical or mental handicaps, 100 million suffer from malnutrition, 200 million are in need of education, and less than 10 per cent have been immunized against the six most frequent and most dangerous infectious diseases.[1] Fifteen per cent of the population in Africa, Asia, and South America are children, but their deaths account for 40–60 per cent of the overall mortality of all age groups.[7]

The most frequent causes of child mortality are infectious diseases (at least 40 per cent)[7]—many of them being commonplace in developed countries—and protein and caloric deficiency whose most common clinical forms are kwashiorkor and atrophy. However, causes of infant mortality vary according to age group: perinatal deaths occur due to obstetric disorders; postnatal (1–12 months) deaths are most often due to diarrhoea, respiratory infections, malaria, protein and caloric malnutrition; and mortality among pre-school children results from kwashiorkor, and infectious and parasitic diseases.

AIDS must be included as one of the great epidemics of the end of this century. Babies born of HIV positive mothers (i.e. those with human immuodeficiency virus (HIV) antibodies) are often premature, with low birth-weight and malnourished between three and six months when compared with babies born of HIV negative mothers. An increase in mortality has been noted during the first three months of life in babies born of HIV positive mothers. At the age of 12 months the mortality rate 23.4 per cent for the former and 10.85 per cent for the latter. At 24 months the mortalities are 31.3 per cent and 14.2 per cent respectively. When taken together with data from the United States and Europe,[8] the rate of transmission of HI from mother to child is 25 per cent.

Diabetes is also one of the main chronic illnesses that affect children worldwide. However, in developing countries the majority of children die in the first few years of their life.[9]

In Nicaragua,[10] while in 1955 infant mortality was 140 in every 1000 live births, in 1986 it was 65 and still it continues to fall. The analyses consider seven different causes for this decrease: better distribution of wealth, improved nutrition, stimulation and prolonged breast-feeding, education of mothers, immunization campaigns, improved health services for the population and the prioritization of public health services. This data clearly show that the education of mothers is directly linked to infant mortality. The average rate of illiteracy among Nicaraguan women was 50 per cent in 1963 and 26 per cent in 1985.[10]

The issue regarding vaccinations, oral rehydration, or breast-feeding is related to the degree of education of the mothers: it is always necessary to secure an infrastructure that allows the population to benefit from an accessible and efficient health care system.

In Africa and Asia, 500000 women die in childbirth every year. The risk of a pregnant woman dying is 100–200 times greater for a woman from a poor country than it is for a woman from an industrialized country.[1]

It is logical that progressive improvement and the increase in highly qualified health cover results in higher costs. In contrast to developing countries with a rate of infant mortality greater than 50 in every 1000, European countries have recorded a negative correlation in the past 10 years between gross national product (GNP) per capita and the rate of infant mortality. However, for a more accurate evaluation, it is necessary to carry out more socio-medical studies to assess the relation between cost and benefit. Only the countries with a high GNP per capita belong to the group with the lowest rates of infant mortality. However, the notable decline in infant mortality registered in European countries during the period 1937–55, occurred even though the highly developed equipment available was not actually put to use. In other words, levels of infant mortality above 50 in 1000 could be reduced as a result of factors other than the application of new technologies—a fall in the level of infant mortality could be achieved by quite simple and cheap methods, acceptable and applicable on a large scale, as happened in Europe 40–50 years ago. Unfortunately, however, many developing countries have opted for a strategy based on advanced technology with the sole aim of reducing neonatal deaths (for example premature births, intrauterine asphyxia, or non-viable malformations). This cannot lead to a noticeable decrease in infant mortality in these countries. It would be better to eliminate the causes of infant mortality, the most important of which are infectious illnesses; but the risks at childbirth must also be reduced to a minimum.[11]

In 1985 a large fall in infant mortality was noted in countries such as Sri Lanka, Costa Rica, the Indian state of Kerala, and China,[10] and in each case this fall occurred in a relatively short period of time. Seven conditions were considered as causes of this phenomenon:

(a) the autonomy of women;

(b) improved education (above all of the mother);

(c) the creation of accessible health centres;

(d) movements to guarantee the efficiency of health services;

(e) an adequate minimum of nutrition;

(f) vaccination of the whole population; and

(g) antenatal and postnatal services.

Morbidity

The world can be divided into the northern hemisphere, with scarcely a quarter of the population, and the southern hemisphere, taking the Tropic of Cancer as the dividing line. In the northern hemisphere, cardiovascular as well as proliferative and degenerative illnesses predominate, as do stress and sedentarism, road accidents, and social conditions leading to depression, violence, delinquency, and alcohol, tobacco and drug abuse. In the south, infectious parasitic disease predominate, with malnutrition and symptoms of insecurity (resulting from wars and natural disasters). Nevertheless there exists a certain overlap: communications and movement bring diseases from the south to the north and industrialization and urbanization as a result of development take diseases from the north to the south.[1]

Disability in the Third World is another important phenomenon: there are 230 million invalids in Asia, 50 million in Africa, and 40 million in South America, almost a third of them being children under the age of 15. In 25 per cent of Third World families there is some form of disability.[1]

To evaluate the extent of need for medical materials, four indicators have been used: diarrhoea, parasitic ulcer, dracunculiasis, and nutritional state, taking into account the fact the there are large differences between morbidity and mortality even within the same geographical area. Children under the age of five can expect to have an average of 3–4 cases of diarrhoea per year and mortality as a result diarrhoea reaches 12 in 1000. It is believed that approximately 1000 million people are infected by *Ascaris lumbricoides*, 900 million by 'hookworms', and 500 million by *Trichuris trichiura*. Although dracunculiasis occurs mainly in rural areas and its incidence is therefore more difficult to calculate, it is estimated that the infected population is about 10 million each year.[12]

The widespread prevalence of malnutrition must be associated with infant mortality since it increases risk of infection. It is the underlying cause of 50 per cent of all deaths in South America.[1,12] The infections most linked to malnutrition are diarrhoea, measles, and malaria.[1]

In a cohort study carried out in Brazil,[13] with a longitudinal follow-up of 6000 children from underdeveloped areas, it showed a relationship between morbidity and family income. The smaller the economic resources the greater the morbidity in the family unit or population.

A factor strongly related to morbidity is the accessibility of health services to the population. To evaluate this factor various constants have been studied:[6]

- The population that receives treatment for illnesses and accidents and regular contributions of essential medicines, at most within an hours' journey.

- Women cared for by trained staff during pregnancy.

- Women cared for by trained staff during childbirth.
- Children cared for by trained staff during the first 12 months of life.

Although data is lacking for 44.2 per cent of the world population, it is estimated that three-quarters of the population do not have access to health care, 38 million women are not looked after during pregnancy, and 46 million give birth without the presence of trained staff.[1,6]

Infection

Diseases preventable by vaccination

Every year 50 million children are not correctly vaccinated against diphtheria, tetanus, whooping cough, polio, measles, and tuberculosis; three million die and a further three million are left handicapped.[6] Approximately 10 per cent of children are infected with diphtheria every year of life: at the age of 10 all the non-vaccinated children have been infected (some 800 million every year). One in 1000 in Africa suffer serious diphtheria and 10 per cent of these children die.[1] Tetanus accounts for between five and 61 per cent of neonatal mortality, depending on the country, and appears in at least 15 per 1000 live births. There are some 500 000 cases every year, with a mortality rate of 80 per cent, it being most frequent in rural areas.[1,7] Eighty per cent of children under five years old are infected with whooping cough[1]; and between one and 18 in very 1000 children with poliomyelitis suffer residual paralysis.[1,4] Measles is another major cause of mortality (five per cent or more in all ages) occurring, above all, in malnourished children.

Gastroenteritis

Nearly 750 million children suffer acute gastroenteritis every year. This illness is responsible for some four million deaths each year in children under the age of five. Neither diarrhoea nor parasites are the direct causes of these deaths, but dehydration and malnutrition.[6] However, oral rehydration can prevent dehydration, which regularly kills two-thirds of children with acute diarrhoea.[6,14]

The infectious disease which is the greatest cause of mortality in developing countries is diarrhoea: a child under five years old suffers between two and 10 cases each year and there are more than 450 million children under the age of five in these countries, which amounts to 1400 cases of diarrhoea each year. Mortality among the poorest and most malnourished children reaches one per cent.[1,7] Diarrhoea causes around 12 000 deaths every day among children in Asia, Africa, and Latin America. Infectious agents are the most common aetiology, either virus, bacteria, or parasites. While *Escherichia coli* and rotavirus predominate as the most common germs in developed countries, in underdeveloped countries *Campylobacter jejuni* and *Clostridium difficile* are predominant. Other types of agent such as *Shigella*, *Salmonella*, *Cryptosporidium*, and *Giardia lamblia* are spread over the whole world. Identification of the agent responsible for a particular disease is important not only for treatment but also for carrying out epidemiological studies.[15] The American National Research Council has highlighted the importance of knowledge of the aetiological agents in infectious diseases among children, and there is a great deal of interest in the study of the relation between the level of antibodies in the mother and passive immunity in children.

Respiratory infections

These cause one-third or more of deaths in children and account for 15 per cent of deaths among all age groups.[1] Four million children die every year from acute respiratory infections; in general, pneumonia. Some of these deaths are due to malnutrition or disease against which people could be immunized. Respiratory infections give rise to half the visits of children to health services worldwide. All children have between four and eight cases of infection each year, generally in the upper respiratory tract, but infections in the lower respiratory tract are more frequent in underdeveloped countries.[6]

Respiratory infections and diarrhoea cause between half and two-thirds of the morbidity and mortality from infectious diseases in developing countries.[1]

Tuberculosis

It is calculated that there are 1600 million people carrying the bacteria and every year there are 10 million new cases, resulting in three million deaths, the risk being 100 times greater in developing countries.[1,4,6] It is one of the most common diseases of the Third World population, whereas in industrialized countries it is controlled by the BCG vaccination.

Sexually transmitted diseases

It is estimated that five per cent of adolescents and young people contract sexually transmitted diseases each year. It must be pointed out that these diseases are caused by more than 20 different microorganisms.[6]

Malaria

According to the latest figures from WHO, in 1987 there were five million cases of malaria worldwide, excluding Africa, although it has been calculated that the total number could exceed 100 million.[1,6] Malaria causes at least 1.5 million deaths each year, mainly in Africa. It must not be forgotten that 43 per cent of the world population lives in areas with risk of infection, in many of which control measures are not taken.[6] Its incidence is less in dry areas and places of high altitude. There are four types of plasmid: malaria, oval, vivax, and falciparum, the latter being the cause of cerebral malaria, with a mortality rate of 50 per cent.[17]

Hepatitis B

Between 10 and 15 per cent of the population of east Asia and west Africa are infected with the hepatitis B virus (HBV)—170 million people are carriers of HBV; 350 000 die each year from cirrhosis of the liver and 150 000 die from hepatic carcinoma.[1]

AIDS

In ten countries studied Africa, the number of children under the age of five infected with HIV that die each year will be between 250 000 and 500 000 by the year 2000. WHO hopes to reduce mortality among children under the age of five, in these ten countries, by 78 in every 1000 live births by the year 2000, but infection by HIV could increase this to more than 150. The increase in mortality resulting from HIV among adults will increase the number of children under the age of 15 whose mothers will die from HIV/AIDS. In 1990 HIV/AIDS caused the death of approximately 1.5 to 2.9 million young women, producing between 3.1 and 4.5 million orphans. This means that between six and eleven per cent of the population under the age of 15 will be orphaned. All this necessitates the rapid and efficient development of appropriate programmes and policies.[18]

Parasites

In Asia, Africa, South America, and The Caribbean 200 million people are infected by Schistosomiasis—a disease transmitted by parasites through water—and another 600 million are at risk of infection.[1,6] In developing countries 25 per cent of the population are infected with worms; 24 million Latin Americans are chronically infected by *Trypanosoma cruzi*;[1] and some 280 million people in underdeveloped countries are infected with amoeba.[1]

Nutrition

Between 450 and 650 million human beings constantly go hungry. In the Sahara area of Africa these figures will increase by the end of the century, although food resources will not—in fact, they could even decrease.[1] The limit of absolute hungry is set at 1450 calories daily per person. Undernourishment is recognized when calorie intake falls to 2000 and malnutrition occurs when the deficit is not in terms of calories but proteins and vitamins.[19] Hunger (including undernourishment and malnutrition) affects 75 per cent of humanity. In Africa it affects 25 per cent, in the Far East 20 per cent and in South America 13 per cent. In absolute terms the starving population is greater in the Far East than in Africa and South America.[19]

Although increases in food production have been achieved, in Africa food production per capita has decreased by one per cent. It is not necessary to develop new technology but rather to spread existing knowledge and to redirect policies towards rural areas. In fact the problem is one of access to food, by not having the money to buy it, or the land to cultivate it, or products which would be exchanged for it. Short-term cheap solutions do not exist.[20]

In Southern Asia there are 50 million undernourished children and in Latin America 25 million, in spite of the food surplus in the region. Above all, malnutrition affects infants, the period in which it is most frequent and most serious. The greater part of mental and physical development is completed during infancy and therefore adequate nutrition should be the priority in these years. The nutritional state of these children depends not only on the availability of food, but also on other factors such as illnesses (especially if they recur); the lack of basic knowledge among parents concerning the nutritional needs of children in their early year (such as the importance of breast-feeding, introduction of weaning foods at 4–6 months, frequent feeding, enrichment of diet with oil or fats, vegetables every day); ensuring that feeding or digestion and liquids intake is not interrupted during illness and that feeding continues during convalescence, with regular weight-checks; and the nutritional state of the mother during pregnancy, the health of the mother, and spacing between pregnancies. Programmes for monitoring the development of infants, as distinct from nutritional programmes—which aim to recuperate undernourished children—seek to avoid malnutrition by means of adequate feeding and prevention of disease.[20]

The knowledge that various symptoms can be linked to inadequate diet and specifically to vitamin deficiency has almost wiped out diseases such as scurvy, beri-beri, pellagra, and others. Even severe forms of protein–caloric deficiency such as kwashiorkor and atrophy have been confined to areas of the Third World. Iron, iodine, and vitamin A deficiency, however, are still seen in developing countries. There are WHO/UNICEF programmes such as 'child survival and development revolution' which try to persuade these countries to introduce immunization programmes, growth and development monitoring, adequate nutrition, gastroenteritis monitoring, and specific campaigns against avitaminosis A or ferropenia. We know about the risk factors which lead to chronic states of deficiency and nutritional problems in rich countries: obesity, cardiovascular diseases, or certain types of cancer, but in the 'fourth world' of the deprived areas of large cities, malnutrition is superimposed on these other problems and principally affects childrens' development.

Grande Covian[21] suggests that underdeveloped and industrialized countries ought to be encouraged to exchange their products more. Whilst the former are cereal consumers, the latter feed these products to their animals—7000 calories of cereals are used to produce 1000 calories of meat. This exchange would balance out the lack of meat in the Third World and the First World would use up their cereal surplus, thus reducing industrial civilization diseases and at the same time providing underdeveloped countries with more meat protein.[22,23]

However, it should not be forgotten that in a study of the prevalence of chronic malnutrition carried out in Massachusetts,[24] this was greater than expected, without acute malnutrition being detected. This suggests that chronic malnutrition is on the increase among children at risk in industrialized areas.

In the case of infection, the nutritional state of the child is more important than the causal agent. In a study carried out in Israel,[25] far more malnourished than well-fed children with diarrhoea were admitted to hospital. However, rotavirus was detected with equal prevalence in both groups, indicating that the state of nutrition is an important indicator of the likely prognosis and gravity of the illness.

Accidents

Injuries and accidents are frequent causes of mortality among children and adolescents in developing countries. Many of the accidents in countries with limited resources are comparable to those occurring in developed countries. Falls constitute the most common cause, with 40–52 per cent amongst minor age groups, whilst mortalities due to traffic accidents have increased (5–24 per cent).[26] It is important to note that apart from the child's age being a risk factor, lack of parental training also contributes.[27]

Prevention of disease

Prevention and cure should always go together, particularly in Third World countries. Despite cure being the demand formulated by the patient, prevention is the more efficient way of raising health standards.

In developing countries millons of children die each year, many from diseases which could be avoided using only limited resources. Amongst the strategies that have been developed are promotion of breast-feeding, personal hygiene, immunization programmes, growth and development programmes, family planning, and monitoring of pregnancy.

Breast-feeding

Breast-feeding and vaccination are two important measures for achieving the survival of children in developing countries, and health professionals in close contact with the population promote both programmes. Breast-feeding does not interfere with the immunization programme according to the timetable recommended by the EPI (Expanded Programme on Immunization) Global Advisory Group for use in developing countries, indeed breast-feeding and EPI are mutually beneficial.[28]

The 'kangaroo-mothers' method[29] has shown itself to be an excellent way of providing low birth-weight newborns with warmth and food on demand—making sure that children remain continuously in contact with their mother's body constitutes a 'technologically autochthonous' resource, useful in those countries with limited resources.

In the decade of 1973–83 in Sao Paolo, mortality rates among the babies of nursing mothers fell by 50 per cent and 70 per cent respectively. However, surveys carried out in 1973–74 and 1984–85 showed no change in the prevalence of protein–caloric malnutrition or in the socio-economic characteristics of the population; but may be that improvements to the water supply system and time spent breast-feeding could explain up to 20 per cent the mortality rate of the babies of nursing mothers'.[30]

Vaccines

Vaccination has been one of the priority means of prevention among infants. Through the efforts of numerous organizations, two-thirds of the world's children have been vaccinated against Diphtheria, Tetanus, Pertussis (DTP) and polio; 72 per cent have received BCG vaccinations and 59 per cent have been immunized against measles. However, only 29 per cent of women have had two anti-tetanus jabs. Vaccines against yellow fever, japanese encephalitis, hepatitis B, rubella, mumps, and meningitis have been used solely in specific regions of the world. It is hoped that over the next decade other vaccines will be available against pneumonia, gastroenteritis, meningitis by *haemophilus influenzae* type b, infection by rotavirus, and meningococcal meningitis. Genetic engineering has been a useful way of finding new vaccines.[31]

The EPI programme (Expanded Programme on Immunization) was created by WHO/UNICEF in the hope that in 1990 the world's children would be immunized before their first birthday against six diseases: measles, poliomyelitis, tuberculosis, whooping cough, diphtheria, and tetanus.[4] In Nigeria, EPI was started in 1979 and has demonstrated its effectiveness, as since 1986 mortality due to measles and whooping cough has fallen. However, the incidence of tuberculosis has increased in this country despite national coverage for BCG being over 80 per cent of the population.[32] This serves to underline the fact that the immunization timetable used in industrialized countries is not always appropriate for underdeveloped countries. Moreover, as infectiousness changes with the weather, immunization programmes should start adapting to circumstances.

In the Gaza strip 13 years ago, there was high infant mortality, with figures of 100–150 per thousand live births, owing to ignorance and poverty. The initiation of vaccine coverage programmes, diarrhoea monitoring, and spread of centres for assisting births has caused mortality to fall to 29 in every thousand. The Palestinian leaders were responsible—they decreed that immunization should be considered as a form of religious precept whose disregard would be seen as a sin. Thus health and religious beliefs evolved together.[33]

Immunization against measles is one of the more useful vaccines, its use having caused the incidence of measles to fall both in developing and in developed countries. However, morbidity and mortality continues to be high despite widespread immunization. This could be due to disregard for the proposed vaccine timetable, lack of vaccine, or deterioration of vaccine due to incorrect storage conditions.[34]

Population growth and the environment

It was thought that in order to reduce the birth rate it was only necessary to reduce infant mortality. In this way, it was reasoned, that when families realize that their children are not going to die, they will proceed to have fewer. However, it is almost impossible to reduce the birth rate with measures intended to reduce mortality by means of vertical programmes imposed on the population which, in the majority of cases, is illiterate.

For deep-rooted customs to change, the reduction of mortality should be accompanied by an improvement in quality of life.[35,36] Reduction of the birth rate seems to require other conditions such as social and economic improvement. As such, it is necessary to reduce poverty and promote socio-economic development, otherwise there is the danger of the community destroying its own ecosystem by overpopulation.[35,36]

Health was originally an individual concern, later a family one, and has now become a collective responsibility, the theoretical framework for which should be based on maintaining the capacity of the ecosystem to sustain quality and diversity of life. This maintenance would entail consideration of the implications of different lifestyles, which should be such that they are in harmony with the environment, in recognition of the fact that our health is unavoidably linked with that of the planet.[35,36]

Populations which survive thanks to technological achievement are on the increase. In 1988 32.4 per cent of children survived because they had been immunized. However, every year approximately 14 million babies and half a million mothers die, even though there are technological resources available to avoid these deaths. This is not an ecological problem but a political one between the developed and developing countries—the World Bank estimated that in 1990 more than 100 million people were living in absolute poverty.[4,36]

In the next 100 years the world population may double or even triple. This could lead to a 'demographic trap' whose progress can be summarized in three sentences. First, human expansion will still be supplied by its ecosystem.

Second, the needs of the population will come to exceed that which can be supplied by the environment so that we will be obliged to use up biological reserves; and human consumption would then be forced to decrease due to the collapse of the ecosystem. Faced with this the possible ways out would be limited to reduction of the population by death due to starvation and disease, or genocide; removal of the population to 'ecological refuges'; or maintenance of the population by food and other resources coming from another location, either as an emergency measure or indefinitely. The 'demographic trap' is therefore a new term for an old idea: destruction of biological support produces an ecological disaster in which man is involved.[35]

Literacy and education

According to data from UNESCO in 1985 27.7 per cent of people over 15 years of age were illiterate: 666 million (75 per cent) in Asia and two per cent in industrialized countries. In Africa the situation is even more alarming since in some countries illiterates comprise more then 50 per cent of the population[20,37,38] (Fig. 5.4).

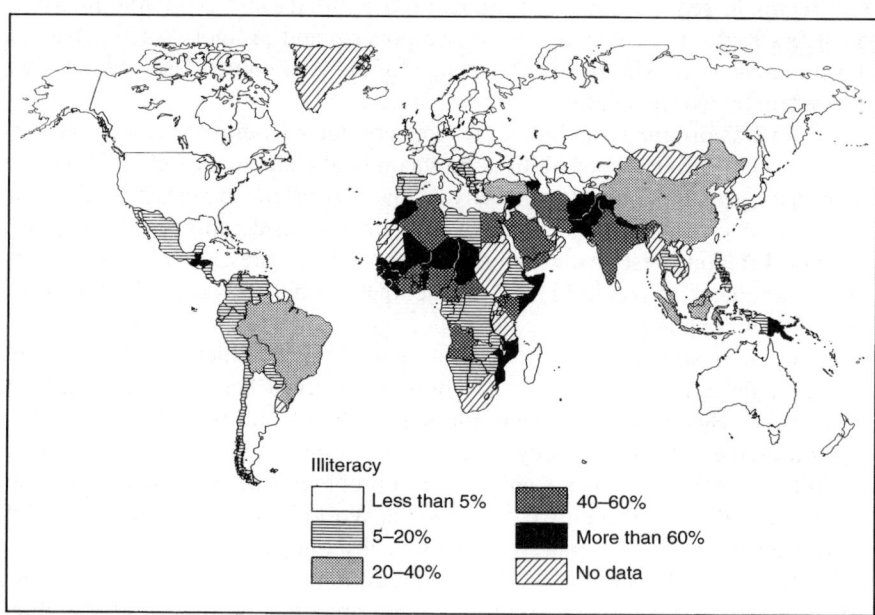

Fig. 5.4 Illiteracy in the world. (Source: reference 37.)

UNESCO aspires to teaching adults to read and write and the basic schooling of all children. Illiteracy needs to be eradicated by the year 2000, but there are still 960 million illiterate adults and 100 million children who have no schooling (a difficult figure to check). The increase of illiterates in industrialized countries has also to be considered.[20,37,38] A great effort has been made to teach people to read and write and the percentage of illiterates has fallen, even though the total number has risen due to population increase. Despite the number of children attending school having risen, there continue to be large numbers of illiterate women and men (20.5 per cent of men and 34.9 per cent of women) and in the poorest developing countries, education spending has fallen.[20,37,38]

One important piece of data is that there are relations between greater agricultural production and more schooling, the number of children in a family and the degree of education, and reduced infant mortality and malnutrition and greater schooling amongst mothers.[20,37,38]

Refugees

Africa is a continent where there are approximately six million refugees (Fig. 5.5). If the displaced population on the borders of each state is added, the figure rises to 15 million.[39] If monitoring health is problematic in underdeveloped countries, the problem of refugees contributes even greater difficulties.

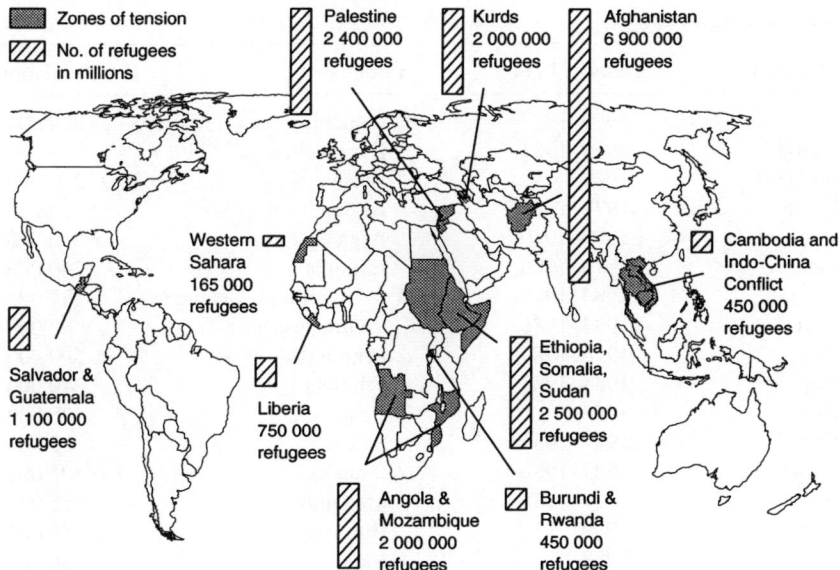

Fig. 5.5 Refugees in Africa (1990). (Source: *El Pais*; reproduced from United States Committee for refugees.)

In developing countries more than 30 million refugees and displaced persons depend on help in order to survive (Table 5.1). A large part of the help comes from the West. In this population, mortality during periods of displacement reaches rates 60 times higher than normal. Although mortality is increased in all age groups, it is greater between the ages of one and 14. The most common causes of mortality are measles, diarrhoea, acute respiratory infections, and malaria. This is influenced by the high prevalence protein–caloric malnutrition and lack of immunization. However, it is difficult to initiate urgent programmes based on balanced and frequent food provision, availability of drinking water, immunization against measles, and control of infectious disease, above all of those illnesses which have to be declared.[39]

A study carried out on children under five,[40] whose characteristic is that of constant moving around either because they belong to nomadic groups or because they are refugees, revealed a low uptake of vaccines in comparison with children from static families. Only 25–30 per cent 'traveller children' had completed the first dose of vaccine against tetanus, diphtheria, and polio, compared with 85.5 per cent overall. Immunization against whooping cough was 15 per cent as opposed to 75.6 per cent overall. Ethnic minority children in Europe experience special problems. These are considered in detail in Chapter 25.

Table 5.1 *Recent refugees influxes, host countries, countries of origin, and populations affected*[39]

Host country	Years of influx	Country of origin	Population
Thailand	1975–1979	Indochina	280 000
Thailand	1979–1981	Kampuchea	300 000
Bangladesh	1977	Burma	200 000
Pakistan	1978–1980	Afghanistan	2 500 000
Iran	1979–1980	Afghanistan	2 000 000
Somalia	1979–1980	Ethiopia	700 000
Honduras	1983–1986	Salvador and Nicaragua	37 000
Mexico	1983–1986	Central America	47 000
Sudan	1976–1984	Eritrea (Ethiopia)	500 000
Sudan	1984–1985	Ethiopia	340 000
Sudan	1985	Chad	120 000
Ethiopia	1987–1988	Sudan	320 000
Ethiopia	1987–1988	Somalia	305 000
Malawi	1987–1988	Mozambique	555 000
Rwanda	1988	Burundi	50 000
Turkey	1988	Iraq	36 000
Guinea	1990	Liberia	80 000
Ivory Coast	1990	Liberia	60 000

Programmes

The European Community Commission responsible for finance has authorized important aid since its initiation in 1957. Aid allocated by the European Development Fund (EDF) has continued to increase. From the 48.4 million to 77.3 million ECUS (1963-1985). Nowadays, aid is allocated to different sectors such as non-governmental organizations projects (NGO), refugees, and special programmes such as assistance for AIDS and programmes on science and technical service development (STD).[42]

In general, programmes directed at the Third World have been subjected to harsh criticism. Inefficient planning and the difficulties involved in monitoring and follow-up have made it necessary to revise aid policies. In fact, despite financial aid, the improvement in Third World health has been nothing more than minimal. This is particularly true of Africa, where in many cases the situation has worsened. Economic crises in developing countries often cause a reduction of the budget assigned to health, in order to be able to pay foreign debts.[42]

European Community (EC) aid to Third World health budgets during the 1960s prioritized investment in infrastructure and equipment which received up to 90 per cent of the total amount. Formerly, loans were allocated to the construction of large hospitals, generally located in capital cities such as Mogadishu, Somalia (600 beds); Nouakchott, Mauritania (450 beds); or Antananarivo, Madagascar (730 beds). This trend coincided with the independence of the countries affected.[42] However, it is evident that these projects entailed serious problems. These were hospitals badly adapted to their environment, they needed a great infrastructure which was not always available, and it was difficult to get them to work. Local health budgets were not sufficient to finance them. These experiences made a revision necessary of the type of aid needed. Experts' reports sent to the EC pointed that far from achieving improvements, these projects had imposed new burdens on poor countries' national budgets, mortgaging the development of other sectors.

All this has allowed the definition and revision of a series of fundamental principles which were subsequently adopted by the ACP (Africa, Caribbean, and Pacific) states in the Freetown Conference of December 1978 and most recently revised in 1986.[42]

The priority objectives of the EC's policy are the following:[42]

- to raise the level of health service coverage, principally at primary level, by means of a rationalization of its structures, implying that hospitals should offer more specialized services;
- to improve cost efficiency, rationalizing the use of financial and local human resources;

- to improve the general support structure of the health system, including demands such as pharmaceutical products and environmental hygiene;
- to rationalize the use of human resources.

In the 'Priority health needs in Central America and Panama' plan[5] one of the fixed aims is to mobilize resources in favour of the more vulnerable sectors of the population, particularly children; those least privileged in cities and rural areas; and those who are displaced due to violence, looking elsewhere to satisfy their needs; that is to contribute to the people's well-being. In the introduction to the 'Programme for immediate action for infant survival in Central America and Panama'[5] reference is made to the problems the region suffers:

- accelerated demographic growth among low income groups;
- massive inequalities in income distribution;
- voluntary and involuntary migration.

This programme's strategy is centred on its principal aspects:

- child growth and control of development;
- oral rehydration therapy;
- breast-feeding;
- immunization;
- prevention and control of high risk pregnancy and regulation of fertility under reproductive and obstetric risk;
- prevention and control of acute respiratory infections.

All these examples make one think that aid rationalization will occur gradually. European Community programmes in the Third World[42] aspire to improve both the human economic elements. They also speak of improving the environment with the aim of enabling it to sustain the physical and psychological development of the population.

Energy and resources

For decades part of the world has lived comfortably thanks to the enormous quantities of energy and resources provided by the Third World.[43] Whilst rich countries use advanced fuel technology, poor countries continue to use traditional fuel. Even now, at the end of the twentieth century, more than 50 per cent of the world's population still uses wood as the only source of fuel, and their population is concentrated in underdeveloped countries. These countries, where three-quarters of the world's population live, produce only 20 per cent of the electricity generated throughout the world.[44]

There is a good correlation between energy consumption and GNP. Modern man expects an enormous quantity of high intensity energy from nature. The daily consumption of food is estimated at 3000 kilocalories, which implies a tonne of foodstuff per individual per year. The expanse of cultivated land is between 13.7 and 15 million square kilometres which provides a sustenance base for human beings. Each person is maintained by 0.4 hectares, which corresponds to a density of 250 people per square kilometre. Evidently, this theoretical distribution does not correspond to reality.[21]

Poverty requires the breeding of frugal and very efficient animals such as the goat, which feeds on roots and shoots, thereby making recultivation of the ground more difficult. Indeed, it is said that 'the bedouin is not the son of the desert but its father'.[21]

However, while some rich countries continue to consume a third of world resources annually, it is very difficult for the Third World even to have access to the absolute necessities.[43]

Conclusion

The child health challenges in developing countries remain huge and daunting. Solutions are as much political and economic as they are medical, requiring genuine improvements in living standards. As in Europe, poverty and its consequences remains the major determinant of child ill-health. Child health workers in Europe can learn from the experience of child health care in developing countries, particularly the importance of public health and primary care programmes and community participation (see Chapter 34). They can contribute to the solutions through advocacy and the further development of concepts of primary child health care and community participation.

References

1. Gentilini, M. (1989). *Médecine tropicale* (4th edn). Médecine-Sciences Flammarion, Paris.
2. Perez, R. (1989). *La infancia y la juventud en los paises en desarrollo*. Documentos para el desarrollo (No 2). Cruz Roja Espa/nola, Madrid.
3. Levene, M.I. (ed.) (1991). *Jolly's diseases of children* (6th edn). pp. 529–75. Blackwell Scientific, Oxford.
4. Olle, J.E. (1990). ¿Hay que vacunar a los ni/nos de los países subdesarrollado? *Med. Clin.* (Barc.), **95**, 454–5.
5. Plan Sanitario (1984). *Necesidades prioritarias de salud en Centroamérica y Panamá*. Costa Rica.

6. *World Health statistics annual* (1989). World Health Organization, Geneva.
7. Warren, K.S. and Mahmoud, A.A.F. (1984). *Tropical and geographical medicine*, McGraw-Hill, New York.
8. Halsey N.A., Boulos, R. Holt, E., Ruff, A.Ø, Brutus, I., Kissuger, P. *et al.* (1990) Transmission of HIV-1 infections from mothers to infants in Haiti. Impact on childhood mortality and malnutrition. The CDS/JHU AIDS Project Team. *J. Amer. Med. Assoc.*, **264**, 2088–92.
9. WHO Diamond Project Group (1990). WHO multinational project for childhood diabetes, *Diabetes Care*, **13**, 1062–8.
10. Sandiford, P., Morales, P., Gorter, A., Coyle, E. and Smith, G.D. (1991). Why do child mortality rates fall? An analysis of the Nicaraguan experience. *Am. J. Public Health*, **81**, 30–7.
11. Stembera, Z. (1990). Perspectivas para una mayor supervivencia infantil. *Foro Mundial Salud*, **11**, 78–85.
12. Huttly, S.R. (1990). The impact of inadequate sanitary conditions on health in developing countries. *World Health Stat. Quart.*, **43**, 118–26.
13. Barros, F.C., Victoria, C.G. and Vaughan, J.P. (1990). The Pelotas (Brazil) birth control study 1982–1987: strategies for following up 6000 children in a developing country. *Paediatr. Perinatal Epidemiol.*, **4**, 205–20.
14. Mota-Hernandez, F. (1990). Estrategias para la disminución de la morbi-mortalidad por diarreas agudas en Am!erica Latina. *Salud Pública Mex.*, **32**, 254–60.
15. Guerrant, R.L., Hughes, J.M. Lima, N.L. and Crane, J. (1990). Diarrhea in developed and developing countries: magnitude, special settings, and etiologies. *Rev. Infect. Dis.* **12** (Suppl. 1), 541–50.
16. Graham, N.M. (1990). The epidemiology of acute respiratory infections in children and adults: a global perspective. *Epidemiol. Rev.*, **12**, 149–78.
17. Phillips, Rev. and Solomon, T. (1990). Cerebral malaria in children. *Lancet*, **ii**, 1355–60.
18. Preble, E.A. (1990). Impact of HIV/AIDS on Africa children. *Soc. Sci. Med.*, **31**, 671–80.
19. Almansa, F. (1990). PROSALUS y la ayuda alimenticia. Seminario sobre politicas de desarrollo y ayudas alimentarias en el Tercer Mundo. Temas de cooperación (No 1). pp. 67–71. Coordinadora de ONG, Madrid.
20. Grant, G.P. (1989). *Estado mundial de la infancia, 1989.* UNICEF, Barcelona.
21. Grande Covian, F. (1989). El Pais, Semanal (15) 47.
22. Scrimshaw, N.S. (1990). Nutrition: prospects for the 1990s. *Ann. Rev. Public Health*, **11**, 53–68.
23. Allen, L.H. (1990). Functional indicators and outcomes of undernutrition. *J. Nutr.*, **120**, 924–32.
24. Dietz, W.H. (1990). Undernutrition of children in Massachusetts. *J. Nutr.*, **120**, 948–54.
25. Dagan, R., Bar-David, Y., Sarov, B., Ketz, M., Kessiz, I., Guttenberg. D *et al.* (1990). Rotavirus diarrhea in Jewish and Bedouin children in the Negev region of Israel: epidemiology, clinical aspects and possible role and malnutrition in severity of illness. *Pediatr. Infect. Dis. J.*, **9**, 314–21.
26. Bangdiwala, S.I., Anzola-Perez, E., Romer, C.C., Schultz, B., Valdtz-Lazo, F.J., *et al.* (1990). The incidence of injuries in young people: I. Methodology and results of a collaborative study in Brazil, Chile, Cuba and Venezuela. *Int. J. Epidemiol.*, **19**, 115–24.

27. Bangdiwala, S.I. and Anzola-Perez, E. (1990). The incidence of injuries in young people: II. Log-linear multivariable models for risk factors in a collaborative study in Brazil, Chile, Cuba and Venezuela. *Int. J. Epidemiol.*, **19**, 125–32.
28. Kim-Farley, R., Collins, C. and Tinker, A. (1990). Linkages between immunization and breast-feeding promotion programs. *J. Hum. Lact.*, **6**, 65–7.
29. Colonna, F., Uxa, F., de Graca, A.M. and de Vonderweld, U. (1990). The 'kangaroo-mother' method: evaluation of an alternative model for the care of low birth weight newborns in developing countries. *Int. J. Gynaecol. Obstet.*, **31**, 335–9.
30. Monteiro, C.A., Pino, H.P., Benicio, M.H.A. and Victoria, C.G. (1989). Mejores perspectivas para la supervivencia de los nin/os. *Foro Mundial Salud*, **10**, 218–23.
31. Bart, K.J. and Lin K.F. (1990). Vaccine-preventable disease and immunisation in the developing world. *Paediatr. Clin. North Am.*, **37**, 735–56.
32. Babaniyi, O.A. (1990). A 10-year review of morbidity from childhood preventable diseases in Nigeria: how successful is the expanded programme on immunization (EPI)? An update. *J. Trop. Pediatr.*, **36**, 306–13.
33. Lasch, E.E. (1990). Child health in a developing population with changing patterns of belief (Gaza 1973–1983). *Harefuah*, **118**, 522–5.
34. Markowitz, L.E. and Orenstein, W.A. (1990). Measles vaccine. *Pediatr. Clin. North Am.*, **37**, 603–25.
35. King, M. (1990). Health in a sustainable state. *Lancet*, **ii**, 664–7.
36. Shoo, R. (1990). Overpopulation and death in childhood. *Lancet*, **ii**, 1312.
37. Garcia, A. (1990). Alfabetizar no es enseñar a leer. *Antena Misionera*, **244**, 6–10.
38. Anon. (1990). Año Internacional de la Alfabetización. *Manos Unidas*, **96**, 9–16.
39. Toole, M.J. and Waldman, R.J. (1990). Prevention of excess mortality in refugee and displaced populations in developing countries. *J. Am. Med. Assoc.*, **263**, 3296–302.
40. McKenzie, A.B. (1990). Traveller mothers and babies. *Br. Med. J.*, **301**, 123.
41. McDonald, C. (1989). *La communauté européene et la santé dans le Tiers Monde Development*. Report of 'Commission des Communautés Européennes', Luxembourg.
42. Rifkin, J. (1990). *Entropia. (Hacia el mundo invernadero)* Ed. Urano S.A., Barcelona.
43. Pichs, R. (1991). Vulnerabilidad tecnológica y crisis energética en el Tercer Mundo. *Informes. Món-3*. **6**, 32–4.

PART II

Social and demographic trends in Europe

Demographic trends are vital to an understanding of changing patterns of child health; this part considers trends in pregnancy, birth-weight, family structure, and child mortality and morbidity. Changes occurring across the European region have had a profound effect on health and well-being of children. The data presented in this part provide an essential backdrop to the discussion of specific aspects of child health in subsequent parts of the book.

6 Demographic trends in pregnancy and birth-weight

Jitka Rychtaříková

As the number of children in the family has continually decreased in European countries this century, more and more attention has been given to reproduction losses in the first year of life. These deaths, mostly closely related to previous intrauterine development, are to a large extent determined not only by biological but also by social factors. Among the biological variables of a demographic nature we usually include the mother's age and parity; among the social ones we include, for example, legitimacy, education, job position, and so on. Before investigating the development of some of these variables and their impact on infant mortality, let us first look at infant mortality within general overall mortality and the structural changes in infant mortality.

Infant mortality in relation to life expectancy

Even today, in advanced countries, infant mortality represents a far from trivial share of the overall mortality and tends to be seen as a significant social and health characteristic. In countries with a very low mortality, the infant mortality rate (i.e. the ratio of the number of deaths of children under one year of age in a given period to the total number of live births registered in the same period) is still substantially higher than in the higher age groups. We find the same mortality rate again only after the fifth decade of life. The fall in infant mortality this century has been greater than in all other age group—from more than 200 per to less than 10 per 1000. This roughly twentyfold decrease has substantially contributed to the prolongation of the life expectancy at birth. The values of specific contributions of the drop in infant mortality to the changes in the life expectancy at birth, since the beginning of this century in Sweden and Czechoslovakia, are given in Table 6.1. The contribution of the change of infant mortality to the increase of life expectancy at birth is given by the equation:

$$d = (e_0^{t+n} - e_0^t) - (e_1^{t+n} - e_1^t)(l_1^{t+n}+l_1^t)/2$$

where d is the contribution of the change of infant mortality to the differential in life expectancy at birth (e_0^t, e_0^{t+n}) from life tables, in the periods t and $t+n$; l_1^{t+n} measures the life table survivors to age 1 with a radix of 1 in a life table from periods t or $t+n$. For example, in Table 6.1, in Sweden 1900 and 1910 the increment in life expectancy at birth was 4.82 years. 2.12 years (contribution d) of this value was due to the decrease in infant mortality rate.

Table 6.1 *The contribution of infant mortality to the prolongation of the life expectancy at birth in Sweden and Czechoslovakia*

period	boys			girls		
		contribution			contribution	
t/t+n	$e_0^{t+n} - e_0^t$	years	%	$e_0^{t+n} - e_0^t$	years	%
			Sweden			
1900/1910	4.82	2.12	43.9	4.70	1.85	39.3
1920/1930	6.06	0.21	3.6	5.40	0.23	4.3
1930/1950	8.02	1.75	21.8	8.65	1.37	15.8
1950/1960	1.51	0.26	17.1	2.46	0.22	9.0
1960/1970	0.45	0.37	81.8	2.03	0.29	14.2
1970/1980	0.76	0.32	42.7	1.56	0.28	17.9
1980/1988	1.39	0.11	7.9	1.15	0.06	4.9
			Czechoslovakia			
1900/1910	3.88	1.80	46.5	4.18	1.59	38.0
1920/1930	5.51	2.59	47.0	5.99	2.06	34.3
1930/1950	9.01	4.04	44.8	10.35	3.62	35.0
1950/1960	6.71	3.96	59.0	7.59	3.58	47.2
1960/1970	−1.41	0.09	–	−0.18	0.07	–
1970/1980	0.55	0.29	52.0	1.02	0.30	29.7
1980/1988	0.98	0.36	36.8	1.33	0.15	10.9

Note: e_0^t is the expectation of life at birth in the period t, i.e. the mean future lifetime (the average number of years lived after birth) under condition of mortality situation of the period t.

We also see from Table 6.1 that from the beginning of the twentieth century until the sixties the decrease in infant mortality substantially contributed to the increments in mean length of life. In Sweden we notice a decrease in relative contributions from 40 per cent around 1900 to five per cent around 1990. In Czechoslovakia, the corresponding values were within a range of 30 to 50 per cent. This development would seem to indicate that the possibilities of reducing overall mortality by a reduction in infant mortality have been exhausted. At present, infant mortality is but little involved in the differences in overall mortality between individual countries.

Trends in infant mortality related to birth-weight

In Europe after the Second World War the substantial reduction in infant mortality passed through several qualitatively different stages. In the first stage we notice that there was primarily a decrease in post-neonatal mortality, while since the sixties, individual countries, at various periods, gradually succeeded in reducing mortality immediately after birth. In this context many countries were able to substantially reduce infant mortality of low birth-weight infants. This was due to the introduction of new perinatological methods and of up-to-date instrumentation into intensive care units looking after high risk neonates.

The values of mortality indicators for the first year of life change considerably with the *age* of deceased infants; moreover, they differ according to *birth-weight*. The process of dying in relation to age may be quantitatively expressed in an infant life table, an analogy of the 'classical' life table. Age groups are usually given in days for the first week of life, in weeks for the first month and in months for the remaining part of the first year of life. The probability of death within a given time interval is given by the equation.

$$q_x = \frac{D_x}{B - \sum_{i=0}^{x-1} D_i}$$

where D_x is the number of deceased infants of age x, and the denominator expresses the number of survivors, i.e. the number of live births, B, less the number of deceased infants up to the age $x - 1$.

The values of probability of death, in Sweden and Czechoslovakia for the years 1986–87, are given in Table 6.2, which show that the risk of death (q_x) rapidly decreases with age. On the first day of life (zeroth completed day) mortality is approximately ten times higher than on the sixth completed day. Even more marked differences exist between the first and last week and between the first and last month. Differences between countries with a very low (Sweden, six per 1000) and somewhat higher (Czechoslovakia, 13 per 1000) infant mortality rate are seen throughout the first year of life—at all ages the values of probability of death in Czechoslovakia are double those for Sweden. But as the absolute differences are greatest immediately after birth, the reduction of this mortality has today in the advanced countries the greatest impact on the final level of infant mortality.

The values of infant mortality indicators conceal a great variability due to birth-weight (Table 6.62). In Czechoslovakia, for the weight category up to 1499 g, we find a high risk of death especially in the neonatal period—approximately fifty times higher than the average, while for the post-neonatal period it is ten- to twentyfold higher. In the weight category 1500–2999 g the excess mortality was twice as high as the average. Infants born with a birth-weight of 3000–4999 g, particularly those nearest to 4000 g, have the best prospects of life.

The reduction of infant mortality in the advanced countries these days follows two directions: mortality reduction of infants in low birth-weight categories; and reduction of the proportion of infants born with a low birth-weight—of importance as a preventive measure. At present the former is more important for the reduction of infant mortality. As infant mortality is being reduced in the groups

Table 6.2 *Probability ($\times$ 10 000) of death according to infant age (q_x) in Sweden and Czechoslovakia for the years 1986–1987*

Age	Sweden	Czechoslovakia	Czechoslovakia (according to birth-weight)		
			< 1499 g	1500–2999 g	3000–4999 g
Days					
0	13.5	23.8	1477.8	46.3	5.4
1	8.0	19.3	1421.1	38.9	3.9
2	4.2	11.9	825.7	27.2	2.6
3	3.1	6.2	480.4	13.3	1.6
4	1.8	4.7	394.4	10.4	1.0
5	1.2	4.3	410.6	9.5	0.8
6	0.8	2.6	277.1	4.8	0.7
Weeks					
0	32.5	72.7	4281.5	149.4	16.0
1	3.5	10.6	965.0	21.8	2.9
2	2.1	3.9	329.7	6.8	1.7
3	0.9	2.8	148.3	6.0	1.2
Months					
0	39.5	90.5	5096.3	184.8	22.2
1	4.9	8.7	226.6	18.5	5.0
2	4.1	6.7	100.5	11.2	5.0
3	3.1	6.1	62.5	13.5	3.7
4	2.5	4.6	23.6	8.0	3.5
5	1.9	3.9	31.5	7.2	2.8
6	1.2	3.0	39.5	6.9	1.7
7	1.1	2.1	23.8	3.5	1.7
8	0.5	2.2	7.9	3.8	1.8
9	0.4	1.5	31.8	2.3	1.1
10	0.7	1.2	8.0	2.2	0.9
11	0.5	1.3	31.9	2.5	0.8
0–11	60.3	131.3	5377.8	262.7	50.0

Note: non-smoothed data; age in completed durations (i.e. age last birthday).

with the lowest birth-weight, the birth-weight structures of the survivors are coming close to the structures of live born infants. This, in turn, means that in individual populations we find an increasingly higher frequency of infants born with a lower birth-weight. It should, however, be noted that the care provided for these threatened neonates has substantially improved—and this includes also a reduction of the risk of permanent damage.

Determinants of birth-weight

On the whole we might say that birth-weight is primarily determined by the length of gestation and that, in turn, depends mainly on the state of health of the woman. The intrauterine maturation of the fetus may be slowed down by biological, social, and other factors. A lower birth-weight is mostly found with multiple pregnancies and in infants born at short inter-pregnancy periods. A simultaneous action of biological and social factors should be considered possible with the age of the mother and parity. In older primiparae the usually lower birth-weight is mostly influenced by the biological condition of the mother, while in young multiparae we find chiefly social causes. The optimum age for childbearing seems to be in the interval 20–29 years, at which age mothers give birth to the smallest proportion of infants with a low birth-weight. A detailed analysis of infant mortality in a birth cohort of children born in 1984 in the Czech Republic reveals that the infant mortality rate among infants born to mothers below the age of 20 years and between the ages of 30 and 34 is roughly four per 1000 higher (15 per 1000) than among infants born to mothers aged 20 to 29 years (11 per 1000). In this study parity was seen as having a considerable effect on infant mortality. In the same age categories infant mortality almost doubled in the transition from the second to the third or higher parity.

Affects of marital and fertility changes on infant mortality

Let us now compare the earlier mentioned situation of infant mortality with the global development of demographic indicators in Europe since the mid-sixties. In the succeeding years new unconventional family forms became relatively widespread in the advanced countries. While we could call the period from the end of the Second World War until the late sixties the 'golden age of the family', with a growing proportion of the inhabitants marrying early and wishing to have several children, later years brought a conspicuous change in the pattern of procreative behaviour. From roughly the late sixties onwards the marriage rate began to drop, above all in the age group 20–24 years, without any noticeable compensation at a higher age. Both first and second marriages became more and more replaced by cohabitation. At the same time the divorce rate went up. The mean number of children per woman often dropped in some places to below 1.5—a value which, on a long-term basis and under conditions of relative economic stability, was recorded in demographic history for the first time (Fig. 6.1). This new, and, in the future, probably ever more widespread pattern of procreative behaviour, shows a clear trend towards shifting the bulk of procreation from the age group 20–24 years to the group 25–29 years, with a simultaneous decrease of procreation in the marginal categories, i.e. below 20

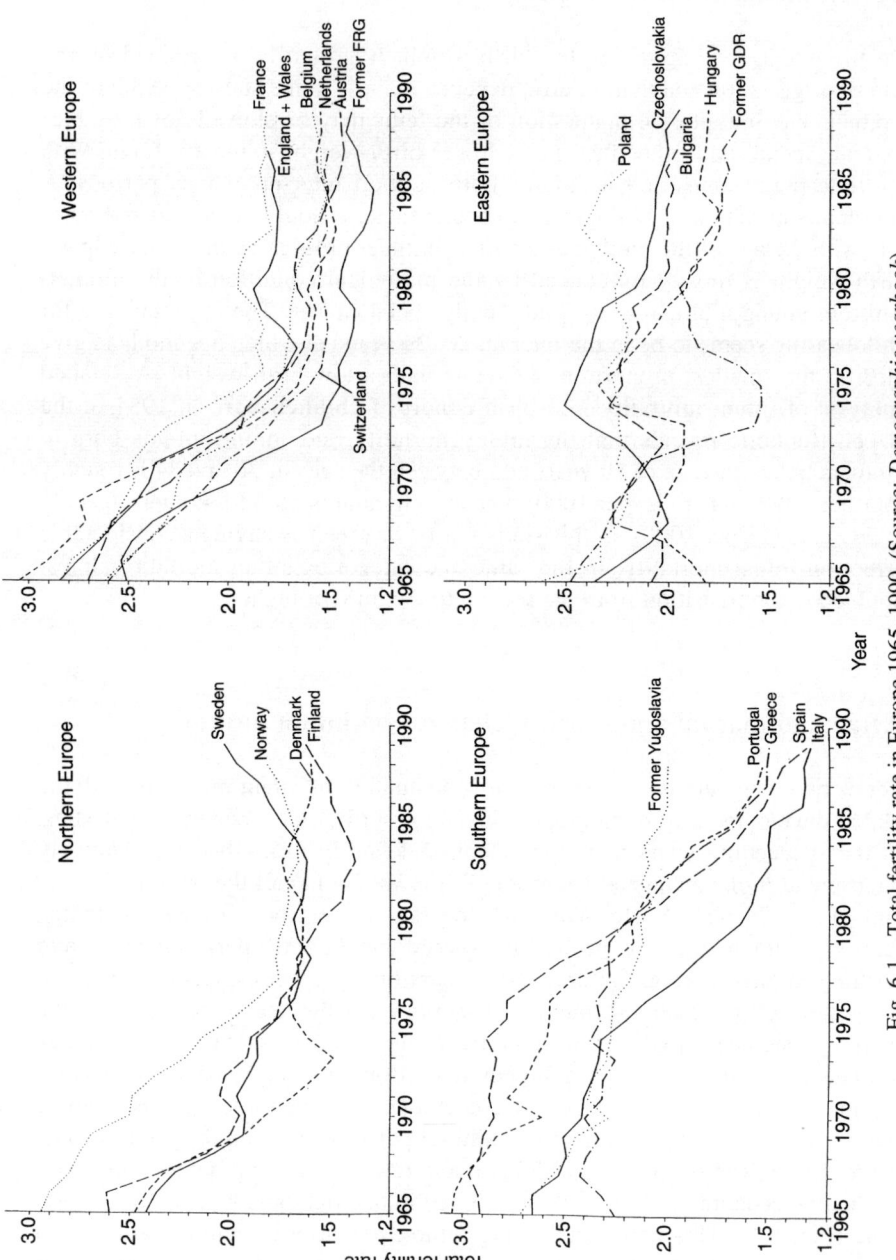

Fig. 6.1 Total fertility rate in Europe 1965–1990. (Source: *Demographic yearbook*)

Table 6.3 *Fertility indicators in Europe in 1965 and 1985*

	TFR		20–24[1]		25–29[2]		Illegitimate[3]	
	1965	1985	1965	1985	1965	1985	1965	1985
Northern Europe								
Denmark	2.61	1.45	0.85	0.36	0.85	0.60	9.5	43.0
England and Wales	2.85	1.78	0.85	0.44	0.93	0.64	7.7	19.2
Finland	2.47	1.64	0.71	0.36	0.76	0.60	4.6	16.4
Norway	2.93	1.68	0.87	0.44	0.91	0.63	4.6	25.8
Sweden	2.42	1.73	0.68	0.37	0.68	0.66	13.8	46.4
Western Europe								
Austria	2.70	1.47	0.79	0.47	0.78	0.51	11.2	22.3
Belgium	2.60	1.49	0.79	0.40	0.85	0.65	2.4	6.5
France	2.84	1.82	0.90	0.49	0.90	0.72	5.9	19.6
Former FRG	2.51	1.28	0.72	0.29	0.80	0.50	4.7	9.4
Netherlands	3.04	1.51	0.64	0.26	1.05	0.65	1.8	8.3
Switzerland	2.61	1.51	0.67	0.29	0.91	0.63	3.9	5.6
Southern Europe								
Greece	2.32	1.68	0.61	0.59	0.76	0.51	1.1	1.8
Italy	2.55	1.41	0.61	0.39	0.86	0.50	2.0	5.4
Portugal	2.07	1.71	0.71	0.50	0.89	0.53	8.3	12.3
Spain	2.97	1.61	0.55	0.36	0.99	0.58	1.7	7.1
Yugoslavia	2.71	2.05	–	–	–	–	8.3	9.1
Eastern Europe								
Bulgaria	2.07	1.95	0.88	0.93	0.52	0.50	9.4	11.7
Czechoslovakia	2.37	2.07	0.95	0.96	0.71	0.60	5.1	7.0
Former GDR	2.48	1.74	0.92	0.79	0.69	0.54	9.8	33.8
Hungary	1.82	1.83	0.73	0.75	0.53	0.57	5.2	9.2
Poland	2.52	2.33	0.92	0.87	0.72	0.75	4.5	4.7
Romania	1.91	2.19	0.70	0.96	0.50	0.61	–	–

[1] Fertility rate at reached age 20–24.
[2] Fertility rate at reached age 25–29.
[3] Out-of-wedlock live births per 100 total live births.

years and above 30 (Table 6.3). A steadily higher proportion of children (more than 20 per cent) are born out of wedlock, while an ever greater proportion of women remain childless by intent. Due to the large-scale introduction of modern contraceptive methods, the number of children conceived before marriage substantially decreased, except in the Eastern European countries. These trends in demographic behaviour are so significant that the expression 'second demographic transition' has been coined to describe them.

Since the late sixties, these changes, especially those in procreative behaviour, began to spread from northern Europe through the west to the south. The south, however, has some specific features—the substantial drop in childbearing did not go hand in hand with a significant rise in illegitimacy and divorce rates. On the demographic map of Europe only one region remained but little affected by these changes, and that is Eastern Europe. The countries of this region differ with regard to infant mortality, having for the most part preserved the demographic patterns of the post-war period. In the European context their procreation rate is relatively high and the age of the mothers low. Apart from a high rate in the former GDR, the rate is low. But as procreation takes place under conditions of low utilization of up-to-date contraceptives, we also find a high abortion index (i.e. number of induced abortions per number of live births) see Table 6.4. Infant mortality in this region (Eastern Europe) is among the highest in Europe.

How can these changes in demographic indicators affect infant mortality, if we leave aside the fundamental and decisive ones—the steadily improving health care provided for pregnant women and neonates? Two fundamental demographic variables, which in fact are closely related, i.e. the mother's age and parity, have moved towards a reduction of procreation in marginal age groups (below 20 and above 30 years) that are burdened with a higher risk and towards a decrease in mean parity, the smaller mean number of children per woman (i.e. total fertility rate or TFR) being primarily the consequence of a radical reduction in the number of large families. From the point of view of minimizing the risk of infant mortality, the new patterns of procreative behaviour are favourable, as procreation takes place in the optimum age interval. Of those women having children, the concentration on two children only is also favourable for infant mortality. Legitimacy as a possible variable influencing birth-weight probably has a different impact in different countries. In Sweden and Denmark, where now more than 40 per cent of children are officially born out of wedlock, such children have a status comparable with legitimate ones. However, in eastern and southern Europe illegitimate children are born to genuinely single mothers, whose pregnancy under external stress may result in the birth of a child with a lower birth-weight, who is thus at greater risk in its subsequent development. We see, for example, in 'former' Czechoslovakia, although for a long time single mothers and their children have had the same legal status as all mothers and their children, in the weight categories below 2499 g we find twice as many illegitimate as legitimate infants. The geographical distribution of countries according to infant mortality tallies with their distribution according to the frequency of low birth-weight newborns. Low infant mortality values bespeak a high quality not only of postnatal but also of prenatal care, the latter acting as prevention against the birth of at-risk babies. These trends in the development of infant mortality, including favourable demographic trends, among which we should place the growing educational standards of women, will in all probability also determine development in regions with an as yet less favourable situation.

Table 6.4 *Selected demographic indicators in Europe in 1965 and 1985*

	Total reduced first marriage rate[1] per 1000				Total reduced divorce rate per 1000[2]		Induced abortion ratio per 100[3]	
	1965		1985		1965	1985	1985	
	Men	Women	Men	Women				
Northern Europe								
Denmark	1026	984	538	572	182	452	37.1	
England and Wales	1038	1002	650	661	107	438	21.5	
Finland	959	930	552	584	137	293	22.0	
Norway	921	872	532	562	102	326	28.5	
Sweden	986	957	490	525	178	455	31.3	
Western Europe								
Austria	923	994	590	599	145	308	–	
Belgium	992	1002	620	650	82	240	–	
France	1013	993	531	540	107	304	22.5	
Former FRG	913	1102	585	598	–	312	14.3	
Netherlands	1131	1132	555	574	72	344	10.7	
Switzerland	892	897	641	663	127	287	–	
Southern Europe								
Greece	1218	1185	889	870	–	110	–	
Italy	998	1024	680	695	–	41	35.7	
Portugal	1105	1008	765	787	–	–	–	
Spain	1008	982	630	640	–	–	–	
Yugoslavia	991	1027	787	–	–	–	99.5	
Eastern Europe								
Bulgaria	951	893	894	939	103	208	94.3	
Czechoslovakia	965	901	867	916	167	309	52.8	
Former GDR	858	1037	701	739	–	383	39.6	
Hungary	986	978	796	857	227	333	63.0	
Poland	–	–	791	881	–	166	20.0	
Romania	910	943	864	846	204	–	84.4	

[1] 'Total reduced first marriage rate' is the sum of age-specific reduced first marriage rates defined as a number of the first marriages to the middle year population in a given age. (It expresses the relative frequency of married people; in the case of cumulating marriages in one year it can exceed 1.)
[2] 'Total reduced divorce rate' is the sum of duration-specific divorce rates according to duration of marriage. (It expresses relative frequency of divorced people in a marriage cohort.)
[3] 'Induced abortion ratio' is the ratio of the number of induced abortions to the number of live births.

Bibliography

Calot, G. (1990). *Project international*. INED, Paris.
van de Kaa, D.J. (1987). Europe's second demographic transition. *Population Bulletin*, **42**, (March) 3–570.
Monnier, A. (1990). La conjoncture démographique. *Population*, **45**, 924–36.
Rychtaříková, J. (1980). La portée de la mortalité infantile dans la reproduction démographique. *Acta Universitatis Carolinae Geographica*, **XV**, (2), 32–52.
Syrovátka, A. and Rychtaříková, J. (1984). Naissances vivantes et décès de moins d'un an selon le poids à la naissance en République socialiste tchèque entre 1950 et 1980. *Population*, **39**, (3), 515–40.
Syrovátka, A. and Rychtaříková, J. (1990). Demografické aktuality pro pediatry. *Pokroky v pediarii*, **11**, 183–207.
Zřobilová, J. (1997). Les tables de la mortalité infantile par cause. Application è la Tchécoslovaquie et à la France, 1968–1972. *Population*, **32**, (1), 555–78.

7 Demographic trends in families in Europe—with particular reference to Poland

Aldona Sito

Families in Europe are undergoing intense demographic changes which are a reflection of wider socio-economic and political transformations. Overall, a general pattern of trends can be observed in family lifestyles across Europe. The extended family has been widely replaced by the nuclear family (parents and children). The trend for a small number of children (one or two) has been established in almost all the European countries. This is reflected by declining fertility rates and low population growth. Since the 60s, a growing popularity of informal unions has taken place especially in Nordic and Western European countries with the result that, at present almost 25 per cent of children in these parts of Europe are born out of marriage (Dencik 1987; Dumon 1989; Kozakiewicz 1985; Leridon and Villeneuve-Gokalp 1988; Munoz-Perez 1986). The sociological and psychological aspects of this phenomenon of cohabitation chosen as a long-term lifestyle have been the subject of numerous studies (Kellerhals and Roussel 1987; Kozakiewicz 1985; Lopez and Cliquet 1984; Munoz-Perez 1986; Rupp *et al.* 1980; O'Neill and O'Neill 1972; Sufin 1988; Trost 1990). In spite of the above, trends in divorce indices are still rising across Europe.

Since 1960, a fall in marriage rates among men and women of all ages has been observed in Western and North European countries (*Demographic yearbook 1989*; Dencik 1987; Kellerhals and Coenen-Huther 1990; Lopez and Cliquet 1984; *Selected demographic indicators by country 1950–2000*). The marriage rates continue to be high in Central and Eastern European countries in which demographic data reflect the more traditional family lifestyles (Avdeyev and Troitskaya 1991; Bozkowa and Sito 1983; David and McIntyre 1981; Dyczewski 1981; Okólski 1988; *Rocznik statystyczny 1990*).

In an ad hoc survey carried out among members of APEE (Association for Paediatric Education in Europe) from Spain, Portugal, Greece, France, United Kingdom, and Sweden (Sito 1985) the following demographic trends were recognized as important in family life in these countries:

- younger age of sexual initiation;
- cohabitation becoming a recognized lifestyle both in the premarital period and as a long-term partnership;
- more full-time working mothers;

- increasing age of getting married;
- increasing age of giving birth to the first child;
- increasing number of children born outside marriage;
- decreasing number of children per family and increasing single-child families;
- increasing use of fertility control;
- more single-parent families;
- decreasing and ambiguous father's role;
- lower age of children leaving home.

It is interesting that although the countries included represent very different socio-demographic problems the trends in family demographic data are similar. It is also significant that all respondents in this small survey stressed a growing social acceptance of premarital sex, extramarital sex, divorce, fertility control, and a partnership style of marriage.

Demographic trends are studied by quantitative data collection, analysis, and research. Such data concerning population, marriage, divorce, fertility rates, desired and real family size, family planning practices, and above all mortality trends exist for almost all countries in Europe (*Demographic yearbook 1989*; Grant 1991; Henshaw 1990; Kellerhals and Coenen-Huther 1990; Lopez and Cliquet 1984; Munoz-Perez 1986 and 1987; *Selected demographic indicators by country 1950–2000*; *World population prospects as assessed in 1980*; *Sytuacja demograficzna Polski*).

To understand the social, health, and political implications of this wealth of data, we must also take into consideration the numerous and diverse factors conditioning the existing trends, facts, and figures (Géraud 1989). For example, in discussing the recent fall in marriage rates in present-day Europe, Kellerhals and Coenen-Huther (1990) bring in the historic perspective and remind us that in 1880, among the Swiss population at the age of 50, 18 per cent of men and 20 per cent of women were never married. In 1980 the figures were 9 per cent and 10 per cent respectively.

Considering more recent times, although there is a reduced influence of orthodoxy in terms of family, religion, social, and economic norms and in current trends in legislation, there are still more questions than answers regarding the reasons for the prevailing family lifestyles in Europe. Does the continuing trend of reduced fertility and the increased number of couples who choose not to have children, as well as the growing number of informal unions, mean that the family is becoming less accepted as the basic social unit? Do young people decline to have a traditional marriage and family because they, as children or adolescents, did not feel secure enough in their own family?

In studying the changes in European family demography some points should be borne in mind. Although the figures might suggest that 'the family' is in decline, in Denmark (Dencik 1987) over 80 per cent of small children live in nuclear families and 75 per cent of the children will live with their biological parents until they are grown up. In comparison, only nine per cent of small children live with a single parent, while another nine per cent live in reconstructed families. It should also be remembered that there have been undulating trends regarding family life throughout history. The demographic situation of today and the predictions for the future may be modified, for example, by conservative attitudes such as the increasing strength of pro-life groups and pressure to introduce more rigid legislation concerning abortion and protection of the unborn child.

Demographic trends and the family in Poland

Poland, once a predominantly rural society, underwent rapid industrialization and urban migration in the 50s and 60s. It is still, in many ways, a traditional society in transition with strong contradicting influences: the state, the Roman Catholic Church, and the luring attraction of 'the West'. By population, Poland ranks sixth in Europe (Tables 7.1 and 7.2). The population pyramid reflects its

Table 7.1 *Selected demographic data on Poland, 1990*

Population (1990)	38 197 012
Population density (persons per square km)	121
Proportion female	54.3%
Proportion urban	62%
Rate of natural increase	4.3
Crude birth rate per 1000	14.4
Crude death rate per 1000	10.1
Infant mortality rate per 1000 live births (according to WHO definition)	19.3
Maternal mortality rate per 100 000 pregnancies	22
Total fertility rate (lifetime live births per woman)	2.08
Life expectancy at birth (years)	
Males	66.8
Females	75.5
Number of physicians (per 10 000 population)	21.4
Number of nurses and midwives (per 10 000 population)	60.6
Economy:	
GNP per capita (1988)	$1850

Data from the Central Statistical Office, Warsaw.

Table 7.2 *Some demographic characteristics of European countries 1989*

	Population (in millions)	Population annual growth rate (%), 1980–89	Total fertility rate, 1989
Eastern Europe			
Bulgaria	8990	0.2	1.9
Czechoslovakia	15 639	0.2	2.0
Former GDR	16 630	–0.3	1.7
Hungary	10 578	–0.1	1.7
Poland	37 963	0.8	2.2
Romania	23 150	0.5	2.1
Northern Europe			
Denmark	5130	0	1.5
Finland	4960	0.4	1.6
Ireland	3510	0.9	2.4
Norway	4230	0.3	1.7
Sweden	8490	0.2	2.0
United Kingdom	57 200	0.2	1.8
Southern Europe			
Albania	3210	2.0	2.9
Greece	10 030	0.4	1.6
Italy	57 525	0.1	1.3
Portugal	10 470	0.6	1.7
Spain	38 810	0.4	1.5
Yugoslavia	23 690	0.7	1.9
Western Europe			
Austria	7260	0	1.4
Belgium	9930	0	1.6
France	56 160	0.4	1.8
Former FRG	61 990	0	1.4
Netherlands	14 830	0.5	1.6
Switzerland	6650	0.5	1.5
Former USSR	286 717	0.8	2.4

(From *Rocznik Statystyczny* 1990 and Grant 1991.)

history and the devastation of the Second World War (Fig. 7.1). Also other demographic fluctuations are seen: in the period 1980–83 there was a transient and natural increase in the birth rate.

Today, in many respects, the demographic trends in Poland are those of a developed European country, i.e. falling birth rate, decreasing nuptiality, rising divorce rate, declining number of children per family (Tables 7.2 and 7.3). No

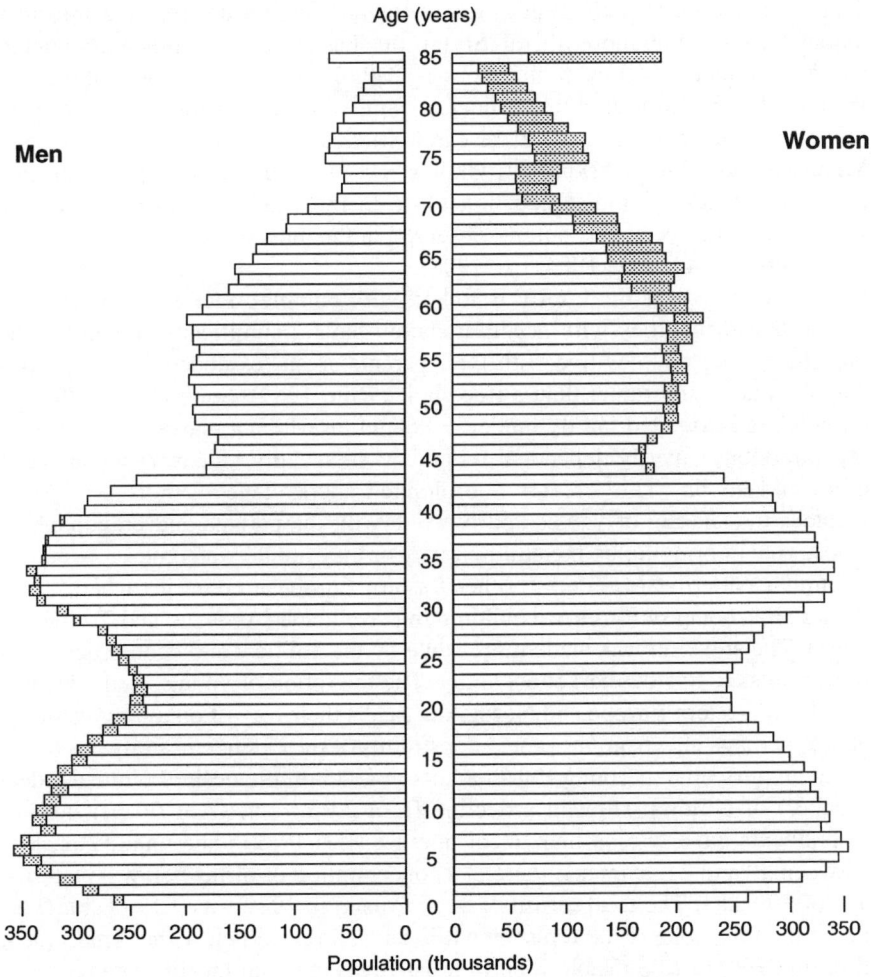

Fig. 7.1 Population pyramid by sex and age, Poland 1989.

Table 7.3 *Trends in vital statistics in Poland*

Rates per 1000 population	1970	1975	1980	1985	1989
Marriages	8.5	9.7	8.6	7.2	6.7
Divorces	1.1	1.2	1.1	1.3	1.2
Births	16.6	18.9	19.5	18.2	14.8

(From *Rocznik Statystyczny* 1990)

data on cohabitation exist, but attitudes towards premarital sex and informal unions have become more liberal. So far, this has not been significantly altered by the stronger position of the Roman Catholic Church in post-communist Poland. However, the traditional nuclear family is the prevailing and accepted model as confirmed by several research studies (Adamski 1984; David and McIntyre 1981; Dyczewski 1981; Okólski 1988). It should be pointed out that the family takes an undisputed first place in the value system of the Polish society. This has been particularly observed in the most critical moments of our recent history (Adamski 1984; Les 1987).

The small size of the family is linked with complex factors: surveys have shown that difficulties with accommodation have a significant influence. The fact that young couples live with their parents as an 'extended family' is frequently a necessity rather than a free choice (Sito 1989). Sufin (1988) refers to the modified extended family model in Poland, in which a married couple lives separately but is partly dependent on parents financially, in caring for the children, and so on. This creates a prolonged 'dependency syndrome' which includes the sharing of values and lifestyle with the parents and grandparents, whose role in bringing up the children may or may not be welcome.

Similar patterns are found in other Eastern European countries where, as in Poland, it is not easy for grown children to leave home (Avdeyev and Troitskaya 1991). The situation was made more acute by the political and economic transition from state to free-market economy. The migration of young, well educated people to Western Europe and North America is their way of obtaining independence, perhaps also from unwanted constraints of the extended family.

An enquiry among young Polish adults in 1985 on the desired number (ideal number) of children showed a decline from 2.7 to 2.4. Over 50 per cent of respondents gave two as their ideal number (Les 1987). The natality peak is between 20 and 24 years and there is a concentration of births below a maternal age of 30 years. The total fertility rate in Poland in 1989 was 2.13 (Table 7.2), i.e. at the threshold of the replacement level; it dropped below the replacement level in 1990, to 2.08 (Table 7.1). In urban areas the total fertility rate has been below replacement level since the 1960s.

The number of children born out of marriage in Poland is not high. About 20 per cent of newly-weds are pregnant. Family planning practice in Poland is an example of contradictory influences and lack of cohesion between the declared attitudes and practices. According to results from large-scale representative surveys (David and McIntyre 1981; Okólski 1983, 1988), 80 per cent of couples use fertility control. (The term 'contraception' has a negative connotation due to the pressures that exist against modern contraceptives.) The methods most often used were withdrawal and rhythm, while the pill and IUDs were used by not more than 10 per cent. As the 1987 World Fertility Survey concluded, the phase of fertility transformation in Poland has culminated in relatively low fertility at present. The quality of this kind of fertility control, however, is unacceptable—reliance on traditional methods or lack of continuity in the use of modern ones lead to unplanned pregnancy and recourse to abortion in cases of failed contraception (Okólski 1983, and 1988).

The 'abortion law' was introduced in Poland as early as 1957. The indications included 'social reasons' which meant that at up to 12 weeks of pregnancy most women could obtain an abortion. Unfortunately, family planning counselling, although integrated into maternal and child health (MCH) services, was not sufficiently implemented. Also, the availability and credibility of contraceptives were inadequate, although it should be added that fertility awareness methods have been taught for many years during pre marital courses organized, as an obligatory preparation for family life, by the Catholic Church.

In post-communist Poland abortion has become a subject of political discussion and an anti-abortion legislation is being prepared within the bill, protecting the unborn child. This corresponds to trends beginning also in former Czechoslovakia and Hungary. Results from surveys (Kozakiewicz 1985; Okólski 1983, 1988) show that Polish society does not approve of abortion as a method of family planning, demonstrating discrepancy between declared attitudes and widespread practices. The figures are incomplete (Table 7.4), but it is

Table 7.4 *Number of abortions and abortion ratio per 100 known pregnancies by completeness of data in European countries*

	Number of abortions	Ratio
Statistics believed to be complete		
Belgium (1985)	10 800	8.7
Bulgaria (1987)	119 900	50.7
Czechoslovakia (1987)	156 600	42.2
Denmark (1987)	20 800	27.0
England and Wales (1987)	156 200	18.6
Finland (1987)	13 000	18.0
Former GDR (1984)	96 200	29.7
Hungary (1987)	84 500	40.2
Netherlands (1986)	18 300	9.0
Norway (1987)	15 400	22.2
Scotland (1987)	10 100	13.2
Sweden (1987)	34 700	24.9
Former Yugoslavia (1984)	358 300	48.8
Incomplete statistics		
France (1987)	161 000	17.3
Former FRG (1987)	88 500	12.1
Ireland (1987)	3700	5.9
Italy (1987)	191 500	25.7
Poland (1987)	122 600	16.8
Romania (1983)	421 400	56.7
Former Soviet Union	6 818 000	54.9

(From *Henshaw* 1990.)

estimated that up to 1989, almost as many induced abortions as live births took place per year (Okólski 1988). Data from the former USSR (Avdeyev and Troitskaya 1991) reveal an even more open form of birth control by induced abortion. Lack of training for professionals and the community, as well as the virtual non-availability of modern contraceptive methods, has provoked the formation of a culture characterized by a liberal attitude to abortion and a low motivation to contraceptive use (Avdeyev and Troitskaya 1991).

Although demographic trends in the former USSR are very difficult to interpret and data are incomplete, Blum and Pressat (1987) analyzed changes in mortality over the past 30 years on the basis of a new life table by sex and years of age (1984–85). Apart from a drop in infant and child mortality rates, there is an increased mortality in older age groups and a marked excess mortality in men above 45 years. A similar pattern is observed only in Poland (Fig. 7.2). The causes of this situation are complex but one of the main factors, mortality due to cardiovascular disease, has risen by 70 per cent since 1965 among males in this age group. Lifestyle factors (smoking, alcohol consumption, lack of physical exercise, and stress) are considered to be the leading underlying causes (Adamski 1984; Bozkowa and Sito 1983).

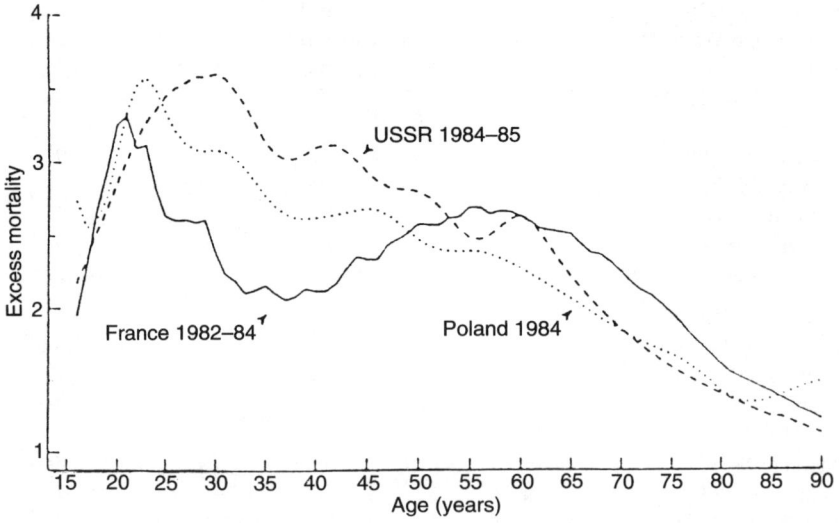

Fig. 7.2 Excess male mortality in the former USSR, Poland, and France. (Source: Blum and Pressat 1987.)

Other Eastern European countries

Some demographic data are presented in Tables 7.2 and 7.4. These indicate that differences between the individual countries are considerable. Compared to Western Europe, the total fertility rate is higher, although it is declining. The other characteristic is the high abortion ratio. In all of these countries there are inadequate family planning services. The restrictive abortion and family planning policy in Romania up to 1990 proved an unsuccessful pronatalistic measure and resulted in an increased maternal mortality rate through illegal abortions.

The lowest fertility rate and negative population growth in this part of Europe is observed in Hungary (Table 7.2). The demographic data concerning the German Democratic Republic was influenced by migration to the West. It is necessary to wait in order to make a demographic analysis of United Germany.

The decline of fertility in southern Europe

Because of the delayed demographic transition, birth rates remained relatively high in Spain, Greece, and Portugal after the Second World War. In the 30 years following, the populations in these countries were under the same influences which shaped the demographic developments in the more industrialized Western Europe (Munoz-Perez 1987). In spite of the falling birth rates due to a desire for smaller families, there was a rise in marriage rates, but the desire for smaller families is the main cause of the recent fall in birth rates, ten years after the Western European countries. The total fertility rate of 1.3 in Italy in 1988 was the lowest in Europe (Table 7.2). This finding is the result of long-term demographic transformations superimposed on the adoption of the Western style of reproductive behaviour.

Implications of demographic trends on family functioning in Europe

The reciprocity of family transformations and demographic changes have already been emphasized. The multiple models of the personal and family lifestyles of today reflect the priority of individual decisions and options, and the reduction of 'expected' behaviour. Studies have explored the factors that are responsible for successful family interactions (Olson and McCubbin 1983). However, the implications of present day trends will be the reality of tomorrow, with particular regard to the increased percentage of children growing up in single-parent or reconstructed families, and the increased number of old people who cannot be cared for by their children. This requires the planning of new approaches at the present time, for future needs, and health education pro-

Table 7.5 *Main demographic indicators for Europe 1991*

Country/ region	Population on 1st January 1992 (000)	Population increase/ decrease 1991 %	Natural increase 1991 %	Net migration 1991 %	Crude marriage rate 1991	Total fertility rate 1991	Infant mortality 1991
Council of Europe member states	511 595.5[3]	0.59[3]	0.39[3]	0.20[3]	–	–	–
Austria	7 860.8	0.90	0.15	0.75	5.6	1.50	7.5
Belgium	10 022.0	0.35	0.21	0.14	6.1	–	8.4
Bulgaria	8 974.9	–0.16	–0.16	–	5.4	1.57	16.9
Cyprus	714.6	1.09	0.99	0.10	10.1	2.45	10.6
Czechoslovakia	15 598.8	0.21	0.19	0.03	6.7	1.92	11.5
Denmark	5 162.1	0.30	0.09	0.21	6.0	1.67	7.5
Finland	5 029.3	0.61	0.33	0.28	4.7	1.80	5.8
France	57 206.2	0.55	0.41	0.14	4.9	1.77	7.4
Germany	80 365.5[3]	–	–0.09	–	–	–	–
Germany, DR	15 569.2[3]	–	0.57	–	–	–	–
Germany, FR	64 796.3[3]	–	0.03	–	–	–	–
Greece	10 168.3[3]	–	–	–	–	–	–
Hungary	10 337.2	–0.17	–0.17	–	5.9	1.86	15.6
Iceland	259.7	1.50	1.06	0.44	4.8	2.19	5.5
Ireland	3 541.7	0.65	0.60	0.05	4.8	2.18	8.2
Italy	57 788.2	0.07	0.01	0.06	5.3	1.26	8.2
Liechtenstein	29.3[3]	–	–	–	–	–	–
Luxembourg	389.8	1.41	0.32	1.08	6.7	1.60	9.2
Malta	359.5	1.01	0.69	0.32	7.3	1.90	8.9
Netherlands	15 128.6	0.79	0.46	0.33	6.3	1.61	6.5
Norway	4 273.6	0.56	0.37	0.19	4.8	1.92	6.2
Poland	38 309.2[3]	0.33	0.37	–	6.1	2.05	15.0
Portugal	9 846.0	–0.12	0.13	–0.25	7.3	1.51	10.8
San Marino	23.6	1.43	0.37	1.06	7.7	1.25	15.6
Spain	39 055.9	0.16	0.12	0.04	5.6	1.28	7.8
Sweden	8 644.1	0.62	0.33	0.29	4.2	2.11	6.1
Switzerland	6 833.8	1.23	0.35	0.88	7.0	1.61	6.2
Turkey	57 972.1	2.23	2.16	0.07	–	3.58	56.5
United Kingdom	57 700.8[3]	–	–	–	–	–	–
Other UN ECE member states	627 925.2[3]	0.74[3]	0.67[3]	0.07[3]	–	–	–
Albania	3 353.1[3]	–	1.81	–	–	–	32.9
Israel	5 077.3[3]	–	3.70	–	–	–	–
Romania	22 749.2	–1.90	0.10	–2.00	7.9	1.56	22.7
Former USSR	291 772.9[3]	0.50[3]	0.54[3]	–0.04[3]	–	–	–

Table 7.5 (cont.)

Country/ region	Population on 1st January 1992 (000)	Population increase/ decrease 1991 %	Natural increase 1991 %	Net migration 1991 %	Crude marriage rate 1991	Total fertility rate 1991	Infant mortality 1991
Former Yugoslavia	24 149.8[3]	0.53[3]	0.46[3]	0.07[3]	–	–	–
Total	1 139 520.7[3]	0.68[3]	0.54[3]	0.14[3]	–	–	–
Total Europe	578 539.8[3]	0.30[3]	0.16[3]	0.14[3]	–	–	–
Northern Europe	84 601.4[3]	0.39[3]	0.29[3]	0.10[3]	–	–	–
Western Europe	177 835.2[3]	0.70[3]	0.16[3]	0.54[3]	–	–	–
Southern Europe	145 459.0[3]	0.24[3]	0.18[3]	0.06[3]	–	–	–
Central Europe	95 967.2[3]	–0.33[3]	0.17[3]	–0.50[3]	–	–	–
Eastern Europe	74 677.0[3]	0.16[3]	0.03[3]	–0.13[3]	–	–	–

[3] = Missing data estimated from growth rates of preceeding years.
(From: *Recent demographic developments in Europe (1993)*. Council of Europe Press, Strasburg.)

grammes should also include this issue of the problems of the shrinking role of the family in social support networks.

To relate family demographic trends with the quality of child health in Europe would be to lose the complexity of factors which influence health in both its positive and negative aspects. On the other hand, if demographic phenomena are regarded as indices of health then the trends presented in this chapter may be regarded as indicative of the changing problems and the increasing challenges for the paediatrician, especially those concerning the psychosocial and promotive aspects of child health.

Concluding remarks

The political, social, and economic upheaval of 1989–92 in Central and Eastern Europe and the former Soviet Union, had, have, and will continue to have a very significant effect on the demographic phenomena in individual countries, as well as throughout Europe.

A report on recent demographic developments prepared by the Council of Europe's Population Committee (1993) provides a comprehensive source of quantitative data on families in Europe, extended to include all European countries: Table 7.5 summarizes the main demographic indicators for 1991.

Monitoring of family data and their trends is essential for our understanding of what is happening to families in Europe. Every effort should be made to obtain reliable data from every country, a task which requires both effort and resources. In the mean time, there is also need for critical interpretation of available data in the light of the wider social and economic context. For example, statistics on extramarital births in Scandinavian countries can not be interpreted in the same way as in Bulgaria or Poland.

Taking into account the fact that Europe comprises countries of extremely divergent demographic characteristics (Table 7.5), monitoring of very basic vital and health statistics such as infant mortality and maternal mortality continue to be relevant and important. Some other important demographic data which can be used for monitoring trends in families are

- life expectancy, birth and death rates;
- marriage rate and women's age at first marriage;
- divorce rates;
- extramarital births;
- total fertility rate;
- mean age of women at birth of first child.

Interpretation of individual indicators can be misleading in the demographic melting pot of European region. Thus, at present, the lowest fertility rates are found in southern European countries such as Italy, Spain, and Greece where the traditional family model (with high marriage frequency, low marriage age, low divorce rate, few extramarital births) prevails.

To understand and follow what really happens in families, the demographic and health data must be supplemented with information on psychosocial aspects of family life. Some appropriate indicators have been studied (Bozkowa and Sito 1983; Dencik 1987; Köhler and Jakobsson 1991; Olson and McCubbin 1983). Other chapters of this book deal more fully with social indicators of child and family health.

Such factors as family lifestyle, cohabitation, and reconstructed family rates, incidence of child abuse, use of birth control, and abortion as well as education, living conditions, physical and social environment all have tremendous bearing on family trends. In recent years the impact of international migrations has had an increasing demographic effect in western and northern European countries, becoming the dominant component of their population growth.

The following concluding statements can be formulated:

- demographic indicators are an important tool for monitoring family trends in Europe;
- the family as a unit is difficult to study;
- the definition of a family in Europe has become hazy;
- families are seldom units of observation and monitoring;
- available information on families is fragmentary and not comparable between countries and systems of data collection;

- social indicators are a necessary supplement for studying family behaviour and the quality of family functioning. They are also important in the interpretation of the ongoing demographic transitions.

References

Adamski, F. (1984) *Socjologia malzenstwa i rodziny.* p. 292. Painstwowe Wydawnictwo Naukowe (State Scientific Press). Warsaw.

Avdeyev, A. and Troitskaya, I. (1991). Family planning and demographic development of the USSR. Paper delivered at the *3rd European Conference on Child Abuse and Neglect, Prague, 23–26 June 1991.* (Unpublished).

Blum, A. and Pressat, R. (1987). Une nouvelle table de mortalité pour l'URSS (1984–1985). *Population,* **6**, 843–62.

Bozkowa, K. and Sito, A. (ed.) (1983). *Zdrowie rodziny* (Family health). Painstwowe Zaklady Wydawnictwo Lekarskich (State Medical Press). Warsaw

David, H.P. and McIntyre, R.J. (1981). *Reproductive behaviour: Central and Eastern European experience.* Springer, New York.

Demographic year book 1989. (1990). United Nations, New York.

Dencik, L. (1987). Danish demographic data. The BASUN project. Paper presented at the Conference *Growing into a Modern World, Trondheim, June 1987.* (Unpublished).

Dumon, W. (1989). Les évolutions des politiques familiales en Europe, en refernce aux transformations de la famille. *Familles d'Europe sans frontieres* (Actes du Congres, Paris, 4–5 December 1989), pp. 51–65.

Dyczewski, L. (1981). *Rodzina polska i kierunki jej przemian.* p. 25. Ośvodek Dblevment·eji i Studiw̄ Socjologicznych (Social Studies and Documentation Centre). Warszawa.

Géraud, R. (1989). *Mamy-boom et baby-flop d'une pilule l'autre.* Contraception, Fertilite, Sexualite, **17**, 479–81.

Grant, J. (1991). *The state of the world's children.* UNICEF, New York.

Henshaw, S.K. (1990). Induced abortion: a world review 1990. *International Family Planning Perspectives,* **16**, 59–65.

Kellerhals, J. and Coenen-Huther, J. (1990). Familles Suisse d'aujourd'hui: évolution récente et diversité. *Cahiers Médico-Sociaux,* **34**, 7–31.

Kellerhals, J. and Roussel, L. (1987). Les sociologues face aux mutations de la famille: quelques tendences des recherches 1965–1985. *L'Année Sociologique,* **37**, 15–43.

Köhler, L. and Jakobsson, G. (1991). *Children's health in Sweden.* Modin-Tryck, Stockholm.

Kozakiewicz, M. (1985). *Mlodziez wobec seksu, malzenstwa i rodziny, Perspektywa europejska.* Instytut Wydawniczy Zwiazkow Zawodowych (Trade Union's Publishing Institute). Warszawa.

Leridon, H. and Villeneuve-Gokalp, C. (1988). Entre père et mère. *Population et societes,* **220**.

Les, E. (1987). Les jeunes en Pologne. *Revue Francaise des Affaires Sociales,* **4**. 111–20.

Lopez, A.D. and Cliquet, R.L. (eds) (1984). *Demographic trends in the European region. WHO Regional Publications, European Series* No. 17. WHO, Copenhagen.

Munoz-Perez, F. (1986). Changements récents de la fécondité en Europe occidentable et nouveaux traits de la formation des familles. *Population*, **3**, 447–62.

Munoz-Perez, F. (1987). Le déclin de la fécondité dans le sud de l'Europe. *Population*, **6**, 911–42.

Okólski, M. (1983). Abortion and contraception in Poland. *Studies in Family Planning*, **11**.

Okólski, M. (1988). *Reprodukcja ludnosci a modernizacja spoleczenstwa* (Reproduction of population and modernization of society). Ksiazka i Wiedza, Warszawa.

Olson, D. and McCubbin, H.I. (1983). *Families: what makes them work?* Sage Publications, Beverly Hills, California.

O'Neill, N. and O'Neill, G. (1972). *Open marriage*. Evans, New York.

Population Committee, Council of Europe. (1991). *Recent demographic developments in Europe*. Council of Europe Press, Luxemburg.

Rocznik Statystyczny 1990. Glówny Utzad Statystyczny (Central Bureau of Statistics). Warsaw.

Rupp, S., Schwartz, K., and Wingen, M. (1980). Eheschlissung und Familienbildung heute. *Deutsche Geschaft für Bevolkerungswissenschaft*. Wiesbaden.

Selected demographic indicators by country 1950–2000. (1980). United Nations, New York.

Sito, A. (1985). Ad hoc survey on trends in family lifestyles in selected European countries. Unpublished data collected from APEE members, Barcelona, September 1985.

Sito, A. (1989). *Ocena ksztalcenia zdrowotnego rodziców i jego rola w promowaniu zdrowia rodziny* (Evaluation of parent education: its role in family health promotion). Institute of Mother and Child, Warsaw. (Docent thesis.)

Sufin, E. (1988). *Les modeles familiaux en France et en Pologne dans la représentation des jeunes* pp. 155–64. Cult. Soc: Est., Paris.

Sytuacja demograficzna Polski. Report. (1990). (Demographic situation in Poland.) Glówny Utzad Statystyczny (Central Bureau of Statistics). Warsaw.

Trost, J. (1990). Les consequences politiques de l'evolution de la famille: l'example Suedois. In *Familles d'Europe sans frontières* (Actes du Congres, Paris 4–5 Decembre 1988), pp. 93–97.

World population prospects as assessed in 1980. (1981). United Nations, New York.

8 Trends in childhood mortality and morbidity
Roy A. Carr-Hill

Many people worry about infant ill-health, including parents, policy makers, and politicians. Whilst the attention to children is welcome it can, however, make it difficult to collect and interpret 'objective' data. The purpose of this chapter is to make some estimates of the trends in childhood mortality and morbidity since the Second World War.

One consequence of increased survival of children after perinatal morbidity, traffic accidents, and so on is an increased number of chronically ill and disabled children. Equally, there appears to be a growth in the incidence of allergies, diabetes, and cerebral palsy. Long-term illness in children has therefore become more important, and these long-term diseases make demands not only on the health care system, but also on the family, on social welfare, and on the community at large.

Definitions of childhood mortality and morbidity

The first point to note is that any age limits are conventional and, in particular, that the notion of childhood is recent (Aries 1969).

Assessing the importance of trends in morbidity, even when they are measured, is extremely difficult. First, advances in treatment affect the likelihood of survival, if the condition is or was life-threatening, and the quality of that survival. The burden of disability (Blaxter and Patterson 1982) and other non-fatal outcomes may show a corresponding increase as mortality declines. Furthermore, a comprehensive assessment of morbidity would need to take into account the duration and severity of variation in access to, and utilization of, health care and the difficulty of assessing severity.

Infant mortality

Overall rates and trends until 1975

The infant mortality rate (IMR), as defined by WHO, has dropped substantially in all European countries (Table 8.1). The quarter-century between 1950 and 1975 has often been considered as the 'golden age' of social development in developed countries. There were spectacular declines in the relatively high

Table 8.1 *Infant mortality rate, per 1000 live births, by country and region for selected years (five-year averages)*

	1950–55	1960–65	1970–75	1975–80	1980–85	1985–90
Northern Europe	28	21	16	12	10	8
Denmark	28	20	12	9	8	7
Finland	34	19	12	9	6	6
Ireland	41	28	18	15	9	9
Norway	23	17	12	9	8	7
Sweden	20	15	10	8	7	6
United Kingdom	28	22	17	14	11	9
Western Europe	44	26	18	13	10	9
Austria	53	32	24	16	12	11
Belgium	45	27	19	13	11	10
France	45	25	16	11	9	8
Germany	48	28	22	15	11	9
Netherland	24	16	12	10	8	8
Switzerland	29	20	13	10	8	7
Southern Europe	79	52	31	23	18	15
Greece	60	50	34	25	15	17
Italy	60	40	26	18	13	11
Portugal	31	76	45	30	20	15
Spain	62	42	21	16	11	10
Former Yugoslavia	128	80	45	35	30	25
Eastern Europe	83	44	28	23	19	17
Bulgaria	92	36	26	22	17	16
Czechoslovakia	54	23	21	19	16	15
Former GDR	58	31	17	13	11	9
Hungary	71	44	34	27	20	20
Poland	95	51	27	23	20	18
Romania	101	60	40	31	26	22
Former USSR	73	32	26	28	26	24

Source: United Nations (1989).

levels of child poverty, infant mortality, and illiteracy which prevailed in the early 1950s. The nutritional status of children improved rapidly in parallel with fast and steady growth of the household economies of the poorest; the major infectious disease were controlled; and the coverage and efficacy of preventative and curative health services was extended, virtually free of charge, to nearly all children in most countries.

In the 1950s and 1960s, health conditions improved in all countries although the rate of improvement varied substantially. Overall there was a convergence of IMR values with the fastest declines in Bulgaria, Finland, Poland, and the former USSR (around 70 per sent) compared with Greece and the United Kingdom (around 40 per cent).

Nevertheless, inequalities remained. In France, for example, although IMRs declined considerably for all social groups between 1950 and 1970, the ratio between the IMRs of unskilled and professional groups moved only from 2.76 to 2.49 (United Nations 1982). The same appears to be true even in countries such as Denmark with more equitable income distribution: whist the overall neonatal mortality rate declined from 11 to 8 per 1000 between 1970 and 1974, the differential between those born to unskilled workers as compared to those born to professionals moved from 2.6 to 3.3 (Townsend and Davidson 1982). A review by Antonovsky and Bernstein (1977) of 26 trend studies on social class and infant mortality for Europe and the USA concluded that, by the mid-1970s, strong class differentials persisted with respect to both neonatal and post-neonatal mortality. By 1975, therefore, a newborn in an unskilled worker's family in Europe (and the USA) still was, on average, two to three times as likely to die during the first year of life as was a newborn from a professional family.

The extent to which these differentials are partly a consequence of the shifts in the relative sizes of the groups at the top and bottom of the occupational scale is difficult to assess because of the many factors involved (see Carr-Hill 1990 for an analysis of UK data). The fact remains that inequality is extraordinarily persistent.

Recent trends

With few exceptions, improvements in infant mortality rates over the past 15 years (measured at five-yearly intervals since 1975) have been smaller than during the 'golden age' (1950–75). This 'slowing down' is not, however, entirely surprising given the low level of mortality already reached in most countries. But it is noticeable that, in some Eastern European countries, the infant mortality rate has not declined during the past decade so that the differentials among countries have widened.

Whilst it is unclear whether or not infant mortality differentials (between social classes, urban vs. rural areas, developed vs. backward areas) have tended to narrow over the past 18 years (since 1975), in many cases they remain quite large. Even in countries with explicit egalitarian policies, like Sweden, there is still a close link between social class and risk and death among children, and among boys in particular (Olsson and Spent 1989). Regional disparities persists: for example, in the USSR in 1988, the IMR varied from a low of 11 per 1000 in Lettonia and Lithuania to highs of 53 in Turkmenistan and 49 in Tagikistan (various authors 1989).

Considerable 'excess infant mortality' still exists in most industrialized countries, with the possible exception of Scandinavia and Japan. Improvements in medical technology, in part giving an improved chance of survival of low birth-weight infants and in part of the identification and eventual termination of high-risk pregnancies, have lowered the 'biological minimum' to about five per 1000 live births.

In the late 1980s, sudden infant death syndrome (SIDS) was the leading cause of post-neonatal mortality in all countries, accounting for between 34 and 52 per cent of deaths in each country studied. It should be noted, however, that the SIDS classification may have 'taken the place' of the 'violent mortality' classification (see Fig. 8.1). 'Congenital anomalies' was the second leading cause of death, accounting for between 16 and 32 per cent of all deaths (see Table 8.2).

Other studies have shown that the largest differentials in infant mortality (and therefore the greatest potential for prevention) occur for post-neonatal death rates among normal birth-weight (2500 g or more) infants (Kleinman and Kiely 1990). Kleinman and Kiely (1990) present an analysis in 500 birth-weight groups, *excluding* deaths where the underlying cause of death was a congenital condition (Table 8.3). Apart from the much lower rates reported in Sweden, there is not much variation in each birth-weight group between the countries.

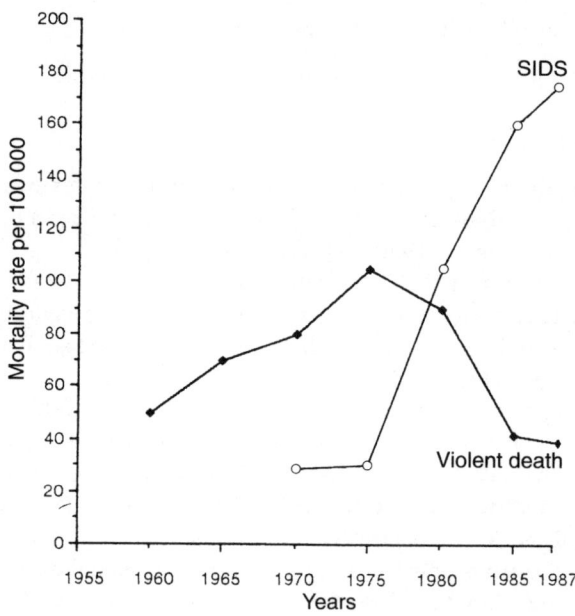

Fig. 8.1 Comparative evaluation of mortality due to SIDS and of violent mortality in infants between 1960 and 1987 (per 100 000 live births), France.

Table 8.2 *Post-neonatal mortality rates (per 100 000 live births) for selected causes of death, 1986*

	England and Wales	France	Netherlands	Norway	Sweden
All causes	427	373	296	369	197
Congenital anomalies	74	63	76	84	64
Perinatal conditions	31	24	20	34	0
Respiratory system disease	47	15	28	19	0
Sudden infant death syndrome	195	158	100	190	75[1]
Residual	80	113	72	46	58

[1] Note that, in Sweden, the 'sudden infant death syndrome' is not distinguished from other 'symptoms and ill-defined conditions'.

Table 8.3 *Post-neonatal mortality rates (per 1000) by birth-weight group (congenital anomaly deaths excluded)*

	Birth-weight (g)				
	2500–2999	3000–3499	3500–3999	4000–4499	4500+
Denmark	3.9	2.5	1.7	1.5	1.0
England and Wales	3.8	2.6	2.1	1.8	2.0
Scotland	3.5	2.4	1.8	1.9	2.7
Sweden	1.8	1.2	1.1	0.9	0.9

Childhood mortality

In childhood, one of the major causes of death is accidental injury (Table 8.4). The overall figures show how infants are much more at risk in France and that the rates for girls remain higher in all age groups. In contrast, whilst Norway has very low injury rates for infants, prompting Williams and Kotch (1990) to suggest that there may be a difference in coding, none of the countries has the lowest rate for both boys and girls in any other age group. Williams and Kotch (1990) present detailed breakdowns of these figures by cause, showing that

- for incidental poisoning (E800–869), children under 10 are most vulnerable in France but over years the 'lead' is taken by England and Wales;
- for falls (E880–888) there is no systematic difference;

Table 8.4 *Injury mortality per 100 000 in selected countries by gender and age group 1984–86*

	Infant <1		1–4		5–9		10–14	
	Male	Female	Male	Female	Male	Female	Male	Female
England and Wales	23.1	16.6	12.8	8.5	9.4	5.5	12.6	5.5
France	54.3	38.3	19.6	13.2	12.9	7.9	15.7	7.5
Netherlands	25.6	18.2	14.6	7.6	9.6	3.7	11.0	5.7
Norway	10.3	1.4	16.3	10.4	16.3	6.5	14.6	5.7

All external causes E800–E999.

- for fire and flames (E890–899), children under 10 are most vulnerable in Norway;
- for drowning (E900), children under 10 are most vulnerable in The Netherlands and Norway;
- there are no systematic differences for firearms (E922);
- for homicide (E960–978), children in Norway are slightly more vulnerable, (as are young adolescents in Norway most vulnerable to suicide).

However, it should be emphasized that prevention, or treatment, has been effective. Accidental mortality rates of children have fallen dramatically in Western European countries following the introduction of safety regulations (Fig. 8.2).

Childhood morbidity

In Sweden, between 15 and 30 per cent of four-year-olds have been found to have important health problems, the corresponding frequency during school age being between 25 and 35 per cent. These results agree, on the whole, with those obtained from similar studies in other Nordic countries (see Kohler and Jakobsson 1987). This means that physical deviations increase up to the age of 10, and decline thereafter. Not so, however, for vision impairments, which continue to increase until the age of 14 to 16. Physical deviations appear to be consistently more common among boys than among girls, with the exception of obesity. Diseases of the eyes and ears, diseases of the respiratory organs, motor disabilities, excess weight, skin disease, and surgical problems predominate during predominate during pre-school age. Allergies and spinal malformations, for example, are added during school age. Psychosocial problems are common among schoolchildren and increase as they grow older.

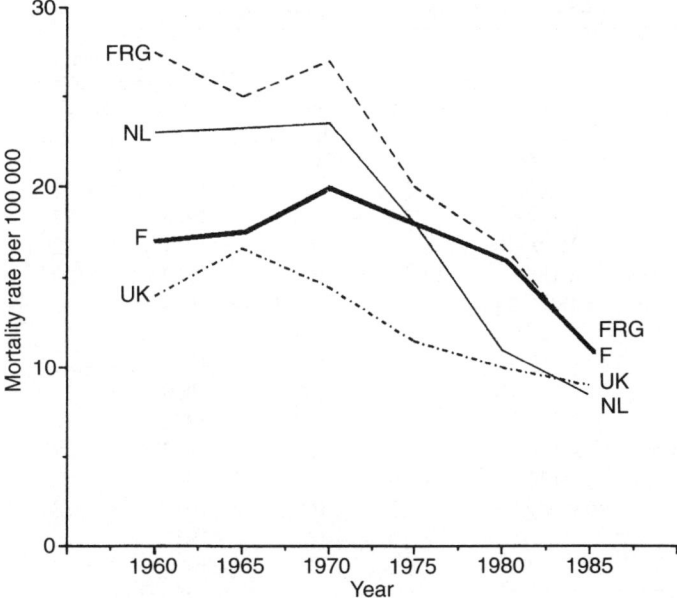

Fig. 8.2 Evolution of accidental mortality rates (per 100 000) of children aged one to 14 years between 1960 and 1985 in France, UK, former Federal Republic of Germany, and The Netherlands.

The focus on the remainder of this section is on the positive indicators of potential health status, and in the following section on the emergence of new morbidity.

Growth and development

The study of human growth or 'auxology' has become a scientific discipline in its own right and has given rise to numerous surveys of growth throughout the world (for example Eveleth and Tanner 1976; Tanner 1981). These studies are based on the presumption that

"A child's growth rate reflects, better than any other single index, his state of health and nutrition; and often indeed, his psychological situation also. Similarly, the average value of children's heights and weights reflect accurately the state of a nation's public health and the average nutritional status of its citizens when appropriate allowance is made for differences, if any, in genetic potential" (Eveleth and Tanner 1976.)

Floud (1983) shows how the heights of recruits to the army have been recorded as early as the first half of the eighteenth century; and also argues that, when conscription was introduced, this involved the inspection of very large sections—if not the whole—of the young male population on a regular basis. Using these data, and standardizing for the age of measurement by relating the mean values to the modern English standard, the following comparisons can be made (Table 8.5).

Table 8.5 *Trends in height among European males*

Country	Earliest data			Recent data		
	Date	Age of men measured	Mean height	Date	Age of men measured	Mean height
Belgium	1834	12	164.0	1969	18	173.9
Denmark	1789	22	165.7	1968	17	175.0
France	1819–26	20	166.0	1971	12	173.3
North Germany	1889	20–22	167.7	1962	20	176.3
West Germany	1887–94	20	165.2	1958	20	173.5
Bavaria	1875	18	164.6	1958	20	171.0
All Italy	1874–76	20	162.2	1952	20	167.4
North Italy	1874–76	20	163.6	1969	18	173.8
South Italy	1874–76	20	163.3	1970	18	174.0
The Netherlands	1865	19	165.0	1975	18	180.1
Norway	1761	18–19	159.5	1962	18	179.3
Portugal	1899	20–21	163.4	1911	18+	163.5
Spain	1860–93	19–22	163.7	1955	18+	166.1
Sweden	1840	21	165.1	1974	17	178.4

There has been a steady increase in mean-achieved height in all countries over the last two centuries. Moreover, in all countries except Sweden, there remains very pronounced differences between the achieved height of socio-economic groups. For example, a reconstructed time trend for the UK, shows (Table 8.6) no clear trend for men: and the suggestion of a trend for women is probably an artefact occasioned by classifying women by their husbands social class (see Carr-Hill and Pritchard 1991).

Table 8.6 *Difference in height between RG social class I & II and IV & V among young adults (aged 20–24) since 1940*

	1940	1945	1950	1955	1960	1965	1970	1975	1980
Men	3.9	3.0	3.9	2.9	3.4	2.4	2.5	3.2	3.1
	(306)	(525)	(421)	(395)	(440)	(460)	(529)	(529)	(493)
Women (Husband's occupation)	3.1	3.1	3.6	3.9	2.2	1.3	3.3	2.4	1.2
	(352)	(450)	(465)	(394)	(449)	(469)	(524)	(530)	(510)
Women (Father's occupation)	0.4	0.8	4.0	2.9	2.4	2.7	1.7	1.2	3.1
	(380)	(371)	(383)	(360)	(417)	(446)	(483)	(416)	(321)

Source: Knight (1985) Table 7; and own calculations from Knight's survey.

Dental caries

Dental health has improved substantially over this period partly, because of flouride (Stecksen-Blicks *et al.* 1989), and partly because of more regular tooth brushing,—whether flouride toothpaste is used or not—(Schroder and Granath 1983). Thus, in Sweden the percentage of children with permanent dentition who are caries-free has risen from 20 per cent of 5-year-olds (47 per cent of 3 years old) in 1974, to 60 per cent (83 per cent) in 1988. Dental caries is decreasing among children due to the fluoridization of toothpaste and, to a lesser extent, water. For example, in the UK the percentage of children aged 6 with decay in either deciduous or permanent teeth dropped from 80 per cent in 1973 to 55 per cent in 1983 (OPCS 1985). However, there are still inequalities between social groups. By their early teens, children from families headed by a parent in a manual occupation are twice as likely to have visited the dentist only because there was something wrong, than those children from families headed by a parent in a non-manual occupation; and the differences, although attenuated, remains when controlling for the mother's pattern of attendance (Table 8.7).

Table 8.7 *Dental care and socio-cultural differences*

	0–4		10–15		Mothers regular		Attendance only when hurt	
	NM[1]	M[2]	NM	M	NM	M	NM	M
Last visit check-up	42	33	87	75	78	71	53	48
Last visit trouble	3	3	11	18	6	9	12	14
Never been	56	63	2	8	16	20	35	38

Source: General Household Survey (1987).
[1] Non-manual. [2] Manual.

A new morbidity for tomorrows children?

The incidence of communicable disease, acute respiratory infections, and disease of the digestive kind has fallen radically in most countries. But a 'new' (or newly recognized) morbidity has emerged. Two sources will be considered: those from environmental problems and those resulting from alienation at a micro level.

Pollution and over consumption

Those due to 'ecological' causes. For example, increases in food poisoning have been registered together with rises in reported food intolerance. Similarly, there have been sharp rises in the number of cases of asthma (Table 8.8a). Whilst there may well have been some changes in definition (Gabbay 1982), environmental change must have played a major part. These could be particularly serious in the industrial and mining areas of Eastern Europe (Illsley, 1990; but see ICN, 1990).

Equally, the reported rates of medically treated eczema have increased substantially; Taylor et al. (1984) suggest once again that there is greater professional and parental recognition of eczema, but also the increased use of agricultural chemicals, household detergents, and soaps are also a partial cause. Moreover, the doubling in cases of obesity cannot be ascribed to changes in definition or reporting and may well indicate a longer term problem.

Table 8.8(a) *Morbidity and risk in the UK among 0–4-year-olds of two generations (per 1000 households)*

	Prevalence of morbidity			Treatment for injuries	
	First generation	Second generation		First generation	Second generation
Medically treated eczema	2.2	12.3	All injuries however treated	216	385
Treatment for asthma	6.2	18.9	All types of hospital treatment	181	233
Obesity relative to age, height, and sex	34	74	Admission to hospital for injury	14	27

Table 8.8(b) *Morbidity and risk in the UK: comparison of three cohorts (per 1000 households)*

	1946 cohort	1958 cohort	1970 cohort
Medically treated eczema by age six years	57	73	122
Juvenile diabetes by age 10–11 years	2	6	13

Child abuse

The reported rise in child abuse cases can have many different causes—differences of definition, of target population, of sampling procedures, response rates, methods of data collection, and the particular questions posed.

Mertens (1989) reviews a number of studies internationally, and finds rates varying between 6 and 62 per cent for women, and 3 and 16 per cent for men reporting sexual abuse during childhood. The wide range is partly due to variations in definitions, etc., used. With common definitions, there is more stability. (see Table 8.9).

Table 8.9 *Percentages of men and women reporting sexual abuse before the age of 18 in Sweden, Norway, and Denmark*

Country	Year	Women	Men
Sweden	1983	9	3
Norway	1985	19	14
Denmark	1987	14	7

Source: Mertens (1989).

(Un)Happiness

A recent international questionnaire study of European school children's health habits, provided good comparative data (Marklund and Strandell 1989). On the whole, Swedish pupils—about 3,000 children in total, aged 11, 13, and 15—were very pleased with life compared with those in Hungary. However, as in other countries, satisfaction declined with increasing age.

Among the 11- and 13-year-olds, it was the Swedish and Norwegian children who liked school the most. Something evidently happens, however, at senior level, because 15-year-olds had come to be a good deal less satisfied, in all countries except Hungary. Could it be, as conjectured by Dencik (1989) and Rydell (1990), that schools themselves play the part of problem-creators and, with their expert-controlled activities, pathologise undesirable forms of behaviour?

Conclusions

Child mortality has declined substantially in all European countries. Because rates of 'accidental death' have not been dropped as much they are now a major cause of death—and of the ensuing traumas for the parents. Nevertheless, social class differences in mortality—whether due to illness or accident—remain, and are at their greatest among small children.

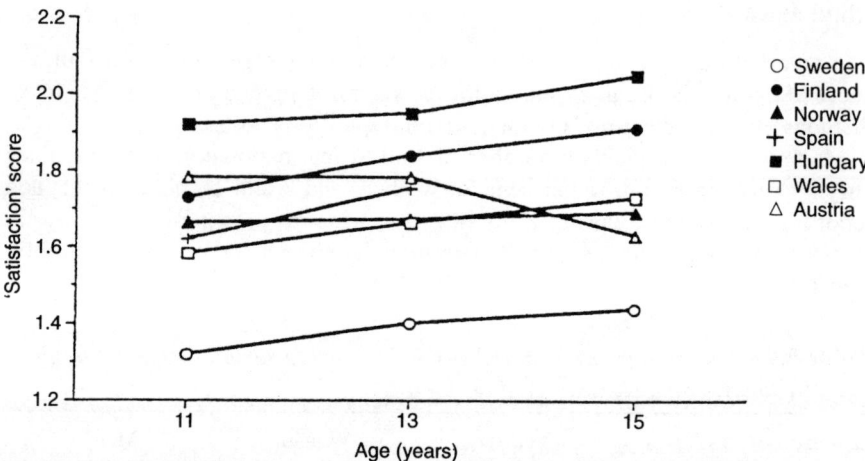

Fig. 8.3 General satisfaction with life, girls. Average score on a scale from 1 = very good to 4 = not at all good. (Source: Marklund and Strandell 1989.)

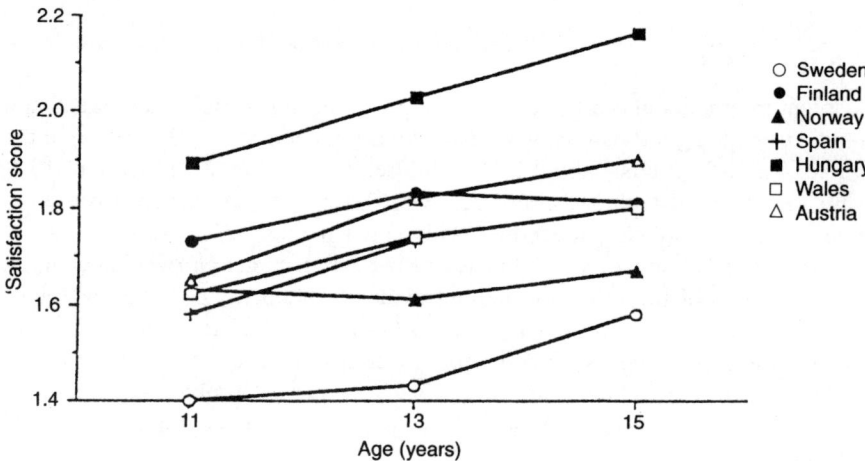

Fig. 8.4 General satisfaction with life, boys. Average score on a scale from 1 = very good to 4 = not at all good. (Source: Marklund and Strandell 1989.)

The data on childhood morbidity is weak. The main source of population data is self-report surveys and, whilst they probably provide reasonably reliable estimates of incidence of common complaints, they are not easily translated into epidemiological data. Moreover, the incidence of such complaints tells us little about the children's health status.

The presentation in this chapter has instead focused on indicators of healthy growth; and the data showed marked improvements over time, although once again, social class differences remain. At the same time, 'new' morbidities have emerged, some linked to the consequences of industrialization, some to affluence.

Acknowledgements

To Paula Press for producing the text; to Raymond Illsley for many productive discussions on trends in inequalities; and to the ESRC for their support to the Centre for Health Economics.

References

Antonovsky, A. and Bernstein, G. (1977). Social class and infant mortality. *Social Science and Medicine*, Vol II. 453–70.
Aries, P. (1969). *Centuries of childhood*. Penguin, Harmondsworth.
Blaxter, M. and Patterson, E. (1982). *The health of the children*. Hienemann, London.
Carr-Hill, R.A. (1989). The measurement of inequities in health: lessons from the British experience. *Social Science and Medicine*, **31**, 393–404.
Eveleth, P.B. and Tanner, J.M. (1976). *Worldwide Variations in Human Growth*. Cambridge University Press, London.
Floud, R., Walter, K., and Gregory, A. (1990). *Height, health and history*. Cambridge University Press, London.
Gabbay, J. (1982). Asthma attacked. In *The problem of medical knowledge*, (ed. P. Wright and A. Treacher). Edinburgh University Press.
Kleinman, J.C. and Keely, J.L. (1990). Post neonatal mortality in the United States: an international perspective. *Pediatrics*, **86** (6), 1091–7.
Kohler, L. and Jakobsson, G. (1987). *Children's health and wellbeing in the Nordic Countries*. Clinics in Developmental Medicine, No. 98, Mackeith Press, Oxford.
Lindgren, G.W. (1988). Genetics of growth and development: the case of Sweden or how old was Jerker. *Coll. Anthrop*, **12**, 23–45.
Mertens, P.L. (1989). Sexualbrott mot bran. Presentation och diskussion ou nagra centrala teman inom forskingsromradet. *Projektet sexualla overgrupp mot barn*, Delrapport 2, Brottsforebyggande radet Stockholm.
Olsson, S. and Spent, R. (1989). *Sweden—heaven or hell? Gulag or Kennel?* UNICEF, Stockholm.
Stecksen-Blicks, C., Holm, A.K. and Mayangi, H. (1989). Dental caries in Swedish four-year-old children *Swedish Dental Journal*, **13**, 39–44.
Tanner, J.M. (1981). *Historical studies of human growth*. Cambridge University Press.
Taylor, B., Wadsworth, J., Wadsworth, M.E.J. and Peckham, C.S. (1984). Changes in the reported prevalence of childhood eczema since the 1939–1945 war. *Lancet*, **ii**, 1255–7.
Townsend, P. and Davidson, N. (1982). *Inequalities in health*. Penguin, Harmondsworth.

United Nations (1982). *Level and trends of mortality since 1950*. United Nations, New York.
United Nations (1989). *World population prospects 1988*. United Nations, New York.
Various authors (1989). *Women and children in the USSR*. Vesnik Statistik, No 1.
Williams, B.C. and Kotch, J.B. (1990). Excess injury mortality among children in the United States: comparison of recent international statistics. *Pediatrics*, **86**, 1067–73.

PART III

Global threats to child health

Two major worldwide threats to child health are considered in this part. The first, war, has reared its head again in Europe and the effect on children has been devastating; in many other parts of the world children have been victims of protracted wars which have ravaged whole countries. The psychological effects on children of the threat of war are considered as well as the direct effects on children of being caught up in war. HIV, the second global threat, is a pandemic of major proportions, the full implications of which, for the child population of the world, are only just becoming evident. Other global threats such as poverty are considered in later parts.

9 Children and war
Tytti Solantaus

Introduction

In every sense, children and war are incompatible. Children represent growth, development, and future for humankind, while war means destruction and death. Yet children, more than any other part of the population, have been and continue to be victimized by war as well as the threat of war.

The two world wars were devastating to children and families. About 30 million families were displaced during the Second World War. About eight million children were left homeless in Germany alone (Langmeier and Matejcek 1975). During the First World War, children suffered from undernourishment and child mortality rose rapidly. Hundreds of thousands of children were drawn into the working force. Juvenile delinquency figures rose all over Europe (Save the Children International Union 1932).

Apart from the world wars, the world has been plagued with local wars and conflicts. Typically, these conflicts are embedded in the society in which they occur and they persist year after year. Military violence and threat is an everyday reality for children and families; for instance, over 70 per cent of Beirut families experienced fighting in their neighbourhoods during one six-month period in 1984–85 (Bryce and Walker 1986).

The ratio of soldiers to civilians dying of war has changed from 9:1 to 1:9 (UNICEF 1986) during this century. Over 90 per cent of causalities in long-term conflicts are civilians, and children and young people are among the first to suffer. In the intifada, the Palestinian uprising in the occupied areas, over 50 per cent of those injured were under 20 years old and 83 per cent were under 25 during a one-year period 1988–89 (Henley and Giacaman 1990). It has been estimated that 150–300 000 children die in the world each year because of military action (Fjaer 1990).

War does not only mean suffering and death from violence. Wars and long-term conflicts impoverish societies and erode their social structures. Conflicts rage in countries that are poor to begin with. Their health systems are underdeveloped, as are other structures of society. The conflicts drain the already limited resources. In the lives of families, this means shortage of goods, warmth, health services, and education resulting in illiteracy, hunger, cold, illness, and premature death. In Mozambique, UNICEF has estimated that about 320 000 under-fives died because of the consequences of the war of destabilization during 1981–86 (UNICEF 1987).

Even in relatively developed countries such as the former Yugoslavia, war is accompanied by the disruption of well-organized and equipped health and education services, and the threat of epidemics. For example, in the Bosnian capital Sarajevo, under siege for more than a year, it is threatened with the total collapse of its services, including electricity and water. Infectious diseases have increased, as well as the number of cases of nutritional anaemia and low birth weight, (Acheson 1993).

The utter disgrace of humanity is the use of child soldiers. This means the recruitment of children to the military, training them to be soldiers, and sending them to the front and combat. It is estimated by the United Nations that there are about 200 000 child soldiers in the world (Standley 1990).

In the world today, children are faced with war in one way or another in every society. Even those children who are not directly exposed to war themselves see war on television and they react readily to the threat of war. When tension in international politics was high in the early 1960s and 1980s and there was a threat of nuclear war, children and young people reacted with worry and anxiety (Escalona 1963; Schwebel 1965; Goldberg *et al.* 1985; Goldenring and Doctor 1986; Chivian *et al.* 1988).

Research on children and war started by documenting war-time statistics (Save the Children International Union 1932) and moved on to describing children's psychological reactions during the Second World War (Bodman 1941; Burbury 1941; Mons 1941; Freud and Burlingham 1942; 1943; Bodman 1944). The developmental and coping processes that operate in war and under threat of war have been studied only very recently. Overall, our knowledge about children and war is still very limited.

This chapter focuses on child development and mental health in times of war and threat of war. Physical consequences, child deaths, injuries and handicaps, as well as the indirect consequences of war, undernourishment, infectious diseases, and lack of education are beyond the scope of this chapter.

Psychological and behavioural symptoms and reactions

Reports on children's psychological reactions in World War II in Britain brought to light a somewhat unexpected finding at the time: the child population seemed to endure the bombings with remarkable resilience and only a small minority suffered from psychological symptoms (Bodman 1941; Burbury 1941; Mons 1941; Freud and Burlingham 1942, 1943; Bodman 1944). On the other hand, first reports from the civil strife in Northern Ireland went to the other extreme. Worries were expressed that the young people were a lost generation morally and psychologically (Lyons 1973; Fraser 1974).

Research has moved on since then and become more analytical and focused. Children growing up in conflict are far from being a lost generation (McWhirter and Trew 1982) and resilience does not mean that traumas leave no marks

(Luthar and Zigler 1991). Neither extreme captures the complexity of life, which is a continuous interplay of resilience and vulnerability.

In the armed conflicts of today children show a diverging picture of emotional, behavioural and psychosomatic problems as well as resilience. Children's reactions depend on how much they and their families are victims of violence themselves. Children's and their families' possibilities of coping with the adversities depend on how intact the societal structures remain and how children's basic needs of care, food, and shelter can be taken care of.

Children's emotional reactions include fear, anxiety, depression, and emotional lability (Fraser 1974; Dawes et al. 1989; Punamäki 1987, 1989; Baker 1990; Raundalen et al. 1987; review of Israeli studies Raviv and Klingman 1983). According to Baker (1990) almost one-third of Palestinian children (28 per cent) were afraid of leaving the house and almost one-half (48 per cent) were terrified at the sight of occupation soldiers. One in ten children (11 per cent) showed signs of depression. The study was carried out in 1989.

Psychosomatic problems include difficulties falling asleep, nightmares, problems in eating, headache, stomach ache, enuresis (Fraser 1974; Raviv and Klingman 1983; Punamäki 1987; Dawes et al. 1989). Rayhida et al. (1986) report a high level of psychosomatic symptoms among Lebanese children (58 per cent).

Children's behavioural reactions include restlessness, aggressiveness, disobedience, fighting, problems with peers, and withdrawal from social contacts (Punamäki 1987; Dawes et al. 1989; Baker 1990). Many children have problems in concentration (Dawes et al. 1989). School attendance is reported to suffer in Northern Ireland (Heskin 1980). In addition to classical truancy, this might be due to fears about the journey to school (Heskin 1980).

Dawes et al. (1989) studied mothers and children in 67 households after a violent burning down of four communities, where 70 000 people were left homeless, in South Africa in 1986. This study is unique in that it analyses the impact of age and sex. The age range was from two to 17. About 40 per cent of the children exhibited psychological symptoms. The most frequent symptom was fear across all age groups and both sexes. The second most prominent symptom was startle reactions to sounds reminiscent of the attack. Children of all ages were described sleeping with clothes on and fleeing the house at a knock on the door. The next most frequent symptom was a change in emotional expression. Small children showed regressive behaviour, weepiness, and clinging to their mother. Older children were reported to be withdrawn, apathetic, listless or irritable, and restless.

Problems with sleeping and eating were more common among under-sevens, while psychosomatic problems such as headache and stomach ache, as well as problems in concentration and memory, were more common in older children. Children between seven and eleven had social difficulties, either in the form of aggressive behaviour or withdrawal from peer relationships. Boys were more prone to these problems than girls. Overall, boys were more vulnerable in their younger years than girls, while this was reversed in adolescence.

Dawes *et al.* (1989) report that nine per cent of children were diagnosed as having post-traumatic stress disorder. This consisted of a cluster of symptoms including marked fear of recurrence of the events, startle reactions, sleep problems and mood changes, clinging behaviour, and fear of being left alone.

Losing a family member

Children who lose a family member become vulnerable to short-term and long-term problems (Kaffman and Elizur 1979, 1983; Elizur and Kaffman 1977, 1982). Raundalen *et al.* (1987) studied displaced children in a Red Cross shelter in Uganda. Over half of the children had experienced either the death (46 per cent) or loss of contact with a parent, death of a sibling (53 per cent), and violence/killing (96 per cent). Children recollected running away with extreme anxiety and horror. In the shelter, the children suffered from emotional arrest, emptiness, shock, anxiety, and depression. Depressive traits were documented in 80 per cent of the children.

In another Ugandan sample from town schools Raundalen *et al.* (1987) were able to study children's experience of death due to different reasons. The study was done by analysing children's essays. Death due to ageing, due to two opposing forces fighting, and death due to blind violence when soldiers take revenge on innocent civilians provoked very different reactions and after-effects. The blind random violence arouses the highest anxiety and persistent fear. The associated feelings were anxiety, depression, and feelings of being unprotected and defenceless.

Torture

Violence becomes even more devastating if it is targeted on identified children, which is the case in torture. The Lawyers' Committee for Human Rights (1986) reports extreme police violence on children in detention in South Africa leading in many cases to psychological and physical damage, and sometimes even death. The majority of children showed signs of extreme stress, disorientation, difficulties in communication, apathy, withdrawal from relationships, anxiety disorders, depression, and psychotic episodes. Straker and Moosa (1988) report post-traumatic stress disorder in tortured children.

Post-traumatic stress disorder is, however, a problematic diagnosis to use in these extreme situations. It covers reactions to trauma in peace time, but the consequences of torture and specified violence often exceed the symptoms described as post-traumatic stress disorder.

Psychiatric morbidity

The impact of armed conflict on psychiatric conditions in children and adults was studied in Northern Ireland (Fraser 1971, 1974; Lyons 1971; MacAuley and Troi

1983), and hardly any correlation with the civil strife was found. This seems to suggest that children's general psychiatric morbidity does not rise in long-term conflicts. However, these studies have methodological problems. No epidemiologically sound studies have been carried out. The Dawes *et al.* (1989) and the Raundalen *et al.* (1987) studies suggest strongly that in the hard-hit areas, children suffer from severe psychological problems including anxiety disorders, depression, and post-traumatic stress disorder.

In conclusion

The research evidence is still very scanty and all conclusions are very tentative. Unfortunately there are no follow-up studies. However, it seems fair to conclude that children react in war and conflict with a diversity of psychological and behavioural symptoms. If violence has not affected the child and his or her family personally, the symptoms seem to be transient. Children become more vulnerable if violence is especially targeted on them and their families. In these circumstances children's psychological symptoms are more severe and persistent.

However, one has to be careful not to make too far-reaching conclusions. Many children do not develop psychological problems. Children are even reported to survive extreme stress psychologically intact (Raundalen and Dyregrov, unpublished manuscript).

On the other hand, children who show very little immediate reaction might develop symptoms later. It is possible that a 'sleeper effect' of early traumatization appears in later life. Lahad and Ayalon (1990) point out that the scars of traumatization might be deeply embedded in the child and the research methods used might not tap them at all. The damage left by war might not be measurable by the conventional techniques and they might even be unnamed by traditional psychology, claim Lahad and Ayalon (1990).

Family influences

In peace time, a well functioning family (Block 1971; Werner and Smith 1982) and good relations with at least one parent (Hunter and Kihlstrom 1979; Rutter 1979) may protect the child in adverse situations. Family discord, parental mental illness, economic deprivation, which leads for instance to overcrowding, are known to be risk factors for children's well-being, especially if they occur together (Rutter 1979). During recent years there has been increasing interest in the impact of parental mental disorder on children. Maternal depression is shown to be linked with developmental problems in small children (Weissman *et al.* 1972; Richman 1976; Zahn-Waxler *et al.* 1990).

These peace-time studies emphasize the importance of the family. The interesting question is, what is the family's role and can the family protect the child also during war? There is very little knowledge here and especially little about the family as a network of relationships. Most studies have only concentrated on the mother–child relationship.

In wartime children orient themselves towards the family and become very attached (Ziv *et al.* 1974). The family relationships are also very important for the adults. Palestinian women rated discord with their husbands as very threatening, even more so than fighting in the streets (Bryce and Walker 1986). Only death or kidnapping of a family member was more threatening. It is understandable that family problems are more threatening in times of war than in peace, because a family in discord might not be able to offer the psychological security and refuge needed for its members. McWhirter (1983), referring to the civil strife in Northern Ireland, goes as far as saying that family discord is a more serious threat to child mental health than violence in the community. There is, however, very little knowledge about this, especially about the interplay of wartime hardships and family discord.

The lack of energy, food, health care, and economical resources bring enormous everyday problems to families, and especially to mothers. These hardships tax the resources of the family members. Bryce and Walker (1986) report how economically and educationally deprived, depressed Lebanese mothers were liable to child abuse, which they regretted themselves, but could not help.

It has been argued (Gustafsson 1990) that if the family can offer the child 'an island of normality' in war and conflict, it supports the child's coping ability. However, when the level of political hardship is very high, a good family life does not seem to protect children from psychological symptoms (Punamäki 1989).

The role of the mother, for example the mother's mental health or separation from the mother, has been one of the major topics in discussing family influences since the Freud and Burlingham (1942, 1943) studies. Freud and Burlingham argued that it is the mother's mental state that determines how the child fares rather than the war experiences, and that separation from the mother was more harmful than the bombings.

Later findings have shed more light on the complexity of these issues. Räsänen (1988) followed up those who were evacuated from Finland to Sweden as children during the Second World War. Their mental health and success in life were studied 40 years later and compared with a matched group of non-evacuees. The striking finding was that there were very small differences between these two groups. In the tosses and turns of life, the early experiences were evened out.

Raundalen and Dyregrov (unpublished manuscript) criticize easy generalizations from one war situation to another. The Freud and Burlingham studies (1942 and 1943) apply only to Britain in World War II. The reality for children in many of the contemporary conflicts is that leaving their homes is their only chance of survival. Raundalen and Dyregrov maintain that child refugees are not necessarily the hardest hit victims of war, but rather, these are the children who have been able to leave. Many parents also send their children away in order to protect them from almost certain death.

As to the impact of the mother's mental health on child well-being, maternal depression was found to be correlated to the child's psychological problems among Lebanese families (Bryce and Walker 1986). In South Africa, if the mother was diagnosed as having post-traumatic stress disorder, the child was likely to suffer from it as well (Dawes *et al.* 1989). Punamäki's results (1987) also support this finding.

Luthar and Zigler (1991) point out that the mother's mental state has often been taken as an 'all or none' phenomenon and one does not know what it is that affects the child. Seifer and Sameroff (1987) argue that the severity and chronicity of the mother's mental problems are a better predictor of the child's problems than the fact of the diagnosis itself. Punamäki (1989) was able to show that when the political hardships increased, only the mother's internal locus of control protected the child, and not her mental health in general. The more the Palestinian mothers confronted violence, the more they employed active coping modes and exhibited an internal locus of control (Punamäki 1987). Also, the more the Palestinian mothers suffered from psychological symptoms, the more the children employed active and courageous coping modes in spite of their mental problems.

The mother–child relationship is mutually interactional. The mother's anxiety can be transferred to the child, but the child also influences the mother. The child's suffering is painful to the mother, as she sees how helpless she is in her efforts to protect her child (Punamäki 1987). The child's sufferings can contribute to the mother's anxiety.

It is striking how little research is available on fathering. It has been documented that the absence of the father preoccupies the child (Ziv *et al.* 1974) and can be one of the reasons for bed-wetting in children (Kaffman and Elizur 1979). The focus should be shifted towards seeing the family as a network of relationships which include the siblings and both parents.

Participating in the conflict

A long-term conflict is not simply an outer reality to the child, but it is his or her world. The child's environment is often actively involved in the conflict and children themselves take part in it. Children's activites are often supported by the community.

During armed conflict, overt anxiety and fear might lead to inappropriate actions in frightening situations, whereas being brave is the only way to survive. Social pressure in the community also supports down playing of overt anxiety as people are expected not to show their fears and anxieties (Ziv *et al.* 1974; Lahad and Ayalon 1990; Punamäki 1987). This kind of situation might leave children with only two options—extreme bravery or withdrawal. Indeed, as to their reactions to the occupation soldiers, Palestinian children fell into one of two extreme groups—about 47 per cent were terrified by the soldiers, while 37 per cent reported no fear at all (Baker 1990). Only 16 per cent fell in between.

In psychological terms, when children throw stones and build road blocks, what they are doing is coping actively in adversity. Politically active children are shown to have an internal locus of control (Baker 1990; Punamäki and Suleiman 1989). An internal locus of control serves as a protective function in children in peace time (Murphy and Moriarty 1976; Werner and Smith 1982). However, in the Punamäki and Suleiman study neither active nor courageous coping modes were effective in protecting children from mental health problems. Furthermore, in the Baker study (1990) children showed both internal locus of control and depression. This goes against the notion that psychological symptoms, especially depression, are linked with helplessness and an external locus of control (Seligman 1975).

To understand this one has to consider the societal situation as well as the individual one. Children's political activity aims not only at mastering the actual situation at hand, but also to contribute knowingly to the national struggle. For them, a better future lies with the success of the struggle (Punamäki and Suleiman 1989; Raundalen and Dyregrov, unpublished manuscript). Because political activity endangers children even more to violence and hardships, they are vulnerable to mental health problems in spite of their active opting. The children are in what Punamäki and Suleiman call a 'psychological dilemma of horror and heroism'. Follow-up studies are needed to document the long-term effects of this dilemma.

Attitudes and antisocial behaviour

There has been a worry that children who live in long-term conflict adopt attitudes that are favourable to war and violence, and racist or hateful attitudes towards other people (Garbarino *et al.* 1991). Although there is some evidence of this (Gal 1990), it seems to be a simplistic generalization on both the human condition and the social complexities in armed conflict.

The situation of war and conflict is full of confusion and complexity; it is not just 'black and white' (Andama 1987). Lahad and Ayalon (1990) talk of continuous contradictions and ambivalences in everyday life. One tries to carry on everyday routines but at the same time be prepared for violence; to promote trust in other people while continuously being aware of suspicious objects or people; educating towards peaceful coexistence while justifying war. Punamäki (1989) has pointed out the dilemma of Palestinian mothers of having to choose to protect the child from war or take action to guarantee his or her future.

These contradictions are part of the life of children, and they show in children's own attitudes. The data from Northern Ireland is interesting in this respect.

The Protestants and Catholics are the counterparts of the civil strife, and, for instance, the school system is, by and large, segregated. It is therefore of interest to see how children perceive and identify with the denominations. Cairns and Duriez (1976) showed that 10–11-year-olds were very sensitive to the cues of their groups of affiliation, and switched off information which came with the dialect of the opposite party. On the other hand, very few children identified themselves by denomination (McWhirter and Trew 1982; Trew 1983). Only a very small minority, comprising mostly boys, saw themselves mainly and foremost as members of their religious group. As to attitudes towards violence, Russel (1973) reports that a majority of schoolboys favoured the use of violence for political ends in Northern Ireland. On the other hand, more than a third of them wanted to move away from the country when older as a reaction to the violence. Lorenc and Branthwaite (1986) found no evidence that the Irish school-children were more tolerant of violence than English children.

It is difficult to make conclusions out of these studies because they are so contradictory, and because there are no baseline data on children's attitudes before the conflict. However, contrary to the stereotypical expectation, children's and young people's attitudes do not seem to be simplistic copies of the divisions of society.

Raundalen *et al.* (1987) report that children are not ready to accept revengeful and hateful attitudes even if they themselves have been victims of violence. A great majority of Ugandan children of 13 to 15 years of age expressed neither aggression (90 per cent) nor revenge (92 per cent) towards their aggressors (Raundalen *et al.* 1987). Highly victimized children in the Red Cross shelter wanted to become doctors, nurses, and relief workers rather than fighters and soldiers. Raundalen *et al.* attribute this to the lack of political socialization towards hatred.

Antisocial behaviour

Juvenile delinquency and antisocial behaviour have been shown to rise during war and armed conflict (Save the Children International Union 1932; Fee 1976; Curran *et al.* 1980). The explanations for this are manifold. It has been argued that in a violent environment children do not learn to control their aggressions (Freud and Burlingham 1943), and that violence and rioting become part of one's way of life and an accepted norm (Lyons 1973). However, these beliefs have been contested (for a review see Heskin (1980) and Mcwhirter and Trew (1982)).

There are other aspects of society, other than war, which support the rise of delinquency in war and conflict. Poverty, overcrowding, poor housing, and poor educational and career prospects are all factors related to the rise of delinquent behaviour (West and Farrington 1973) and these prevail in societies living in a long-term military conflict. The persistence of juvenile delinquency also depends on how quickly the other social problems of the society are solved after the conflict is over.

Child soldiers

It is estimated by the United Nations that there are 200 000 child soldiers in the world (Stanley 1990). There is very little systematic knowledge on these children and their fates. Anecdotal evidence tells that child soldiers are used in dangerous and mortal tasks such as combat (Irandokhte 1984; Stanley 1990).

The Renamo rebels in Mozambique are known to kidnap school-aged boys and take them to their military bases. After being trained to kill, the children are sent back to the areas they came from, even to their own villages, to kill people, including their own family. These children show many kinds of psychological and social problems when they are captured and returned to their communities. The experience disrupts their normal development of identity. Identification with the oppressor, which leads to violent and brutal behaviour, is one of the most problematic sequelae (UNICEF Intercom 1990; Richman 1991).

Once again, however, it has to be remembered that not all children are damaged by the experience. Raundalen and Dyregrov (unpublished manuscript) report how a cognitive understanding of what is happening in society helps children overcome the atrocities of their captivity in the Renamo bases.

The threat of nuclear war

In the early 1960s during the Berlin and Cuban crises and in the early 1980s as part of the Euro-missile crisis the world faced a threat of nuclear war. Schwebel (1965) and Escalona (1963) studied children's reactions to the threat in the early 1960s and found that children were both aware and worried of it. The same was found in the 1980s.

The threat of nuclear war was one of the top worries among young people throughout the industrialized world in the early 1980s (Goldberg et al. 1985; Solantaus et al. 1985; Goldenring and Doctor 1986; Chivian et al. 1988) For a review see Solantaus (1991). It was expressed by boys and girls alike and by children of all social classes (Diamond and Bachman 1986; Solantaus et al. 1985). Socially well adjusted children and those with better school achievement were more worried about nuclear war than others (Goldenring and Doctor 1986). The worry about nuclear war increased with age until early adolescence, at about 11 to 13, and declined after that.

Although boys and girls were equally worried about the nuclear threat, girls expressed stronger fears and anxiety (Goldberg et al. 1985; Solantaus et al. 1985). Girls are socialized to express their anxieties more than boys, and this might explain some of the gender difference. The differences in male and female traditions regarding war and peace might also contribute to the observed gender difference. The political, technological, and military knowledge of war is traditionally a male reserve, while there is no active mastery of military affairs in women's tradition. On the contrary, women have always been victims of warfare. Women have also mended the wounded and buried the dead. It is no wonder, then, that the image of war in the minds of girls is suffering, while boys connect it more with adventure and heroism (Engeström 1978).

One of the concerns of the researchers when undertaking their studies was the possible adverse effect of the threat of nuclear war on children's mental health. However, the expression of worry was not related to any measures describing mental ill-health. It was not related to personality characteristics like self-esteem (Wahlstöm 1988) or the child's general anxiety level and his or her proneness to react with anxiety (Goldenring and Doctor 1986). Rather it was related to interest in government and social issues (Diamond and Bachman 1986). Worry about nuclear war reflected the awareness of the young people of the threat, rather than it being a pathological anxiety amongst most of the children and young people.

However, there was a small group (about five per cent) of young people who were more troubled and whose state resembled depression (Goldberg *et al* 1985, Diamond and Bachman 1986). They felt worthless and alienated from their communities and dissatisfied with life in general. They showed no interest in social issues, felt deeply pessimistic about the future, and they despaired about the nuclear threat. Diamond and Bachman (1986) call them the nuclear despair group. The threat of nuclear war did not seem to play a decisive aetiological role in their condition, but it was one of the contributing factors.

Children became aware of the threat through the mass media. The role of parents and school was minor compared with television (Beardslee and Mack 1982; Goldberg *et al.* 1985; Sheffet *et al.* 1988). However, television cannot educate children on complex issues like this, it can only inform about the details. It was no wonder then that the level of knowledge about nuclear weapons was very low among children and young people (Zweigenhaft 1985; Roscoe and Goodwin 1987). Solantaus (1989) suggests that if communication and joint activity with adults on global issues are lacking, the world remains impossible to understand for children and young people. This might lead to a turning away from global issues towards the private sphere of life. The image of the world might remain fragmented and the youngster does not take responsibility for global issues. However, there is very little knowledge about the developmental processes involved. There is a great need for research on these issues.

Protection of children

In spite of all the adversity and suffering in armed conflicts and threat of war, most children seem to develop without major psychological damage. For the sake of intervention, it would be important to tease out those factors that protect children and those that make them especially vulnerable in armed conflict. This is the main objective in research on children and war.

There is a group of children who are at special risk, and who should receive special attention. They are the children who are more vulnerable generally: handicapped children, children who have experienced desertion, abuse, or loss of a parent, and children who have been uprooted from their homes (Lahad and Ayalon 1990). Unfortunately, this group grows as long as the conflict continues.

Children's experiences of violence often elicit defensive avoidance in children as well as on the part of adults, parents, and teachers. However, traumatized children should be encouraged to talk about their experiences and express them in creative forms (Ayalone 1983; Raviv and Klingman 1983; Richman 1991; Raundalen and Dyregrov, unpublished manuscript). Teachers and parents can be encouraged to help traumatized children by recognizing the children's distressed past and finding ways for them to express their experiences in play, music, and other creative activity (Richman 1991).

Understanding what is happening in society helps children see the world as a predictable place, where things can be influenced, rather than it being a state of total chaos without any scope for intervention (Gustafsson 1990; Lahad and Ayalon 1990). Schools and the family carry the responsibility for explaining the world to children. Many teachers in conflict areas try to give the children a frame of reference into which even the worst violence can be fitted, so as to counteract the impact of atrocities on the children (Gustafsson 1990; Ayalon 1983; Lahad and Ayalon 1990; UNICEF Intercom 1990; Raundalen and Dyregrov, unpublished manuscript).

An understanding of the world is not necessary only for children in armed conflict, but also for children in more peaceful countries. If children are not helped to understand what the world is about, they might proceed to shut it out of their consciousness and not learn to take responsibility for it (Solantaus 1989). Peace education is a necessary part of school education.

Poverty and lack of education bring additional risks. Bryce and Walker (1986) recommend that interventions in Beirut should not be planned according to geographical areas, except for the hardest hit areas, but rather, directed towards the poorest part of the community. Mothers with very little education had only a limited repertoire of coping skills (Bryce and Walker 1986).

Global measures

The *UN Convention on the rights of the child*, approved by the United Nations General Assembly in November 1989, spells out children's rights to survival, development, and protection. Its 38th article deals with children in war. It is based on the international humanitarian law and it obliges the state parties to ensure protection and care of children who are affected in armed conflict.

UNICEF has voiced a principle that children should have first call on society's concerns and capacities in both good times and bad. If at all, this should be applied to children in war and conflict. As an encouraging, albeit small step forward, both sides in the war in El Salvador agreed on a cease-fire in

1985, to allow children to be immunized against infectious diseases. Since then this has been repeated over five years, and three million doses of vaccine have been administered (Grant 1990).

Paragraphs two and three in article 38 in the *Convention on the rights of the child* deal with child soldiers. The state parties are obliged to take 'all feasible measures to ensure that persons under 15 years do not take direct part in hostilities' and refrain from recruiting any person who has not reached the age of 15. When recruiting those between 15 and 17, priority should be given to those who are oldest.

The article has weaknesses, however. First, it is not clear what 'all feasible measures' mean, and neither is it clear what is meant by taking a 'direct part in hostilities'. It leaves open the possibility of children taking an indirect part in hostilities. Furthermore, recruiting under-fifteens is forbidden, but the article does not say anything about volunteering. Another problem is that most of the armies that have children as soldiers are rebel groups, which do not respect international law. However, they are often supported by full states. It should be universally agreed that these states be held responsible for the use of child soldiers by the respective rebel groups.

War is not good for children, nor is it good for anyone. As long as there is war, children will suffer. Disarmament and striving for a lasting peace are necessary for the world. Disarmament releases an enormous amount of both psychological and economic resources. Many global and national problems which now create tension could be solved with these resources. The ultimate aim must be a just world, which does not give rise to war, where human values prevail, and where nations have the resources and skills to solve problems without violence.

References

Acheson, D. (1993). Health, humanitarian relief, and survival in former Yugoslavia. *British Medical Journal*, **307**, 44–8.
Andama, J.W.H. (1987). The parents' dilemma. In *War, violence and children in Uganda* (ed. C.P. Dodge and M. Raundalen), pp. 53–82. Norwegian University Press, Oslo.
Ayalon, O. (1983). Coping with terrorism: the Israeli case. In *Stress reduction and prevention* (ed. D. Meichenbaum and M. Jaremko), pp. 293–339. Plenum, New York.
Diamond, G. and Bachman, J. (1986). High school seniors and nuclear threat, 1975–84: political and mental health implications of concern and despair. *International Journal of Mental Health*, **15**, 210–41.
Baker, A. M. (1990). Psychological impact of the intifada on Palestinian children in the occupied West Bank and Gaza: an exploratory study. *American Journal of Orthopsychiatry*, **60**, 496–505.
Beardslee, W. and Mack, J. (1982). The impact on children and adolescents of nuclear developments. *Task force report No 20.* American Psychiatric Association, Washington DC.
Block, J. (1971). *Lives through time.* Bancroft, Berkeley, CA.

Bodman, F. (1941). War conditions and the mental health of the child. *British Medical Journal*, **2**, 486–8.

Bodman, F. (1944). Child psychiatry in war-time Britain. *Journal of Educational Psychology*, **35**, 293–301.

Bryce, J. and Walker, N. (1986). *Family functioning and child health: a study of families in West Beirut*. Final report submitted to UNICEF, December 31, 1986. UNICEF, New York.

Burbury, W.M. (1941). Effects on education and air raids on city children. *British Medical Journal*, **2**, 660–2.

Cairns, E. and Duriez, B. (1976). Influence of speaker's accent on recall by catholic and protestant school children in Northern Ireland. *British Journal of Social and Clinical Psychology*, **15**, 441–2.

Chivian, E., Robinson, J.P., Tudge, J.R.H., Popov, N.P., and Andreyenkov, V.G. (1988). American and Soviet teenagers' concerns about nuclear war and future. *New England Journal of Medicine*, **319**, 407–13.

Curran, D., Jardine, E.F., and Harbison, J. (1980). Factors associated with deviant attitudes in Northern Ireland school boys. In *A society under stress* (ed. J. Harbison). Open Books, Somerset.

Dawes, A., Tredoux, C., and Feinstein, A. (1989). Political violence in South Africa: some effects on children of violent destruction of their community. *International Journal of Mental Health*, **18**, 16–43.

Diamond, G. and Bachman, J. (1986). High school seniors and nuclear threat, 1975–84: political and mental health implications of concern and despair. *International Journal of Mental Health*, **15**, 210–41.

Elizur, E. and Kaffman, M. (1977). *Infants who become enuretics: a longitudinal study of 161 kibbutz children*. (Monographs of the Society for Research in Child Development.) University of Chicago Press, Chicago.

Elizur, E. and Kaffman, M. (1982). Children's bereavement reactions following death of the father, II. *Journal of the American Academy of Child Psychiatry*, **21**, 474–80.

Engeström, Y. (1978). War in the imagination of Finnish school children. *Current Research on Peace and Violence*, **1**, 91–103.

Escalona, S. (1963). Children's responses to the nuclear war threat. *Children*, **10**, 137–42.

Fee, F. (1976). *Reading and disturbance in Belfast schools*. Education and Library Board, Belfast.

Fjaer, R.B. (1990). Primary health care to children in war. In *Wartime medical services, Proc. 2nd Int. Conf.* (ed. J.E. Lundeberg, U. Otto, and B. Rybeck), pp. 39–43. Försvarets forskningsanstalt, Stockholm.

Fraser, R., M. (1971). The cost of commotion: an analysis of the psychiatric sequelae of the 1969 Belfast riots. *British Journal of Psychiatry*, **118**, 257–64.

Fraser, R.M. (1974). *Children in conflict*. Penguin, Harmondsworth.

Freud, A. and Burlingham, D. (1942). *Young children in wartime*. Allen and Unwin, London.

Freud, A. and Burlingham, D. (1943). *War and children*. Ernst Willard, New York.

Gal, R. (1990). The impact of intifada on Israeli youth. In *Wartime medical services, Proc. 2nd Int. Conf.* (ed. J.E. Lundeberg, U. Otto, and B. Rybeck), pp. 130–43. Försvarets forskningsanstalt, Stockholm.

Garbarino, J., Kostelny, K., and Dubrow, N. (1991). What children can tell us about living in danger. *American Psychologist*, **46**, 376–83.

Goldberg, S., LaCombe, S., Levinson, D., Ross Parker, D., Ross, C., and Sommers, F. (1985). Thinking about the threat of nuclear war: relevance to mental health. *American Journal of Orthopsychiatry*, **55**, 503–12.

Goldenring, J. and Doctor, R. (1986). Teen-age worry about nuclear war: North American and European questionnaire studies. *International Journal of Mental Health*, **15**, 72–92.

Grant, J.P. (ed.) (1990). *The state of the world's children*. UNICEF and Oxford University Press, Oxford.

Gustafsson, L.H. (1990). In case of war—how can we make reality of children's rights? In *Wartime medical services, Proc. 2nd Int. Conf.* (ed. J.E. Lundeberg, U. Otto, and B. Rybeck), pp. 31–8. Försvarets forskningsanstalt, Stockholm.

Henley, D. and Giacaman, R. (1990). Injuries of the uprising: a study of disabilities sustained through violence in the Israeli occupied territories 1988–89. In *Wartime medical services, Proc. 2nd Int. Conf.* (ed. J.E. Lundeberg, U. Otto, and B. Rybeck), pp. 153–5. Försvarets forskningsanstalt, Stockholm.

Heskin, K. (1980). Children and young people in Northern Ireland: a research review. In *A society under stress* (ed. J. Harbison and J. Harbison). Open Books, Somerset.

Hunter, R. and Kihlstrom, N. (1979). Breaking the cycle in abusive families. *American Journal of Psychiatry*, **136**, 1320–2.

Irandokhte,? (1984). Children of war in Iran. In *Child and war* (ed. M. Kahnert, D. Pitt, and I. Taipale). Gummerus, Jyväskylä. (In Finnish.)

Kaffman, M. and Elizur, E. (1979). Children's bereavement reactions following death of the father. *International Journal of Family Therapy*, **1**, 203–31.

Kaffman, M. and Elizur, E. (1983). Bereavement responses of kibbutz and non-kibbutz children following the death of the father. *Journal of Child Psychology and Psychiatry*, **24**, 435–42.

Lahad, M. and Ayalon, O. (1990). Children and war. In *Wartime medical services, Proc. 2nd Int. Conf.* (ed. J.E. Lundeberg, U. Otto, and B. Rybeck), pp. 47–54. Försvarets forskningsanstalt, Stockholm.

Langmeier, J. and Matejcek, Z. (1975). *Psychological deprivation in childhood*. Halsted Press, New York.

Lawyers' Committee for Human Rights. (1986). *The war against children: South Africa's youngest victims*. Lawyers' Committee, New York.

Lorenc, L. and Branthwaite, A. (1986). Evaluations of political violence by English and Northern Irish school children. *British Journal of Social psychology*, **25**, 349–52.

Luthar, S.S. and Zigler, E. (1991). Vulnerability and competence: a review of research on resilience in childhood. *American Journal of Orthopsychiatry*, **61**, 6–22.

Lyons, H.A. (1971). Psychiatric sequelae of the Belfast riots. *British Journal of Psychiatry*, **118**, 265–73.

Lyons, H.A. (1973). Violence in Belfast—a review of psychological affects. *Public Health*, **87**, 231–8.

MacAuley, R. and Troi, M. (1983). The impact of urban conflict and violence referred to a child psychiatry clinic. In *Children of the troubles* (ed. J. Harbison), pp. 33–43. Stranmills College Learning Resources Unit, Belfast.

McWhirter, L. (1983). Northern Ireland: growing up with the 'troubles'. In *Aggression in global perspective* (ed. A.P. Goldstein and M. Segall). Pergamon, New York.

McWhirter, L. and Trew, K. (1982). Children in Northern Ireland: a lost generation? In *The child in his family,* Vol 7. *Children in turmoil: tomorrow's parents* (ed. E.J. Anthony and C. Chiland), pp. 69–82. Wiley, New York.

Mons, W.E.R. (1941). Air raids and the child. *British Medical Journal*, **2**, 625–6.
Murphy, L.B. and Moriarty, A.E. (1976). *Vulnerability, coping and growth*. Yale University Press, New Haven.
Punamäki, R.-L. (1987). Psychological stress of Palestinian mothers and their children in conditions of political violence. *The Quarterly Newsletter of the Laboratory of Comparative Human Cognition*, **9**, 116–19.
Punamäki, R.-L. (1989). Factors affecting the mental health of Palestinian children exposed to political violence. *International Journal of Mental Health*, **18**, 63–79.
Punamäki, R.-L. and Suleiman, R. (1989). Predictors and effectiveness of coping with political violence among Palestinian children. *British Journal of Social Psychology*, **29**, 67–77.
Raundalen, M. and Dyregrov, A. How war effects children—how to reach children in war. Examples from Uganda, Mozambique, Sudan and the West Bank. Unpublished manuscript.
Raundalen, M., Lwanga, J., Mugisha, C., and Dyregrov A. (1987). Four investigations of stress in Uganda. In *War, violence and children in Uganda* (ed. C.P. Dodge and M. Raundalen), pp. 83–108. Norwegian University Press, Oslo.
Raviv, A. and Klingman, A. (1983). Children under stress. In *Stress in Israel* (ed. S. Breznitz), pp. 138–62.Van Nostrand Reinhold, New York and London.
Rayhida, J., Shaya, M., and Armenian, H. (1986). Child health in a city at war. In *Wartime: the state of children in Lebanon* (ed. J. Bryce and H. Armenian). American University of Beirut, Beirut.
Richman, N. (1976). Depression of mothers of preschool children. *Journal of Child Psychology and Psychiatry*, **17**, 75–6.
Richman, N. (1991). A letter from Mozambique. *Newsletter of the Association for Child Psychology and Psychiatry*, **13**, 33–5.
Roscoe, B. and Goodwin, M.P. (1987). Adolescents' knowledge of nuclear issues and effects of nuclear war. *Adolescence*, **22**, 803–12.
Räsänen, E. (1988). *The effect of the separation experiences during childhood on the mental and physical health and social well-being in adulthood. A psychosocial study of the later effects of war-child separation experiences*. Publications of Kuopio University, original reports, 2. Kuopion yliopiston painatuskeskus, Kuopio. (In Finnish.)
Russel, J. (1973). Violence and the Ulster schoolboy. *New Society*, **25**, 204–6.
Rutter, M. (1979). Protective factors in children's reactions to stress and disadvantage. In *Primary prevention of psychopathology:* Vol. 3. *Social competence in children* (ed. M.W. Kent and J.E. Rolf), pp. 49–74. Lawrence Erlbaum, Hillsdale, New Jersey.
Save the Children International Union (1932). The impact of war on children and young people. In *Child and war* (ed. M. Kahnert and I. Taipale), pp. 59–84. Gummerus, Jyväskylä. (In Finnish).
Schwebel, M. (1965). Nuclear cold war: student opinions and professional responsibility. In *Behavioral science and human survival* (ed. M. Schwebel). Science and Behaviour Books, Palo Alto, CA.
Seifer, R. and Sameroff, A.J. (1987). Multiple determinants of risk and invulnerability. In *The invulnerable child* (ed. E.J. Anthony and B.J. Cohler), pp. 51–69. Guilford Press, New York.
Seligman, M.E.P. (1975). *Helplessness: on depression, development and death*. W.H. Freeman, San Francisco.

Sheffet, A.M., Zutz, N.M., Titelbaum, J.M., and Louria, D.B. (1988). Adolescence and the nuclear arms race. *Social Science and Medicine*, **27**, 995–8.

Solantaus, T. (1989). The global world—a domain for development in adolescence? *Journal of Adolescence*, **12**, 27–40.

Solantaus, T. (1991). Young people and the threat of nuclear war, 'Out there is a world I belong to': a literature review. *Medicine and War* (Suppl.) 1: 5–95.

Solantaus, T., Rimpelä, M., and Rahkonen, O. (1985). Social epidemiology of the experience of the threat of war among Finnish youth. *Social Science and Medicine*, **21**, 145–51.

Stanley, A. (1990). Child warriors. *Time*, June 18, pp.

Straker, G. and Moosa, F. (1988). Post-traumatic stress disorder: a reaction to state-supported child abuse and neglect. *Child Abuse and Neglect*, **12**, 383–95.

Trew, K. (1983). Group identification in a devided society. In *Children of the troubles. Children of Northern Ireland* (ed. J. Harbison). Learning resources unit, Stranmillis College, Belfast.

UNICEF (1986). *Children in situations of armed conflict*. UNICEF, New York.

UNICEF (1987). *Children in the front line. The impact of apartheid, destabilization and warfare on children in southern Africa*. UNICEF, New York.

UNICEF Intercom (1990). *Mozambique's education battleground*. No 56, April 1990, UNICEF, New York.

Wahlström, R. (1988). The relationship of self-esteem and moral development to the fear of war and desire for peace among young people. Department of Education, Jyväskylä University, Jyväskylä (In Finnish).

Weissman, M.M., Paykel, E.S., and Klerman, G.L. (1972). The depressed woman as mother. *Social Psychiatry*, **7**, 98–108.

Werner, E.E. and Smith, R.S. (1982). *Vulnerable but invisible: a study of resilient children*. McGraw-Hill, New York.

West, D. and Farrington, D. (1973). *Who becomes delinquent*. Heinemann, London.

Zahn-Waxler, C., Kochanska, G., Krupnick, J., and McKnew, D. (1990) Patterns of guilt in children of depressed and well mothers. *Developmental Psychology*, **26**, 51–9.

Ziv, A., Kruglanski, A. W., and Schulman, S. (1974). Children's psychological reactions to wartime stress. *Journal of Personality and Social Psychology*, **30**, 24–30.

Zweigenhaft, R.L. (1985). Students surveyed about nuclear war. *Bulletin of the Atomic Scientists*, **41**, 26–7.

10 Children and HIV infection
Marie-Louise Newell and Catherine Peckham

Global impact of AIDS

The growing magnitude of HIV infection in women and children has been recognized, and by the beginning of this decade more than three million women, most of childbearing age, were estimated to be infected with HIV. About 80 per cent of these infected women live in sub-Saharan Africa (Chin 1990), but the problem is not restricted to this region and increasing numbers are being reported in the USA, Europe, Asia, and South America. Based on the numbers of reported AIDS cases, the results of prevalence studies of HIV infection in pregnant women, local fertility rates, and assuming a vertical transmission rate of 25 per cent, WHO has estimated that by the end of 1992, there will be one million children with AIDS worldwide. By the end of the decade there could be at least 10 million HIV infected children (Chin 1990; Chin and Mann 1990; Hunter 1990; Preble 1990). These WHO estimates are likely to be conservative, as reporting of AIDS cases is incomplete, particularly where diagnostic facilities are not widely available and political circumstances mitigate against it. Within a relatively short time period, the AIDS epidemic has emerged as a major health problem with enormous social, political, medical, and economic implications.

In Africa, where most HIV infections are acquired heterosexually, approximately equal numbers of men and women are infected. However, this situation may be changing and in a recent review of three population studies an infection rate 1.4 times higher in females than in males was demonstrated (Berkley *et al.* 1990). In the USA and Europe heterosexual transmission is increasing in importance, although the majority of AIDS cases are in homosexual men, and the male–female ratio is about 10:1. In certain Latin American countries, many bisexual men became infected early in the epidemic and acted as a link for infection between the homosexual and heterosexual communities. As a result, the pattern of infection in these countries is changing, with increasing numbers of women infected heterosexually (Quinn *et al.* 1989). In parallel with the rise in heterosexual transmission there has been an increase in the number of children with AIDS. By the end of 1990, about 3000 children under the age of 13 had been reported with AIDS in the US, and more than 2000 in Europe (Centers for Disease Control 1991*a*; European Centre for the Epidemiological Monitoring of AIDS 1990) (Fig. 10.1).

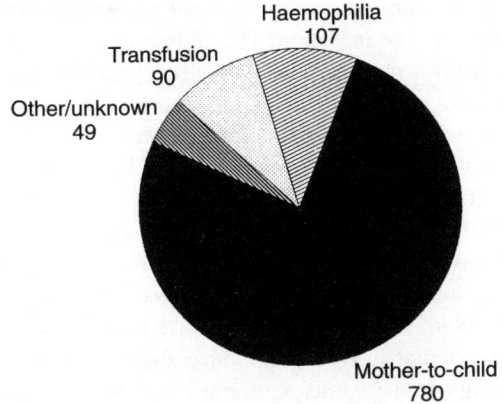

Fig. 10.1 Paediatric AIDS in Europe, by mode of acquisition of infection (1990; excluding 1094 Romanian cases).

Mode of acquisition

Most children acquire HIV infection vertically from their mother (Table 10.1). This may occur before, during, or shortly after birth, but the relative importance of each of these routes is unknown. Intrauterine infection has been demonstrated by the identification of virus in fetal tissue, placenta, and in cord blood. The very early onset of AIDS in some children also suggests intrauterine acquisition of infection. Because of the increased exchange of blood between mother and child at the time of delivery, and because the virus has been detected in cervical secretion, transmission during delivery is a possibility. Although Lindgren *et al.* (1991) showed a small but insignificant trend favouring caesarian delivery, prospective studies published to date have not been able to confirm this and no significant difference in the rate of vertical transmission according to mode of delivery has been reported (Blanche *et al.* 1989; European Collaborative Study 1988). Transmission of HIV through breast milk has been described in situations where the mother acquired the infection shortly after birth, following a contaminated blood transfusion (Oxtoby 1988) or through heterosexual contact (van de Perre *et al.* 1990). In the acute phase of primary infection, these women will be

Table 10.1 *Mode of acquisition of HIV infection in children*

Vertically: before/during/after birth
Contaminated blood or blood products
Contaminated needles/syringes
Sexual contact

more viraemia than those who were antibody positive before delivery and therefore more likely to transmit the infection. The added risk of transmission of HIV through breast milk from a mother who was already antibody positive during pregnancy is in the region of 15 per cent (Dunn et al. 1992).

Acquisition of HIV infection through contaminated blood remains a problem in countries where blood donors at increased risk of infection are not excluded and where blood is not screened for HIV antibodies (Greenberg et al. 1988; N'Tita et al. 1991). In these countries there has been a concerted effort to make the indications for blood transfusions more stringent thereby limiting the number of transfusions given. Shaffer et al. (1990) evaluated 1100 children seen in the paediatric emergency ward of a large hospital in Kinshasa, Zaire, and found a relatively stable, high paediatric HIV prevalence and a decreased but continued risk of infection through transfusions. Contaminated needles and syringes and micro blood transfusions remain a risk, as demonstrated by the recent discovery of nearly 1000 children with AIDS in Romania, most of whom acquired infection in this way (European Centre for the Epidemiological Monitoring of AIDS 1990). This sad experience highlights the need to ensure the use of clean equipment. Scarification and circumcision, which is common in certain parts of Africa, have also been implicated as possible routes of transmission, although definitive evidence is lacking (Hrdy 1987).

Many haemophiliacs, both children and adults, acquired HIV infection through contaminated blood components used in the treatment of haemophilia. There have been no new infections in haemophiliac children in the UK since 1985, with the introduction of routine screening of blood for HIV antibodies and heat treatment of clotting factors.

Intravenous drug use, with sharing of needles and syringes contaminated with infected blood, is a major mode of acquisition of infection in many countries. This provides an entry of infection into the heterosexual population, either through prostitution to finance the drug habit or through sexual contact with non-drug-using partners.

Although HIV has been found in saliva, sweat, tears, and urine, there is no evidence that infection can be acquired from these sources. Indeed, it is not transmitted by touching someone who is infected, through droplets coughed or sneezed into the air, nor from sharing utensils such as cups and plates, or from swimming pools or toilet seats, nor via insects. Information on the lack of casual transmission from children to their close household contacts is accumulating and there have been no reports of transmission of HIV acquired from children in family, day, or foster-care settings, or schools (Rogers et al. 1990).

The potential for occupational transmission of HIV was appreciated early in the course of the AIDS epidemic and has been a persistent professional and public health issue. The risk depends on: the probability of infection occurring following a particular incident; the probability of that incident occurring; and the prevalence of HIV infection in the population concerned. Blood is the only body fluid implicated in occupational HIV infection to date, which may relect the low virus load in other body fluids. The risk of infection after parenteral exposure to infected blood is estimated to be approximately 0.4 per cent (95 per cent confidence interval: 0.0–0.9 per cent) (Henderson et al. 1990). The risk of infection from mucous membrane exposure or contamination of non-intact skin with HIV-infected blood remains a possibility but is too low to be quantified in prospective studies currently under way. Contamination of unbroken skin with HIV-infected blood has not been implicated in HIV transmission, despite the high frequency of this mode of exposure.

Precautions taken to prevent the spread of hepatitis B virus, which is much more infectious than HIV, should be more than adequate to prevent transmission of HIV (Centers for Disease Control 1988; Royal College of Obstetricians and Gynaecologists 1990).

Prevalence of HIV infection

AIDS is the end-point of HIV infection and the incubation time from infection to the development of symptoms can be long. Although a few people develop AIDS soon after they have become infected, most remain asymptomatic for prolonged periods. Studies of groups of people with known time of infection (Schechter et al. 1989; Goedert et al. 1989; Biggar 1990) suggest that about 50 per cent of infected people develop AIDS within 10 years. It is important to emphasize that many people, particulary those without symptoms, may be unaware that they are infected, or even that they are at risk of infection. Even during this early stage, they can transmit the infection to a sexual partner.

Knowledge of the prevalence of HIV infection in specific populations within a country provides more accurate information of the current situation than reports of AIDS cases, but is difficult to obtain. Information available is based on studies in well defined populations such as prostitutes, pregnant women, attenders of genito-urinary clinics, army recruits, hospital admissions, or laboratory reports of positive HIV tests. HIV prevalence based on such studies may not necessarily reflect the true situation in the general population.

Unlinked anonymous testing of blood taken for other purposes has provided the most useful information in the monitoring of the epidemic (Gill et al. 1989), although even this is limited to those people who have their blood taken for other purposes. An increasing number of anonymous, unlinked studies are now in progress (Ippolito et al. 1990; Ades et al. 1991; Novick et al. 1989; Gwinn et al. 1991; Hankins et al. 1990). The prevalence of HIV infection in pregnant women is important, because this has implications for infection in the child, vertical transmission from mother to child being the main mode of acquisition of infection in children. Table 10.2 shows the prevalence of HIV infection in pregnant women, identified in screening programmes. In all studies, HIV prevalence is highest for women from large, inner city areas. For example, in New York (Novick et al. 1989) the prevalence per 1000 pregnant women increased from

Table 10.2 *HIV-1 seroprevalence in antenatal populations, rate per 1000*

Population	Source	Prevalence
Neonatal screening		
London, UK, 1991	Ades *et al.* 1991	0.59
London, UK, 1988–91	Ades *et al.* 1991	0.40
Scotland, 1990	Tappin *et al.* 1991	0.29
US, 38 states, 1989	Gwinn *et al.* 1991	1.50
Quebec, Canada, 1989	Hankins *et al.* 1990	0.61
Sydney, Australia, 1989	McLaws *et al.* 1990	<0.45
New York, USA, 1987/88	Novick *et al.* 1989	6.57
Italy, 1988	Ippolito *et al.* 1990	1.19
Massachusetts, USA, 1987	Hoff *et al.* 1988	2.10
Antenatal screening		
Sweden, 1988		0.13
Malawi, 1989		230.70
Nairobi, 1989		70.80

1.6 in up-state New York to 12.5 in New York City; in London (Ades *et al.* 1991) the rate was 0.42 per 1000 in outer London and 1.02 per 1000 in inner London; and in Quebec (Hankins *et al.* 1990) the rate increased from 1.8 per 1000 to 4.6 per 1000 respectively.

However, the results of unlinked, anonymous testing are difficult to interpret, since no information is available on maternal risk factors, such as intravenous drug use. The strength of such studies is that they are population based and so do not suffer from bias due to refusal to be tested or the failure to identify an individual at risk. Nevertheless, they only include women whose pregnancies result in a live birth.

Antenatal screening

In any named antenatal screening programme, it is important to decide the target population and to weigh the benefits of knowledge of HIV infection status for a woman and her child against any disadvantages that may accrue. For example, a decision will need to be reached as to whether screening should be restricted to women identified to be at hight risk or to all women, irrespective of identification of risk behaviour. Women at increased risk of infection may not be aware of this and those who already know that they are infected may not wish to divulge this information (Barbacci *et al.* 1991; Ades *et al.* 1991). Studies have shown that those opting out are at increased risk of being infected. As the epidemic continues and the prevalence of HIV infection in pregnant women rises, fewer women will realize that they are at increased risk of being infected.

In areas where the prevalence of HIV infection is high, it may be justifiable to offer screening to all women, provided sufficient resources are available for pre-test counselling by adequately trained staff, post-test counsellors, and the provision of educational material. The success of a universal screening programme is likely to depend on the motivation of those offering the test (Sherr and Hedge 1990; Temmerman et al. 1990a).

HIV infection is a family disease and there is a need to recognize this in the context of an antenatal, named screening programme. The benefits of such a programme for the mother include the early recognition of her infection leading to the earlier detection of HIV-related symptoms at a time when management and treatment may be more effective (Table 10.3). In addition, it provides the opportunity to discuss issues relating to spread of HIV infection, and advice on birth control. It is important that she be given information about the risk of vertical transmission of infection, and offered the opportunity of termination of the pregnancy. There is increasing evidence that knowledge of the HIV infection status of the mother may benefit the child, as a result of earlier diagnosis and, although there is no cure, more appropriate management, prophylaxis, and treatment leading to a better quality and prolongation of life. One of the major drawbacks of widespread testing relates to confidentiality issues.

Pregnancy and HIV infection

It has been suggested that pregnancy could accelerate the course of HIV infection in an infected woman and as a result women have been offered termination of pregnancy to protect their own health. However, recent prospective studies (Johnstone et al. 1988; Schoenbaum et al. 1988) do not support this view for asymptomatic women. Symptomatic women who become pregnant have not been adequately studied and further information is needed to clarify this issue.

Research in Africa (Ryder et al. 1989; Temmerman et al. 1990b; Miotti et al. 1990) has shown an increase in adverse pregnancy outcomes in HIV-infected

Table 10.3 *Issues to be addressed in post-test counselling in the antenatal period*

Effect of HIV on pregnancy outcome
Risk of infection in child
Effect of pregnancy on course of HIV infection
Natural history of HIV infection in mother and child
Breast-feeding
Prevention of spread of HIV infection
Social support
Care issues
Availability of voluntary agencies

---

women. Although Ryder et al. in Kinshasa (1989) found no difference in rates of abortion or stillbirths, infants of seropositive mothers were more likely to be premature, of low birth-weight, and to have a higher neonatal mortality rate than infants of seronegative mothers. Temmerman et al. (1990b) presented results from Nairobi suggesting an association between maternal HIV infection and stillbirth, and confirmed the association with low birth-weight. In Malawi (Miotti et al. 1990), HIV infection was shown to be correlated with spontaneous abortion. Separately, Braddick et al. (1990), Halsey et al. (1991), and Lepage et al. (1991) presenting results on cohorts in Nairobi, Haiti, and Kigali, also showed low birth-weight to be associated with maternal HIV infection.

In contrast, European and North American prospective studies of HIV infection in pregnancy have not shown an increased risk of adverse pregnancy outcome (Selwyn et al. 1989; Johnstone et al. 1988). In a study in New York, of 39 seropositive and 58 seronegative pregnant women enrolled in a methadone programme, there was no difference in the frequency of spontaneous or elective abortions, ectopic pregnancies, preterm delivery, stillbirth, or low birth-weight, nor was there a difference between the groups in antenatal, intrapartum, or perinatal complications. In the European prospective studies where birth-weight was related to the mothers' intravenous drug use rather than to the HIV infection in the child, there was no difference in the birth-weight between infected and non-infected infants born to HIV-seropositive women. Those mothers who injected drugs during pregnancy had smaller babies (Blanche et al. 1989; European Collaborative Study 1988).

The adverse outcome found in studies in Africa and Haiti could reflect the social and health status of the mother, rather than the direct effect of HIV infection on the fetus or infant. The higher prevalence of illness in the mothers and other adverse AIDS-related family factors could affect the nurture and care given to the child (Braddick et al. 1990). Maternal health is a strong predictor of child survival, and, although low birth-weight has been found to be associated with advanced HIV disease, it is not clear whether this is the direct effect of HIV infection in pregnancy or a general effect of illness in the mother.

Vertically acquired infection

The proportion of children acquiring the infection through vertical transmission in Europe and the US in about 80 per cent.

Early diagnosis

Because maternal HIV antibody crosses the placenta, the presence of HIV antibodies in a young child does not necessarily indicate that the infant is infected, but may merely reflect maternal infection. As maternal antibodies may persist well into the second year of life, the diagnosis of HIV infection in a child born to an HIV-positive woman based on the presence of HIV antibodies may have to be delayed until the second year of life. Of course, HIV infection can also be diagnosed by the detection of virus or viral antigen from lymphocytes or free viral antigen in serum. However, these tests are expensive, can only be done in specialized laboratories, and are not widely available for routine diagnostic purposes. Also, not all cells will carry the virus and free antigen may not be present in an infected child. A failure to detect virus or antigen in a young, antibody-positive child does not exclude infection, but a positive virus or antigen test is likely to indicate infection. Hopefully, the polymerase chain reaction method of diagnosis of HIV infection, which amplifies viral genetic material, thus facilitating the detection of minute quantities of virus, will lead to an earlier diagnosis of infection. At present this remains a research tool and in infants (De Rossi *et al.* 1991; Tudor-Williams 1991), transplacental contamination from maternal blood may be a problem. Further evaluation is required before this method can be widely used.

This difficulty in establishing an early diagnosis of HIV infection poses many problems. Parents and health professionals live with the uncertainty of diagnosis—every common cold could be indicative of infection. Living with this uncertainty could affect bonding between mother and child. Until proven otherwise, the child is likely to be considered infected. It also has important implications for treatment decisions, since many HIV-associated symptoms and signs are non-specific, and treatment of non-infected children with potentially toxic drugs, which could have long-term sequelae, should be avoided.

Vertical transmission rates

Estimates of the rate of vertical transmission of HIV infection from mother to child, from published papers of prospective studies, range from seven to 39 per cent (Newell *et al.* 1990) (Table 10.4). The recent findings of the European Collaborative Study (1991) indicate a vertical transmission rate of 13 per cent for a largely asymptomatic, white, intravenous-drug using population, with a 95 per cent confidence interval from 9.5 to 16.3 per cent. There was no difference in rates between centres in Europe, nor over time. Although this rate applies to Europe, the vertical transmission rates from mother to child reported from Africa appear to be higher, in the order of 30 per cent. The reason for the difference is not clear, but could well be partly explained by differences in maternal disease status, both clinical and immunological, as this could relate to viral load and infectivity. Other factors influencing viral load, such as primary infection, or factors stimulating the immune system such as other chronic infections and drug use, could also be important. There is a paucity of information on maternal risk factors for vertical transmission and this is an area currently under study (Newell and Peckham, 1993).

Table 10.4 *Rates of vertical transmission*

Location	Source	Rate (%)	95% confidence interval (%)
USA	Scott et al. (1989)	36	(11–69)
	Goedert et al. (1989)	29	(18–43)
	Andiman et al. (1990)	16	(7–31)
Zaire	Ryder et al. (1989, 1991)	39	(29–50)
Zambia	Hira et al. (1989)	39	(30–49)
Rwanda	Lepage et al. (1991)	33	(27–39)
Italy	Gabiano et al. (1992)	33	(23–44)
France	Blanche et al. (1989, 1990)	27	(19–28)
Europe	European Collaborative Study (1988, 1991)	13	(9–16)
Haiti	Halsey et al. (1991)	25	

(From Newell *et al.* 1990)

Natural history

The initial presentation of HIV infection in children is usually non-specific and includes generalized lymphadenopathy, hepato/splenomegaly, diarrhoea, fever unexplained by other causes, failure to thrive, and parotitis. Other more serious manifestations include persistent oral candida, chronic parotitis, lymphoid interstitial pneumonitis, progressive encephalopathy, and serious bacterial and other opportunistic infections. Without a definitive diagnosis of HIV infection it is usually not possible to determine whether these symptoms or signs are HIV related, particularly in populations with a high background prevalence of intercurrent infections.

In the European Collaborative Study (1991), based on follow-up from birth, the initial clinical manifestations in symptomatic infected children were a combination of persistent lymphadenopathy, hepatomegaly, and splenomegaly, although in 30 per cent of these children the initial presentation was AIDS or oral candida rapidly leading on to AIDS. Using survival methods, this study showed that an estimated 83 per cent of infected children exhibited signs of HIV infection within six months of age, either hypergammaglobulinaemia, clinical signs, or a low CD4:CD8 (T4:T8) ratio. By 12 months, 26 per cent had developed AIDS and 17 per cent had died of HIV-related disease. The rate of progression of HIV-related disease declined after 12 months, and the condition of most children remained stable or even improved over the second year. The clinical manifestation and the progression of the disease were closely related to the immunological status of the child; for example, neurological problems became apparent only when the immune system was depressed, and were not usually presenting symptoms. The clinical presentation of HIV disease may be different in Africa, probably due to a different spectrum of potential opportunistic pathogens, such as tuberculosis and cytomegalovirus.

The incubation period from initial exposure to the onset of AIDS is variable, with a third of children presenting with a rapid progression to AIDS in the first year of life. At this stage, little information is available on the long-term prognosis for the remainder.

Scott et al. (1989) described the natural history of a group of HIV-infected children most of whom were first identified because of symptomatic disease. The most common manifestations were lymphoid interstitial pneumonitis (LIP), encephalopathy, recurrent bacterial infections, and candida oesophagitis. The median age of presentation of symptoms was eight months, and 21 per cent presented after two years. Mortality was high in the first year of life, largely due to Pneumocystis carinii pneumonia (PCP), and the long-term survival was short. In contrast, the median survival time of children with LIP was 70 months. Connor et al. (1991) reported that the majority of perinatally HIV-infected children with PCP were six months or younger and 50 per cent were previously unknown to be infected.

Blanche et al. (1990) analysed 94 consecutive infected children followed up after their first clinical symptoms. One third suffered from the early onset of an opportunistic infection. LIP occurred at a mean age of 29 months, significantly later than opportunistic infections or severe encephalopathy. Laboratory results at initial examination, such as low numbers of CD4 cells, correlated with clinical symptoms. A subgroup of patients expressed very early signs of severe immunodeficiency and encephalopathy, whereas the majority had a longer survival and less severe clinical symptoms during their first years of life. Children are at risk of acquisition of PCP at levels of CD4 cells well above the cut-off levels defined for adults (Kovacs et al. 1991; Connor et al. 1991).

Any child born to an HIV-infected mother should be followed regularly from birth, both to establish infection and to initiate treatment at the earliest possible stage. In Europe and the USA, AZT is increasingly used in paediatric HIV infection, but there is no consensus of opinion about when to start AZT treatment, or on the most appropriate dose (Pizzo and Wilfert 1990). Prophylaxis for PCP is recommended for HIV-infected children who are immunosuppressed (Centers for Disease Control 1991b), and management of persistent oral candida, for example, has been facilitated by the introduction of fluconazol. New anti-retroviral treatments are being introduced, and it is likely that combination therapy, such as that used in cancer treatment, will become the treatment of choice. However, these are costly drugs and it is unlikely that they will become available in those parts of the world where the majority of inflected children live, and where health resources are extremely limited.

Immunization

The immunological abnormalities associated with HIV infection have raised concerns about immunization of infected children, especially with live vaccines.

Asymptomatic HIV-infected infants respond normally to immunizations, although immunocompromised and HIV-symptomatic children may not mount an appropriate and satisfactory immune response and may show a decline in antibody levels. To date, no increase in adverse reactions to immunizations has been reported in HIV-infected children. WHO recommends routine immunization for HIV-infected children, but withholding BCG vaccination from those who are symptomatic and from all HIV-infected children whose risk of acquiring tuberculosis is low. As oral polio-vaccine virus is excreted in the faeces and could be dangerous if acquired by an immunosuppressed individual, substitution of inactivated polio vaccine for oral polio vaccine may be considered for children living in households where someone may be immunosuppressed or have symptomatic HIV infection. Theoretical concerns that immunization might accelerate the course of the HIV infection are not supported by the available evidence (Lallemant-Le Coeur *et al.* 1991).

Breast-feeding

Postnatal transmission of infection through breast milk can occur in a child whose mother acquires the infection after the infant's birth (Oxtoby 1988), and the risk of infection through breast milk in an infant born to a woman who was HIV positive before the birth is also recognized. A meta-analysis of 6 large prospective studies suggests that in these circumstances, the additional risk of transmission is in the region of 15 per cent (Dunn *et al.* 1992).

Howie *et al.* (1990) showed clearly the protective effect of breast-feeding against gastrointestinal infections, a protection which persists beyond the period of breast-feeding itself. Pabst and Spady (1990) provide evidence that breast-feeding enhances the active immune response in the first year of life. The estimated number of infant deaths associated with bottle-feeding by an HIV-positive mother appears to greatly outweigh the comparable number associated with breast-feeding, especially in settings with high baseline levels of infant mortality (Kennedy *et al.* 1990). Breast milk is important in preventing intercurrent infections which could accelerate progression of HIV-related disease in already infected infants, and could delay progression of disease in HIV-infected children (Ryder *et al.* 1991; Tozzi *et al.* 1990).

In the light of all information available, WHO has again reiterated the importance of continued breast-feeding (World Health Organization 1987).

Identification of HIV infection after birth

Where there is a universal programme of antenatal screening, most children born to HIV-infected mothers will be identified at birth. However, in low prevalence areas or where HIV testing in pregnancy is not routine, the majority of women with asymptomatic HIV infection will not be identified; some women will be unaware that they are at risk and others will not wish to disclose this information. In this situation, HIV infection may not be diagnosed until the child presents with HIV-related manifestations.

This may have two consequences: one, that because of the lack of a specific syndrome, HIV is not considered in the differential diagnosis, which can lead to unnecessary investigations, multiple referrals, and considerable delay in initiating appropriate treatment. Second, is that when the child presents with symptoms, the diagnosis of HIV infection may be the first recognition of infection in the family. This could have serious consequences for inter-family relationships and decisions that have to be made regarding testing of other family members. This highlights the absolute necessity of counselling before a child is tested, and family support throughout.

Mortality from HIV infection

Maternal mortality

Adult AIDS cases and deaths could equal or exceed the expected number of deaths from all other causes in the most severely affected sub-Saharan African cities by the early 1990s (Chin 1990). Consequently, several million uninfected children born to infected parents will be orphaned, and the breakdown of families and social structure will result in an increased mortality risk for this group. In most central African cities and in some inner-city areas in the developed world, such as New York City, AIDS has become the leading cause of death for women aged 20–40, and there has been a parallel rise in infant and child mortality (Chu *et al.* 1990). If current mortality trends continue, HIV/AIDS can be expected to become one of the five leading causes of death in the USA, in women of reproductive age, by 1991. HIV-related deaths accounted for 11 per cent of deaths in black women aged 25–34 and three per cent of all such deaths in white women in the USA in 1988 (Chu *et al.* 1990; Centers for Disease Control 1990).

Increasing HIV-related adult mortality is creating a large and growing number of children under the age of 15 whose mothers have died of HIV. It is predicted that during the 1990s, between 1.5 and 2.9 million women of reproductive age in sub-Saharan Africa will die as a result of HIV infection, resulting in between 3.1 and 5.5 million AIDS orphans. This means that between six and 11 per cent of the population under age 15 will be orphaned (Preble 1990). Hunter (1990) reports that estimates from a study in four Ugandan districts indicate that the total number of orphans ranges between 620 000 and 1 200 000. Although extended family networks are absorbing these children according to traditional rules, they may be vulnerable to increased mortality due to economic and health stresses on their caretakers, many of whom are elderly persons.

Child mortality

The recent progress made in ensuring child survival through the expanded programme of immunization and the oral rehydration programme are already being negated in regions with a high prevalence of HIV-1 infection (Valleroy et al. 1990). Based on 1987 maternal seroprevalence data, Valleroy and colleagues (1990) have estimated that in Kampala, Uganda, by 1992 between one-tenth and one-third of all under-five mortality will be attributable to HIV-1 infection.

Quinn et al. (1990), reporting on work undertaken by Boulos et al., state that HIV infection would result in a proportional increase in the child mortality rate of 5–10 per cent (assuming 80 per cent mortality for HIV-infected children in the first five years of life, a seroprevalence rate among pregnant women of 0.5 per cent, and a vertical transmission rate of 33 per cent). An increase in seroprevalence to one per cent would result in an increase in child mortality by 15–20 per cent.

Preble (1990) estimates that in 10 African countries studied, HIV in children under five will cause between a quarter and half a million child deaths annually by the year 2000. The enormous stress that HIV-related child morbidity and mortality put on already overstretched health systems will make it increasingly difficult for health ministries to provide wide-reaching preventive and curative health care to children. There is evidence that the morbidity and mortality of young African orphans are higher than among African infants and children who are in the care of their natural mother, especially if they are orphaned before they are weaned.

In addition to mortality directly due to HIV infection, excess mortality will occur in all children born to HIV-infected mothers. The European Collaborative Study (1991) highlights the high mortality in a group of children born to HIV-positive mothers, irrespective of HIV infection in the child. Several African studies (Lepage et al. 1991) report lower birth-weights among the children born to HIV-positive mothers compared with children born to HIV-negative controls. Lower birth-weight carries with it an increased risk of mortality. Indeed, children born to intravenous-drug using mothers in Europe have been shown to have lower birth-weight, to be at increased risk of sudden infant death, and to have higher infant mortality (Deren 1986).

Infection acquired after birth

Haemophilia

For HIV-infected children and adolescents with haemophilia, the problems are augmented by the fact that they already have a serious chronic disorder, and, because of the sex-linked inheritance of their disorder, other male members of the family may have haemophilia too.

For many haemophiliacs HIV infection forces dependence on others at precisely that time of life normally associated with increasing independence. All infected adolescents need time to express their views and concerns in private, and they need regular informal appointments for both counselling and physical examination. The normal vulnerability of adolescent boys and girls can be made intolerable by the difficulties imposed by HIV infection on the establishment of normal relationships (Jones 1990). Society is well aware of the link between haemophilia and HIV infection and this has posed problems for children at school, where children with haemophilia may be perceived to be infected, even if they are not.

AIDS incubation time may differ in different exposure groups, probably because of different exposures to potential opportunistic pathogens. Among those with haemophilia, children developed AIDS more slowly than adults; and haemophiliac adults developed AIDS more slowly than homosexual men (Biggar 1990). Haemophiliac children are less likely to develop LIP than vertically infected children, although the case fatality rate is equally high in both groups (Jason *et al.* 1988). Most HIV-infected haemophiliacs developing AIDS will present with PCP. Oral candida, herpes simplex and herpes zoster are earlier manifestations. HIV infection seems to have little effect on the growth of asymptomatic, haemophilic children (Jones 1990).

Acquisition from blood transfusion

A Swedish study (Blaxhult *et al.* 1990) showed that age at transfusion significantly influenced latency period from infection with HIV to development of AIDS, but this was not influenced by the sex of the recipient or health at the time of transfusion. Overall, the younger the age the longer the period of latency. However, rapid onset of HIV-related illness has been reported in infants infected by transfusion at birth (Saulsbury *et al.* 1987), with clinical illness in one child as early as four months (Krasinski *et al.* 1989). Donegan *et al.* (1990) reported a 90 per cent seroconversion rate after transfusion with contaminated blood with a progression rate to AIDS of 13 per cent by three years, similar to that described by others.

Adolescence

Adolescence is a time of experimentation, a time of change, a time of vulnerability, in which behaviour patterns are being established. Adolescents are a group at increased risk of HIV infection, through sexual exposure or through intravenous drug use. There has been an increase in adolescent sexual activity over the last two to three decades with both a declining age at first intercourse and increasing number of partners over time (Gayle and D'Angelo 1991). The impact of the increasing proportion of adolescents who have had intercourse is heightened by the relatively few who consistently use contraceptive methods that could also prevent HIV infection and other sexually transmitted diseases. Other features of adolescent sexual behaviour may influence the risk of HIV transmission in this population: receptive anal intercourse may be more common since homosexual adolescent males who have intercourse tend to have older male partners. Curtis *et al.* (1989) found that although sexual intercourse was common among adolescents, they apparently refused to acknowledge their personal risk of HIV infection. Hein in the USA (1989) reported a male:female ratio among adolescents with AIDS closer to equality than among adults, implying that heterosexual transmission was the major route of infection. Burke *et al.* (1990) also reported an approximately equal seroprevalence of HIV infection among male and female applicants for US military service aged less than 20 years.

The poverty, violence, and culture of inner cities resulting from social deprivation may make adolescents turn to drugs, although the extent of this is unknown. Crack (a form of cocaine) use by itself has not been directly linked to the spread of HIV, but prostitution and the increased high-risk sexual behaviour that often accompanies crack use has been associated with an increase in sexually transmitted diseases rates and will undoubtedly have a similar effect on HIV transmission (Fullilove *et al.* 1990). Studies of drug-using adolescents in the US revealed that AIDS prevention messages have been heard but not heeded. Sexual encounters are approached with high AIDS awareness but low HIV protection (Helquist 1990). Additionally, injectable forms of cocaine and heroin may accompany crack use and increase the risk of HIV transmission (Chaisson *et al.* 1989).

In Brazil, and undoubtedly inner city areas of other countries, HIV infection has become a problem among street children who, living below subsistence level, prostitute themselves and may get involved in drug-trafficking. An anonymous seroprevalence study of homeless 13 to 18-year-olds in New York City showed rates of HIV positivity of seven per cent in males and 5.5 per cent in females. It strongly suggests that heterosexual transmission of the virus is spreading rapidly (Rogers 1989; Stoneburner *et al.* 1990). Wang *et al.* (1991) reported the increased risk of hepatitis B and HIV infection in street youths in Canada, and showed that adolescents who live on the street are at increased risk, in this case due to their sexual behaviour involving multiple partners and anal intercourse.

Family/social issues

There is clear evidence from prevalence studies that HIV infection, although occurring in all populations, is particularly prevalent among minority groups. As far as women and children are concerned, HIV infection is very much associated with poverty and social disadvantage. The problem is confounded by lack of access to medical care and support. The rise of tuberculosis and syphilis in

New York supports this (Centers for Disease Control 1989). Most HIV-positive women in Edinburgh, for example, have been infected by intravenous drug use and come from areas of the city with problems of multiple deprivation (Brettle *et al.* 1987).

The problems for children born to HIV-infected mothers in these circumstances do not solely relate to their HIV infection. Exposure to other infections such as tuberculosis, cytomegalovirus, and gastroenteritis in an HIV-infected child may alter the progression to disease.

HIV infection in a child must be considered as part of a family problem, since other family members may also become infected; the whole family will need support and guidance. Many of these families experience alienation by their neighbours, friends, relatives, by schools, and, indeed, medical professionals. For these reasons, confidentiality must be respected and limited to a 'need to know' policy. There is no justification for staff to insist on knowing of specific children with HIV infection. The only reason that the head of a school or centre should know of a child's HIV status is in order to avoid the spread of common childhood infections to an HIV-positive child.

In addition to the clinical management, there is a need for social support and advice, such as guidance to entitlements, or the possibility of respite care. Many hospital-based clinics have set up home-support teams, interdisciplinary groups which permit discussion and feedback and also provide an opportunity to inform, educate, and modify entrenched and often hardened attitudes to marginalized groups. A pivotal role for the team is in liaising with the voluntary sector, which can provide residential care, volunteer support, and hardship awards.

When children from a background of social deprivation, in areas where HIV infection is prevalent, are taken into care, issues relating to testing for HIV are raised. The need to clarify risk to improve the possibility of an adoptive or foster-care placement should be tempered by an understanding of the complexity and limitations of HIV antibody testing in identifying the HIV status of the very young child, and awareness of the ethical issues posed by the fact that a positive result on an HIV antibody test of the infant identifies the biological mother as having HIV infection. The widespread testing of all infants and children awaiting adoption or foster placement is not warranted, given the variability of prevalence of HIV infection in childbearing women; each case should be considered on its own merit and the likelihood of infection assessed.

HIV-infected children should be allowed to attend normal schools when their health permits. No case of HIV infection has been transmitted in the school setting (Rogers *et al.* 1990). The HIV-infected child should be allowed to lead a normal life, and not treated differently from others. Parents of HIV-infected children should be aware of the potential for social isolation should the child's condition become known to others in the care or educational setting. School, day-care, and social service personnel and others involved in education and caring for these children should be sensitive to the need for confidentiality and the right to privacy in these cases.

Conclusion

Not only is management of the infected child and the family of primary importance, but emphasis should be given to primary prevention of HIV infection. This is no easy task, and will involve changing people's sexual behaviour through education and the availability of condoms; and acceptance that there is a problem of intravenous drug use and trying to limit spread through this route by all possible approaches (Hartgers 1990). Clean blood and adequate infection control (Department of Health 1990) remains of paramount importance.

Beyond the year 2000, the eventual level of HIV/AIDS in any specific population or country will be a measure of both the commitment and the effectiveness of AIDS prevention programmes in the 1990s (Chin and Mann 1990).

References

Ades, A.E., Parker, S., Berry, T., Holland, F.J., Davison, C.F., Cubitt, D., *et al.* (1991). Prevalence of maternal HIV-1 infection in Thames regions: results from anonymous unlinked neonatal testing . *Lancet*, **337**, 1562–4.

Andiman, W., Joyce Simpson, B., Olson, B., Denver L., Silva, T., Miller, G. (1990). Rate of transmission of human immunodeficiency virus type 1 infection from mother to child and short-term outcome of neonatal infection. *American Journal of Diseases in Children*, **144**, 755–66.

Barbacci, M., Repke, F.T., and Chaisson, R.E. (1991). Routine prenatal screening for HIV infection. *Lancet*, **337**, 709–11.

Berkley, S., Naamara, W., Okware, S., Downing, R., Konde-Lule, J., Wawer, M., *et al.* (1990). AIDS and HIV infection in Uganda—are more women infected than men? *AIDS*, **4**, 1237–42.

Biggar, R.J. (1990). International registry of seroconverters. AIDS incubation in 1891 HIV seroconverters from different exposure groups. *AIDS*, **4**, 1059–66.

Blanche, S., Rouzioux, C., Guihard Moscato, M.-L., Veber, F., Mayaux, M.-J., and Jacomet, C. (1989). A prospective study of infants born to women seropositive for human immunodeficiency virus type 1. *New England Journal of Medicine*, **320**, 1643–8.

Blanche, S., Tardieu, M., Duliege, A., Rouzioux, C., Le Deist, F., Fukunaga, K., *et al.* (1990). Longitudinal study of 94 symptomatic infants with perinatally acquired human immunodeficiency virus infection. *American Journal of Diseases in Children*, **144**, 1210–5.

Blaxhult, A., Granath, F., Lidman, K., and Giesecke, J. (1990). The influence of age on the latency period to AIDS in people infected by HIV through blood transfusion. *AIDS*, **4**, 125–9.

Braddick, M.R., Kreiss, J.K., Embree, J.E., Datta, P., Ndinya-Achola, J.O., Pamba, H., *et al.* (1990). Impact of maternal HIV infection on obstetrical and early neonatal outcome. *AIDS*, **4**, 1001–5.

Brettle, R., Bisset, K., Burns, S., Davidson, J., Davidson, S., Gray, J., *et al* (1987). Human immunodeficiency virus and drug misuse; the Edinburgh experience. *British Medical Journal*, **295**, 421–4.

Burke, D.S., Brundage, J.F., Goldenbaum, M., Gardner, L. I., Peterson, M., Visintine, R., and Redfield, R.R. (Walter Reed retrovirus research group) (1990). Human immunodeficiency virus infections in teenagers: seroprevalence among applicants for US military service. *Journal of the American Medical Association*, **263**, 2074–7.

Centers for Disease Control (1988). Update: universal precautions for prevention of transmission of human immunodeficiency virus, hepatitis B virus, and other bloodborne pathogens in health-care settings. *Morbidity and Mortality Weekly Report*, **37**, 377–88.

Centers for Disease Control (1989). Congenital syphilis—New York City, 1986–1988. (Editorial.) *Morbidity and Mortality Weekly Report*, **38**, 825–9.

Centers for Disease Control (1990). AIDS in women—United States. (Editorial.) *Morbidy and Mortality Weekly Report*, **39**, 845–6.

Centers for Disease Control (1991*a*). Table 3. United States AIDS cases by age group, exposure category, and race/ethnicity reported to the Centers for the Centers for Disease Control through December 1990. *AIDS*, **5**, 352.

Centers for Disease Control (1991*b*). Guidelines for prophylaxis against *Pneumocystis carinii* pneumonia for children infected with human immunodeficiency virus. *Journal of the American Medical Association*, **265**, 1637–44.

Chaisson, R.E., Bacchetti, P., Osmond, D., Brodie, B., Sande, M.A., and Moss, A.R. (1989). Cocaine use and HIV infection in intravenous drug users in San Francisco. *Journal of the American Medical Association*, **261**, 561–5.

Chin, J. (1990). Epidemiology. Current and future dimensions of the HIV/AIDS pandemic in women and children. *Lancet*, **336**, 221–4.

Chin, J. and Mann, J.M. (1990). HIV infections and AIDS in the 1990s. *Annual Review of Public Health*, **11**, 127–42.

Chu, S.Y., Buehler, J.W., and Berkelman, R.L. (1990). Impact of the human immuodeficiency virus epidemic on mortality in women of reproductive age, United States. *Journal of the American Medical Association*, **264**, 225–9.

Connor, E., Bagarazzi, M., McSherry, G., Holland, B., Boland, M., Denny, T., *et al.* (1991). Clinical and laboratory correlates of *Pneumocystis carinii* pnuemonia in children infected with HIV. *Journal of the American Medical Association*, **265**, 1693–7.

Curtis, H., Lawrence, C., and Tripp, J. (1989). Teenage sexuality: implications for controlling AIDS. *Archives of Disease in Childhood*, **64**, 1240–5.

Department of Health (1990). *Guidance for clinical health care workers: protection against infection with HIV and hepatitis viruses*. HMSO, London.

Deren, S. (1986). Children of substance abusers: a review of the literature. *Journal of Substance Abuse Treatment*, **3**, 77–94.

De Rossi, A., Ades, A.E., Mammano, F., Del Mistro, A., Amadori, A., Giaquinto, C., *et al.* (1991). Antigen detection, virus culture, polymerase chain reaction, and *in vitro* antibody production in the diagnosis of vertically transmitted HIV-1 infection. *AIDS*, **5**, 15–20.

Donegan E., Stuart, M., Niland, J.C., Sacks, H.S., Azen, S.P., Dietrick, S.L., *et al.* (1990). Infection with human immunodeficiency virus type 1 (HIV-1) among recipients of antibody-positive blood donations. *Annals of Internal Medicine*, **113**, 733–9.

Dunn, D., Newell, M., Ades, A., and Peckham, C. (1992). Risk of HIV-1 transmission through breast feeding. *Lancet*, **340**, 585–8.

European Centre for the Epidemiological Monitoring of AIDS (1990). *AIDS surveillance in Europe* (Quarterly Report No. 28). ECEMA, Paris.

European Collaborative Study (1988). Mother-to-child transmission of HIV infection. *Lancet*, **ii**, 1039–42.
European Collaborative Study (1991). Children born to women with HIV-1 infection: natural history and risk of transmission. *Lancet*, **i**, 253–60.
Fullilove, R.E., Fullilove, M.T., Bowser, B.P., and Gross, S.A. (1990). Risk of sexually transmitted disease among black adolescent crack users in Oackland and San Francisco, California. *Journal of the American Medical Association*, **263**, 851–5.
Gabiano, C., Tovo, P., de Martino, M., Galli, L., Giaquinto, C., Loy, A. et al. (1992). Mother-to-child transmission of HIV-1: risk of infection and contacts of transmission. *Pediatics*, **90**, 369–74.
Gayle, H.D. and D'Angelo, L.J. (1991). Epidemiology of acquired immunodeficiency syndrome and human immunodeficiency virus infection in adolescents. *Paediatric Infectious Disease Journal*, **10**, 322–8.
Gill, O.N., Adler, M.W., and Day, N.E. (1989). Monitoring the prevalence of HIV. *British Medical Journal*, **299**, 1295–8.
Goedert, J.J., Kessler, C.M., Aledort, L.M., Biggar, R.J., Andes, W.A., White, G.C., et al. (1989). A prospective study of human immunodeficiency virus type 1 infection and the development of AIDS in subjects with haemophilia. *New England Journal of Medicine*, **321** (No. 17), 1141–8.
Greenberg, A.E., Nguyen-Dinh, P., Mann, J.M., Kabote, N., Colebunders, R.L., Francis, H., et al. (1988). The association between malaria, blood transfusions, and HIV seropositivity in a paediatric population in Kinshasa, Zaire. *Journal of the American Medical Association*, **259**, 545–9.
Gwinn, M., Pappaioanou, M., George, J.R., Hannon, H., Wasser, S.C., Redus, M.A., et al. (1991). Prevalence of HIV infection in childbearing women in the United States. *Journal of the American Medical Association*, **265**, 1704–8.
Halsey, N.A., Boulos, R., Holt, E., Ruff, A., Brutus, J.–R., Kissinger, P., Quinn, T.C., Coberly, J.S., Adrien, M., and Boulos, C. (CDS/JHU AIDS project team) (1991). Transmission of HIV-1 infections from mothers to infants in Haiti. *Journal of the American Medical Association*, **264**, 2088–92.
Hankins, C.A., Laberge, C., Lapointe, N., Lai Tung, M.T., Racine, L., and O'Shaughnessy, M. (1990). HIV infection among Quebec women giving birth to live infants. *Canadian Medical Association Journal*, **143**, 885–93.
Hartgers, C. (1990). Drug user interventions. *AIDS Care*, **2**, 399–402.
Hein, K. (1989). Commentary on adolescent acquired immunodeficiency syndrome: the next wave of the human immunodeficiency virus epidemic. *Journal of Paediatrics*, **114**, 144–9.
Helquist, M.J. (1990). Public policy issues. *AIDS*, **4**, S35–7.
Henderson, D.K., Fahey, B.J., Willy, M., Schmitt, J.M., Carey, K., Koziol., D.E., et al. (1990). Risk for occupational transmission of human immunodeficiency virus type 1 (HIV-1) associated with clinical exposures. *Annals of Internal Medicine*, **113**, 740–6.
Hir, S., Kamanga, J., Bhat, G., Mwale, C., Tembo, G., Luo, N. et al. (1989). Perinatal transmission of HIV-1 in Zambia. *British Medical Journal*, **299**, 1250–2.
Hoff, R., Berardi, V.P., Weiblen, B.J., Mahoney-Trout, L., Mitchell, M.L., and Grady, G.F. (1988). Seroprevalence of human immunodeficiency virus among childbearing women. *New England Journal of Medicine*, **318**, 525–30.
Howie, P.W., Forsyth, J.S., Ogston, S.A., Clark, A., and du V Florey, C. (1990). Protective effect of breast feeding against infection. *British Medical Journal*, **300**, 11–16.

Hrdy, D.B. (1987). Cultural practices contributing to the transmission of human immunodeficiency virus in Africa. *Reviews of Infectious Diseases*, **9**, 1109–19.

Hunter, S.S. (1990). Orphans as a window on the AIDS epidemic in sub-Saharan Africa: Initial results and implications of a study in Uganda. *Social Science and Medicine*, **31**, 681–90.

Ippolito, G., Stegagno, M., Angeloni, P., and Guzzanti, E. (1990). Anonymous HIV testing on newborns (letter to editor). *Journal of the American Medical Association*, **263**, 36.

Jason, J.M., Stehr-Green, J., Holman, R.C., and Evatt, B.L. (Haemophilia–AIDS collaborative study group) (1988). Human imunodeficiency virus infection in haemophilic children. *Journal of Paediatrics*, **82**, 565–70.

Johnstone, F.D., Maccallum, L., Brettle, R., Inglis, J.M., and Peutherer, J.F. (1988). Does infection with HIV affect the outcome of pregnancy? *British Medical Journal*, **296**, 467.

Jones, P. (1990). HIV infection and haemophilia. *Archives of Disease in Childhood*, **65**, 364–8.

Kennedy, K.I., Fortney, J.A., Bonhomme, M.G., Potts, M., Lamptey, P., and Carswell, W. (1990). Do the benefits of breastfeeding outweigh the risk of postnatal transmission of HIV via breastmilk? *Tropical Doctor*, **20**, 25–9.

Kovacs, A., Frederick, T., Church, J., Eller, A., Oxtoby, M., and Mascola, L. (1991). CD4 T-Lymphocyte counts and Pneumocystis carinii pneumonia in paediatric HIV infection. *Journal of the American Medical Association*, **265**, 1698–703.

Krasinski, K., Borkowsky, W., and Holzman, R.S. (1989). Prognosis of human immunodeficiency virus infection in children and adolescents. *Paediatric Infectious Disease Journal*, **8**, 216–20.

Lallemant-Le Coeur, S., Lallemant, M., Cheynier, D., Nzingoula, S., Drucker, J., and Larouze, B. (1991). Bacillus Calmette–Guérin immunization in infants born to HIV-1-seropositive mothers. *AIDS*, **5**, 195-9.

Lepage, P., Dabis, F., Hitimana, D., Msellati, P., Van Goethem, C., Steven, A., *et al.* (1991). Perinatal transmission of HIV-1: lack of impact of maternal HIV infection on characteristics of livebirths and on neonatal mortality in Kigali, Rwanda. *AIDS*, **5**, 295–300.

Lindgren, S., Anzen, B., Bohlin, A. Lidman, K. (1991).HIV and child-bearing: Clinical outcome and aspects of mother-to-infant transmission. *AIDS*, **5**, 1111–16.

Mclaws, M., Brown, A. R. D., Cunningham, P. H., Imrie, A. A., Wilcken, B. and Cooper, D.A. (1990). Prevalence of maternal HIV infection based on anonymous testing of neonates, Sydney 1989. *Medical Journal of Australia*, **153**, 383–6.

Miotti, P.G., Dallabetta, G., Ndovi, E., Liomba, G., Saah, A.J., and Chiphangwi, J. (1990). HIV-1 and pregnant women: associated factors, prevalence, estimate of incidence and role of fetal wastage in central Africa. *AIDS*, **4**, 733–6.

Newell, M., and Peckham, C.S. (1993). Risk factors for vertical transmission of HIV-1 and early markers of HIV-1 infection in children. *AIDS*, **7**, S591–7.

Newell, M., Peckham, C.S., and Lepage, P. (1990). HIV-1 infection in pregnancy: implications for women and children. *AIDS*, **4**, S111–17.

Novick, L.F., Berns, D., Stricof, R., Stevens, R., Pass, K., and Wethers, J. (1989). HIV seroprevalence in newborns in New York State. *Journal of the American Medical Association*, **261**, 1745–50.

N'Tita, I., Mulanga, K., Dulat, C., Lusamba, D., Rehle, T., Korte, R., *et al.* (1991). Risk of transfusion-associated HIV transmission in Kinshasa, Zaire. *AIDS*, **5**, 437–9.

Oxtoby, M.J. (1988). Human immunodeficiency virus and other viruses in human milk, placing the issues in broader perspective. *Paediatric Infectious Disease Journal*, **7**, 825–35.

Pabst, H.F. and Spady, D.W. (1990). Effect of breast-feeding on antibody response to conjugate vaccine. *Lancet*, **ii**, 269–70.

Pizzo, P.A. and Wilfert, C.M. (1990). Treatment considerations for children with human immunodeficiency virus infection. *Paediatric Infectious Disease Journal*, **9**, 690–9.

Preble, E.A. (1990). Impact of HIV/AIDS on African children. *Socal Science and Medicine*, **31**, 671–80.

Quinn, T.C., Zacarias, F. R. K., and St. John, R.K. (1989). AIDS in the Americas: an emerging public health crisis (letter). *New England Journal of Medicine*, **320**, 1005–7.

Quinn, T.C., Narain, J.P., and Zacarias, F. R. K. (1990). AIDS in the Americas: a public health priority for the region. *AIDS*, **4**, 709–24.

Rogers, D.E. (1989). Federal spending on AIDS—how much is enough? (letter). *New England Journal of Medicine*, **320**, 1623–4.

Rogers, M.F., White, C.R., Sanders, R., Schable, C., Ksell, T.E., Wasserman, R.L., *et al.* (1990). Lack of transmission of human immunodeficiency virus from infected children to their household contacts. *Journal of Paediatrics*, **85**, 210–14.

Royal College of Obstetricians and Gynaecologists (RCOG) (1990). *HIV infection in maternity care and gynaecology*. (Revised Report of the RCOG Sub-Committee on Problems associated with AIDS in Relation to Obstetrics and Gynaecology.) RCOG, London.

Ryder, R.W., Nsa, W., Hassig, S.E., Behets, F., Rayfield, M., Ekungola, B., *et al.* (1989). Perinatal transmission of the human immunodeficiency virus type 1 to infants of seropositive women in Zaire. *New England Journal of Medicine*, **320**, 1637–42.

Ryder, R.W., Manzila, T., Baende, E., Kabagabo, U., Behets, F., Batter, V., *et al.* (1991). Evidence from Zaire that breast-feeding by HIV-1-seropositive mothers is not a major route for perinatal HIV-1 transmission but does decrease morbidity. *AIDS*, **5**, 709–14.

Saulsbury, F.T., Raldolph, F., Wykoff, M. P. H., and Boyle, R.J. (1987). Transfusion-acquired human immunodeficiency virus infection in twelve neonates: epidemiologic, clinical and immunologic features. *Paediatric Infectious Disease Journal*, **6**, 544–8.

Schechter, M.T., Craib, K. J. P., Le, T.N., Willoughby, B., Douglas, B. *et al.* (1989). Progression to AIDS and predictors of AIDS in seroprevalent and seroincident cohorts of homosexual men. *AIDS*, **3** (No. 6), 347–54.

Schoenbaum, E.E., Davenny, K., and Selwyn, P.A. (1988). The impact of pregnancy on HIV-related disease. In *AIDS and obstetrics and gynaecology* (ed. C.N. Hudson and F. Sharp), pp. 65–75. Royal College of Obstetricians and Gynaecologists, London.

Scott, G.B., Hutto, C., Makuch, R.W., Mastrucci, M.T., O'Connor, T., Mitchell, C.D. *et al.* (1989). Survival in children with perinatal acquired human immunodeficiency virus type 1 infection. *New England Journal of Medicine*, **321**, 1791–6.

Selwyn, P.A., Schoenbaum, E.E., Davenny, K., Robertson, V.J., Feingold, A.R., Shulman, J.F. *et al.* (1989). Prospective study of human immunodeficiency virus infection and pregnancy outcomes in intravenous drug users. *Journal of the American Medical Association*, **261**, 1289–94.

Shaffer, N., Hedberg, K., Davachi, F., Lyamba, B., Breman, J.G., Masisa, O.S., *et al.* (1990). Trends and risk factors for HIV-1 seropositivity among outpatient children, Kinshasa, Zaire. *AIDS*, **4**, 1231–6.

Sherr, L. and Hedge, B. (1990). The impact and use of written leaflets as a counselling alternative in mass antenatal HIV screening. *AIDS Care*, **2**, 235–45.
Stoneburner, R.L., Chiasson, M.A., Weisfuse, I.B., and Thomas, P.A. (1990). The epidemic of AIDS and HIV-1 infection among heterosexuals in New York City. (Editorial Review). *AIDS*, **4**, 99–106.
Tappin, D.M., Girdwood, R. W. A., Follett, E. A. C., Kennedy, R., Brown, A.J., and Cockburn, F. (1991). Prevalence of maternal HIV infection in Scotland based on unlinked anonymous testing of newborn babies. *Lancet*, **337**, 1565–7.
Temmerman, M., Moses, S., Kiragu, D., Fusallah, S., Wamola, I.A., and Piot, P. (1990*a*). Impact of single session post-partum counselling of HIV infected women on their subsequent reproductive behaviour. *AIDS Care*, **3**, 247–52.
Temmerman, M., Plummer, F.A., Mirza, N.B., Ndinya-Achola, J.O., Wamola, I.A., Nagelkerke, N., *et al.* (1990*b*). Infection with HIV as a risk factor for adverse obstetrical outcome. *AIDS*, **4**, 1087–93.
Tozzi, A.E., Pezzotti, P., and Greco, D. (1990). Does breast-feeding delay progression to AIDS in HIV-infected children? (letter). *AIDS*, **4**, 1293–4.
Tudor-Williams, G. (1991). Early diagnosis of vertically acquired HIV-1 infection. *AIDS*, **5**, 103–5.
Valleroy, L.A., Harris, J.R., and Way, P.O. (1990). The impact of HIV-1 infection on child survival in the developing world. *AIDS*, **4**, 667–72.
van de Perre, P., Simonon, A., Msellati, P., Hitamana, D.G., van Goethem, C., A. Bazubagira, *et al.* (1990). Transmission postnatale du VIH-1 de la mere a l'enfant dans une cohorte de meres ayant seroconverti a Kigali (Rwanda). In Proc. *5th Int. Conf. on AIDS in Africa, Kinshasa, Zaire, October 1990*.
Wang, E.E., King, S., Goldberg, E., Bock, B., Milner, R., and Read, S. (1991). Hepatitis B and human immunodeficiency virus infection in street youths in Toronto, Canada. *Paediatric Infectious Disease Journal*, **10**, 130–3.
World Health Organization (1987). Breast-feeding/breast milk and human immunodeficiency virus (HIV). *Weekly Epidemiological Record*, **33**, 245–6.

Further reading

P.A. Pizzo and C.M. Wilfert (eds) (1990). *Paediatric AIDS: the challenge of HIV infection in infants, children and adolescents*. Williams and Wilkins, Baltimore, USA.
AIDS 1990: a year in review. Current Science, London.

PART IV

Children and the environment

This part considers two environmental issues related to child health: pollution and accidents. Accidents are the most important cause of mortality and morbidity in children over the age of one year in Europe; strategies for child accident prevention and the promotion of child protective environments are considered. Pollution and its effects are increasingly recognized as important in child health though the full extent of the effects of pollution are yet to emerge; the potential effects on children are comprehensively reviewed.

Chapter 11 ('Pollution and child health') was completed before the UN Conference on the Environment and Development, the so-called 'Earth Summit', was held in Rio de Janiero in June 1992. The themes and recommendations of the chapter are broadly in line with those of the Rio Declaration.

11 Pollution and child health
Sheena Nakou

The well-being of man is influenced by all environmental factors: the quality of the air, water and food; the winds and the topography of the land; and the general living habits.
Hippocrates, *Airs, waters and places*

As mankind enters the twenty first century, the precept of the Hippocratic writings that human well-being is influenced by environmental factors continues to be fundamental to our understanding of health, and particularly the health of children. Our medical predecessors of the Hippocratic school could not have foreseen the extent to which human 'living habits' have themselves influenced the environment. Many of the man-made environmental changes have resulted in improved health, well-being, and life expectancy of human populations. Improved housing, better hygiene and more efficient methods of food production have increased the likelihood of survival of children and achievement of their potential. The endeavours of mankind to improve living conditions have, however, also introduced new environmental health hazards, including pollution of the air, water, and soil by a wide variety of agents; chemical, physical, and biological. These agents may be directly harmful to human health or exert an indirect effect on the quality of life by upsetting the ecological balance of an area.

Chemical agents

It is estimated that in addition to the naturally occurring elements and compounds, the world's chemical industry has introduced more than five million compounds, many of which are potentially toxic. Toxic chemicals belong to a diverse range of substances—solids, liquids, gases, particles, and fibres, alone or in mixtures. Some are toxic in the elemental state, others only as compounds, inorganic or organic. Some are stable and accumulate in the environment, others are short-lived, decomposing or combining with other substances to produce new forms which may be less or more toxic.

The toxic properties of the heavy metals lead and mercury were recognized in ancient Greece and Rome from effects on metal workers and miners. Subsequently, many of the adverse health effects of other toxic chemicals were first demonstrated in the workplace, but chemical hazards are not confined to those who are occupationally exposed. Other sections of the population, including children, may be in contact with dangerous quantities of toxic substances released into the environment during the manufacture, transport, storage, use, and disposal of chemical products.

Physical agents

Human life evolved with natural exposure to ionizing radiation, ultraviolet rays, extremes of temperature, and noise. More than one-half of natural radioactivity comes from radon, a gaseous decay product of radium. Release of radon into the rooms of well-sealed buildings constitutes a hazard which could be considered natural but modified by man. Human activity has increased the radioactivity level overall by about one fifth, but local levels may exceed the acceptable range. New technology has also introduced new forms of non-ionizing radiation with unknown risks.

Chemicals released into the atmosphere, notably chlorofluorocarbons used as coolants and aerosol propellants, destroy the ozone in the upper layer of the earth's atmosphere, allowing greater penetration of the sun's ultraviolet rays. Increased ultraviolet exposure is associated with an increase in skin cancers and cataracts. Combustion of fossil fuels has resulted in an atmospheric build-up of carbon dioxide and other gases which allow sunlight to pass through, but trap the heat, causing global warming, (the greenhouse effect). Anthropogenic noise levels may be great enough to cause hearing loss, and the background noise in city streets and in the vicinity of heavy machinery may be a source of stress.

Biological agents

Contamination of water and food by viruses, bacteria, and parasites has always been a hazard of human settlements, and one of the major successes of national public health services is the establishment and maintenance of systems to ensure the provision of clean water and uncontaminated food. Persistent vigilance is essential as Europe still sees outbreaks of water-borne infections and foods are found to contain dangerous levels of pathogenic organisms. Contamination of drinking water is a special danger when mass population movements put a strain on sewage disposal and water supply systems, as when a region is subject to an influx of refugees or tourists.

Sewage effluent in lakes, rivers, and coastal waters, and organic refuse on beaches, can result in eutrophication, contamination of edible shellfish, and the direct threat of infection to bathers and participants in other aquatic recreational activities (Shuval 1986) many of whom are children. As family holidays and children's water sports become increasingly popular and more adventurous, the importance to child health of the quality of recreational waters is apparent.

Exposure to pollution

In the cities of Northern Europe, the cradle of the industrial revolution of the nineteenth century, several generations of children have already been conceived, born, and grown up in surroundings heavily polluted by a wide variety of chemicals emitted by the factories, foundries, and furnaces. Southern Europe became industrialized somewhat later, but in their haste to catch up, safety measures which were belatedly being brought into effect in the older established units were often bypassed. Vehicular and home-heating fuels added to the volume of air pollutants. Even the countries which did not build their own nuclear power plants came within the range of their neighbours'. The use of agricultural and household chemicals burgeoned in rural and urban areas alike. The volume of sewage emptied into Europe's lakes, rivers, and seas multiplied. Toxic waste was buried or dumped at sea.

Probably none of Europe's children are exposed to no form of pollution, and most are exposed to several forms, yet pollution is hardly touched upon in the training of paediatricians and child care personnel. The risk of exposure of children to pollutants is related to their stage of development as well as to the scale of pollution and the environmental levels reached, which are in turn dependent on the sources of the pollutants, their physical state, their stability in the environment, and the means of spread.

Scale of pollution

The scale of pollution can vary from being confined to a small localized area to being global in extent. Indoor pollution may affect one house only or even a single room and its source may be building materials, paints, heating or cooking fuels, household chemicals, cigarettes, or particulate matter transferred from the workplace on clothes or hair. Infants who spend a substantial part of their day inside the home are likely to be the most affected.

Point sources of specific pollutants may exert primarily a localized effect as exemplified by the distribution and uptake by children of lead in the vicinity of lead smelters (Benetou-Marantidou *et al.* 1988; Hatzakis *et al.* 1989). Even in such cases a certain amount of the pollutant may be dispersed more widely to contribute to the global pool (Ducoffre *et al.* 199). Similarly, water-borne pollutants such as methylmercury, although more concentrated close to the polluting source, may also accumulate in distant marine organisms (MAP 1987). Gaseous airborne pollutants from industrial sources (Suess *et al.* 1984) and vehicular exhaust (Kohler and Jackson 1987) may constitute a direct health hazard to populations at the point of emission but also become widely distributed in the atmosphere, with the potential to threaten the ecological balance through acid rain deposition and the greenhouse effect. Widespread dispersal occurs of radioactive material released into the atmosphere following accidents in nuclear power plants or atomic bomb explosions (WHO 1987a).

Level of pollution

Acute high-level exposure to toxic agents occurs in a variety of situations involving children. Exposure of parents at the workplace may influence conception or intrauterine development (Savitz et al. 1989). Industrial accidents may result in heavy pollution of the surrounding area, as occurred in Seveso, Italy in 1976 with dioxin; in Bhopal, India in 1984 with methyl isocyanate; and with the Chernobyl nuclear reactor core meltdown in 1986 with radioactive iodine, caesium, and other products. Ingestion of heavily contaminated food also constitutes acute high-level exposure. Examples are the consumption of bread made from wheat treated with an organic mercury fungicide in Iraq in 1971–72 (Weiss and Clarkson 1982), and rice-bran cooking oil contaminated with polychlorinated biphenyl in Taiwan and Japan (Cordero 1990). Immersion in water highly contaminated with untreated sewage is another such risk, which may occur during floods, boating accidents, or simply, unwise bathing.

Long-term, relatively high exposure may occur at the workplace, in the immediate vicinity of metal smelters and other point sources, from lead-based paint in old house, and in neighbourhoods built on toxic waste dumps, and it is important to identify such 'hot spots'. Long-term consumption of food with a high content of toxic chemicals may provide a very high intake. Fish which had ingested and concentrated methyl mercury from factory effluent in the Minamata and Niigata areas of Japan were consumed over the years by the fishermen and their families, a high proportion of whom developed neurological symptoms (Weiss and Clarkson 1982). Again in Japan, renal damage resulted from long-term consumption by populations of rice irrigated with factory effluent with a high cadmium content. Japan offers extreme examples, but in Europe there have been incidents of lead poisoning from food and drink prepared or stored in utensils containing lead, and babies have developed methaemoglobinaemia following consumption of well water with a high concentration of nitrites from fertilizers.

The most pervasive form of exposure is long-term contact with low levels of pollutants, and most children are in daily contact with multiple chemicals, biological agents, and physical hazards through air, soil, water, and food.

Sources, routes and pathways of environmental pollutants

Multiple factors affect the introduction and dispersal of pollutants in the environment and the extent of exposure of populations and individuals.

Air pollution

Since mankind started using fire for cooking and heating, combustion has been a major source of air pollutants, both indoor and out. Burning of wood, charcoal, and other biological products at the domestic level, followed later by coal, paraffin, and gas, filled countless generations of Europe's residences with smoke. Industrial processes requiring heat and energy, the development of electrical power, and the introduction of steam and petroleum-powered transport all combined to elevate combustion to the position of a public health concern. In spite of increased public awareness of the problem and the introduction of ever more stringent regulations, European cities are all subject to fluctuating levels of combustion-related fumes. The composition varies according to the source, the efficiency of combustion, and the prevailing climatic conditions, but there is generally a combination of vehicle exhaust and smoke from industrial power plants, domestic fires, and oil-fired central heating. These sources put out a mixture of carbon monoxide and dioxide, nitrogen and sulphur oxides, hydrocarbons (from unburned fuel, which in city driving may amount to 15 per cent), and particulates. The soot etc. may contain traces of toxic matter such as arsenic, from some types of coal, or lead, from petrol enriched with tetraethyl lead as an 'antiknocking' agent. In the southern cities, characterized by bright sunlight, the nitrogen oxides undergo photochemical conversion to ozone, which along with vaporized hydrocarbons, is the basis of photochemical smog, considered to be carcinogenic. The cities of northern and eastern Europe tend to have a higher output of sulphur dioxide from coal and diesel and fuel oils. The wetter climate predisposes to solution of sulphur and nitrogen oxides to form acid rain and fog.

Mining and smelting of metal ores have generated an increased load of atmospheric pollutants since the processes were discovered, but in the past two centuries in Europe, a wide variety of other industries have produced toxic chemicals or radioactive substances, either as end products or by-products, some of which escape into the air. Apart from metals such as lead, mercury, manganese, cadmium, nickel, and chromium, a variety of inorganic materials such as asbestos, and organics such as benzene, toluene (methylbenzene), styrene (phenylethene), polyvinyl chloride and tri- and tetrachloroethane may reach hazardous levels, and some, such as carbon disulphide and hydrogen sulphide, are foul smelling (Suess *et al.* 1984; WHO 1987*b*). Indoor air may become heavily polluted with cigarette smoke or fumes from cooking or heating fuels.

Some atmospheric pollutants break down rapidly, some filter upwards to the upper atmosphere to produce global effects, or are dispersed over a wide area by wind currents, and others are deposited on the surface of the earth. Surface pollutants may be redistributed as dust into the air under dry, windy conditions, or they may add to the soil or water load and enter the food chain. Leafy plants have the capacity to remove some gaseous and suspended pollutants from the air.

Soil pollution

Soil around smelters, power plants, and factories may become polluted by deposition of air-borne particulate matter. Irrigation of fields with polluted water or use of sludge from industrial or domestic waste may result in increases in toxic substances such as metals. Soil acidity may be changed by acid rain, causing the release of trace elements such as aluminium. Buried toxic waste may work its way to the surface soils. Indiscriminate and careless use of agricultural chemicals results in build-up of herbicides, insecticides, fungicides, and fertilizers in the soil and surface waters.

Soil pollutants constitute a direct hazard to children playing in fields and adjacent areas. Also, deposited in dust on fruit and foliage or absorbed into certain plants via the roots, they are consumed as part of the human food intake, either direct or after consumption by animals and transfer to meat, milk, and dairy products. 'Food chain' routes were publicized during the Chernobyl episode (WHO 1987a) but are followed by non-radioactive pollutants also.

Water pollution

The routes for pollution of drinking water parallel those of soil pollution. In addition, domestic sewage and industrial effluent may drain into lakes, rivers, and wells used as sources of drinking water, introducing chemicals but also microbial contamination. Enforcement of stringent control measures has ensured that such dangers occur less in Europe than in some other parts of the world, but they may be increasing due to competition for decreasing supplies of water between domestic needs and agricultural, industrial, and recreational demands. Natural disasters such as flood and earthquakes, and anthropogenic catastrophes such as the pollution of the Rhine following fire in a chemicals factory in 1987, put an increased strain on water facilities. Pollutants may also be introduced during the storage and distribution of water. Lead from water pipes has been shown to be dissolved in soft water and certain kinds of plastic and asbestos piping may be hazardous.

Discharge of untreated sewage and industrial effluent, dumping of ships' cargoes, and accumulation of miscellaneous solid refuse in seas, lakes, and rivers results in increased uptake of pollutants by aquatic organisms. This may have untoward effects on the organisms themselves, but also, when they are part of the food chain, constitutes a hazard for humans of, for example, increased mercury intake from fish consumption (MAP 1987) or infection by pathogenic microorganisms from shellfish (Shuval 1986; MAP 1991). It is becoming increasingly evident that bathing and other forms of recreational activity in polluted waters are associated with risk of infections.

Food

Pollutants may be incorporated in food from dust, soil, and water and concentrated at succeeding stages of the food chain. Pesticide residues may not have been eliminated before harvesting. Further substances may be introduced during storage, processing, or cooking, from utensils, additives, and careless handling. The food of nursing infants, i.e. breast-milk, may contain pollutants excreted from the mother's burden.

Miscellaneous sources

The utilization of manufactured products may be the most hazardous stage of the cycle, particularly for children. Building materials used in the home or schools have been incriminated in childhood pollution-related conditions, e.g. lead-based paints, formaldehyde, radon, and there is a possibility that asbestos and chromium-rich cement dust from buildings may be unsafe. Many household products are poisonous to children when ingested, and may not be innocuous at the levels of everyday use. Some toys have been found to contain toxic substances, usually pigments, as have cosmetics, which also may be allergens.

It must be remembered that small children normally exhibit behaviour which puts them in direct contact with their immediate physical environment to a greater degree than adults. Infants crawl around on the floor, they play in the dirt and sand and even eat it, they suck their dirty fingers and toes, and explore objects with their mouths. Older children play out of doors in dusty dirty surroundings and eat with unwashed hands. When they go bathing or boating, they often swallow large volumes of water. They do not read instruction labels on containers of potentially toxic products. When their parents are self-employed, children may also be exposed to workplace hazards. In short, children have easier access to pollution pathways than most adults.

Many forms of pollution are linked with social inequity. The poorer families live in the districts with higher pollution, near the factories, in ageing homes where dust control is more difficult. Parental workplace exposure is greater as the poorest paid jobs are often the dirtiest.

Absorption

Environmental pollutants, including microorganisms, may enter the body by inhalation, by ingestion, and, to a lesser extent, by percutaneous absorption. Some pollutants exert topical effects by direct contact with the skin or mucosal surfaces, without appreciable absorption. In the fetus the main portal of entry is the placenta.

Inhalation

The uptake of toxic gases, vapours, and particulate matter from inhaled air is determined by the rate and depth of ventilation and the concentration of the pollutant. The absorption of gases depends on the solubility and reactivity of the gas. Water-soluble gases, such as sulphur dioxide and formaldehyde, are absorbed in the nose and pharynx; less soluble gases, such as nitrogen dioxide and ozone, penetrate into the lower respiratory passages; and carbon monoxide is absorbed by haemoglobin into the bloodstream from the alveoli.

Inhaled particles larger than 10 μm in diameter are filtered out by the nose and nasopharynx and eliminated or swallowed along with the nasal secretions. Smaller particles are deposited in the trachea and the bronchi from where some are cleared to the pharynx by ciliary action. The smallest particles, 1–2 μm or less in diameter reach the alveoli, from where they may be transferred by direct permeation or by the alveolar macrophages into the blood or the pulmonary lymphatics.

Conditions which impair ciliary action result in less effective clearing of the lower respiratory tract. Exercise, which increases the rate and depth of respiration, results in greater intake of pollutants. Children have a higher respiratory rate and a greater volume of inspired air in proportion to their size than adults. In children who are mouth-breathers, the filter of the nasal passages is bypassed. Small children are less likely to eliminate nasal and tracheopharyngeal sputum, which is instead swallowed, adding to the ingested pollutant load.

Ingestion

In addition to the transfer to the stomach of some of the pollutants cleared from the respiratory tract, toxic substances are ingested in food and drink. Polluted dust and dirt may be carried to the mouth on dirty hands and other objects. This route is particularly apparent in smokers and in small children who suck their fingers, mouth a variety of objects which are dirty or have toxic contents, and may even eat dirt (pica). Ingestion also occurs during submersion in polluted water. The site, rate, and degree of absorption of pollutants from the digestive tract is dependent on their concentration, state, chemical or biological nature and solubility, and on the mode of handling by the enzyme systems. The nutritional status and the dietary constituents may enhance or impede intestinal absorption due to competition at transfer sites, alterations in intestinal motility, and other means. Thus, for example, children who are iron and calcium deficient tend to absorb a greater proportion of the lead they ingest.

Children have a proportionally higher food intake, weight for body weight, than adults. They also absorb a higher proportion of some ingested pollutants, for example absorption of ingested lead is about 10 per cent in adults and 30–40 per cent in young children.

Skin contact and percutaneous absorption

The intact skin constitutes an effective barrier against many environmental hazards. This cutaneous defence mechanisms, physical, chemical, and cellular, are not, however, completely impregnable to the passage of various forms of radiation and chemical and infective agents, and the injured skin is more easily penetrated. The skin itself is a target organ for many forms of pollutant. Small children, through their play habits, come into skin contact with polluted dust and soil and they tend to have proportionately greater expanses of skin exposed than adults.

Placental transport

The fetus is susceptible to intrauterine exposure and a variety of pollutants freely cross the placental barrier to enter the fetal circulation directly. Some, such as mercury, attain a higher level in the fetal than in the maternal circulation (Marsh *et al.* 1980) and others are partially blocked by the placenta. Some, such as cadmium, appear to be preferentially deposited in the placenta.

Fate of pollutants in the body and modes of action

Accounts of the pharmacodynamics and toxicology of specific chemical pollutants and the mechanism of action of radiation may be found in relevant textbooks. There is wide variety in the behaviour of pollutants in the body, in their circulation, their metabolism, their accumulation at different sites, their breakdown, and their elimination, and therefore in the intensity and duration of their effects. The concept of dose–response relations is complex even in the case of a drug administered in a planned dosage for therapeutic purposes. The complexity increases when the chemical, or combination of chemicals, is introduced inadvertently in an unknown dosage over an indefinite period of time.

The 'dose' may be taken in by one route only, as with methyl mercury from fish in the diet (Kjellstrom *et al.* 1986) or carbon monoxide in the lungs. In the case of atmospheric pollution with lead or other dust-borne pollutants, some may be inhaled by small children, but most will be ingested as dust and soil (Winnecke and Kramer 1984). The total dose from atmospheric radioactivity comprises external, from the air; internal from inhalation of the air; external from the soil; and internal from the ingestion of contaminated food. The relative contribution of the various routes varies with the duration of the polluting episode (WHO 1987a). The total body intake may be estimated, but the concentration of different pollutants at different sites will vary. Radioactive iodine, for example, accumulates in the thyroid gland; certain kinds of asbestos accumulate in the pleura.

The effective dose depends on the means and the rate of removal from the target sites and from the circulation in general, and in this respect the concept of 'half-life' is useful as a measure of the persistence of effect. Some of the toxic agents are bound or broken down and rendered inactive in the body. Detoxification takes place in the liver and immaturity or damage of the liver result in prolongation of toxic effects. Excretion may be effected via the kidneys, gut, or lungs, and, in nursing mothers, in the breast-milk. Some pollutants, especially metals, are deposited in the hair, nails, and teeth, from where they are eventually eliminated. Storage in the bones or body fat may result in re-entry of pollutants into the circulation. For most pollutants the effective dose at the target organ can only be inferred from other measurements, such as levels of the pollutant in the air or water, or in samples of blood, urine, hair, fingernails, or tooth enamel. Total body burden of some pollutants such as metals can be estimated by neutron-activation techniques.

The 'response' part of the dose–response relationship may be even more difficult to assess. The toxic agents may be metabolic poisons, enzyme inhibitors, or allergens, they may be cytotoxic or genotoxic or they may have one or more of these effects on one or more organs or types of tissues (Goldstein and Gochfeld 1990). The effects of a specific pollutant on an individual or a population are often delayed or modified. Some of the most representative examples of modifying factors are drawn from adult populations but the principles apply also in childhood.

Genetic predisposition puts some individuals at a higher risk of developing pollution-related malignancies (e.g. lung cancer from exposure to cigarette smoke) or allergic manifestations (e.g. chromium-induced dermatitis or asthma from environmental allergens). Certain Mediterranean populations are characterized by a high prevalence of glucose-6-phosphate dehydrogenase deficiency which results in haemolysis in some affected individuals who come into contact with naphthalene in the environment. The nutritional state affects not only the absorption but also the distribution and activity of toxic substances. In iodine-deficient individuals, radioactive iodine is more readily taken up into the thyroid gland. Calcium-deficient post-menopausal women are more susceptible to the osteomalacia induced by cadmium.

Concomitant exposures to more than one substance may result in an increase or a decrease of toxic effects. Smokers are much more likely than non-smokers to develop asbestos-related lung cancer, demonstrating a form of synergism, whereas selenium appears to exert a protective effect against mercury toxicity.

Sex-related differences exist in the manifestation of toxic effects. For example, evidence of impairment of haemoglobin synthesis by lead appears at lower levels of blood lead in females than in males.

Age differences in susceptibility are a function of the level of maturity of the target systems. High intake of methyl mercury by pregnant women may result in fetal neurological damage in the absence of detectable effects in the mother (Marsh et al. 1980) and intrauterine exposure to, among other agents, ionizing radiation, lead (Cordero 1990), and polychlorinated biphenyls (Jacobson et al. 1990) may be associated with impairment of brain development and intellectual deficit, at levels not apparently harmful in later development. Much has been written about 'threshold' levels of exposure to environmental agents, below which no untoward effects are detected, and which therefore may be considered 'safe' levels. Development of more sensitive testing invariably shows that there is probably no 'no effect' level for most pollutants.

Effects of environmental pollutants on target organs and systems

No tissue is exempt from possible effects of some kind of environmental agent, but tissues characterized by high rates of cellular turnover and metabolic activity are more susceptible to damage. Children have a greater risk of being affected, at the same tissue levels of exposure, than adults, for a variety of reasons. Firstly, the developing tissues and enzyme systems of the fetus and infant are more susceptible to impairment. Secondly there is a greater likelihood of children surviving the 20–30 years required for some of the delayed clinical effects to develop. In addition, mutagenic action on the gonads in previous generations is expressed as congenital abnormalities in the offspring.

A detailed catalogue of possible effects would not be appropriate here, but a few examples will illustrate the range of environmental hazards, some of which have multiple effects.

The nervous system

Many environmental chemical and physical agents cause neurological damage, centrally or peripherally, resulting in motor or sensory impairment, intellectual deficit, or behavioural problems. Notable examples are heavy metals such as lead and mercury, pesticides such as the organophosphates which inhibit acetylcholinesterase, and the carbamates, organic solvents, carbon monoxide, and radioactivity. Intrauterine exposure to certain agents such as mercury and ionizing radiation may result in mental retardation or spasticity.

The respiratory system

Inhaled pollutants may provoke immediate respiratory distress due to local irritation, as with tobacco and wood smoke, sulphur and nitrogen dioxides, ozone, and formaldehyde which may also produce irritation of the eyes. Some immediate effects may also be due to an allergic response and bronchoconstriction may be observed. Respiratory function has been found to be impaired in populations of children living in heavily polluted urban areas. Inhaled pollutants may predispose to respiratory infections in children, and ultimately, chronic obstructive lung disease. Long-term exposure to environmental cigarette smoke, photochemical oxidants, and other agents may be associated with subsequent development of lung cancer.

The urinary tract

Renal damage is a not uncommon side-effect of certain drugs and is also a known hazard of excessive work-place exposure to certain agents such as, for example, lead, cadmium, and volatile hydrocarbons, and bladder cancer has been caused by aniline dyes. Environmental levels of exposure would need to be high to cause appreciable damage.

The skin

The skin is susceptible to damage from all kinds of environmental agents and is particularly prone to radiation and ultraviolet and chemical burns. Cutaneous manifestations are multitudinous. They include local irritation, allergic and photosensitive reactions, and pigmentation disorders, and, in the long term malignant change.

The immune system

Some of the skin and respiratory effects are due to xenobiotic-mediated hypersensitivity reactions to pollutants. Other pollutants may produce a xenobiotic-mediated immunosuppression response which may also be associated with myelosuppression affecting red or white blood cells or both. The inhibition of immune function decreases resistance to infections and also appears to be one of the factors involved in carcinogenesis.

The reproductive system

Environmental exposures interfering with reproduction may go unnoticed because of the complexity of the reproductive process. It is likely that a variety of agents impair reproductive function in one or both partners by actions on enzymes or hormonal balance. Agents may impede conception or provoke damage or death of the germ cells or conceptus. Teratogenesis is a term which originally denoted abnormal morphogenesis, but it has been extended to encompass growth retardation, developmental disability, and impairment of cognitive ability and behaviour patterns. Periconceptual exposures of both parents constitute a hazard to conception, maintenance of pregnancy, and optimal development of the fetus. Hazards at some or all stages of the reproductive process include metals and organometallics, organochlorine pesticides, polyhalogenated biphenyls, anaesthetic gases, cigarette smoke, and ionizing radiation (Cordero 1990). The periconceptual stage is particularly dangerous because of workplace exposures.

Mutagenicity and carcinogenicity

Mutagenicity is the result of exposure to external agent(s) and endogenous factors. In the susceptible individual, exposure to radiation or certain viruses or chemicals causes DNA damage, which in the germ cell may result in transmission of congenital abnormalities in successive generations or non-survival. In the somatic cell, DNA damage is the first step towards tumour development which is further controlled by endogenous modifying factors such as oncogenes, tumour suppressor genes, the immune state, and enzyme systems. Children are exposed to combination of potential carcinogens throughout life and their effect is cumulative, contributing to the development of adult cancer. Some childhood cancers may be related to parental exposures and some childhood leukaemias may be the outcome of individual exposure to, for example, ionizing radiation in a genetically susceptible child.

Psychological effects

Apart from the adverse biological effects, known or suspected exposure to hazardous environmental agents is associated with varying degrees of stress and anxiety in segments of the population. Ecological disasters, such as nuclear accidents and oil spills, trigger a flood of rumours and misinformation which may culminate in mass panic. Children and adolescents, alarmed by observing the reactions of the adults, are especially likely to experience fear and feelings of insecurity and helplessness. Even in non-disaster periods, their heightened concern about ecological problems may result in intolerable levels of anxiety.

Assessments of health effects of pollutants

The health effects of exposure to low-level environmental pollutants may be difficult to detect, at both the individual and the population level, for a variety of reasons.

Firstly, the disease entity resulting from the exposure may be very common, or associated with other possible aetiological factors. One example is that of childhood respiratory infections which are so common that in the individual child the cause–effect interaction may not be clear, and only an epidemiological study can demonstrate that having parents who smoke, or living in a neighbourhood with air pollution, increases the incidence (Douglas and Waller 1966). The same applies to bathing in polluted coastal waters and gastrointestinal infections (Shuval 1986) and exposures which may increase the risk of pregnancy loss or the birth of low-weight infants (Savitz *et al.* 1989).

Second, the effects may be so subtle that they are not recognized in the individual but only identified in population studies, such as hearing deficits from arsenic (Bencko and Simon 1977) and intelligence deficits from mercury

(Kjellstrom et al. 1986) and lead (Hatzakis et al. 1989). 'Subclinical' exposure may be detected only on special testing.

Third, the adverse effects may be the outcome of a multifactorial process in which the exposure to an environmental pollutant is only one of the factors. In this case the effects are seen in only a few of the exposed population, as in allergic responses and in some forms of congenital malformation (Rokicki et al. 1989).

Fourth, the disease produced is so rare that at first an environmental cause is overlooked. An example is hepatic angiosarcoma due to contact with polyvinyl chloride. However, this kind of rare effect, once the correlation has been made, can be considered a 'sentinel' event indicating exposure to a specific agent. Thus, when pleural mesothelioma was diagnosed in residents of an isolated Greek rural area, a search for a source of asbestos was made. It was found to be the local rock used for making whitewash for painting the homes (Langer et al. 1987).

Fifth, the development of effects may be widely separated, in time and place, from the exposure incident, so that the connection is obscure. Parental exposure to mutagens comes into this category, as does exposure to environmental carcinogens when the time-lag to diagnosis of cancer may be so long that the exposure is not remembered, or as in the case of childhood exposure, not even known.

Clinical studies

The clinical model of history, symptomatology, and investigation has an important place in the diagnosis of pollution-related disease, especially in the handling of the individual case. Exposure history should be an integral part of every investigation, especially of symptoms known to be associated with pollution or in unusual clinical manifestations. In the case of children, history of prenatal exposure is important, including possible workplace contact with toxic substances (Savitz 1989; Cordero 1990).

In the event of known exposure to specific pollutants, such as radioactivity or lead, the measurement of a range of biological indicators provides an estimate of the body burden and constitutes the basis for therapeutic decisions and monitoring the course of the damage and the efficacy of treatment (WHO 1987a; Vivoli et al. 1989).

Many pollutant-mediated diseases are clinically indistinguishable from those of other aetiology, e.g. respiratory and skin manifestations, but specific allergens may be identified. Clinical investigations may be helpful in the event of suspected exposure to neurotoxins (Pearson and Dietrich 1985), and documentation of unusual disease entities may lead to the identification of new forms of environmental hazard. However, by the time one individual in an exposed population is diagnosed as having clinically detectable effects, it is likely that many others will also be affected to a greater or lesser degree. In such a case, a search for the source, along with investigation of the rest of the population, is indicated.

Epidemiological studies

In the elucidation of health effects of environmental hazards, the clinical approach alone is insufficient. In order for causal relationships to be verified, subtle changes to be detected, rare expressions to be recognized, dose–effect relationships to be quantified, and long-term outcomes to be measured, epidemiological methods are needed. Much information has been gathered on populations exposed to workplace hazards, and also case–control studies have indicated the danger of some forms of occupational exposure. Findings from such studies indicate the possibility of toxic effects occurring in non-occupationally exposed populations, but they are not necessarily applicable to children who have different modes of exposure and different degrees of susceptibility due to developmental and maturational factors. Thus, specific epidemiological studies need to be designed for the investigation of the effects of prenatal and childhood exposures.

Case–control studies have been made for rare forms of malignancy and specific congenital abnormalities, 'clinical trial' types of studies may be suitable for looking at the effects of known specific exposures, and cohorts have been used in a variety of studies. Inappropriate sample selection and other methodological problems have reduced the value and impaired the comparability of many studies. Guidelines have been laid down to minimize epidemiological methodological defects (WHO 1983, 1987a), but there are still many problems inherent to the design, execution, and interpretation of environmental studies such as the need for large samples, the role of social background variables (Winneke and Kramer, 1984), mixed exposures, and other, unrecorded, possible aetiological agents such as viral infections in the case of childhood malignancies (Little and Boyle, 1991).

Residence in a polluted area is a factor which is often associated with other potentially detrimental influences, including poor living conditions and parental occupation and smoking habits. The confounding effect makes difficult the interpretation of findings (Sterling and Weinkam 1990), especially when passive smoking in the home is also associated with maternal smoking during pregnancy. A recent prospective study of 1260 babies in two Greek communities, one with heavy industrial pollution, showed different relative risks of respiratory infection from various environmental factors at different ages (Nakou *et al.* 1992). Residence in the polluted community carried a higher risk of lower respiratory infection in pregnancy and in the second year of life. Smoking in pregnancy was associated with increased lower respiratory infection in pregnancy and in the first year of life, but in the first year poor general living conditions and smoking in the home also had an effect. No additional effect was detected from gas cooking or paraffin heating.

One of the most extensively investigated environmental pollutants is lead, and many earlier studies of its effects on the fetus and on children were subject to methodological problems. More recent attention to comparability in study design, sample selection, laboratory quality control, use of standardized tests, and close collaboration between study groups has resulted in the assembly of detailed dose–response data for a wide range of toxic effects of lead on children (Smith 1989).

The children who are most heavily exposed to industrial pollution are often those who are subject to a wide variety of other adverse life experiences, such as poverty, poor parental education, and inadequate housing. A study in a community surrounding a lead smelter in Greece showed that the children living in the immediate vicinity of the smelter had the highest blood lead levels and performed poorest on neurological testing. However, their living conditions were also the poorest and their families the most deprived, lacking the means to move from the polluted area (Benetou-Marandidou *et al.* 1988).

Experimental exposure of populations to pollutants, is, of course, unethical, but there have been occurrences of 'natural experiments' such as the Chernobyl nuclear accident and it is important that the opportunity for accurate documentation of effects is not missed (WHO 1987*a*). Introduction of new measures such as reduction of the lead content in petrol (Colombo *et al.* 1990) or the closing down of a factory may result in a dramatic reduction of environmental pollutant levels, and population response may be monitored.

Toxicological studies

Epidemiological studies are based on the identification of untoward effects already produced in exposed populations. Certain effects can be anticipated and even quantified by the use of toxicological studies of chemicals and other possibly hazardous environmental agents, either before populations are exposed or when the question of toxicity has been raised. Methods include animal bioassay and *in vitro* testing on cell cultures, studying mutagenicity, carcinogenicity, and cell death. Animal studies are expensive and the species differences in metabolism make extrapolation to the human response uncertain. Human cells can be used for *in vitro* testing, eliminating the species variation. It is more economical and gives quicker results, but may not be predictive of behaviour in the intact living organism. Molecular epidemiology, a method which identifies individual risk according to exposure and genetic predisposition, is still at an early stage of development and validation.

Pharmaceuticals are routinely tested before they are put on the market, but many other chemicals are manufactured and put into use, or released during the manufacture or use of other products, with no adequate checks on their possible adverse health effects.

The management of pollution

Certain measures may be taken for the restriction of pollution and the prevention of untoward effects. These measures are based on information available at a given time, which in many instances is incomplete. The information is derived from a process of hazard identification and quantification and risk characterization, with an attempt to determine the 'acceptable' human exposure (Roberts and Hayns 1989; Hogan et al. 1990).

General measures

European governments have acknowledged state responsibility for ensuring certain standards of environmental safety. This is expressed in national legislation covering a variety of aspects of air, water, and food quality. Much of the legislation is based on recommendations from supra-governmental bodies such as the relevant committees of the EU, and from various international agencies such as those listed below.

- United Nations Environmental Programme (UNEP) concerned with environmental protection. The UN organized the 1992 'Earth Summit'*.

- Food and Agriculture Organization (FAO) concerned with agriculture and fishing practices and food safety.

- World Health Organization (WHO) concerned with health effects and health promotion.

- International Labour Office (ILO) concerned with workplace safety.

- International Atomic Energy Commission (IAEC) concerned with effects of ionizing radiation.

Some of these agencies have programmes specifically related to Europe, e.g. the European Office of WHO, and the Mediterranean Action Plan (MAP) which represents collaboration between UNEP, WHO, and FAO for matters concerning pollution and protection of the waters and coastline of the Mediterranean sea. In addition, European agencies exist, such as the European Standards Centre (Centre Européenne de Normalization, CEN) which recommends safety criteria for consumer products, including chemical safety of toys.

Governments run monitoring programmes to check the quality of drinking water and coastal recreational waters (using indicator organisms), food safety, and ambient air levels, in cities, of certain toxic emissions (usually sulphur and nitrogen oxides and particulate matter, along with ozone and carbon monoxide in some places). There are regulations concerning the sulphur content of fuel oils, the lead content of petrol, and the allowable levels of toxic constituents in

---

* The 'Earth Summit', i.e. the UN Conference on Environment and Development, took place in Rio de Janeiro, Brazil, 3–14 June 1992. Agreements negotiated by most of the world's governments resulted in two mains documents, the Rio Declaration on Environment and Development, and Agenda 21, a programme of action for sustainable development. Agenda 21 comprises forty programme areas, of which six confront the problems of pollution directly. These are the areas concerning protection of seas and freshwater resources, and the management of toxic chemicals and hazardous wastes. Particular attention was given to environmental measures dealing with international traffic of hazardous materials, and transboundary pollution.

fluid effluent and airborne emissions. All these measures have a definite but limited impact on health effects of environmental pollution.

Local authorities or other agencies involved in assessment and control of pollution have various strategies at their disposal. Monitoring of levels of pollutants in air, water, soil, food, etc. is an important part of the assessment process, but it is insufficient on its own, and the impact on the population must also be measured. Population monitoring also provides the first indication of health effects from agents not being measured. Disease surveillance is a public health strategy used for watching large populations for increased incidence of particular diseases (Goldstein and Gochfeld 1990). Medical surveillance refers to the periodic evaluation of biological indicators in individual or populations at risk. For example, trends in blood lead levels, followed after the introduction of control measures, show clear evidence of a decreasing trend of blood lead in several European countries (Schultz *et al.* 1989; Ducoffre *et al.* 1990; Colombo *et al.* 1990).

Research on possible adverse health effects of specific pollutants and combinations of pollutants helps in the anticipation of problems in exposed populations and assists in the delineation of protective measures.

Most areas of Europe can expect an ecological emergency of some nature, and contingency plans should be made for the control of pollutants and the management of the populations affected. Paediatricians should be informed of the potential dangers in their community and they should be involved in the planning and execution of the contingency measures. The need for psychological intervention during and after such emergencies should be anticipated.

Health and environmental education and dissemination of information regarding the dangers of pollution constitute an important component of prevention and protection programmes. People are more likely to conform to legislation and to adopt safety conscious behaviour and conservation techniques if they are well informed of the risks and benefits (Weterings and Van Eijndhoven 1989).

Children themselves are particularly sensitive to environmental issues and their enthusiasm for planting trees, collecting waste materials for recycling, and not littering beaches can be cultivated through educational programmes and helped to persist into adult life, despite the teenage passion for motorized transport. Well informed populations are less likely to panic in the event of an ecological accident and will respond to appeals for practical help and cooperation in the institution of special measures, whereas poorly informed people tend to be suspicious, uncooperative, and alarmist.

Specific measures

Specific episodes of pollution in a community may be indicated by increased environmental levels or heralded by clinical effects in a person or persons, children being likely to be the first to show adverse effects.

Management strategies include identification and removal of the source, or if justified by the level of exposure, evacuation of the population; investigation and treatment of clinical effects in those affected and search for and management of sub-clinical effects in those not obviously affected; design and implementation of specific preventive measures on a community and an individual basis.

Public health teams have a major role to play in the monitoring and management of health effects of pollution in a community, but the primary health care workers, with their intimate knowledge of the living conditions and habits of the children they care for, are in a unique position both to observe possible pollution-related effects and to educate families about risks and prevention measures (Institute of Medicine 1988). Many of the hazards are home-based and the family doctor, paediatrician, or health visitor should be alert to dangers and to education opportunities. Parents will often take greater care if they believe the health of their children is threatened, and will adjust their occupational practices, handling of household and agricultural chemicals, household dust control, etc., to protect their offspring. Health workers at the community level have a responsibility to be informed about local sources of pollution and to be on the alert for new hazards. They can exert informed pressure on policy makers and participate in planning for local solutions.

References

Bencko, V. and Symon, K. (1977). Test of environmental exposure to arsenic and hearing changes in exposed children. *Environmental Health Perspectives*, **19**, 95–101.

Benetou-Marantidou, A., Nakou, S., and Micheloyiannis, J. (1988). Neurobehavioural estimation of children with life-long increased lead exposure. *Archives of Environmental Health*, **43**, 392–5.

Colombo, A., Leyendecker, W., Versino, B., Nakou, S., Hatzichristidis, D., Papadopoulou, S., and Chartsias, B. (1990). *Impact of gasoline lead on human blood. The Athens lead experiment.* ECSC, EEC, EAEC, Brussels and Luxembourg.

Cordero, J.F. (1990). Effect of environmental agents on pregnancy outcomes: disturbances of prenatal growth and development. In *Environmental medicine* (Medical Clinics of North America, Vol. 74, No. 2) (ed. A.C. Upton), pp. 279–90. W.B. Saunders, Philadelphia.

Douglas, J.W.B. and Waller, R.E. (1966). Air pollution and respiratory infections in children. *British Journal of Preventive and Social Medicine*, **20**, 1–8.

Ducoffre, G., Claeys, F., and Braux, P. (1990). Lowering time trends of blood lead levels in Belgium since 1978. *Environmental Research*, **15**, 25–34.

Goldstein, B.D. and Gochfeld, M. (1990). Role of the physician in environmental medicine. In *Environmental medicine* (Medical Clinics of North America, Vol. 74, No. 2) (ed. A.C. Upton), pp. 245–61. W.B. Saunders, Philadelphia.

Hatzakis, A., Kokkevi, A., Maravelias, C., Katsouyianni, K., Salaminios, F., Kalandidi, A., *et al.* (1989). Psychometric intelligence deficits in lead-exposed children. *In Lead exposure and child development* (ed. M.A. Smith, L.D. Grant, and A.I. Sors), pp. 211–23. Kluwer Academic, Dordrecht.

Hogan, M.D., Fouts, J.R., McKinney, J.D., and Rall, D.P. (1990). Disease-causing effects of environmental chemicals. In *Environmental medicine* (Medical Clinics of North America, Vol. 74, No. 2) (ed. A.C. Upton), pp. 461–73. W.B. Saunders, Philadelphia.

Institute of Medicine (1988). *Role of the primary care physician in occupational and environmental medicine.* National Academy Press, Washington DC.

Jacobson, J.L., Jacobson, S.W., and Humphrey, H.E.B. (1990). Effects of *in utero* exposure to polychlorinated biphenyls and related contaminants on cognitive functioning in young children. *The Journal of Pediatrics,* **116**, 38–45.

Kjellstrom, T., Kennedy, P., Wallis, S., and Mantell, C. (1986). *Physical and mental development of children with prenatal exposure to fish. Stage 1 preliminary tests at age 4.* Report 3080. National Swedish Environmental Protection Board, Solna, Sweden.

Kohler, L. and Jackson, H. (1987). *Traffic and children's health.* Report 2, 1987. NHV, Gothenburg, Sweden.

Langer, A.M., Nolam, R.P., Constantopoulos, S.H., and Moutsopoulos, H.M. (1987). Association of Metsovo Iung and pleural mesothelioma with exposure to tremolite-containing white wash. *Lancet,* **i**, 965–7.

Little, J. and Boyle, P. (1991). Some aspects of the epidemology of cancer in children. In *Children and families with special needs: the right to hope,* (ed. E. Petridon and S. Nakou). Proc. ESSOP Conf., Athens.

MAP (Mediterranean Action Plan) (1987). *Assessment of the state of pollution of the Mediterranean sea by mercury and mercury compounds.* MAP Technical Reports Series No. 18. UNEP, Athens.

MAP (Mediterranean Action Plan) (1987). *Assessment of the state of pollution of the Mediterranean sea by pathogenic organisms.* UNEP (OCA)/MED WG.25/Inf. 7. UNEP, Athens.

Marsh, D.O., Myers, G.J., Clarkson, T.W., Amin-Zaki, L., Tikriti, S., and Majeed, M.A. (1980). Fetal methylmercury poisoning: clinical and toxicological data on 29 cases. *Annals of Neurology* **7**, 348–53.

Nakou, S., Antoniadou-Koumatou, I., and Sarafidou, E. (1992). Means of domestic heating and cooking, cigarette smoking in the home, and pregnancy outcome and infant health. In *Quality of the indoor environment* (ed. J.N. Lester, R. Perry, and G.L. Reynolds), pp. 409–16. Selper, London.

Pearson, D.T. and Dietrich, K.N. (1985). The behavioural toxicology and teratology of childhood: models, methods and implications for intervention. *Neurotoxicology,* **6**, 165–82.

Roberts, L.E.J. and Hayns, M.R. (1989). Limitations on the usefulness of risk assessment. *Risk Analysis,* **9**, 483–94.

Rokicki, W., Latoszkiewicz, K., Krasnodebski, J. (1989). Congenital malformations and the environment. *Acta Paediatrica Scandinavica* (Suppl. 360), 140–5.

Savitz, D.A., Whelan, E.A., and Kleckner, R.L. (1989). Effect of parent's occupational exposures on risk of stillbirth, preterm delivery, and small-for-gestational-age infants. *American Journal of Epidemiology,* **129**, 1201–18.

Schultz, A., Attewell, R., and Skerfving, S. (1989). Decreasing blood lead in Swedish children, 1978–1988. *Archives of Environmental Health,* **44**, 391–4.

Shuval, H.I. (1986). *Thalassogenic diseases.* UNEP Regional Seas Reports and Studies No. 79. UNEP, Nairobi.

Smith, M.A. (1989). The effects of low-level lead exposure on children. In *Lead exposure and child development* (ed. M.A. Smith, L.D. Grant, and A.I. Sors), pp. 3–48. Kluwer Academic, Dordrecht.

Sterling, T. and Weinkam, J. (1990). The confounding of occupation and smoking and its consequences. *Soc. Sci. Med.*, **30**, 457–67.

Suess, M.J., Grefen, K., and Reinisch, D.W. (eds) (1984). *Ambient air pollutants from industrial sources: a reference handbook*. Elsevier, Amsterdam.

Vivoli, G., Bergomi, M., Borella, P., Fantuzzi, G., Simoni, L., Catelli, D. *et al.* (1989). Evaluation of different biological indicators of lead exposure related to neuropsychological effects in children. In *Lead exposure and child development* (eds M.A. Smith, L.D. Grant, and A.I. Sors), pp. 224–39. Kluwer Academic, Dordrecht.

Weiss, B. and Clarkson, T.W. (1982). Mercury toxicity in children. In *chemical and radiation hazards to children* (ed. L. Finberg), pp. 52–9. Ross Laboratories, Columbus, Ohio.

Weterings, R.A.P.M. and Van Eijndhoven, J.C.M. (1989). Informing the public about uncertain risks. *Risk Analysis*, **9**, 473–82.

Winneke, G. and Kramer, V. (1984). Neuropsychological effects of lead in children: interactions with social background variables. *Neuropsychobiology*, **11**, 195–204.

WHO (1983). *Guidelines on studies in environmental epidemiology*. Environmental Health Criteria, Document 27. WHO/IPCS, Geneva.

WHO (1987a). *Nuclear accidents and epidemiology*. WHO Environmental Health Series, No. 25. WHO, Copenhagen.

WHO (1987b). *Air quality guidelines for Europe*. WHO Regional Publications, European Series, No. 23. WHO, Copenhagen.

12 National inequalities in accident mortality among children and adolescents in the European countries

Bjarne Jansson and Leif Svanström

Introduction

Accidents are the leading cause of death among children and adolescents in the industrialized countries (World Health Organization 1991). We can see the beginning of a similar development in many of the pre-industrialized countries. The question is whether there are still differences in mortality between European countries in the same way as there are differences between economically strong and weak groups in one and the same country (Baker *et al.* 1984; Vågerö and Östberg 1989).

Historically, the child health care services and social medicine have had a strong influence in this area as pressure groups. They played an important role, for example, in the initiation of a nationwide child safety programme which has led to reduced mortality among children in Sweden during the postwar period (Berfenstam 1970). This example illustrates the important role that the people engaged in child health care play as policy makers and initiators of local preventive measures.

The aim of this chapter is therefore to describe the nature and magnitude of the problem in Europe in order to stimulate continued and intensified efforts to reduce accidents among children and adolescents in Europe.

Taxonomy

The concept of injuries and accidents

The distinction between accidents and injuries is important and there is a general shift in many countries from using the concept of accident towards using injury as the overall term. However, an accident is an event that results or could result in an injury. One unfortunate connotation of the term accident is that such an event and its outcomes can be interpreted as being unpredictable or random and therefore uncontrollable or not preventable at all. The determinants of these events can be studied and understood and this new understanding can be used to prevent accidents. A new concept of '*accidentology*' has therefore been developed. (Svanström 1988; Andersson 1991). One characteristic feature is that an accident is regarded as a process instead of a single event. The coding of the sequence of events preceding an injury is thereby more reliable and supports adequate countermeasures. For a programme of injury control to succeed, everyone must have a sense of predictability of accidents. Analogous concepts have already been accepted, such as traumatology and suicidology.

Classification systems

Injuries can be classified according to the place or environment where they occur. The main environments include, traffic, home, school, and sports activities. This increases the possibilities of directing preventive measures at major deficiencies.

For a number of years, it has been clear that the International Classification of Diseases (ICD) and its E code system is not sufficient for the needs of local and regional preventive programmes. Many suggestions for improvements have been made and the last revision of the ICD was substantially influenced by the NOMESCO (Nordic Medico-Statistical Committee 1991).

To achieve a better understanding of the accident phenomenon, the Nordic classification of injuries is now being introduced in the Nordic countries (The National Board and Health and Social Welfare 1989). The classification has basically the following construction, divided into specific codes:

(i) cause of contact;

(ii) place;

(iii) injury mechanism;

(iv) activity; and

(v) a description of the sequence of events and the circumstances connected with the injury. Additionally, supplementary classification modules have been developed for more detailed studies on traffic, and sports injuries, and those related to particular products such as toys.

The Nordic Classification is used for investigative purposes and prevention, research, and epidemiological comparisons at the local, regional, national, and international levels.

There are several scales for rating the severity of injuries. The abbreviated injury scale (AIS) is most widespread and was first introduced in 1971 (Committee on Injury Scaling 1985). The AIS is a numerical scale ranging from one (minor injury) to six (maximum injury—virtually unsurvivable). The scores are based on five criteria: threat to life, permanent impairment, treatment period, temporary disability, and energy dissipation. Injuries are grouped in the AIS manual by body region.

Lack of data

Some general limitations have been observed in registry data. Under-reporting is a problem that has attracted attention as it limits the possibilities of planning appropriate measures and determining priorities. The lack of comprehensive statistics for all types of accidents complicates intersectoral analyses. Some national registries can only with difficulty, if at all, be broken down to the county or local level. The present system for classification of the external cause of injuries, the E code, has major taxonomic deficiencies (Jansson 1988).

A number of European countries keep records of morbidity data but in developing countries, there is mostly no or very limited information available. There is a need for improvement in the availability and quality of basic epidemiological data in Europe as well as developing countries.

Mortality data are available from all countries but due to the taxonomic deficiencies of the E code, the data are of limited use as a basis for prevention. Injuries occurring at work and during leisure activities cannot be separated, the place and time of the accident is not stated, and different types of accident such as falls, burns, and road accidents are not given separate categories.

However, the data available are adequate for a rough estimation of the trends and the current situation concerning accident mortality among children in Europe. The WHO *Health for all indicator data base* comprises statistics from all WHO countries (World Health Organization 1990), and mortality data for the period 1970 to 1988 or the latest available year in each country have been used, together with statistics presented annually (World Health Organization 1991). The figures are based on the average population in each country and are presented per 100 000 children in the age groups 0–14, 15–19, and 20–24 years.

Injury mortality among children and adolescents

The worldwide perspective

Accidental injuries are the leading cause of death under the age of 24 years in more than half of the nearly 60 countries that report statistics on injuries (World Health Organization 1991). The overall injury mortality based on available data from all WHO regions was, according to the latest available figures, at least 75 359 fatalaties per year among children aged 0–14 years (World Health Organization 1991). The figures are divided per WHO region as follows: the Americas, 16 943; South-East Asia, 985; Europe 39 987, Eastern Mediterranean region 2667; and the Western Pacific region 14 777. For the age group 15–24 years, the total number of deaths reported worldwide was 88 922. In the Americas there were 29 138 deaths; in South-East Asia 484; in Europe 40 192; in the Eastern Mediterranean 1691; and in the Western Pacific there were 17 417 deaths.

However the figures are missing from the African region and from various countries in several of the regions as well. China reports only data from selected areas, approximately ten per cent of the population. In 1989 China reported approximately 12 000 deaths, half of which is due to drowning. In Japan the number of deaths is about 2000 per year and 25 percent are due to drowning. The number of deaths is therefore heavily underestimated in the world. There are also fluctuations from year to year.

There are considerable differences between countries. For example, Sweden reports seven deaths per 100 000 and Uruguay 35 deaths per 100 000 inhabitants 0–14 years of age (World Health Organization 1991).

In both developed and developing countries, injuries account for 10–30 per cent of all hospital admissions and in the USA injury represents the first cause of primary contact with physicians (World Health Organization 1991). In Thailand, for example, the primary causes of mortality or morbidity are traffic accidents and homicide (Karolinska Institute 1989).

In an extensive study of the mortality among children up to 15 years of age in Sweden, children of parents with manual occupations were found to be over-represented (Vågerö and Östberg 1989). The biggest difference in mortality between children with different social backgrounds was due to accidents. The accident rate among children in areas with high proportions of socio-economically disadvantaged groups was higher than in other areas (Nathorst-Westfelt 1982). Comparisons in the USA showed, for example, that the accident rate in low income areas was higher for all types of accidents excepts falls and air disasters (Baker *et al.* 1984). When adjustment was made for urban and rural areas, the differences persisted to the disadvantage of rural areas. Further research is therefore needed in order to clarify in more detail the background and triggering factors involved.

Trends and differences in Europe

Age 0–14 years

At least 40 000 children aged up to 14 years die every year in Europe owing to accidents. Data are lacking from several countries, however (Albania, Monaco, and Turkey). The former Soviet Union accounts for most of these deaths with 30 000 children per annum. In the USA, which has a comparable population, 8000 children die each year.

According to the latest available data from WHO (1990), the average mortality owing to unintentional injuries and poisoning in Europe among children aged up to 14 years is 15.9 per 100 000. The mortality in Eastern and central European countries is almost twice as high as in Western Europe: 23.7 compared to 12.6 per 100 000. One country differs essentially from all the others—Romania, with 57.4 deaths per 100 000 children (Table 12.1). Four of the Western European countries had a mortality exceeding the average for Europe. Portugal had twice as high a mortality as the whole of Europe in 1988—32.0 compared to 15.9.

Table 12.1 *Childhood mortality at age 0–14 years per 100 000 inhabitants due to unintentional injuries and poisoning in countries with above the European average rate (1988)*

Western Europe	Rate	Eastern Europe	Rate
France	18.1	Bulgaria	27.7
Greece	19.5	Czechoslovakia	24.5
Israel	21.3	Former GDR	16.7
Portugal	32.0	Poland	20.6
		Romania	57.4
		Former USSR	16.1
All Europe	15.9		

Countries with a very low mortality—less than half the European average—are Luxemburg (3.9), Iceland (3.9), Sweden (7.3), and Malta (7.9). Other countries with a low mortality are Holland (8.1), Norway (8.4), Finland (8.8), Italy (9.3), Denmark (10.1), and the United Kingdom (10.1). During the period 1970–88, the overall mortality has decreased in most countries, by 27 per cent in the Eastern and central European countries and by 50 per cent in Western Europe (World Health Organization 1990). Four countries show the opposite trend, however, with an increased mortality (Table 12.2) in Israel (+8 per cent), Malta (+11 per cent), Spain (+18 per cent), and the former Soviet Union (+5 per cent).

Age 15–24 years

The total number of deaths in this age group in Europe according to the latest figures was 40 192: 32 795 boys (82 per cent) and 7397 girls (18 per cent). Data for these age groups are also lacking from several countries. More than half of these deaths occurred in the former Soviet Union.

The average mortality for the age group 15–19 years in the whole of Europe is 40.4 deaths per 100 000 and for the age group 20–24 years 54.5 per 100 000. The incidence is thus considerably higher than for the age group 0–14 years. For the age group 15–19 years, two of the Eastern European countries—Bulgaria and Hungary—are above the average for Europe. Eight Western European countries—Switzerland, Portugal, Norway, Luxembourg, Iceland, Finland, Belgium, and Austria—also have a higher mortality than the average for Europe. Countries in which the mortality has increased during the period are Bulgaria, Iceland, Ireland, Luxembourg, Portugal, and Spain.

The situation for the age group 20–24 is similar. Hungary, Poland, and Romania are over-represented in the East and Austria, Belgium, Finland, France, Greece, Luxembourg, Norway, Portugal, and Switzerland in the West. Countries

Table 12.2 *Mortality due to unintentional injuries and poisoning in the 0–14 years age group per 100 000 in European countries*

Country	Rate (Year 1970)	(1988)	Difference (per cent)
Austria	33.2	11.6	−65
Belgium	43.1	14.3	−67
Bulgaria	38.3	27.7	−28
Czechoslovakia	30.3	24.5	−19
Former GDR	29.6	16.7	−44
Denmark	24.6	10.1	−59
West Germany	39.0	11.8	−70
Finland	29.9	8.8	−71
France	35.9	18.1	−50
Greece	22.9	19.5	−15
Hungary	21.4	12.9	−40
Iceland	30.8	3.9	−87
Ireland	34.9	11.9	−66
Israel	19.7	21.3	+8
Italy	16.9	9.3	−45
Luxembourg	42.3	3.9	−91
Malta[1]	7.1	7.9	+11
Netherlands	28.9	8.1	−72
Norway	29.2	8.4	−71
Poland	30.0	20.6	−31
Portugal	35.6	32.0	−10
Romania[2]	62.4	57.4	−8
Spain	13.4	15.8	+18
Former USSR[3]	15.4	16.1	+5
Sweden	17.6	7.3	−59
Switzerland	42.9	13.0	−70
United Kingdom	27.9	10.1	−64
Former Yugoslavia	27.4	13.6	−50

[1] Small population base;
[2] all E numbers
[3] Only 1986 and 1987 available.

which have reported an increase are Bulgaria, Belgium, Greece, Luxembourg, Portugal, Spain, Switzerland, and the UK.

The social and structural similarities and differences behind these large differences between Eastern and Western Europe and between countries within these two regions require more detailed studies. Differences which may be related to types of child care, resources, and 'know-how' for designing safer products and environments and more or less openly declared policies for giving priority to safety issues in different communities also warrant further study. *However, countries that have managed to reduce the mortality considerably show what can be done under favourable conditions.* The results can stimulate countries with a high mortality to intensify their safety efforts.

Injuries and child development

Accident risks among children are strongly correlated to how the child develops and functions at different ages. It is important that we know this in order to be able to compensate for children's inability to detect or cope with hazards to which they are exposed, i.e. when the requirements exceed their abilities.

Attempts have been made to estimate the proportion of accidents related to children's learning and development. About 30 per cent of childhood accidents are so strongly related to these factors that preventive measures may retard children's development. The risk of recurrence is also slight, owing to the learning effect. However, we restrict ourselves here to accidents only resulting in mild injuries which in most cases only require self-treatment or outpatient treatment, e.g. grazes, superficial cuts, bruises, or sprains and strains. In a further 37 per cent of cases, the accident can be prevented with relatively simple measures, e.g. by removing dangerous products from the child's immediate environment and by increased supervision of the child (Berfenstam 1970). The remaining accidents require more extensive and expensive changes to adapt the environment more adequately to the child's physical and cognitive limitations. Examples of measures to further reduce the number of deaths in road accidents are general improvement of the internal safety of motor vehicles and continued construction of separate cycle lanes. The use of children's car seats and cycle helmets should be increased by making these items available on loan or at subsidized prices.

Like the risks, the preventive measures are strongly related to the child's age and development (Bäckström 1979). During the neonatal period, when the child has a strong need to suck, the risk of suffocation is great. Examples of risks that are easy to eliminate are, for example, small objects (parts of toys, etc.), plastic material, and poorly made dummies. During the first year of life, when the child starts to learn to move around, the risk of poisoning increases owing to the child's curiosity and desire to taste and feel everything. Alkaline dishwashing detergents, for example, should be placed high up in the kitchen as they may cause severe corrosive injuries to the oesophagus.

When the child has learnt to walk, the risk of falls arises. They are usually trivial but gates and window-catches can prevent falls with more serious consequences. Electric accidents are another problem, but there are now 'earthing error switches' available which break the current before it reaches the body.

Two-year-olds move fast and the need for supervision or removal of hazards in their immediate environment therefore increases. To let them out to play on their own is to overrate their abilities, for example. Drowning accidents may occur even in ditches or deep puddles. Animal bites on the face are another problem. In certain environments, e.g. on farms, where the home and working environment coincide, the need for supervision is naturally particularly great.

At the age of three, the child's interest in tools and implements increases. Burns, cuts, crush injuries, etc. are therefore common hazards.

The four-year-old is typically reckless and often plays at a hectic pace. Playing with matches starts to be exciting. Many children are given a two-wheeled bicycle at this age. The child can only concentrate on one thing at a time and therefore does not detect hazards in his environment, e.g. traffic. According to Sandels' studies, it is not until the age of 12 that children are able to cope with the demands of the traffic environment (Sandels 1975). The alternative is to separate different traffic groups from one another but that is expensive. A five-year-old should not be allowed to go out alone near busy roads. The child's instinct for discovery may take him a long way from home.

At older ages, the combination of recklessness, neglect of natural laws, and certain activities, e.g. skateboarding, downhill skiing, tobogganing, cycling, and motor cycling increases the need for safety equipment and measures to compensate for environmental hazards. In certain cases, prohibition may unfortunately be necessary, especially when other people's lives are jeopardized, e.g. on skislopes or in road traffic.

Check-lists of the most common accident hazards at different ages for use by people working in the child care service have been used in the Falköping project (Svanström and Svanström 1989). The lists are based on authentic child accidents in the municipality (Schelp and Svanström 1987).

Main external causes

Age 0–14 years

About half of the deaths in Europe are due to traffic accidents. The proportion is higher in Western Europe (Table 12.3). Drowning is the next largest single cause of death, about 10 per cent of the total, with a higher proportion in Eastern Europe. The proportion of drowning accidents is highest in the former Soviet Union and Bulgaria, 23 per cent in both cases. Other large groups are poisoning (five per cent), falls (five per cent), and domestic fires (five per cent). A relatively large number of cases are classified as miscellaneous, 30 per cent on average. It is not possible to give any examples from the WHO material as the cases are only reported as miscellaneous without any subgroups. Some examples from the Swedish cause-of-death statistics may give some indication of what is included in this group. Children have been killed by falling objects, crushed between objects, accidentally shot dead, died in accidents with explosives, and been crushed by or fallen off horses.

Table 12.3 Mortality due to unintentional injuries and poisoning by external cause (percentages) among children 0–14 years of age in the European countries (1988)

Country	Total number	Traffic	Poisoning	Falls	Fire	Drowning	Machine	Miscellaneous
Austria	156	41	–	5	3	13	7	28
Bulgaria	375	23	5	8	3	23	–	37
Czechoslovakia	419	30	4	7	4	18	–	36
Denmark	94	52	1	–	3	12	1	12
Finland	82	63	1	1	1	12	2	17
France	1302	43	1	5	3	10	–	27
Former GDR	355	36	3	9	3	16	–	33
Former FRG	835	46	–	5	8	16	1	24
Greece	222	48	1	4	2	11	3	26
Hungary	265	50	3	6	3	13	1	24
Iceland*	8	(5)	–	(1)	–	(2)	–	–
Ireland	99	51	5	4	10	7	6	15
Israel	183	37	3	4	3	9	–	44
Italy	695	50	2	7	2	11	3	24
Luxemburg*	7	(6)	–	–	–	–	–	(1)
Malta*	2	–	–	–	–	–	–	(2)
Netherlands	202	50	1	2	4	20	2	21
Norway	63	48	–	1	13	11	3	19
Poland	1533	40	6	5	3	19	1	26
Portugal	327	49	3	6	4	12	3	22
Spain	847	48	3	5	2	16	1	35
Sweden	109	47	1	3	6	14	2	27
Switzerland	116	41	9	7	12	2	7	40
Former USSR	30 255	17	9	4	6	23	1	41
United Kingdom	845	54	2	4	13	10	1	17
Former Yugoslavia	680	45	3	4	3	12	1	30
Total	39 987							

* Only absolute numbers presented.

Age 15–24 years

More than three-quarters of the roughly 40 000 reported deaths occur in road traffic. Proportionally more deaths are reported in Western Europe. Poisoning is more common in Denmark, Switzerland, the former USSR, Poland, Finland, and former East Germany. Once again, drowning is more common in Eastern European countries.

Public policy for child safety

UN Convention on the rights of the child

According to article 19 in the United Nations charter of children's rights, states, parties shall take all appropriate legislative, administrative, social, and educational measures to protect the child from all forms of physical or mental violence, injury, or abuse (United Nations 1989):

> Such protective measures should, as appropriate, include effective procedures for the establishment of social programmes to provide necessary support for the child and for those who have the care of the child, as well as for other forms of prevention and for identification, reporting, referral, investigation, treatment, and follow-up of instances of child maltreatment described heretofore, and, as appropriate, for judicial involvement.

UNICEF child health programme

The basic initiatives aimed at affecting a child health revolution supported by the UNICEF board are a series of executive actions in four priority areas (United Nations 1983). First, to increase the effectiveness of UNICEF assistance in improving child health and survival. Second, strengthening the capacity of UNICEF to deliver programmes in the most affected, least developed countries, particularly in Africa. Third, to increase the efficiency of UNICEF internal operations. Fourth, to consolidate and increase the financial resources of UNICEF.

Economic depression has three major impacts on children. Disposable family income falls sharply, which has disproportionately severe consequences for poor people and their families. Government budgets for social services—particularly those for nutrition, health, and education—are often the first to be cut back. One particularly worrying consequence of these conditions is that infant mortality is no longer declining at rates previously achieved in the majority of developing countries and there are new fears that infant mortality rates might in fact be rising in many places.

It has been recommended that indicators to be considered when analysing children's needs should include perinatal and neonatal mortality rates, child death rates, maternal mortality and population, life expectancy and literacy rates, the 'physical quality of life' index, school enrolment and literacy rates, as well as per capita income, child population, and infant mortality rates.

UNICEF should intensify its efforts to assess the needs of the most disadvantaged groups and areas, work with governments, and, as appropriate, with non-governmental organizations and other agencies to reinforce activities which help disadvantaged communities to develop their active participation in the development process and attach high priority to helping governments develop and improve their administrative capacity.

WHO target for accident prevention

Target 11 states that deaths from accidents in the European regions should be reduced by at least 25 per cent by the year 2000 (World Health Organization 1981). This target could be achieved if no country had a mortality rate from traffic accidents of more than 20 per 100 000; if countries below that level reduced it to less than 15; if all countries reduced the differences between the sexes, and age and socio-economic groups, if the occupational accident mortality in the region were lowered by at least 50 per cent; and if the mortality from home accidents were significantly reduced.

WHO has stated in target 11 that safety measures to prevent accidents occurring at home and at play to the people most at risk, children and the elderly, deserve particular attention. In its eighth general programme, WHO set the following targets for the year 1995:

- 60 per cent of countries will have assessed the magnitude and determinants of domestic and traffic accidents in their populations based on epidemiological studies;

- 50 per cent of countries will have developed policies and programmes, incorporating intersectoral action, for the prevention of domestic and traffic accidents, and the mitigation of their consequences.

The eighth general programme of WHO and its global programme for accident and injury prevention have their main thrust on developing policy principles and supporting action programmes that are community oriented, particularly at the district or more local level, focusing on prevention from the perspective of the local community.

As part of the WHO global programme, the WHO collaborating centre on community safety promotion was established in the autumn at 1989 at the Karolinska Institute, Department of Social Medicine, in Sweden. The centre is responsible for developing the WHO programme entitled 'community safety promotion'.

A safe community for all

The safe community concept derives from the health policy principle of everyone's right to grow up and live in a community that guarantees its citizens' health and physical and social security. How this should be organized and achieved depends on the political and economic conditions in different cultures and communities. The principle is based on mutual responsibility for equal distribution of the community's resources so that accident hazards can be reduced overall and unequal distribution of risks and injuries eliminated.

Many countries have introduced child safety programmes and Sweden is one of the countries where this work has been successful. The new element is the approach used, the whole community being involved and everyone contributing in his or her particular sphere of responsibility. Emphasis is placed on local action in collaboration with the people living in the community. The strategy derives its inspiration and methods from public health work in developing countries.

What is a 'safe community'? The planning of the WHO community programme involved the development of indicators for a safe community. This work was carried out during preparation of the first 'travelling seminar', and also in collaboration with Dr. Jerry Moller, Flinders University, Adelaide, Australia. The indicators are still used at the international level for determining the progress of community work (Karolinska Institute 1989). They are:

- there should be an intersectoral reference group working with accident/injury prevention;

- the local community network should be involved in the programme;

- the programme should include all ages, environments, and situations;

- the programme should take account of high risk groups and high risk environments;

- the programme should aim at justice for disadvantaged groups;

- the community should be able to document the frequency and nature of accidents and injuries.

A national network of 'safe communities' has been set up on the basis of the Swedish national programme for injury prevention. These municipalities generally have the indicators for safe communities and have also agreed to participate in the exchange of information and experience gained. But, also, a global network is under development. For example, agreements have been reached between the WHO collaborating centre at the Karolinska Institute, and the Ministry of Public Health in Thailand, including Wang Khoi Village; the city of Toulouse, France; Esbjerg, Denmark; and Lidköping, Motala, and Falköping in Sweden. More centres will be involved in the network of safe communities during the next few years.

At the First World Conference on Accident and Injury Prevention, in Stockholm, Sweden a manifesto was adopted on 20th September 1989 (Karolinska Institute 1989). It stated that a public health approach with community-level programmes for accident and injury prevention—'safe community programmes'—is the key to reducing and preventing injuries. The general statements formulated in the Stockholm manifesto concerned equity, community participation, and national and international participation, as detailed below.

1. *Equity*. All human beings have an equal right to health and safety. This principle of social policy is a fundamental premise of the WHO's *'Health for all'* strategy and of the WHO global programme on accident prevention and injury control.

2. *Community participation*. Some communities in developed and developing countries have begun to take community action which has led to safe communities. Therefore, research and demonstration projects for injury prevention and control must include community-level programmes.

3. *National and international participation*. As part of its national health plan, each government should formulate a national policy and a plan of action to create and sustain safe communities. All national health authorities urgently need to develop national safety goals and plans to achieve these goals.

The Stockholm conference has also identified four 'safe community' action areas:

(i) formulate public policy for safety;

(ii) create supportive environments;

(iii) strengthen community action; and

(iv) broaden public services.

These four recommendations were backed up by specific comments.

- Accident and injury prevention should be part of every child survival and primary health care programme. Community level programmes for accident and injury prevention—safe community programmes—are the key to reducing and preventing childhood injuries.

- Those involved in programmes to prevent and control injuries and accidents must first identify and characterize the injury problem and determine which groups are most vulnerable. Accident and injury prevention programmes must then focus on the vulnerable groups, which usually include children, the elderly, and the disadvantaged.

- Governments should strengthen any existing community action programmes and coordinate the work of health and safety agencies, social and economic authorities, professional and voluntary organizations, private industry, and the news media.

- Local accident and injury prevention programmes should include information for safety personnel and the public, training for voluntary and paid personnel, and checklists and other tools that help identify behavioural changes and environmental modifications.

A 'safe community' involves not only the health and safety sector, but also many other sectors, including agriculture, industry, education, housing, sports and leisure, public works, and communications. These sectors must coordinate their efforts to achieve optimum results.

Additionally, injury surveillance systems should be developed in close cooperation with clinicians responsible for hospitals and emergency services, those responsible for surveillance of chronic and infectious diseases, and those responsible for public and community safety.

Guidelines on how to develop 'safe communities' have been developed in an interdisciplinary group, with representatives from both developing and industrialized countries (Karolinska Institute 1989). They could be used as a tool by governments and local groups for developing demonstration programmes on 'safe communities' for children.

Results and opportunities concerning child safety

Successful programmes

A review of the literature shows that action programmes for specific types of accident risks, for example in the USA, have contributed to a reduction of both risks and mortality (Rice *et al.* 1989). A programme including counselling by paediatricians aimed at identifying and eliminating risks for falls led to a reduction of fall injuries by 41 per cent. Another trial concerned the risk of drowning accidents among small children in private swimming pools. The number of drowning accidents in the study area fell by 65 per cent. Compulsory installation of smoke detectors (fire alarms) in dwellings led to a reduction of the number of deaths in connection with fires by 25 per cent. After installation of special window-catches in high-rise apartment blocks, fall accidents from apartments decreased by 90 per cent.

A voluntary child safety campaign which later grew into a national programme was started in Stockholm, Sweden, in the 1950s (Berfenstam 1970). The initiators were a paediatric surgeon and a paediatric physician and specialist in social medicine. The child welfare clinics formed the base for the work. A special child accident committee was created for coordination of the work. The committee also came to play an important role in the national child safety programme. Deaths among children due to accidents have decreased greatly during the last 30 years.

The Falköping trial

That working via the child welfare clinics yields rapid and good results is also shown by a controlled trial in connection with a local intervention programme in a town in central Sweden, Falköping. The number of child injuries registered at the borough's health centres and casualty departments fell by 43 per cent after an intervention period of two years (Schelp and Svanström 1987). A corresponding reduction could not be demonstrated in the control area.

The preventive programme was based on intersectoral contacts between basic societal service sectors like primary care, social service, etc. as well as on involvement of the population individually or through organizations. A reference group was created and came to be the governing body for the project. The group included the chairman of the borough council, the assistant social welfare manager, the heads of the highway department, the police, the environmental health agency, a Red Cross officer, the chairman of the tenants association, the pensioners association, the local media, occupational health care services, a GP, personnel from the casualty department and the child welfare clinic, and a health planner from the primary care organization.

A health plan was adopted by the county council in 1972 as a basis for expansion of broad public health activities in the county. In order to achieve the objectives specified in the plan, a department of community health was set up. Personnel from the department started the injury control trial in the middle of 1970. For example, continuous collection of injury data at the casualty department from 1978 in both the trial and control areas was of great importance both for the planning work and for the evaluation of the intervention programme.

The introduction and planning of the programme was based on a one-year survey of the injury and accident pattern in the community. Before the first meeting of the reference group, informal contact with each member of the group was made one year before the start of the intervention phase in 1979–81. The preventive programme comprised four interdependent phases: mass communication, health education, surveillance of environmental hazards, and modification of risks, both indoor and outdoor.

A permanent exhibition on accident hazards in childhood was displayed at all child welfare clinics. Safety products were demonstrated and distributed in a local shop. Age-standardized guidelines and checklists on hazards in relation to child development and maturation were handled by the nurses at the child welfare clinics. The lists were used as a basis for information and screening of hazards in connection with home calls, visits to the clinic, and via the media. The lists were based on authentic accident cases from the local community reported from the casualty department. A safety file on consumer information was updated regularly at each clinic. A car-seat scheme for newborns and children was started and is now being spread throughout the county. Regular meetings and conferences were held to provide information and education about safety matters for all personnel involved.

Safety inspections of different environmental hazards have been carried out in residential areas, at schools and at day nurseries. Traffic hazards for children, with priority for cycle lanes, were reviewed by all eight local associations in the community. Also, in connection with projection of new housing estates, the accident hazards in adjacent areas were considered.

The active participation of the staff of the child health clinics has created new possibilities for reducing accident and injury hazards among children. The details of the programme have been described in international journals and books.

The role of child health care

What can the child health organization do to increase children's safety? It is a matter of both sustaining what has already been achieved and improving safety in areas in which there are still many and serious accidents.

1. *Influencing.* Both the general public and decision-makers have great confidence in health service personnel as regards their knowledge and expertise on health issues. This confidence should be exploited through information on how the community can help to increase child safety. Not least important is that families with children have a 'spokesman' who protects their interests in a situation where the introduction of preventive measures could be exploited for profit. It should be self-evident that a paediatrician must be present whenever child safety issues are discussed at the municipal level.

2. *Counselling.* Child health care personnel have extensive knowledge and experience of risks and injuries that can be utilized in the planning of children's immediate environment. This knowledge should be systematized and be readily available in connection with routine local planning work.

3. *Lobbying.* Paediatric associations and the child health care organization should act as a pressure group to ensure that child safety is given high priority.

4. *Education.* Everyday routine work requires that the organization invest in continuous education for its personnel. This provides an opportunity for exchange of experience and discussion on how to improve or revitalize their own educational activities. This is necessary in order to maintain the personnel's enthusiasm and efforts to continuously develop and improve their own work.

5. *Injury registration.* Epidemiological collaboration with physicians working at casualty departments and general practitioners gives a better picture of the overall situation in the community. More systematic collection of patient data in combination with the personnel's knowledge of the population and environment provides a better basis for determination of priorities in relation to demographic differences and specific risks, e.g. streets with through traffic or high average speeds. There are now ready made packages for registration and analysis of injury data.

6. *Product development*. Closer collaboration with manufacturers of child safety products and retailers should be established. This not only facilitates product development but also generates ideas on how the use of the products can be increased, through personal contact with families via parental education, etc.

7. *Initiate 'safe kids' and 'safe community' programmes*. The child health care organization should have a central role in the preventive work for children by initiating and maintaining safety programmes together with parents, authorities, and voluntary organizations.

References

Andersson, R. (1991). The role of accidentology in occupational injury research, Ph.D. thesis. Karolinska Institute, Department of Social Medicine, Kronan Health Centre, Sundbyberg, Sweden.

Baker, S., O'Neill, R., and Karpf R.S. (1984). *The injury fact book*. Lexington Books, Lexington, MA.

Berfenstam, R. (1970). Prevention of childhood accidents in Sweden. *Acta Paediatrica Scandinavica* (suppl.) **275**, 88–95.

Bäckström, K. (1979). *Barns och ungdomars beteende och förmåga*, No. 28. Statens Offentliga Utredningar (SOU), Stockholm.

Committee on Injury Scaling (1985). *The abbreviated injury scale* (1985 revision). American Association for Automotive Medicine, Morton Grove, IL.

Jansson, B. (1988). *A system for injury surveillance in Swedish emergency care as a basis of injury control*. (Ph.D. thesis). Karolinska Institute, Department of Social Medicine, Kronan Health Centre, Sundbyberg, Sweden.

Karolinska Institute (1989) *WHO travelling seminar on community safety promotion to Thailand 1989*. Department of Social Medicine, Kronan Health Centre, Sundbyberg, Sweden.

Nathorst-Westfelt, J.Å.R. (1982). Environmental factors in childhood accidents. A prospective study in Gothenburg, Sweden. *Acta Paediatrica Scandinavica* (suppl.) *291*, 1–75.

The National Board of Health and Social Welfare (NBHSW) (1989). *Classification of injuries*. NBHSW, Stockholm.

Nordic Medico-Statistical Committee (1991). *Classification for accident monitoring*. (NORD 1990:100 E, 2nd revision). Nordic Council, Copenhagen.

Rice, D.P., McKenzie, E.J., Jones, A.S., Kaufmann, S.R., Dehissovoy, G., et al. (1989). *Cost of injury in the United States: a report to congress*. Institute for Health and Ageing, University of California and Injury Prevention Center, San Francisco, CA.

Sandels, S. (1975). *Varför skadas barn i trafiken?* (Skandiarapporten nr 2). Stockholm.

Schelp, L. and Svanström, L. (1987). *Community intervention and accidents*. Folksam, Sundbyberg, Sweden.

Svanström, L. (1988). Accidentology—Why?—The need for a scientific approach to reducing injuries for the elderly. Paper presented at WHO working group 'Elderly

Persons' Safety'; Toulouse, France 9–10 September 1988. Karolinska Institute, Department of Social Medicine, Kronan Health Centre, Sundbyberg, Sweden.
Svanström, K. and Svanström, L. (1989). *A safe community—how to prevent accidents at the local level*, WHO travelling seminar, Sweden-Thailand. Karolinska Institute, Sweden.
United Nations (1983). *United Nations children's fund. Report of the executive board* (Suppl No. 10). UN, New York.
United Nations (1989). *Convention on the rights of the child*. UN, New York.
World Health Organization (1981). *Global strategy for health for all by the year 2000*. (Health for all series, 3). WHO, Geneva.
World Health Organization (1990). *Health for all indicator data base*. WHO, Copenhagen.
World Health Organization (1991). *World health statistics annual*. WHO., Geneva.
Vågerö, D. and Östberg, J.A.R. (1989). Mortality among children and young persons in Sweden in relation to childhood and socio-economic *group. J. Epidem. Comm. Health*, **43**, 280–4.

PART V

Concepts of normality

Knowledge of the normal is an essential prerequisite of recognition and management of abnormality. Concepts of normality, both lay and professional, undergo constant change; the concept of childhood itself is relatively new and profoundly influences our view of normality. Normal development is considered from an historical perspective and risk-taking, with particular reference to adolescence, is examined in the light of a changing view of risk.

13 Historical perspectives on childhood
Chris Jenks

Childhood as a recent concept

Despite the obvious fact that children have been and will continue to be omnipresent in human society both across space and through time, it is nevertheless the case that childhood is a relatively recent phenomenon in medicine and in the social sciences. As Mead and Wolfenstein (1955) tell us:

> Although each historical period of which we have any record has had its own version of childhood ... childhood was still something that one took for granted, a figure of speech, a mythological subject rather than a subject of articulate scrutiny.

It is as if the category of childhood only emerged at a comparatively late stage in the historical process. This is an idea supported by many theorists including Hoyles (1979) who plainly states that 'Both childhood and our present day nuclear family are comparatively recent inventions'. This contemporary topicality is itself an instance of the thesis that this chapter will seek to propound. That a state of being, such as childhood, should become formulated through the 'analytic gaze' within a particular epoch must tell us as much about the condition of our society as it does about our children.

Today children are everywhere thought of as normal. Common sense is redolent with images and understandings that contrive to produce the child not just as normal but also as utterly natural. Yet, as Hoyles (1979) demonstrates, 'Childhood is a social convention and not just a natural state'. The absolute necessity of children as real presences throughout history, as opposed to the transitory nature of other phenomena, such as capitalism, HIV, global warming, and feminism—however serious their impact on human beings—has rendered childhood completely mundane; we simply take it for granted (see Jenks 1982). Unlike the poor, children are always with us. As an event childhood is not even different enough to specify a mode of experience that is unique to certain groups of people; it is what everybody does or has done at a stage in their lives. Beyond this, childhood is a passing phenomenon, we 'grow out of it', it is routinely disregarded on our way to achieving our proper destiny—rational adult life. This normative assumption is reflected in our chastisement of people for 'acting childishly'. Being grown up must surely be the purpose of being! Now such an elaboration of what everyone knows about childhood is not peculiarly informative. My intention in rehearsing such ideas is to indicate the embeddedness of our 'knowing' about children in conceptions of the 'normal' and the 'natural'. We must shift our perspective to another site.

Childhood as an historical and cultural experience

Childhood is not the brief physical inhabitation of a lilliputian world owned and ruled by others, childhood is rather an historical and cultural experience and its meaning, its interpretations, and its interest resides within such contexts. These contexts, or social structures, become our topic. It is here where normative expectations arise and it is to an analysis of such structures that we shall proceed.

What I cannot aspire to, in a work of this scale, is a chronology of the changing images of the child and patterns of child care through history; this is a major task which has been attempted in a number of sources. The leading figure in producing such an archaeology of images is Ariès (1962) whose ideas are influential in all subsequent theorizing about the child. To this extent they are worthy of some elaboration for their implications are quite radical in relation to the common-sense view of the child. We should note that Ariès argues from material drawn largely from French culture but he would regard his conclusions as generalizable in regard to the development of the modern Western world.

Primarily, Ariès is informing us that there was a time before which children were invisible. Up to and including the Middle Ages it would seem that there was no collective perception of children as being essentially different to anyone else. People populated the world but their status was never established in terms of their lack of years nor their physical immaturity. At first, hearing this is a difficult proposition to accept, we have already conceded that children are a fact, the truism that they have always been with us. However, what Ariès is pointing to is that the manner of their recognition by adults and thus the forms of their relationships with adults have altered through the passage of time. This is not such a taxing idea to grasp once we think of the more contemporary case of the invention of the 'adolescent' or 'teenager' over, say, the past fifty years. Here we have a quite clearly distinguishable group of people within our society (albeit only within the Western world) who occupy a now firmly established twilight zone of the quasi-child or crypto-adult. Their space is marked out in relation to both the provision of formal education and the condition of the labour market, and the public content of their identity is both provided for and exploited through a whole industry of popular culture and mass consumption. The adult relation with adolescence further contrives in institutionalizing its subjective ambiguity through a complex set of newly, yet firmly established attitudes in relation to legal responsibility, sexual activity, enfranchisement, the ability to drive a car, or go to war, and so on. Yet the adolescent identity, a relative newcomer in our vocabulary of social types, has become a reality. It would be absurd to point to the exact historical moment of adolescence being brought into being but one could speculate that its emergence might well be related to the 1944 Education Act providing compulsory secondary education for all people—its existence is that brief.

To return from this example to Ariès, he is arguing that children have not always existed in the way that we now know them, they have not always been the same thing. In the Middle Ages, he asserts, there was no concept of childhood and it is from this absence that our current view of the child has evolved. Ancient society, we are told, may well have understood the difference of children and grasped the necessity of their development, whereas medieval civilization seems to have either abandoned or mislaid such a recognition. The reason for this loss is unexplained but the evidence of its impact Ariès derives from a study of painting and iconography.

Medieval art until about the twelfth century did not know childhood or did not attempt to portray it. It is hard to believe that this neglect was due to incompetence or incapacity; it seems more probable that there was no place for childhood in the medieval world. (Ariès 1962.)

The art of the Middle Ages does exhibit an extraordinary dearth of depictions of children, they were apparently considered of such little importance that they did not warrant representation in this form. Where such images do occur, as by necessity in the madonna and child, the baby Jesus appears uniformly, from example to example, as a small man, a wizened homunculus without the rounded appeal and vulnerability of the latter-day infant. This then is our baseline, we have to imagine a world of people differentiated only by whether they are being weaned or are working. Ariès now takes us on a journey to the present.

Following in the wake of the Middle Ages, children, in history, emerged initially as playthings. They were not separate from the adult world but provided it with delight or entertainment. Thus, although through the sixteenth and into the seventeenth century people took pleasure in pampering or 'coddling' their children, they were only gradually beginning to realize their presence as a different way of being in the world. Neither was this a universal response to the condition of infancy. Only particularly privileged groups or classes could afford the luxury of childhood with its demands on time and emotion and its paraphernalia of toys and special clothing. For most people children were potential sources of contribution to the economy of the family, and large families were both an investment and a hedge against infant mortality.

Ariès locates the genesis of the modern conception of the child in the eighteenth century and this is a view that is shared throughout the body of the literature on this topic. Robertson (1976) for example, tells us that

If the philosophy of the Enlightenment brought to eighteenth century Europe a new confidence in the possibility of human happiness, special credit must go to Rousseau for calling attention to the needs of children. For the first time in history, he made a large group of people believe that childhood was worth the attention of intelligent adults, encouraging an interest in the process of growing up rather than just the product. Education of children was part of the interest in progress which was so prominent in the intellectual trends of the time.

Children, through this period, had, it would seem, become perceived as different. We witness the arrival of a new category of being, one that is fresh and frail and consequently a target for correction and training by the growing standards of rationality that came to pervade the time. Once a concern with the child's physical health and well-being had been institutionalized along with an attention to their moral welfare then our model for modernity was almost complete. The child moved through time from obscurity to centre stage. The child is forever assured the spotlight of public policy and attention and also a primary place in the family. Indeed one might argue that the family has come to be defined in terms of the child's presence.

We should note that the thesis provided by Ariès is both persuasive and formative and although alternative and critical accounts have been presented, and well gathered by Pollock (1983), they rarely succeed in achieving more than a modification of his central ideas. For Ariès the history of childhood is a transition from darkness into light and he sets not just a pattern for future analysis but also an optimism and a justification of modern-day child rearing that we might properly treat with caution.

DeMause (1976), in similar vein, is most expressive of the dark side and thus somewhat overenthusiastic concerning the illuminating potential of today's parenting. DeMause describes the history of childhood as 'a nightmare from which we have only recently begun to awake' and continues that 'The further back in history one goes, the lower the level of child care, and the more likely children are to be killed, abandoned, beaten, terrorized and sexually abused'. He puts forward what he calls a 'psychogenic theory of history' which revolves around the notion that history consists in the evolution of the human personality brought about through successive and positive developments in the relationship between parents and children. The stages in this process that he puts forward begin with the routine infanticide of antiquity and conclude with the partially realized 'helping mode' of the late twentieth century; the latter being a kind of systematic facilitation of the child's unique intent throughout maturation.

Last in my inventory of child evolutionists, though there are many more, is Shorter (1976). He appears extremely congratulatory of the humane achievements in child rearing that have come to be crystallized in the forms of today's nuclear family. Our changing attitudes have apparently transformed children from the status of object, worthy only of disregard, into the status of subject, and subject of our central attention and self-sacrifice. 'Good mothering ...' we are informed 'is an invention of modernization.' (Shorter 1976). The point, I trust, is clear. The child in history has metamorphosed into an ontology, a subjectivity in its own right, a source of identity and more than this, a promise of the future good. The child has come to symbolize all that is decent and caring about a society, it is the very index of a civilization—witness the outrage and general moral disapproval at the revelations concerning Romanian orphanages, an obvious signifier of the corruption of Communist social structures!

Childhood and the necessity of control

In the examination of childhood that follows I concur with the thesis so far stated, but only so far. It is a theory not with tropes and a process laden with ironies. The modern image of child is one that is clear, visible, and in need of containment. The historical liberation of the child from adulthood has lead, in turn, to the necessity of its constraint by collective practice. The obvious high profile of children in our contemporary patterns of relationship has rendered them subject to new forms of control. As Rose (1989) asserts:

> Childhood is the most intensively governed sector of personal existence. In different ways, at different times, and by many different routes varying from one section of society to another, the health, welfare, and rearing of children have been linked in thought and practice to the destiny of the nation and the responsibilities of the state. The modern child has become the focus of innumerable projects that purport to safeguard it from physical, sexual, and moral danger, to ensure its 'normal' development, to actively promote certain capacities of attributes such as intelligence, educability and emotional stability.

Similarly, just as the delineation of the child's particularity has given rise to specially fashioned forms of control, so also has the diminution of public ignorance and disdain of the child led to new and intrusive forms of violence occurring within the family, from neurotic families to parental sexual abuse.

Changing patterns of normality

What I will produce is a framework for an analysis of the shifting patterns of normality that have been applied to the child through the massive turbulence, upheaval, and transformations that occurred in Europe with the advent of the modern age. This is the period that brought sociology itself into being and was marked by the acceleration of a number of significant structural processes such as the division of labour, industrialization, urbanization, the market economy, and a secularization of belief systems away from the consensual obedience to the deity towards an allegiance to the necessities of science, technology, and progress through growth.

The analysis will depend, as does all sociological theory, on the assumption that its subject, in this case childhood, emerges from a particular structuring of social relationships and that its various meanings derive from the forms of discourse that accompany those relationships. As an example of such an assumption at work let us look at art as a social phenomenon. Although critical aesthetics might argue for the intrinsic quality that is art in terms of say 'beauty' or 'goodness', the sociologist would see art as a practice of production that attained its meaning, its place, and its status within a particular field of symbolic representation and its structures of reception and appreciation. Thus one discourse providing for art as a social phenomenon would be criticism. In the same way childhood appears in different forms in different cultures in relation to structural variables such as rates of mortality and life expectancy, organizations of family life and structure, kinship patterns, and different ideologies of care, and philosophies of need and dependency. A discourse providing for childhood in modern western society might be that of a paediatrician, a parent, a teacher, or an educational psychologist, or equally those of a television producer and an advertising executive (see Jenks 1989).

These different forms of discourse clearly do not have an equivalence. They move in and out of focus according to the different aspects of the subject that are being considered. Sometimes this occurs in parallel but sometimes in competition, and often such discourses are arranged hierarchically, for example—in specific contexts the child-discourse of social workers or juvenile magistrates have a power and efficacy in excess of those of the sibling or parent. But all such discourses contribute to and, in turn, derive from the dominant cultural image of the 'normal' child. This, of necessity, implies that the child is part of and functional within a network of relations, a matrix of partial interests, and a complex of forms of professional knowledge that are beyond the physical experience of being a child.

Hillman (1975), writing in relation to analytical psychology, states that 'Whatever we say about children and childhood is not altogether really about children and childhood'. He is, in the original context, referring to childhood as a causal repository for the explanation of self and the progress of the psyche, but he may equally be read as suggesting that theories of the child are always pointers towards the social construction of reality. Just as I have argued that the child is neither simply 'natural' nor merely 'normal', we may claim to have established, in addition, that the child is not neutral but rather always moral and political. Thus the way that we treat our children is indicative of the state of our social structure, a measure of the achievement of our civilization or even an index of the degree to which humanism has outstripped the economic motive in everyday life. Similarly, the way that we control our children reflects, perhaps as a continuous microcosm, the strategies through which we exercise power and constraint in the wider society. For Durkheim (1961), quite clearly, the purpose of pedagogic theory and practice, as the formal mode of socialization, is to ensure the quality and achievement of a society through the necessary process of cultural reproduction. For others, like Bourdieu and Passeron (1977), socialization is the mechanism through which we continue to confer power and privilege through the investment of 'cultural capital' by virtue of the unnecessary process of social stratification.

Two dominant themes

Throughout the historical and cross-cultural literature on childhood what seem to emerge are two dominant ways of talking and thinking about children; two traditions of conceptualizing the child that although practically supported and reinforced, at different times, by various religious beliefs, political ideologies, or scientific doctrines, are too old and pervasive to be explained by such cultural regimes. For this reason I shall formulate them as images arising from mythology—myths being the devices that people have always employed to account for anomalies or the inexplicable within their cosmologies. These two images I shall refer to as the *Dionysian* and the *Apollonian* views of childhood. To add to the complexity of these configurations I shall suggest that although they are competitive to the point of absolute incompatibility, within cultures they are used to understand childhood, primarily through history but also synchronically, that is, in parallel at the same time.

The Dionysian image

What I am calling the Dionysian image rests on the assumption of an initial evil or corruption within the child—Dionysus being the prince of wine, revelry, and nature. A major buttress to such imagery can be found in the doctrine of Adamic original sin. Children, it is supposed, enter the world as a willful material force, they are impish and harbour a potential evil. This primal force will be mobilized if, in any part, the adult world should allow them to stray away from the appropriate path that the blueprint of human culture has provided for them. Such children must not fall into bad company, establish bad habits, or develop idle hands—all of these contexts will enable outlets for the demonic force within, which is, of course, potentially destructive not just to the child but of the adult collectivity also. The child is Dionysian inasmuch as it loves pleasure, it celebrates self-gratification and it is wholly demanding in relation to any object, or indeed subject, that prevents its satiation. The intrusive noise that is childhood is expressive of a single-minded solipsistic array of demands in relation to which all other interests become peripheral and all other presences become satellites to enabling this goal.

Christianity has provided a major input to this way of regarding the child even though, as Shipman (1972) has pointed out, the fall in infant mortality through modernity has reduced our urgency and anxiety about their state of grace at an early age. Ariès (1962) has pointed to the sixteenth century view of the child as weak, which was accompanied by the practice of 'coddling', but this was not weak in the sense of vulnerable so much as weak in the form of susceptibility to corruption and being 'easily led'. Parenting consequently consisted in distant and strict moral guidance, through physical direction. Stemming from this period, in the tradition of this image, a severe view of the child sustained, one that saw socialization as a form of combat where the headstrong and stubborn subject had to be 'broken', but all for their own good. This harsh campaign of child rearing persisted through the puritanism of the seventeenth century, and even on into the nineteenth century with an evangelical zeal that sought out and waged war on the depravity of drunkenness, idleness, or childhood wherever it was found. Dickens is a great source of such tales of our institutionalized violence towards the young and Coveney (1957) provides a fine collection and analysis of the exercise of this image of the child throughout literature. In practical terms the Dionysian child was being deafened, blinded, and exploited in factory labour and still being sent up chimneys with brushes as late as 1850—in Britain alone.

It would be convenient to regard what I am calling the Dionysian child as an image of a former time, a set of ideas belonging to a simpler, more primitive people than our own, and to some degree this is so. However, we must not disregard the systematic secular exploration of the soul that has been practised and recommended by psychoanalysis throughout the last century. It was Freud who most recently and forcefully formulated this image of the child through his concept of the *id* and in relation to this theory of childhood sexuality. Of the triumvirate that comprise the self for Freud the *superego* is the possession of the collectivity, the *ego* the realm of the adult, and the *id* the special province of the child (and its immature adult counterpart, 'neurosis'). The *id*, as we know, is that libidinal repository of insatiable desire. It is the dark, driving force which acts as the source of all creativity yet which requires to be quelled or 'repressed' such that people can live in relation to one another and have some regard for the mutual incompatibility of their systems of desire. The social bond resides in this repression; the story and its implications for child rearing are familiar, if more subtle.

The Apollonian image

What now of the Apollonian image of the child, the heir to the sunshine and light, the espouser of poetry and beauty? This does appear much more the modern, Western, but only 'public', way of regarding the child. Such infants are angelic, innocent, and untainted by the world which they have recently entered. They have a natural goodness and a clarity of vision that we might 'idolize' or even 'worship' as the source of all that is best in human nature (note these two metaphors often used to denote the love relation between parent and child). Such children play and chuckle, smile and laugh, both spontaneously but also with our sustained encouragement—we cannot abide their tears and tantrums, we want only the illumination from their halo. It is within this model that we honour and celebrate the child and dedicate ourselves to reveal its newness and uniqueness. Gone are the strictures of uniformity, here with romantic vision, we explore the particularity of the person. Such thinking has been instructive of all child-centred learning and special-needs education from Montessori, the Plowden report (1967), A.S. Neill, and the Warnock report (1978), and indeed much of primary teaching in the last three decades. This Apollonian image lies at the heart of attempts to protect the unborn through legislation concerning voluntary termination of pregnancies and endeavours in the USA to criminalize certain 'unfit' states of motherhood, that is, in the transmission of AIDS or drug addiction to the fetus.

Children in this image are not curbed nor beaten into submission, they are encouraged, enabled, and facilitated. The formalization of the Apollonian child occurs with Rousseau, he is the author of their manifesto *Emile*. It is in this work that he reveals the child's innate and immanent capacity for reason and he instructs us that they have natural virtues and dispositions which only require coaxing out into the open. Rousseau provides a rationale for the idea that children are born good and beyond showing us that each child has a unique potential he states something completely new for its time and formative of the future—that children are different from adults, they are an ontology in their own right and as such they deserve special care and treatment.

Let us be clear, these two images of the child that I have designated as the Dionysian and the Apollonian are not literal descriptions of the way children intrinsically differ from adults, they are no more than images. Yet these images are immensely powerful, they live on and give force to the different discourses that we have about children, they constitute summaries of the ways that we have, over time, come to treat and process children 'normally'. What I am pointing to here is that these images are informative of the shifting strategies that Western society has exercised in its increasing need to control, socialize, and constrain people in the historical transition towards modernity. For this part of the analysis I shall draw on the work of Foucault (1977) in his genealogy of discipline and punishment in modern society which, though not specifically about children, has profound implications for our changing ways of thinking about the child.

Foucault's 'anatomy of power'

Foucault offers us a breakdown of the changes in what he calls the 'anatomy of power' in Western culture, and the pivotal change, he suggests, occurs in the mid-eighteenth century—parallel with Rousseau's announcement of the modern child. What we are offered is a description of two images of discipline, which reflects two modes of control, which are, in turn, aspects of two forms of social integration shifting from an old European order to the new order of modern industrial society. These two images resonate strongly with my depictions of the Dionysian and the Apollonian child. Foucault sets out from the mode of imprisonment characteristic of the 'ancien régime' in France, one rooted in the barbarities of medieval times, and he proceeds to unravel the new penology of the post-revolutionary state, a style of punishment that is premised on very different ideas concerning the nature of correction. The year 1789 did not provide an immediate and dramatic break in continuity, but there was then what might be described as a pre-paradigmatic stage of penology when the more advanced thinkers of the age set out to defame and undermine the old systems of punishment and establish a new system theorized much more in terms of dissuasion. The newly emergent methods of discipline show similarities with and influences from other areas of social life, like the armed forces and the schooling system. So as Sheridan (1980) points out in relation to Foucault's thesis; 'there is an astonishing coincidence between the new prison and other contemporary institutions: hospital, factory, school, and barracks', and for our purposes, regimes of child care.

Foucault's essay begins with an account of the appalling violence and degradation publicly inflicted upon a man found guilty of attempting to murder Louis XV of France. It consists in plucking of the flesh, burning with oil and sulphur, dismembering, and drawing-and-quartering. From this hyperbole of retributive punishment Foucault informs us that this kind of awful spectacle diminishes as we move into the nineteenth century. Through this historical period attention moves away from the execution of punishment to the mechanism of trial and sentence. In essence, excessive symbolism is replaced by rational process. This transition in punishment is taken to reflect an overall change in collective attitudes into a society where there seems to be more kindness and at least an appearance of public humanism. This is matched by a diminution in brutality and a recognition of the impropriety of pain. In terms of judicial regimes this instances a shift from retribution to restitution. Violence against the physical body is gradually transformed into a more subtle and intrusive correction and training of the very soul. The government of the individual in modernity has moved from the outside to the inside.

Clearly the implementation of discipline at the societal level cannot be random and spontaneous, it requires a number of concerted strategies to ensure a uniform application and result. Primary among these is the exercise and manipulation of space. People are controlled in relation to the different spaces they inhabit; discipline works through the division and subdivision of action into spatial units. Think of children having a seat at the table or in the car, being sent to their room, playing outside, going to school, attending school assemblies, working in classes, gymnasia, and, of course, being seated at desks, in rows, in groups, or whatever. The 'reading corner' takes on a new significance. Foucault tells us that the original model for spatial control was the monastery cell or indeed the dungeon—this cellular metaphor extends out into other social institutions. The logistics of modernity turn masses of soldiers into rows of tents or barracks, factories become production lines with workers isolated by task within the division of labour, and hospitals become the classification of sickness on a ward system.

The other major strategy of control is temporal. The whole being of a child is delineated and paced according to a timetable. This too, Foucault tells us, is of monastic origin. The child's rising and sleeping, eating and entertainment, all are prescribed in time. The very idea of a school curriculum is an organization of activities around a political economy of form in relation to content. What people learn is scheduled in relation to decisions about relevance and compulsion. The very practice of being a child is marked out in stages, solidified and institutionalized by Piaget (1932), and conceptualized as 'development'. The implications of an individual's response to such an organization of time is critical to his/her placement on existing hierarchies of merit and achievement, which ultimately relate to the existing system of social stratification and the distribution of life-chances in the wider society. Even the child's body is organized temporally in terms of its ablution, nutrition, excretion, exercise, etc. and all this is homologous to the drilling that occurs in the armed forces and the specialization on the factory floor—these are the modern ergonomics of fitting people to functions.

Power is organized through the combination of strategies, barrages of controlling mechanisms are arranged in tactics, subjects become objects to be gathered, transported, and located through collective action. Foucault agrees with Durkheim before him that the individual emerges from patterns of constraint. Indeed, the character of social structures provides for the possibility of personal expression. The individual, whether adult or child, when rendered object, itself becomes instrumental in the exercise of power—such is the force of ideology, the impersonal impact of ideas upon action. As Deleuze and Guattari (1983) tell us, the modern nuclear family structure is one of the foremost devices for shaping the individual and restricting desire in capitalist societies, and it is psychoanalysis in adulthood that helps to reinforce that restraint.

Childhood and the exercise of power in modern times

Modern power does not exercise itself with the omnipotent symbolism of the scaffold; no longer are we witness to the excessive and triumphant zeal that was directed towards the supposed evil of the Dionysian child. Modern power is calculating, it is suspicious, and it appears always modest in its application. It operates through scopic regimes, through observation that is organized hierarchically, through judgements rendered normative within social structures, and through scrutiny and examination. Observation has become a primary metaphor in the social sciences as it reflects the dominant form of the relations between people, and certainly between adults and the new, visible, Apollonian child. The crudity of the old regime of control in social relations gives way to the modern disciplinary apparatus, the post-Rousseauian way of looking to and monitoring the child in mind and body. Surveillance, in the form of child care, proliferates in its intensity and penetration through the agencies of midwives and health visitors, nurses and doctors, postnatal clinics, schools and teachers, psychometric tests, examinations, educational psychology, counselling, social workers, and so on and on through the layers of scrutiny and isolation; all for the child's own good. The Apollonian child is truly visible, it is most certainly seen and not heard.

Such a social structure Foucault epitomizes through the symbol of the ideal prison, Jeremy Bentham's 'panopticon' (see Foucault 1977). The panopticon, unlike the more familiar 'star' prison, was circular with cells arranged in layers of rings around a central observation tower. Each cell would contain one isolated inmate, illuminated by natural lighting from behind and wholly exposed, through the complete cage of the frontage, to the gaze from the observation tower. The surveillance from the central tower takes place through slots, not illuminated from behind, thus the inmates did not know when, or if, they were being watched. Effectively then, they were being watched all of the time. One might properly suggest that the constant surveillance became a feature of the inmates self-presentation; they watched themselves. The 'panopticon' presents itself at a variety of levels; it was a reality, such institutions were built. Symbolically it is the embodiment of an ideal for maximizing scrutiny and control while minimizing the response or intervention of the controlled; and it stands as an apt metaphor for the exercise of power in modern society—in terms of our interests, socialization, education, child care, and provision. There is a delicacy and rapidity in the management of persons through panopticism.

We might suggest that the Dionysian child is an instance of a social structure where the rules and beliefs are external and consensual, where people are less different, and it is the reaffirmation of their similarities that is at the basis of views on child rearing. The offending or evil child has to be beaten into submission; an external, public act that celebrates and reaffirms the shared values of their age. Any transgression in the form of childish behaviour threatens the very core of the collectivity. To be socialized is to become at one with the normative social structure and so the idea of evil that is projected out into the image of the Dionysian child is in fact providing a vehicle for expunging all sentiments that threaten the sacred cohesion of the adult world. To this end real children in such a society sacrifice their childhood to the cause of the collective adult good. Through such control the growing individual learns a respect for society through the experience of shame.

The Apollonian child, on the other hand, may be seen to occupy a social structure permeated by panopticism. The rules and beliefs are more diffuse, people are more different and isolated, and it is consequently more difficult for them to operate within a sense of shared values. Within such a world people manifest their uniqueness and children must be reared to express what is peculiarly special about their personalities. All of this difference is, of course, subversive and must be policed if collective life is to sustain at all. The control moves subtly in response to such a potentially fragmented social structure; as few symbols are shared externality is an improper arena in which to uphold the sacred. Consequently the control moves inside, from the public to the private, and so we monitor and examine and watch the Apollonian child; he or she in turn learns to watch over themselves and shame is replaced by guilt. The panopticon dream is now complete through the internalization of surveillance in the formation of our children's psyches. The Apollonian projection into childhood now appears as a way of resolving the loss of freedom and creativity in adult life.

Bernstein (1975), drawing on Durkheim's (1964) analysis of simple and complex forms of social organization, provides a further complementary model for an examination of different kinds of relationship between adults and children in the form of different ways of organizing schooling. This, like the ideas of Foucault, is also instructive of different visions of society. Bernstein's work is important in this context because he is precisely addressing the transition that has occurred in our image of the learner (the child) and treating it as indicative of changing standards of normality in modern society. In line with my conception of the Dionysian child and Foucault's 'ancien régime' of punishment, Bernstein describes the 'closed' curriculum, and for the Apollonian/Panopticon the 'open' curriculum. In the transition towards modernity from one form of schooling to another Bernstein tells us that there is a weakening of the symbolic significance and ritualization of punishment. Control in schools becomes more personalized, children are confronted more as individuals, and there is a reduced appeal to shared loyalties. A child's activities are less likely to be prescribed by formal categories such as gender, intelligence, and age but rather by the individual's needs and special qualities. There is an alteration in the authority structure between adult and child, the teacher becomes a problem-poser and the authority resides within the learning material. Thus the act of learning through self-discovery celebrates choice and difference. Overall, the learning child has greater autonomy, higher levels of personal aspiration, and more available choice. Bernstein concludes his analysis by saying that

'None of this should be taken in the spirit that yesterday there was order today only flux. Neither should it be taken as a long sigh over the weakening of authority and its social basis. Rather we should be eager to explore changes in the forms of social integration in order to re-examine the basis of social control.'

This is a significant imperative for any sociological understanding of childhood, that the child is always revealing of the grounds of social control. Thus in one sense we get the children we deserve, or to put it more formally, our historical perspectives on normality in childhood reflect changes in the organization of our social structure.

Therefore when Donzelot (1986) tells us that the child has become the interface between politics and psychology, he is developing a wider argument about the functioning of control in modern life. The contemporary state no longer addresses the polity as a whole but rather treats the family as its basic unit of control. All ideas and practices concerning care, justice, and protection of the child can be seen to be instrumental in the ideological network that preserves the status quo. The 'tutelary complex' that Donzelot describes is one that has become established through the practices of social workers and professional carers, and this complex intrudes into 'difficult' families but treads a careful line between repression and dependency such that the family is preserved as the unit of attention and the house of the child.

Concluding thoughts

I shall conclude this examination of normative perspectives on childhood through the historical process with a useful summary provided by Pollock (1983) in her exhaustive study of histories of childhood. She says that the reasons for the modern view of the child, for the reduction of adults' cruelty towards children, and for the emergent informality of child–adult relationships are fivefold: first, the development of an education system; second, the transformation in the structure of families; third, the expansion of capitalism; fourth, the increasing sophistication of parents; and finally the emergence of a spirit of benevolence.

I am interested to hear this distillation of a whole body of literature on our topic, it does not, however, provide me with a cause for satisfaction. Our next topic has already emerged in the staggering contradiction that is provided amidst this period of enlightenment by the unprecedented boom in reported cases of psychological, physical, and sexual abuse of the same children that we have sought here to understand.

References

Ariès, P. (1962). *Centuries of childhood*. Cape, London.
Bernstein, B. (1975). Open schools, open society. In *Class, codes and control*, Vol. 3. Routledge, London.
Bourdieu, P. and Passeron, J.C. (1977). *Reproduction: in education, society and culture*. Sage, London.
Coveney, P. (1957). *Poor monkey*. Rockcliff, London.
Deleuze, G. and Guattari, F. (1983). *Anti-oedipus*. Viking, New York.
DeMause, L. (ed) (1976). *The history of childhood*. Souvenir, London.
Donzelot, J. (1986). *The policing of families*. Hutchinson, London.
Durkheim, E. (1961). *Moral education*. Free Press, New York.
Durkheim, E. (1964). *The division of labour in society*. Free Press, New York.
Foucault, M. (1977). *Discipline and punish*. Allen Lane, London.
Hillman, J. (1975). *Loose ends*. Spring Publications, New York.
Hoyles, M. (1979). *Changing childhood*. Writers and Readers, London.
Jenks, C. (1982). *The sociology of childhood*. Batsford, London.
Jenks. C. (1989). Social theorising and the child: constraints and possibilities. In *Early influences shaping the individual* (ed. S. Doxiades) NATO Advanced Studies Workshop). Plenum, London.
Mead, M. and Wolfenstein, M. (eds) (1955). *Childhood in contemporary cultures*. Chicago University Press, Chicago.
Piaget, J. (1932). *The language and thought of the child*. Routledge and Kegan Paul, London.
Plowden Report (1967). *Children and their primary schools*. A report of the Central Advisory Council for Education (England) HMSO, London.

Pollock, L. (1983). *Forgotten children*. Cambridge University Press, Cambridge.
Robertson, P. (1976). Home as a nest: middle class children in nineteenth century Europe. In *The history of childhood*. Souvenir, London.
Rose, N. (1989). *Governing the soul: the shaping of the private self*. Routledge, London.
Sheridan, A. (1980). *Michel Foucault: the will to truth*. Tavistock, London.
Shipman, M. (1972). *Childhood: a sociological perspective*. National Foundation for Educational Research, Slough.
Shorter, E. (1976). *The making of the modern family*. Collins, London.
Warnock Report (1978). Committee of inquiry into the education of handicapped children and young people. HMSO, London.

14 Concepts of normality in growth and development

Jean-Claude Vuille and Claes Sundelin

Johan Heinrich Pestalozzi (1746–1827), Charles Darwin (1809–1882), and Sigmund Freud (1856–1939) devoted a scientific interest to children's development during the eighteenth and nineteenth centuries, but true scientific perspectives, conceptual models, and methods for systematic studies of growth and development were established only in this century. Arnold Gesell (1880–1961) introduced studies of child development over time with scientific methods. He was the first to use the expression 'child development' when he described the different age-related stages in development (Gesell 1928).

Studies of growth and development today belong to one or more of six main areas: (1) statistical studies of normality, variation, and deviation related to age; (2) longitudinal cohort studies where the questions of stability and continuity over time of different phenomena are often in focus; (3) studies of learning and behaviour, e.g. modelling through positive and negative reinforcement, the child's way of dealing with intellectual problems in different ages, and the special needs of handicapped children in school; (4) interpretation of behaviour in terms of individual motivation and understanding; (5) the importance of human interaction and transactional processes for normal and abnormal growth and development; (6) holistic or ecological models where growth and development are viewed as phenomena under the influence of a variety of sociocultural, institutional, and family factors.

The different research domains overlap, and there are still many controversial questions about the aetiologic mechanisms of deviations and variations. However, there is also an established knowledge of children's growth and development with relevance across the boundaries of traditional research areas. The following statements express some important aspects of this universal knowledge.

- The general basis of growth and development is closely linked to biological maturing on the cellular level and especially the maturing of the central nervous system. Growth and development of *the child* thus follow a basic plan specific for the human species, but there is also a pattern of growth and development in the individual case which is characteristic of *this* child.

- Different dimensions of development (psychomotor, vision, hearing, speech, and language) interact with each other directly in ways which are easy to understand but also indirectly in ways difficult to detect and understand.

- As a result of constitutional and environmental interaction, development is determined both by internal organizing forces and by personal history and experience.

- The same developmental level may be reached along different developmental paths.

- Growth and development cannot be understood as pure quantitative processes. The changes are in many ways of a qualitative nature.

- There is an intraindividual continuity in both growth and development, but in the individual case the prediction of developmental outcome is as a rule insecure, especially concerning social, emotional, and cognitive development. The possibility of reaching high predictive values is inversely proportional to the length of the observation period covered.

- Factors in the family such as emotional support, level of stimulation, human contact, and affection are of utmost importance for cognitive and social development. Serious social and emotional disadvantages (e.g. family dysfunction with violence, neglect, and sexual abuse) produce developmental abnormalities and/or vulnerabilities. The outcome of vulnerabilities in terms of psychosocial problems depends on the load of precipitating factors (e.g. stress, lack of support and security) in later periods of life (Rutter 1979).

To summarize, development can be looked upon as a question of biological maturation, as a learning process, as a resolution of interactional problems and conflicts, as a cognitive change, and as manifestations of cultural or ecological adaptation. An understanding of different perspectives on growth and development is useful to the clinician striving to understand parent–child adaptation and the parent–child relationships. The clinician must elicit parents' attitudes, concerns, and expectations and their behavioural responses to their child. Support to the family in these respects must be built on a differentiated knowledge of developmental and behavioural paediatrics and close teamwork with child psychologists, child psychiatrists, social workers, etc.

Concepts of normality

In the minds of *parents in general* the terms 'normal' and 'abnormal' are heavily loaded. Most parents hate the idea that their child should not belong to the group of 'normal' kids—even when they are assured that the deviation is slight and of minor importance. For most parents, the concept of 'developmental abnormality' means a life-long condemnation with serious consequences. Health professionals must be aware of their capacity to cause parental anxiety and of the risk of blocking the line for further communication by using normality terms in an uncritical and/or a tactless way. The risk of causing harm is of course much smaller with doctors and nurses who are conversant with a wide normal variation.

Normative data provide information about central tendencies and the range of variables in a specific population. They define what is common and what is uncommon, not what is normal and abnormal. For each set of growth measurements taken from the asymptomatic population, it can be expected, for statistical reasons, that some children will be unusually short and some unusually tall. This occurs in part because the range of normality is defined by somewhat arbitrary statistical limits. If the limits are narrow, the measurements will direct attention to a large number of children, many of whom will prove to conform to the 'norm' on further investigation. If they are wide, the measurements will direct attention to very few 'abnormal' children.

However, most children grow along a predictable pathway mainly determined by the individual genetic endowment. This brings us into contact with the concept of *individual normality* which differs from normality based on cross-sectional population statistics. What is normal for one child is abnormal for another child. In practice, this means that it is usually necessary to have at least two or more serial measurements to make it possible to determine if growth and development are normal for a certain child.

It is necessary to realize that the concept of normality, from other and very important perspectives, has a close connection with *function*. A child is usually quite normal from the functional point of view in spite of 'abnormalities' such as amblyopia or one-sided hearing loss, and even a child with a clear handicap may have a normal function in daily life if the handicap is compensated for through environmental adaptations.

Critical periods

Human anatomical, functional, and psychosocial development is not a steady, linear process. Physical growth is characterized by spurts, separated by periods of apparent stagnation, a process in which every organ has its own growth pattern. Extreme examples include the brain, which reaches 90 per cent of its adult size by six years of age, and the reproductive organs, which remain at an infantile size and shape until puberty. These different patterns result in a unique composition of the human body at every stage, as well as unique characteristics of every developmental period. The particular sensitivity of every organ, during rapid growth, to promoting and disturbing external influences forms the biological basis for the concept of 'critical periods'; periods of increased vulnerability which also offer special chances for the promotion of health and development in a specific area and for the repair of earlier damage.

Examples of specific critical periods

Determinants of the special characteristics of critical periods are the biological programme on the one hand, and nutrition and social influences on the other.

Whereas the former is similar for all human beings—modified by individual genetic equipment—the latter may vary considerably between cultures.

Periods determined mainly by the process of biological maturation

The development of the visual cortex. From animal experiments we know that a disruption of sensory input stops the development of the functional architecture of the respective brain area. Untreated squint in a child leads to amblyopia because the sensory signals from one eye are suppressed in order to avoid double images, with similar consequences on the developing brain as cutting the optic nerve. After the age of eight years, amblyopia is hardly treatable, but before the age of five, the prospects for active intervention are excellent.

Acquisition of language and speech. The immigrant family with children of various ages may serve as a model for the demonstration of critical age for language acquisition. The older the children when moving to a foreign country, the greater the difficulties of incorporating new idioms and the greater the need for formal teaching.

In infants and young children the general speech ability and native language are acquired more or less spontaneously by 'endogenous' production of words and sentences, comparison with and imitation of the corresponding expressions used by adults or other children, through positive reinforcement and meaningful communication, but without any knowledge of grammatical rules (Wells 1981). The clinical importance of disturbances and omissions during this critical period will be further discussed later (see p. 216).

Bladder control. Population studies on bladder control show that the percentage of children still wetting their pants or their bed decreases steeply from the age of two to four years and then flattens out (Largo and Gianciaruso 1978). Active training during the critical period is easy and successful in most cases, whereas the treatment of enuresis after the age of five years is a time-consuming and often frustrating procedure. It is not known, however, whether enuresis at school age actually may be prevented by active training between two and four years of age.

Maternal–infant bonding. The formation of a strong bond between mother and child is thought by most psychologists and paediatricians to constitute an extremely valuable stock to start life with. For human beings it is not an absolute prerequisite for normal development, but it increases the chances for continuity of care and good relationships, and it helps in managing the inevitable crises. In certain animal species, such as the goat, ethologists have demonstrated the existence of a very short critical period just after delivery for this bonding to take place. If the mother is unable to lick the newborn during the first fifteen minutes or so, she will reject him. The famous experiments by Kennell and Klaus

(Kennell et al. 1975) and others have given evidence for similar yet much less dramatic interactions during the first postnatal hour(s) in the human species. This is a rare example of the results of scientific studies having immediate consequences for care practices all over the world. There are probably few delivery rooms left where mothers are not offered the opportunity to caress their children immediately after birth, and few obstetric hospitals without accommodation for mother and baby to be together.

Critical periods mainly determined by social factors

Development of basic trust. Some authors would certainly prefer to insert this section in the group of biologically determined critical periods, because some analogies can also be seen in animals. According to psychoanalytical theory, basic trust (in life, in oneself, in other human beings) constitutes the very fundament of psychological health and is established during the first year(s) of life (Eriksson 1950). Maternal deprivation during this critical period is believed to create irreversible damage with lifelong consequences, for instance on the ability to engage in stable relationships and to assume the role of a mother or a father (Bowlby 1951). Extreme variants of this theory state that even temporary absence of the mother may be harmful. In recent years, however, the foundations of this theory have been questioned in the light of modern epidemiological studies. According to Ernst and von Luckner (1985), it is not the loss of the mother in the first year(s) of life nor any other single traumatic event or institutional care *per se* which predispose to long-lasting psychological damage, but rather continuous or repeated frustrations and abuse during the whole period of childhood. Repair is always possible, love never comes too late.

Periods of transition from one social role to another. One example is the age at which a child enters school. This is a critical point in the life of every child, and causes an immediate restriction of liberty, a change of the daily rhythm, a new challenge in having to cope with social pressure, etc. The age chosen for this dramatic event which may have long-lasting positive and negative effects (e.g. joy of learning and development of new coping skills and hence a positive self-image, but also failure with all its tragic consequences), is not determined by nature, but is rather a political decision.

Another example is the well known acceleration of sexual maturation, the causes of which are not well understood. In the course of a century, the duration of childhood has decreased by about four years, i.e. by one-quarter of its original length. At the same time, the age of entrance into adult life with the acceptance of full social responsibility has been postponed for a couple of years, so that a new 'critical period', occupying about ten years, with its own biological, psychosocial, and cultural characteristics has been created. The health problems of this period are so specific in nature that a new medical specialty, 'adolescent medicine', has been created.

Periods of turmoil and periods of latency. Periods characterized by rapid changes of physical appearance (infancy and puberty) and/or by an increased frequency of vehement conflicts (the stubborn toddler and the turmoil of adolescence) are acknowledged as critical by everybody. It is questionable, however, whether the apparently more harmonious intermediate phases really are periods of latency. Possibly they are just as critical as other segments, but concern the internal processes, as is suggested, for instance, by the finding of a peak in the incidence of depression around the age of nine years (Högberg *et al.* 1986). As yet it is not known whether this is a culture-specific phenomenon or whether it has to be considered as a maturational event.

Family factors

Children's development is affected by the economic resources and welfare of their society, by the cultural and religious values of their immediate community, and by prejudice and discrimination from other groups in society. However, the most powerful effects on development are linked to the resources, attitudes, and values of the family. The family is the most important social system in society. Its requirements and function provide the framework for the development of the young.

The child's attitudes towards himself and his environment are established during the first years of life in relation to those who care for him. Assistance to parents who prove to have difficulties in managing the early contact phase with their children is therefore especially important for child development.

Schools, child care institutions, paediatric clinics, and school medical care units reach virtually all children with various activities. Teachers, preschool teachers, paediatric nurses, and so on observe early signs of problems in the family and discover needs, but as a rule they do not have the means of providing assistance. To promote health and development in all children, it is necessary to establish cooperation between institutions with responsibility for children and structures such as the social security system and adult psychiatry.

From the point of view of equality, some groups of children and young people in all European countries show more unfavourable growth and development than others. The general pattern is such as to make it justifiable to refer to the persistence of the old class society, i.e. the disparities are related to the socioeconomic status of the family and to differences in living conditions (Black 1980). If the parents are unemployed, most studies show that the children's living conditions are less favourable and thereby their growth and development have a tendency to be suboptimal.

In the area of school achievement, children from affluent and well educated families have consistently been observed to surpass the performance of children from poor homes. This difference is related to parental values and behaviour which influence children's intellectual development and achievement motivation.

Middle class and professional class parents have a tendency to assimilate the educational oriented values of society. They themselves have often succeeded in society by virtue of intellectual skills. They are therefore likely to reinforce their children's achievement, to criticize school failures, and to stress goals such as curiosity, consideration, and self-control rather than obedience.

It has been observed that first-borns and only children of preschool age are generally more advanced than others in verbal and intellectual skills. As infants, first-borns are given more attention and affection and interact more with their parents, who generally are also more demanding and more involved with the first-born child. Parental attitudes of this kind, however, enhance the risk of the child developing a more dependent and insecure personality.

Some decades ago, a single-parent family was usually a consequence of birth out of wedlock or parental death. Today divorce is the most common reason for children growing up with one parent, and in many affluent countries the divorce rate is around 30–40 per cent. These days the shaping of a family is obviously not a life project in the same sense as it used to be. The fact that 15 per cent of all Swedish families with children under 17 years of age are one-parent families as a consequence of separation, points in this direction (Swedish Save the Child Foundation and Swedish National Bureau of Statistics 1991).

Clinical data suggest that children's upset over parental disagreement and family disruption is most pronounced during the first year after divorce when poor parenting is also usual. During the next two years most children grow in competence and feeling of control, but hostility and opposition are not uncommon in the longer term, especially among boys. Availability of the male parent, who usually does not have custody, seems to be critical for the child's development, effective school functioning, and self-respect, especially for boys. Previous studies have suggested that growing up in a one-parent family negatively affects intellectual growth and performance and physical and socioemotional development. However, later studies with more sophisticated methods, taking into account confounding factors such as the reason for the father's absence, child care-taking, economic factors, etc. have generally led to the conclusion that the correlation between single parenthood *per se* and developmental deviations and adjustment problems is weak (Wallerstein and Kelly 1980).

The development of speech and language

The development of speech and language is a representative example of the narrow relationship between most complex developmental dimensions and factors in the child's environment. The acquisition of language follows a predictable sequence like other developmental phenomena but speech and language development is one of the dimensions most vulnerable to environmental disadvantages. The rate and progression through linguistic development is sensitive to care-taking practices, emotional atmosphere, and interactional patterns between the child and the care-takers (Tetzchner et al. 1989).

Parents and infants start to produce the base for further development in communication long before the baby can understand or produce a single word or even vocalize. Immediately after birth the child and the care-takers start learning to direct each other's attention to interesting environmental subjects and events, to signal needs and feelings, and to interpret each other's intentions.

True delay in the acquisition of language constitutes a serious developmental dysfunction. During physical examinations doctors and nurses should try to develop a model for communication even with the youngest infant. The information received from the child is of highest diagnostic value even when it is non-verbal.

The clinician in a 'well baby' clinic can help parents to understand that their role is to provide a useful model for communication—not to act as teachers demanding the correct pronunciation and grammar.

When a child fails to speak at two years of age, parents often bring their child to a child health care organization. These concerns should never be dismissed since the parents' observations are almost always relevant and communication skill is central to all human relationships and learning.

Disorders of communication result from a wide variety of causes. More serious delay is often an expression of general developmental delay and an indicator of cerebral dysfunction. The prevalence of communication disorders is difficult to estimate, but seven to ten per cent of the general population are below the norm in one or more aspects of communication, according to population studies (Silva 1980). In a national child development study in England it was reported that 1.4 per cent of children aged seven years had largely unintelligible speech, while a large proportion had some speech disorder (Peckham 1973).

Socially disadvantaged groups with low income, unsatisfactory housing, etc. show higher pervalences of communication disorders in most studies, and boys are generally more often affected than girls, who seem to manifest a certain developmental advantage in communication during early childhood (Silva 1980).

Non-organic failure to thrive (N-FTT)

N-FTT is presented here because it provides an example of the significance of the complex interaction between growth, development, and environmental factors.

Non-organic failure to thrive is defined as a failure of growth without diagnosable organic disease. It is a chronic, potentially life-threatening disorder of infancy and early childhood and a possible diagnosis in all children whose weight (or more specifically weight for height) is below the third percentile when birth weight and mean parental height are within normal limits. The social cost of N-FTT is high because it produces a significant cognitive and behavioural morbidity and contributes significantly to the utilization of paediatric medical care. N-FTT is associated with a significant biological illness—malnutrition—but the aetiology is multifactorial. Among the risk factors known today for developing N-FTT the following are prominent:

- temperament disorders and sickness in the child (affective withdrawal, ambivalence, unpredictability, 'difficult child') (Bithoney and Newberger 1982);
- parental social and psychological problems (social isolation, lack of social network, mental retardation, marital dissatisfaction, misuse of drugs);
- infant feeding problems and other interactional abnormalities between child and care-taker (poverty in interaction, understimulation, overstimulation, asynchronous interaction);
- psychosocial family stress (financial problems, marital strain, major losses, health problems).

A comprehensive medical assessment should include a detailed medical examination but also concurrent nutritional, social, and behavioural evaluations. Developmental assessment and follow-up is an important part of the investigation because developmental delays are very common in connection with N-FTT. Speech, language, and reading delays are most striking (Elmer *et al.* 1969).

Adequately controlled longitudinal follow-up studies of N-FTT suggest that a high percentage of the children will suffer from growth retardation, behavioural and affective problems as well as cognitive impairments.

Treatment of malnutrition is the first goal, but N-FTT cannot be treated successfully without remediation of interactional, behavioural, and social patterns. In contrast to children with malnutrition due to organic disease, children with N-FTT often gain weight rapidly when admitted to hospital and given adequate nutrition and emotional and social care.

Obesity—is pronounced accumulation of fat abnormal?

In contrast to specific diseases such as diabetes or mucoviscidosis, obesity is not a clear cut diagnosis of a disease. Therefore, we must ask who decides whether the accumulation of body fat is to be considered and treated as a disease, and on which criteria this decision should be based.

Statistical aspects. For scientific studies it is necessary to define the subjects as precisely as possible, preferably with quantitative criteria. Popular indices like Broca's or Quetelet's cannot be applied in childhood because of the constant change of body shape during growth. Instead, the standard weight for actual height is determined from a growth chart and the percentage deviation of actual from standard weight is calculated. Usually, a deviation of 20 per cent or more is taken as the criterion for obesity. A more valid but less reliable estimate of the amount of body fat is provided by skin-fold thickness measures.

Medical aspects. From the medical point of view, a condition should be considered as pathological if it predisposes to premature death, to the development of specific diseases, or to serious impairment of the quality of life. The latter criterion is difficult to assess. Some aspects can be described objectively, like performance in sports or participation in social activities, but the concept of quality of life is essentially subjective in nature (see below). Adult obesity in men has been shown to represent a risk factor for hypertension, diabetes, coronary heart disease, and premature death, and since the majority of obese children remain obese into adulthood, many paediatricians consider childhood obesity as a potentially dangerous condition (Mossberg 1989). During childhood, fat children are not more often sick than thin children (Börjesson 1962) with the exception that epiphyseolysis of the hip seems to occur more often with overweight subjects. The indication for a strict medical intervention is thus rather weak. Everybody would agree that the higher the degree of obesity the more urgent the necessity to intervene, but there is no demarcation limit beyond which the indication for intervention is absolute. Some obese children suffer from a latent or overt depression, but it seems as if the depression is as often the cause as it is the consequence of being overweight (see below), so even from the psychiatric point of view, obesity is rather a symptom than a cause of disease.

Subjective aspects. The majority of obese children do not feel sick or even deviant. They may suffer from mobbing (bullying) and from constant reproaches, but if left in peace, many of them feel perfectly happy. During puberty the subjective perception changes. Girls especially begin to notice the deviance of their appearance from the general ideal, and this may cause considerable suffering and a deep wish for change. In boys, the corresponding problems are seen less often. Many obese boys are not only heavier but also taller than their peers, which can provide them with a kind of power which often compensates for the deviation. Many obese adolescents avoid the truth; seeming to prefer to adhere to the wishful image they bear within them. What is normal in all these struggles, what is a healthy and balancing reaction, and what is pathological, unfortunate, or just bad? Should the physician try to destroy the obese adolescents' illusions and educate them towards a more realistic attitude and greater personal responsibility? Or should he respect their right to set their own personal goals, even if we know (or assume) that life could offer them more enjoyment and social participation if they lost weight? Since long-term success of therapeutic interventions is rare, yet not impossible, the answer can only be found individually in every single case. For most obese children, however, the harm produced by being labelled as a patient and not being able to reach the expected goal exceeds the achievable benefits, so the degree of actual (not potential) suffering from the consequences of obesity should be the primary criterion for the medicalization of this variant of physical appearance.

Aetiology

Twin studies, epidemiological surveys, and experimental investigations have identified a number of aetiological factors, pathogenetic mechanisms, and contributory social conditions. The relative importance of each of these contributing factors is not well established. Clinical and scientific evidence suggests that aetiology varies considerably between individuals. The hierarchical connections between the various factors are represented in the four-level model proposed by Vuille and Mellbin (1979), see Fig. 14.1. Of special interest in the present context is the importance of psychological and social factors. Scientific studies have produced conflicting results, which led Leon and Roth (1977) to conclude that 'the evidence strongly suggests that obesity is not a unitary syndrome. It

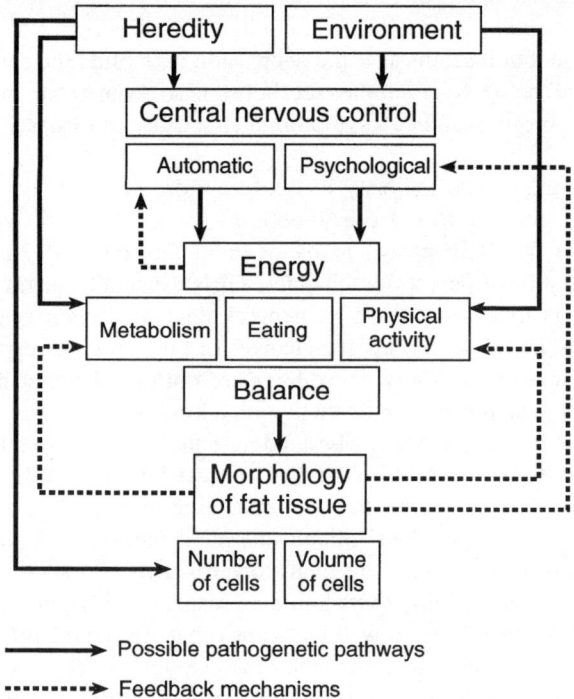

Fig. 14.1 A four-level model for the aetiology of obesity in children.

appears that research efforts would be more profitable if the type of obese person being studied were carefully specified'. As Mellbin and Vuille (1989 a, b) have shown, one important aspect to consider is the pattern of fat accumulation during school age. In children who became overweight very rapidly, significantly more signs of psychosocial stress of various kinds were found than in children with normal weight, constant overweight of early onset, or overweight developing slowly during school age. Evidence was presented suggesting that the association between psychosocial stress and rapidly developing overweight is causal. A recent study from the USA, where a dramatic increase in the prevalence of childhood obesity was observed, demonstrated a strong association with the number of hours spent watching television. None of the other environmental factors studied were able to explain the trend (Dietz et al. 1990). These studies open important avenues towards prevention, even if the basic causal mechanisms are genetically determined.

Interventions: indications, strategies, open questions

In the section on obesity, the dilemma of medical intervention in a condition which is neither clearly pathological nor absolutely normal has been discussed. Here the main problem was the insufficient therapeutic effectiveness along with the possible harmful effects of being labelled as abnormal. Similar considerations may apply in other disturbances of growth and development.

Linear growth

The availability of biosynthetic growth hormone has created the possibility for medical treatment of an increasing number of children with 'linear growth retardation'. The treatment requires medication, with repeated injections over many years, so that the originally healthy child becomes a true patient. In view of these consequences and the potentially harmful pharmacological side-effects of the treatment, 'growth on demand' can certainly never become a service to be offered by paediatricians. On the other hand, children who suffer from true growth hormone deficiency should have the right to receive the substitution which is now available. Unfortunately, there are no tests which enable a reliable distinction to be made between normal and insufficient growth hormone secretion, so very careful overall evaluation has to be made in every case, including the height of the parents, pre-treatment growth velocity, bone age, predicted height, exclusion of other possible medical causes (chromosome anomaly, hypothyroidism, etc.) (Girard 1990). In most cases, even this will not yield an unequivocal answer, and the paediatrician has to face the difficult task of evaluating the motivation of the parents and the child and of balancing the child's capability of adapting against the possibly harmful pharmacological and psychological side-effects of the medication.

Early intervention with developmentally retarded children

During the last three decades, a variety of different national and local programmes for the early identification of children with retarded motor and/or mental development have been created, based on the established knowledge that the development of a child is dependent on the amount and kind of environmental stimuli, and on the assumption that these stimuli can be shaped and adapted to the needs of the individual child by means of professional intervention. An attempt to review the background, the content, the mode of operation, and the outcome of all these programmes would result in a book of its own, and therefore, only a few very general statements can be presented here.

- It is indisputable that every child should be given the *chance for optimal development* of his or her inherent potential. Early identification and promotion measures may help to increase this chance. However, experience and research have revealed a number of problems.

- The correct *diagnosis and prediction* of a child's developmental progress is difficult. Screening tests have been found to be of limited value when long-term perspectives are taken as criteria for validation. An excellent review of this problem has been presented by Dworkin (1989), who recommends, instead of formal screening tests, a system of continuous health surveillance, using all available information, including parent's reports, health visitor's observations, general health status, overall developmental assessment, and tests in questionable cases.

- With respect to the *outcome* of systematic early training programmes, available evidence is conflicting. For some specific forms of developmental delay, such as motor disturbance, including early signs of cerebral palsy, or retardation of speech development, supporting measures have been arranged and become generally accepted before their effectiveness had been demonstrated in controlled studies. After several years of operation and general satisfaction among professionals and parents, it is considered unethical to conduct controlled studies in which the possible beneficial effects of such a programme would be withheld for certain children. The results of those studies that have been performed do not give definite answers. Greater progress than that expected without intervention is achievable, but not every training action offers a clear benefit to every child. In general, however, parents are satisfied that somebody is really caring and working actively with their child, thus sharing the responsibility with them. This is especially important in cases where the disability is obvious or where the child's behaviour is a source of constant irritation and frustration in the family. The situation is much more difficult if a developmental delay is suspected by professional only, but the parents perceive their child as normal. In such cases, only programmes of proven value should be recommended.

- One of the most important factors for the maintenance of achieved progress appears to be the *active involvement of the parents* (Bronfenbrenner 1970). Possible negative effects of parent training have been observed, however. Care has to taken that parents of retarded children are not trained just to execute a plan designed by professionals, because this would make them more directive and less observing and responsive in their interaction with the child. This is undesirable in the light of results of observational studies showing that the development of children is enhanced if parents are able to respond to and reinforce the children's own initiatives.

- *Early identification and training programmes may be misused in a competitive society* to increase the pressure on children performing below the official standard, and their parents. Politicians may assign high priority to such measures as a promising solution to the problem of inequality of chances, thereby disengaging society from the responsibility of providing opportunities for a meaningful and enriching life for all human beings, including those with poor mental capacities.

As a general conclusion it can be stated that modern social or community paediatrics cannot do without deliberate intervention for early identification and treatment of children with special developmental needs. For those cases where these needs are obvious to everyone, the community should provide a variety of treatment and training programmes including support, advice, and cautious training of the parents. The best available methods should be selected, but the requirements, with respect to proven effectiveness in terms of enhanced developmental progress, should not be set too high. On the other hand, specific individual developmental stimulation of children with only a suspected developmental delay should, whenever possible, take place within the mainstream of health and education support in order to avoid the possible negative effects of labelling. If special programmes are started for this purpose, their effectiveness, with respect to the outcome promised to the parents, has to be proven.

References

Bithoney, W. and Newberger, E. (1982). Non-organic FTT; developmental and familial characteristics. *Pediatr. Res.* **16**, 84A.
Black, D. (1980). *Inequalities in health* (Report of a working group chaired by Sir Douglas Black). Department of Health and Social Security, London.
Bowlby, J. (1951). *Maternal care and mental health* (WHO Monograph Series). WHO, Geneva.
Brofenbrenner, U. (1970). *Two worlds of childhood.* Russel Sage Foundation, New York.
Börjesson, M. (1962). Overweight children. *Acta Paediatr. Scand.* **51** (Suppl. 132).
Dietz, W.H.B., Bandini, L.G. and Gortmaker, S. (1990). Epidemiologic and metabolic risk factors for childhood obesity. *Klin. Pädiatr.* **202**, 69–72.

Dworkin, P.H. (1989). British and American recommendations for developmental monitoring: the role of surveillance. *Pediatrics* **84**, 1000–10.

Elmer, E., Gregg, G.S., and Ellison, P. (1969). Late results of the 'failure to thrive' syndrome. *Clin. Pediatr.* **8**, 584.

Eriksson, E.H. (1950). *Childhood and society*. W.W. Norton, New York.

Ernst, C. and von Luckner, N. (1985). *Stellt die Frükindheit die Wiechen?* Forum der Psychiatrie. F. Enke, Stuttgart.

Gesell, A. (1928). *Infancy and human growth*. Macmillan, New York.

Girard, J. (1990). Grandir à la demande? *Med. et Hyg.* **48**, 2931–6.

Högberg, G.L., Langerheim B., and Sennerstam, R. (1986). 9-årskrisen speglad på habiliteringen, barnläkarmottagningen och PBU. *Lakartidnigen*, **83**, 2038–42.

Kennell, J.H., Trause, M.A., and Klaus M.H. (1975). Evidence for a sensitive period in the human mother. In *Parent–infant interaction* (ed. R. Porter and M. O'Conner). Associated Scientific Publishers, Amsterdam.

Largo, R.H., Gianciaruso, M. and Prader, A. (1978). Die Entwicklung der Darm- und Blasenkontrolle von der Geburt bis zum 18, Lebensjahr. *Schweiz Med. Wschr.* **108**, 155–60.

Leon, G.R. and Roth, L. (1977). Obesity: psychological causes, correlations, and speculations. *Psychol. Bull.* **84**, 117–39.

Mellbin, G.R. and Vuille, J.-C (1989*a*). Rapidly developing overweight in school children as an indicator of psychosocial stress. *Acta Paediatr. Scand.* **78** 568–75.

Mellbin, T. and Vuille, J.-C. (1989*b*). Further evidence of an association between psychosocial problems and increase in relative weight. *Acta Paediatr. Scand.* **78**, 576–80.

Mossberg, H.O. (1989). 40 year follow-up of overweight children, *Lancet*, 491–3.

Peckham, C.S. (1973). Speech defect in a national sample of children aged seven years. *Br. J. Dis. Comm.* **8**, 2.

Rutter, M. (1979). Maternal deprivation: 1972–1978. New findings, new concepts, new approaches. *Child Devel.* **50**, 283.

Silva, P. (1980). The prevalence, stability and significance of developmental language delay in preschool children. *Dev. Med. Child Neurol.* **22**, 768.

Swedish Save the Child Foundation and Swedish National Bureau of Statistics (1991). *Facts about Sweden*. Swedish Save the Child Foundation, Stockholm.

Tetzchner, S., Siegel, L.S., and Smith, L. (1989). *The social and cognitive aspects of normal and atypical language development* (Progress in cognitive development research). Springer, New York.

Wallerstein, J. and Kelly J. (1980). *Surviving the breakup: how children and parents cope with divorce*. Basic Books, New York.

Vuille, J.-C. and Mellbin, T. (1979). Obesity in 10-year-olds: an epidemiologic study. *Paediatrics.* **64**, 564–72.

Wells, G. (1981). *Learning through interaction*. Cambridge University Press.

15 Risk and risk-taking in adolescents
Vivien Igra and Charles E. Irwin, Jr

Risk-taking behaviour in adolescents

The second decade of life is a time of exploration and growth. Experimentation during the adolescent years establishes competence and confidence. Experimentation in a potentially hazardous context, however, may jeopardize the adolescent's future.

This chapter is concerned with risk-taking behaviour in adolescents. Specifically, the chapter will review the theoretical structure underlying the study of these behaviours, the nature of particular risk-taking behaviours, the prevalences and consequences of risk-taking behaviours, and how some of these behaviours co-vary. In addition, populations of adolescents who are engaging in particularly high rates of risk-taking behaviours will be considered, as will efforts to prevent and curtail risk-taking behaviours and their consequences for adolescents.

In the context of the chapter, adolescence refers to the chronologic period between 12 and 20 years. Primarily data from the USA are presented in a variety of age intervals depending on available statistical breakdowns. Every effort will be made to give prevalences that pertain specifically to the adolescent age group. However, some data will necessarily include young adults (up to 24 years of age). Data provided by ethnicity or race should be interpreted with caution as they are not, as a rule, stratified by socio-economic status and therefore may actually reflect class, geographic, or other differences rather than ethnic or racial distinctions.

A definition of risk-taking behaviour

In the course of healthy adolescent development, competence is enhanced through experimentation and taking chances within a controlled or positive context. These adaptive, exploratory behaviours can be distinguished from what has been traditionally known as risk-taking behaviour in that the latter is associated with negative health-related consequences (Irwin 1987). Examples of such risk-taking behaviours include sexual activity, substance use, and behaviours causing unintentional injury.

Negative consequences of substance use include academic failure, addiction, curtailed employment opportunities, AIDS, and increased risk of acquiring other sexually transmitted diseases (STDs). Sexual activity during adolescence may result in unintended pregnancy and STDs. Injury risk behaviours may result in permanent disability or death. These behaviours tend to co-vary in complex ways depending on age, gender, and ethnicity or race.

For purposes of this chapter, risk-taking behaviours will refer to volitional behaviours and not behaviours that are the result of psychopathology (e.g. suicide or eating disorders) or environmental forces that are beyond the patient's control (e.g. homicide). The chapter is based mainly on US data but, whenever possible, European data will be presented for comparison.

Theoretical models

Problem behaviour theory

A number of theories have been developed to explain adolescent participation in risk-taking behaviours and to predict those at greatest risk. Jessor's (Jessor and Jessor 1977) 'problem behaviour theory' relates conventionality to decreased 'proneness' to risk behaviour. The theory suggests that adolescents whose values and behaviours conform to conventional societal norms are less likely to engage in risk-taking behaviour. Jessor further suggests that problem behaviour represents a syndrome such that adolescents who engage in one type of risk behaviour are more likely to engage in others.

The theory encompasses three systems of explanatory variables: personality, perceived environment, and behaviour. In the personality system, unconventionality is reflected by a lower value on achievement compared with independence, greater attitudinal tolerance for deviance, and lower religiosity. In the perceived environmental system, unconventionality involves the relative predominance of peer influence over parental influence, lower disapproval by parents of problem behaviour, and greater involvement of peers in problem behaviour.

Unconventionality in the behaviour system is determined by a greater involvement in problem behaviours and less involvement with school activities and church attendance. The greater the unconventionality across the three systems, the greater the proneness to engage in problem behaviour, such as substance use and sexual activity. Recently, Jessor (1991) has expanded his model to include biological factors such as genetic predispositions and protective factors that may mitigate risk 'proneness' in otherwise moderate to high risk youth.

The biopsychosocial model

The 'biopsychosocial model' of risk-taking behaviour suggests that there are biological, psychological, and social factors that contribute to the propensity toward risk behaviours (Irwin and Millstein 1986). Specific biological variables include pubertal timing, hormonal effects, and genetic predispositions. A number of studies have noted, for example, that earlier maturing girls are more likely to initiate sexual activity than their age-matched peers (Shafer et al. 1984; Phinney et al. 1990). In addition, Udry (Udry and Billy 1987; Udry 1988) has suggested that testosterone levels may be related to sexual behaviour in adolescent boys. Finally, recent studies support the role of genetic predisposition to substance abuse, particularly alcohol (Newcomb and Bentler 1989).

Psychological variables include self-esteem, sensation seeking, cognitive and affective states. Orr and others (1989) found that sexual experience was associated with a decrease in self-esteem for adolescent girls. Gaines (1981; in Werner 1991) found that individuals drink alcohol to alter their present condition and make it congruent with a desired condition. Cognitive functioning as measured by decreased school performance is associated with initiation of sexual activity (Irwin 1993). Depression has been associated with substance use in both girls and boys (Werner 1991; Covey and Tam 1990).

Social variables include the roles that peers, parents, and school play in the adolescent's life. Adolescent risk-taking behaviour may be influenced by family structure, communication, emotional closeness, and accepted norms. Adolescents from single-parent families may be less likely to use car seat-belts (Saucier and Ambert 1983), more likely to use substances (Turner et al. 1991), and more likely to initiate intercourse than youth from two-parent households (Newcomer and Udry 1987).

Close relationships between adolescents and their parents seem to deter risk-behaviour. Adolescents who report poor communication with their parents are more likely to initiate intercourse, smoking, and drinking at earlier ages than are adolescents who report good communication (Jessor and Jessor 1977). Parental influence appears to decrease with increasing age of the adolescent and peer influences predominate in later adolescence. Adolescents who remain in school are less likely to engage in risk-taking behaviours than their peers who drop out.

Risk-taking and development

Both the biopsychosocial and problem behaviour theories are developmentally based. They assume that risk-taking behaviours evolve over time and may fulfil developmental needs such as autonomy, mastery, and intimacy (Irwin and Millstein 1986).

According to Jessor, problem behaviour in adolescence should be seen as being 'purposeful, meaningful, goal-oriented, and functional rather than arbitrary or perverse' (Jessor 1982). Further, Jessor asserts that these behaviours may serve as (a) an instrumental effort to attain goals that are blocked or seem otherwise unattainable; (b) a way of expressing opposition to adult authority and conventional society whose norms and values are no longer shared by the younger generation; (c) a way of coping with anxiety, frustration, and failure, or with the anticipation that failure is likely; or (d) a way of expressing solidarity with peers, of gaining access to the peer group, and of demonstrating identification with the youth subculture.

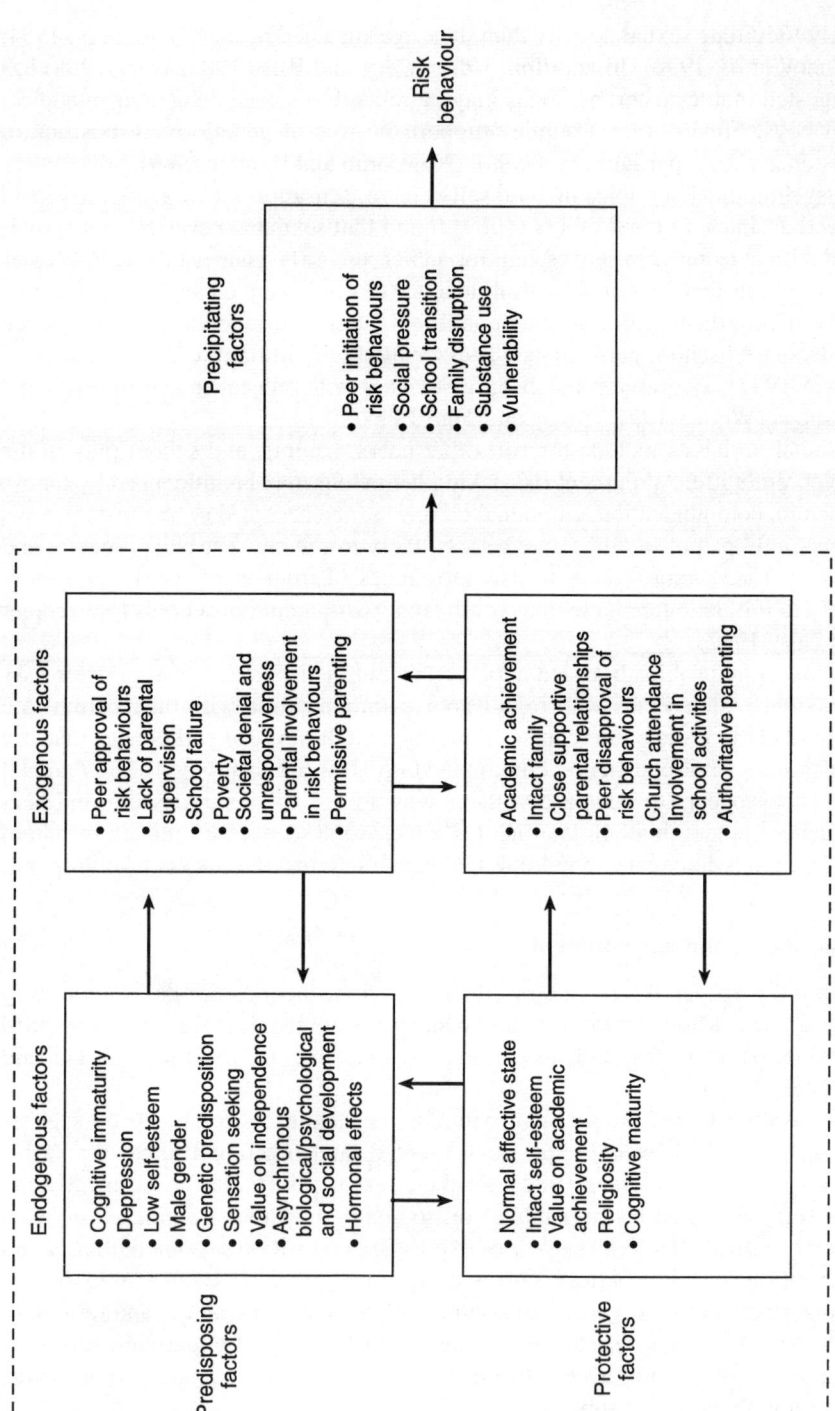

Fig. 15.1 A hypothetical model for adolescent risk-taking behaviour.

Normal adolescent development encompasses increasing independence, autonomy from the family, greater peer affiliation and importance, sexual awareness, and identity formation as well as physiologic maturation. In the context of the above developmental theoretical framework, these changes help explain the rise in risk-taking behaviour observed with advancing chronologic age during adolescence.

Figure 15.1 illustrates a hypothetical model for risk-taking behaviour in adolescents. The model highlights critical factors both endogenous (biopsychosocial) and exogenous (environmental) that are protective or predisposing toward risk-taking behaviour.

Individual risk-taking behaviours

Unintentional injury related behaviour

Unintentional injuries are the leading cause of 'years of productive life lost' (YPLL) for all ages in the US. The United States experiences a higher YPLL rate associated with injury than Japan, France, West Germany, and the United Kingdom (Guyer and Ellers 1990). Accidental injuries were the leading cause of death for adolescents 15 to 19 years in 48 of 58 countries surveyed for males and 31 of 58 countries for females (Taket 1986).

Injury accounts for 77 per cent of the total fatalities among adolescents and young adults 15 to 24 years of age in the US (National Center for Health Statistics 1992). Death rates in adolescents and young adults due to all other causes declined between 1930 and 1980; but deaths due to injuries increased (Paulson 1988). The overwhelming majority of these fatal injuries involved motor vehicles.

Motor vehicles

Injuries to motor vehicle occupants are the major cause of childhood injury resulting in death in the United States. The death rate for motor vehicle occupants aged 15 to 19 years is 10 times greater than the other paediatric age groups (Centers for Disease Control 1990c). Twice as many male as female adolescents are killed in motor vehicle crashes (Centers for Disease Control 1990b).

As drivers, teenagers contribute disproportionately to motor vehicle fatalities, having the highest rates per licenced driver. In 1987, 16 to 19 year olds constituted eight per cent of the population and 14 per cent of drivers in fatal crashes in the US (Williams and Carsten 1989). Adolescent drivers are more likely to be in single-vehicle crashes than are other drivers. In addition, 50 per cent of crashes involving adolescent drivers occur between 9 p.m. and 6 a.m., 58 per cent occur on weekends, and, because adolescents tend to carry more passengers than older drivers, 63 per cent of fatally injured adolescent passengers sustain their injuries in cars driven by other adolescents (Agran *et al.* 1990). Motor vehicle injury mortality rates among adolescents 15 to 19 years of age in the US exceed rates in France, Canada, Norway, and England and Wales, and are twice those of The Netherlands (Williams and Kotch 1990).

Although death rates from motor vehicle injuries are higher in the US than in most developed countries, when mortality rates are adjusted for injury exposure, the US is among the safest countries in which to drive. Large numbers of vehicles travelling greater distances result in a higher aggregate risk. This suggests that decreasing the number of 'person-miles' driven could have a positive impact on the rising motor-vehicle related mortality in the US (Rockett and Smith 1989).

Motorcycles

Ninety per cent of all motorcycle accidents in the US, result in injury or death, compared with nine per cent for all motor vehicle accidents. Fifty-five per cent of all motorcycle deaths occur in 15 to 24-year-olds. Males have a death rate that is 20 times that of females. Most motorcycle fatalities occur on Friday and Saturday in the late afternoon and early evening (Paulson 1988). Compared to a rider with a helmet, the bare-headed motorcyclist involved in a collision is twice as likely to sustain a head injury and three times as likely to die as a result of the injury (Halperin *et al.* 1983).

Bicycles

Death rates for bicyclists peak at 11 to 15 years of age (Paulson 1988). Males outnumber females 2:1 among those injured in bicycle accidents. In one study, a third of bicycle accident victims admitted to riding in a hazardous manner (riding too fast or doing tricks or stunts on the bicycle). In that same study, a third of the victims suffered head and neck trauma and fewer than one per cent were wearing any protective gear (including helmets) at the time of the accident, even though eight per cent said they owned such equipment (Selbst 1987).

Drowning

Drowning, the fourth leading cause of childhood fatal injury in the US, is most common in children under four years and males aged 15 to 19 years (Centers for Disease Control 1990*c*). Males comprise 92 per cent of drowning deaths among 15 to 19 year old adolescents (Centers for Disease Control 1990*b*). Adolescent drownings are distinguished from drownings in younger children in that the former seldom occur in swimming pools. They are more likely to occur in rivers, canals, and lakes. Even in states in the US with substantial coastlines, the vast majority of adolescent drownings occur in fresh water (Wintemute 1990). Many involve boating incidents, and alcohol use has been implicated in 40–50 per cent of drownings among male adolescents (Centers for Disease Control 1990b).

Drowning rates for males aged 15 to 19 years in the US exceed drowning rates for Canadian male youth by 50 per cent and are two to five times greater than rates among adolescent males in other European countries including The Netherlands, France, England and Wales, and Norway (Williams and Kotch 1990).

Firearms

From 1984 to 1988 the firearm death rate for 15- to 19-year-olds increased 43 per cent to 17.7 deaths per 100 000, the highest level to date. Increases were concentrated among black males for whom both the firearm death rate and the firearm homicide rate more than doubled. Although homicide and suicide predominate as causes of firearm mortality, unintentional firearm death remains a significant threat with its highest incidence among 15 to 19-year-old males (National Center for Health Statistics 1991).

Unintentional firearm mortality rates among 15- to 19-year-olds in the US are almost twice those of Canadian youth and at least five times the rate found among 15- to 19-year-old youth in France, England and Wales, Norway, and The Netherlands (Williams and Kotch 1990).

Sexual behaviour

Heterosexual sexual activity

In 1988, in the US, approximately one-quarter of adolescent females of all races and white adolescent males had experienced heterosexual intercourse at least once by their 15th birthdays. A third of Hispanic males and two thirds of black males were sexually experienced by age 15 (Centers for Disease Control 1991a; Sonenstein et al. 1989). The proportion of adolescents 15 to 19 years of age in the US who reported being sexually experienced increased steadily from 1982 to 1988. Among adolescent females the proportion reporting premarital intercourse increased from 47 per cent in 1982 to 53 per cent in 1988 (Forrest and Singh 1990). Approximately a third of that increase occurred between 1985 and 1988 (Centers for Disease Control 1991a).

The largest increases in rates of sexual activity occurred among the youngest adolescent females, white, and non-poor adolescents. The disproportionate increase in sexual activity among white and non-poor adolescent women narrowed the racial and income differences with respect to sexual activity.

In 1988, adolescent females who claimed to have had sexual intercourse earlier in life reported greater numbers of sex partners. Among 15 to 24 year old women who initiated intercourse before age 18, 75 per cent reported having had two or more partners and 45 per cent reported having had four or more partners.

By contrast, only 20 per cent of women initiating intercourse after age 19 years reported having had more than one partner (Centers for Disease Control 1991*a*).

Among young males aged 17 to 19 years, the proportion claiming to have had sexual intercourse increase from 66 per cent in 1979 to 76 per cent in 1988 (Sonenstein *et al.* 1991). Black adolescent males aged 15 to19 years were more likely to report younger ages at first intercourse than were white or Hispanic adolescent males. Thirty-five per cent of black males had had intercourse by their 14th birthday, compared to seven per cent of whites and six per cent of Hispanics (Sonenstein *et al.* 1991).

Sexually experienced males 15 to 19 years of age reported having had an average of five lifetime partners. Black males reported having had significantly more partners both in the previous 12 months and in their lifetimes than white or Hispanic male youth. However, these differences largely disappeared when the number of years since initiation of intercourse was taken into account.

In 1988, 21 per cent of sexually active young males reported more than one partner in any month in the prior year and only five per cent reported multiple partners for six months or more out of the past 12. Male youth were more likely to have a series of monogamous relationships than to have multiple concurrent partners (Sonenstein *et al.* 1991).

Little is known about sexual behaviour among adolescents other than heterosexual vaginal intercourse. Rates of heterosexual anal intercourse among youth ranged from 12 to 26 per cent in several small samples, with rare if any condom use reported (Irwin and Shafer 1992).

Homosexual sexual activity

There is no national data on same-gender sexual behaviour among adolescents in the US. A study conducted in a New York City high school found that ten per cent of females and nine per cent of males reported same-gender sexual behaviour (Reuben *et al.*1988). In addition, retrospective data from adult homosexual and bisexual men indicate that half had initiated same-gender sexual behaviour by age 16 (Haverkos *et al.* 1989).

Contraception

Age at first intercourse is closely related to the use of contraception. In 1988, only 39 per cent of women 15 to 44 years who had first intercourse before age 15 reported using any method of contraception, compared to 56 per cent of those who delayed intercourse until they were 19 years or older (Mosher and McNally 1991). In 1982, 48 per cent of sexually experienced women 15 to 19 years of age reported using a contraceptive method at their first intercourse. This proportion increased to 65 per cent in 1988 almost entirely as a result of increased condom use (Forrest and Singh 1990).

White adolescent females and those who were non-poor were more likely than any other group to have partners who used condoms at first intercourse—52 per cent in 1988 compared to 42 per cent among poor and Hispanic adolescent females. Among black females only 35 per cent had first intercourse with partners who used condoms (Forrest and Singh 1990).

In 1988, 57 per cent of sexually active males aged 15 to 19 years reported that they had used a condom the last time they had intercourse. Twenty per cent of sexually active male youth said that their partner had used an effective female method of contraception (oral contraceptives, IUDs, diaphragms, or spermicide) without a condom and 23 per cent reported either use of an ineffective method or no method of contraception the last time they had intercourse. Black youth had higher rates of condom use at last intercourse than white or Hispanic youth (Sonenstein *et al.* 1989).

In Italy in 1990, 23 per cent of high school students 14 to 19 years of age in a semi-urban area (13 miles south of Rome) reported that they were sexually active, a proportion significantly lower than among adolescents in other European countries and in the US (Centers for Disease Control 1991*c*). Fifty-four per cent of male Italian adolescents and 37 per cent of female Italian adolescents reported always using condoms.

Tobacco, alcohol, and substance use

Use of illicit substances among adolescents has declined in the US since the late 1970s. However, alcohol and tobacco use has remained high. In 1990, half of 15–19-year-olds surveyed reported that they had used an illicit substance at sometime in their lives. A third had used marijuana and one in ten had used cocaine. Ninety per cent of high school seniors reported having consumed alcohol and two-thirds of 15–19 year olds reported smoking cigarettes at some time in their lives.

Tobacco use is the single most preventable cause of death in the US. The majority of adult smokers began smoking cigarettes before 18 years of age. The age at initiation of cigarette smoking has declined for every successive birth cohort in the US since 1930. Those who begin smoking at younger ages are more likely to become heavier smokers and are at increased risk of smoking-attributable illness or death (Centers for Disease Control 1991*d*).

International rates of smoking experience among adolescent men range from a low of approximately ten per cent in Tahiti and Brazil to more than 70 per cent in Japan, Senegal, Nigeria, and Greece. Smoking-experience rates among adolescent women are lowest in Korea, China, and Ethiopia and highest in Greece and Uruguay (Blum 1991).

In Greece in 1988, 70 per cent of students 14 to 19 years of age had smoked cigarettes in the past. Ninety-five per cent of Greek high school students had consumed alcohol in the past year. Almost half of Greek students 17 to 18 years of age reported drinking heavily within the past month. Alcohol consumption by Greek youth declined between 1984 and 1988. However, lifetime prevalence of illicit substances including marijuana, cocaine and heroin increased by 20 per cent among male Greek youth and rates of current use (in the previous month) of illicit substances doubled for both sexes from 1984 to 1988 (Kokkevi and Stefanis 1991).

Alcohol is the drug most often abused by the largest number of children and adolescents. Alcohol has been implicated in deaths from motor vehicle accidents, drowning, fire-related mortalities, and fatal falls (American Academy of Pediatrics 1987).

Rates of adolescent substance use are lower in Sweden than in the US and Greece. In a recent survey of 3500 Swedish youth aged 13 to 18, 35 per cent reported using alcohol, 14 per cent reported using cigarettes, and one per cent reported using illicit drugs (Kelly et al. 1991).

Experimentation with substances commonly begins in early adolescence with the greatest proportion of substance use initiated in the mid to late teens. The major risk for initiation of cigarette, alcohol, and marijuana use is completed for the most part by age 20 and for illicit drug use by 21. Those who have not experimented with any of these substances by age 21 are unlikely to do so thereafter (Kandel and Logan 1984).

For adolescent substance use, past behaviour is often the best predictor of future behaviour. Specifically, similar but less serious substance use has been found to predict subsequent use of more serious substances (Newcomb et al. 1986). Longitudinal studies of adolescent substance use initiation and progression have demonstrated fairly consistent sequences of drug involvement. Adolescent tobacco and/or alcohol use precedes marijuana use. (The impact of cigarette smoking on the progression to higher stages of substance use is greater for adolescent females than for male youth.) Furthermore, few adolescents will try other illicit substances without prior use of marijuana (Yamaguchi and Kandel 1984a).

The influence of alcohol and tobacco use on subsequent marijuana use is independent of age. However, the earlier adolescents begin using marijuana the more likely they are to use other illicit substances (Yamaguchi and Kandel 1984a).

In a study involving initiation of cocaine use over a five-year period in Los Angeles, Newcomb and Bentler (1986) found that alcohol use preceded marijuana use by a year. Marijuana use was an important predictor of cocaine use in the following year.

Factors associated with individual risk-taking behaviour

In the preceding sections, many of the factors associated with risk-taking behaviour have been considered. They are briefly summarized here.

Gender

Boys are more likely than girls to engage in risk-taking behaviour. There are twice as many boys as girls killed in motor vehicle accidents during adolescence. The ratio rises to 1 in 10 for drownings and 1 in 20 for motorcycle fatalities.

Adolescent boys become sexually active earlier and report more partners than girls, though there is evidence for an increase in rates of sexual activity in girls relative to boys. Smoking, alcohol consumption, and use of illicit substances are all higher in adolescent boys. However, there is a trend in Europe for increasing numbers of adolescent girls to take up smoking (Chollet-Traquet 1992).

Age

Risk taking in adolescence increases with age. The 1990 US Youth Risk Behaviour Study showed that the proportion of the high school students drinking alcohol increased sharply with age, as did the proportion using marijuana and other illicit substances. Sexual activity is influenced by the age of physical maturation: girls who mature earlier have earlier menarche and are more likely to be sexually active at younger ages (Phinney *et al.* 1990; Shafer *et al.* 1984). Among males, sexual debut has been associated with increasing levels of testosterone (Udry and Billy 1987).

Adolescents initiating coitus at earlier ages are less likely to use effective contraception and to have multiple partners, with the result that they are at increased risk of sexually transmitted diseases and unwanted pregnancy.

Socio-economic status and ethnicity

As previously stated, differences between ethnic groups should be interpreted with caution, as they may reflect the influence of socio-economic status. Lower socio-economic status is associated with higher levels of risk-taking behaviour, though the increased rate of sexual activity in non-poor adolescent girls suggests that the differences, at least in sexual activity, may be narrowing.

In 1988, 25 per cent of 15–19 year old girls from poor families in the US did not use any contraceptive methods, compared with 17 per cent of girls from families with higher incomes. In the UK, teenage pregnancy is strongly correlated with low income (Smith 1993). However, part of the difference may be accounted for by higher abortion rates among girls from families with higher incomes (Smith 1993). The increase in smoking among adolescent girls in northern Europe affects particularly girls from low income families (Chollet-Traquet 1992).

In the US, black adolescents have an earlier mean age at sexual debut than white or hispanic youths. The differences between the groups, however, have narrowed in recent years. Contraceptive choices also differ by ethnicity. Hispanic males between 15 and 19 years old were far more likely to report the used of an ineffective method, or no method of contraception, at their most recent intercourse, than either black or white youth (Lowenstein *et al.* 1989). For substance use, the pattern is quite different. Bachman *et al.* (1991) found that native Americans had the highest prevalence rates for cigarettes, alcohol, and most illicit drugs. Rates for white students were only slightly less than black, and Asian-American youth had consistently lower rates of substance use.

Family structure and function

Adolescents with close supportive relationships with their parents characterized by good communication, are more likely to delay the onset of sexual activity (Brooks-Gunn and Forstenberg 1989). Close parental supervision is also associated with later sexual debut among adolescents. Though adolescents from single-parent homes are more likely to initiate intercourse, and are less likely to use contraception on sexual debut, (Mosher and McNally 1991; Wyatt (1989) found that if there was consistent parenting; defined as parenting figures who were consistently in the home of origin prior to the age of 18, there were no differences in age of sexual debut.

Close supportive relationships with their parents appear to protect adolescents from substance use. Family disruption, divorce, or separation of parents, is associated with adolescent substance use (Turner *et al.* 1991). Adolescents are protected from the effects of family structural problems by a close relationship with a parent and close parental supervision (Richardson *et al.* 1989).

A relationship between parenting styles and adolescent substance use has been suggested by Baumrind (1991). Adolescents whose parents use an 'authoritative' (demanding and responsive) style are less likely to use substances than either youth whose parents use an 'authoritarian' (demanding but unresponsive) or 'permissive' (non-demanding but responsive) style of parenting. Adolescent children of parents using a 'rejecting–neglecting' style were the most likely to engage in substance use.

Peers

The role of peers in adolescent decision-making about sexual behaviour is complex. In their longitudinal style involving 'transition from virginity to non virginity', Jessop *et al.* (1982) found that young men and women who valued their peers' influence and had friends who were sexually active were more likely to initiate sexual activity. Little is known of the role of peers in contraceptive decision-making. Parents and relatives are the leading source of referral for young American women, attending private practitioners for family planning advice but, for those attending clinics, friends are the leading referral source (Mosher and Horn 1989).

Peer approval of substance use and susceptibility of adolescents to peer pressure have been associated with substance use (Newcomb *et al.* 1987; Dielman *et al.* 1987), and the relatively greater influence of peers relative to parents increases the likelihood of substance use (Jessor and Jessor 1977; Jessor 1991).

School academic aspirations

Adolescents who have lower academic aspirations and perform poorly in school are more likely to become sexually active and less likely to use effective contraception (Hayes 1987); Di Blasio and Benda 1990). Adolescents who value academic achievement over independence were more likely to delay initiating intercourse (Jessor *et al*. 1983).

The initiation of marijuana use and heavy alcohol consumption among adolescents has been associated with a lower value placed on academic achievement, lower expectations of academic achievement, and poor performance grades in school (Newcomb *et al*. 1986). In one study, students attending continuation schools were more likely to use substances than those attending regular schools (Newcomb *et al*. 1987).

A German study looking at smoking behaviour among 12–13-year-olds found that 30–40 per cent of those attending a vocationally-oriented public school (*Hauteschule*) compared to only six per cent of those attending a college preparatory public school (*Gymnasium*) were regular smokers (Centers for Disease Control 1987). Haupteschule students, compared to Gymnasium students, not only smoked more but also had more friends who were smokers and had less positive self-images and higher expectations of positive affective consequences of smoking.

A similar distribution of substance use was found in Greece where high school students in technical–vocational schools had substantially higher rates of both alcohol and tobacco use than students in other public or private high schools (Kokkevi and Stefanis 1991).

Religion

A number of studies have shown that 'religiosity' as measured by increased importance placed on religion or by church attendance is associated with later sexual debut (Jessor *et al*. 1983; DiBlasio and Benda 1990). The effect of particular religious affiliation on sexual activity among adolescents has not been extensively studied. Studer and Thornton (1987) found, however, that rates of sexual experience among 18 year old women was not related to their being Catholic or Protestant.

Studer and Thornton also found that among sexually active 18 year old women, those who attended church more frequently were less likely to use contraceptives than those who seldom attended church. Finally, data from the 'national survey of family growth' indicated that Jewish women are more likely to use contraception at first intercourse than either Protestant or Catholic women. Fundamentalist Protestants are even less likely to use contraception at the time of their first intercourse than either Catholic women or other Protestant women (Mosher and McNally 1991).

Psychological factors

In a recent study of early adolescents (under 14) Orr and others (1989) found that young females who reported having had intercourse had lower self-esteem than those who did not. The self-esteem of sexually experienced male youth did not differ from those who were not sexually experienced.

Adolescent girls who have high self-esteem and feel in control of their lives are generally more effective users of contraception than those who have a low sense of competence and believe that events in their lives are largely beyond their control (Hayes 1987). Among boys, those who are impulsive, socially irresponsible, and are risk-takers tend to be poor users of contraception (Cvetkovich and Grote; in Hayes 1987).

Psychological factors that have been associated with early initiation of substance use include low self-esteem, anxiety, and depression (Dielman *et al.* 1987; Kaplan *et al.* 1984). Some gender differences exist with respect to psychological factors associated with specific substances used by adolescents. For example, adolescent females who subsequently develop a drinking problem have been characterized as anxious, depressed, vulnerable, pessimistic, and submissive. Male adolescents who later develop a drinking problem are described as outgoing, sociable, dominant, and relatively free of symptoms of depression (Werner 1991).

A recent study demonstrated a significant relationship between cigarette smoking and depression among adolescents in the 11th grade (Covey and Tam 1990). In addition, adolescent marijuana users who were depressed were more likely than those who were not depressed to initiate use of other illicit drugs. Furthermore, the depression seemed to abate over a six month period with continued use of these illicit drugs, suggesting that illicit drugs served a self-medicating function for some youths (Mellinger and Balter 1981, in Yamaguchi and Kandel 1984*b*). Furthermore, in a recent longitudinal study of adolescent substance use, depression was associated with increased cocaine use (Newcomb and Bentler 1986).

Finally, cognitive ability as measured by school performance is negatively associated with substance use (Newcomb *et al.* 1987). Baumrind (1987) has noted, however, that high achieving adolescents may also be at risk. Because 'popular' peer groups often devalue academic achievement, high achievers may feel compelled to engage in substance use in order to be accepted by their peers.

Biological factors

A number of studies involving twins and adoption have suggested that predisposition to alcohol abuse may be genetically mediated. Children of alcoholics are four times as likely to abuse alcohol as children of non-alcoholics (Marlatt *et al.* 1988; Adger 1991). Children of alcoholic biological parents are more likely than other children to misuse alcohol, even when they have been separated from their biological parents since infancy and placed in stable adoptive homes (Cloninger 1987). On the other hand, children who are reared by alcoholic adoptive parents are no more likely than other children to become alcoholic themselves. The relatively high heritability is seen most clearly in male children of male alcoholics and less strongly in female children when either parent is an alcoholic (Peale 1986, cited by Marlatt *et al.* 1988).

Cloninger (1987) has suggested that there are two types of alcoholism with different heritability patterns. 'Type 1' involves onset of problem drinking after age 25, and is characterized by binge drinking, periods of abstinence, and 'harm avoiding' behaviour. 'Type 2', according to Cloninger, has onset in adolescence and is characterized by inability to abstain from drinking, fighting and arrests while drinking, and 'novelty seeking' behaviour. A large Swedish study found that adopted sons and daughters of type 1 alcoholic fathers were not more likely to become alcoholics themselves unless they were exposed to heavy drinking in their adoptive environments. Type 1 is also known as 'milieu limited alcoholism'.

On the other hand, adopted sons whose biological fathers were type 2 alcoholics were at increased risk of alcoholism irrespective of their adoptive environments. Adopted daughters of type 2 alcoholic fathers were at increased risk of somatoform disorders rather than alcoholism. Type 2 is also known as 'male limited alcoholism'. It is likely that genetic predispositions play a role in some types of alcohol abuse. Genetic effects are thought to be polygenic, interacting with environmental factors in complex ways (McClearn 1983; in Marlatt *et al.* 1988).

Co-variation

A number of studies have demonstrated that certain risk-taking behaviours in adolescents are associated in predictable ways and that involvement in one type of risk behaviour increases the likelihood of becoming involved in other risk behaviours (Irwin and Shafer 1992; Osgood *et al.* 1988). Jessor and Jessor (1977) have documented an association of early sexual activity with substance use. According to Jessor and Jessor, these behaviours co-vary as a result of similar antecedents and an underlying predisposition to unconventionality (Donovan *et al.* 1991). He found that adolescents who value independence over achievement are influenced more by peers than parents, are less religious, and are more likely to participate in all types of problem behaviour.

Osgood *et al.* (1988) found that co-variation among various types of substance use and delinquent behaviour among older adolescents and young adults is due, in large part, to a general tendency toward 'deviance' and, to a lesser extent, to unique antecedents of individual behaviours and the influence of one behaviour on another.

In a recent study of early adolescents 11 to 14 years of age, Millstein and others (1992) found that adolescents who were sexually active were more likely to report driving or riding in a car under the influence of substances than adolescents who were not sexually active. As mentioned above, adolescent alcohol use has been implicated in all types of injury-related fatalities. In San Francisco, for example, Friedman (1985) found that half of the 12 to 24-year-old victims of fatal accidents of all kinds and one quarter of those dying as a result of homicide or suicide were alcohol intoxicated. In addition, in 1989 in the US, 37 per cent of adolescents aged 15–17 years and 53 per cent of young adults aged 18–20 years involved in fatal automobile crashes had an elevated blood-alcohol concentration (Centers for Disease Control 1991b).

Substance use and injury-related behaviours reported by white adolescent females have been positively correlated with their intentions to become sexually active in the following year (Kegeles *et al.* 1987). In a nationally representative cohort of young men and women in the US, adolescents who had used marijuana and/or were using alcohol were more likely to become sexually active within the year than those who were not using these substances. Conversely, adolescents who were sexually active at any given age were more likely to use alcohol and marijuana during the following year than those who had not had intercourse (Mott and Haurin 1988). For both males and females, the younger the reported age at first use of drugs and the higher the stage of drug involvement, the greater the risk of precocious sexual activity (Rosenbaum and Kandel 1990).

The use of alcohol and illicit drugs is associated with sexual behaviours that place adolescents at increased risk of unintended pregnancy and sexually transmitted diseases. Adolescent females who smoke cigarettes are less likely to use effective contraception than those who do not smoke (Zabin 1984). In Scotland, adolescents who frequently combined alcohol use with sexual activity were seven times less likely to report consistent condom use than adolescents who did not use alcohol when having intercourse (Bagnall *et al.* 1990).

Young women who use illicit drugs other than marijuana are twice as likely to experience a premarital pregnancy as young women who never used these drugs (Yamaguchi and Kandel 1987). This is due in part to an association between substance use and inadequate use of contraceptives. In addition, Biglan and others (1990) found that cigarette smoking, alcohol consumption, and illicit drug use in adolescents were associated with sexual behaviours which placed them at increased risk of sexually transmitted diseases, including HIV. These behaviours included sexual intercourse with multiple partners, intercourse with promiscuous partners and partners who used intravenous drugs, intercourse with not-well-known partners, and non-use of condoms.

A number of studies have linked substance use with an increase in sexually transmitted diseases including syphilis, gonorrhoea, and HIV (Marx *et al.* 1991; Hibbs and Gunn 1991). Despite recent declines in rates of gonorrhoea infection in the general population, the Centers for Disease Control reported a 35 per cent increase in cases of gonorrhoea among adolescents 15 to 19 years of age in San Francisco between 1987 and 1988. The CDC noted that the proportion of cases was greatest in those neighbourhoods that reported the greatest number of 'crack cocaine' related arrests (Fullilove *et al.* 1990).

Crack is a smokeable form of cocaine hydrochloride that has been associated with high-risk sexual behaviour, (including the exchange of sex for drugs or money), and a high rate of sexually transmitted disease, particularly among black adolescents (Fullilove and Fullilove 1989). Among black adolescents 13 to 19 years of age who reported smoking crack, 41 per cent had a history of STD and only 23 per cent reported using condoms at the most recent intercourse. Having a history of STD did not increase the likelihood of condom use in this population.

Consequences

The potential consequences of risk-taking behaviour include unintended pregnancy, sexually transmitted diseases, school failure, disability, and premature death.

Unintended pregnancy

Approximately one million adolescent females, 19 years of age or less, become pregnant each year in the US, and most of these pregnancies are unintended (Fielding and Williams 1991). Forty per cent of the pregnancies occurring among adolescents in this age group are terminated by therapeutic abortion (Centers for Disease Control 1990e, National Center for Health Statistics 1990c).

The ages at initiation and level of sexual activity among US adolescents are comparable to those in most other developed countries. Rates of adolescent childbearing and abortion, however, are higher in the US than in most of the developed world (Blum 1991; Jones et al. 1985). In 1985, for example, the abortion rate for Canadian adolescent females was one third the abortion rate for adolescent females in the US (Wadhera and Silins 1990).

The 1988 birth rate for adolescent females aged 15 to 17 in the US was 34 per 1000, higher than in any year since 1977. The birth rate for older adolescents 18-19 years of age increased by two per cent from 1987 to 1988, to 82 per 1000 (National Center for Health Statistics 1990c). By comparison, birth rates for Canadian women 15 to 19 years of age declined 36 per cent from 35 per 1000 in 1975 to 23 per 1000 in 1987 (Wadhera and Silins 1990).

In the US, a female less than 15 years of age is four times as likely to give birth as is her peer in Canada, the developed nation with the next highest pregnancy rate (Jones et al. 1985). In 1988, 428 000 infants were born to adolescents 15 to 19 years of age in the US. Eighty-seven per cent of these were the result of unintended pregnancies (National Center for Health Statistics 1990b).

Infants born to younger adolescents are at increased risk of adverse neonatal outcomes (McAnarney 1987). In 1988, infants born to adolescent women under 15 years of age were twice as likely as infants born to older women to have low birth-weight and birth asphyxia with five minute AGPAR scores of five or less (National Center for Health Statistics 1990c). The effects of young maternal age on neonatal outcomes are due in large part to inadequate prenatal care, poor nutrition, and substance use (McAnarney 1987).

In 1988, of pregnant adolescents under 15 years of age, 20 per cent had either late (third trimester) prenatal care or prenatal care compared with only four per cent of pregnant women 25 to 29 years of age (National Center for Health Statistics 1990c). In a study of adolescent females less than 19 years of age seen for prenatal care at Boston City Hospital, more than half of the young women used alcohol during their pregnancies, a third used marijuana, and 14 per cent used cocaine (Amaro *et al.* 1989). Data on use of cigarettes was not collected.

Adolescent parenthood has adverse effects on the lives of youth and their offspring. However, the factors that lead some youth to become parents may be as influential in the course of events as the early childbearing itself. Adolescent mothers are more likely to drop out of high school compared with women of similar socio-economic backgrounds and academic aptitude who postpone childbearing. Adolescent mothers and their children are more likely to live in poverty than are older mothers. This is in part because the majority of adolescent mothers are unmarried and in part because their educational deficits make them less likely to find stable remunerative employment and more likely to rely on public assistance than women who begin childbearing later in life (Furstenberg *et al.* 1989).

High school drop-out rates are higher for adolescent fathers than other youth and are not affected by marital status. At least half of children born to adolescent mothers were fathered by men over 20 years of age (Furstenberg *et al.* 1989). However, regardless of age, fathers of children born to adolescent mothers are at a disadvantage with respect to education and employment compared to fathers of children born to older women. In the Baltimore longitudinal study of teenage parenthood, Hardy and Duggan (1988) found that 42 per cent and 23 per cent of black and white fathers, respectively, of babies born to adolescent mothers were neither in school nor employed 18 months after the birth of their child. Children of adolescent mothers are more likely to have cognitive delays, to fail in school, to engage in delinquent acts, and to become parents in their adolescence than are children of older mothers (Brooks-Gunn and Chase-Lansdale 1991).

Sexually transmitted diseases

Inconsistent use of condoms, early age at sexual debut, and multiple partners place adolescents at increased risk of sexually transmitted diseases, including HIV. Three million adolescents are affected with an STD in the US each year (Centers for Disease Control 1991e). Sixty-three per cent of all cases of STD occur in persons less than 25 years of age. A higher proportion of adolescents are sexually inexperienced and of those who are experienced, a higher percentage are inactive for prolonged periods compared with older populations. As a result, given the appropriate denominator, age-specific rates of STD are among the highest of any age group.

Overall reported rates of gonorrhoea have declined since 1981. Rates of gonorrhoea for adolescents 15 to 19 years of age in the US in 1990, however, were essentially unchanged from 1981 at approximately 1100 per 100 000 (Centres for Disease Control 1991e). *Chlamydia trachomatis* causes more lower genital infections among adolescents than does *N. gonorrhoeae*. Adolescent females have the highest age-specific rates of *C. trachomatis* genital infections (Schydlower and Shafer 1990). The prevalence of cervical chlamydia infections has been found to be between eight per cent and 40 per cent of young women from whom specimens were cultured during pelvic examinations (Cates 1990).

Ten to 17 per cent of women with endocervical gonorrhoea infection and 10–30 per cent of women with endocervical chlamydia infection develop pelvic inflammatory disease (PID) (Washington *et al.* 1985). Of the one million cases of PID in the US each year, approximately 20 per cent occur in adolescent females. Young women between 15 and 19 years of age have the highest age-specific rates of PID (Cates 1990). Acute PID increases the adolescents' risk of ectopic pregnancy, infertility, recurrent PID, and chronic pelvic pain.

Herpes simplex type 2 and human papilloma viruses (HPV) cause chronic, recurrent, sexually and perinatally transmissible infections for which there is no known cure. The number of doctors' office visits for women 15 to 19 years of age for Herpes simplex 2 and human papilloma virus genital infections increased dramatically from 1966 to 1988 (Cates 1990). HPV is of particular concern because it has been linked to early neoplastic changes in the cervices of young women.

To date, adolescents represent less than one per cent of all reported AIDS cases in the US. However, 20 per cent of cases of AIDS have been reported among young adults in their twenties. In light of the variable duration of the latency period preceding the development of AIDS following HIV infection, it is likely that many young adults with AIDS contracted the virus during adolescence.

HIV seroprevalence rates among adolescents vary in different populations. Among adolescents 13 to 19 years of age attending the National Medical Center in Washington DC for routine care, 3.7 per thousand were HIV seropositive (D'Angelo *et al.* 1991). In a recent study involving adolescents 15 to 20 years of age at a facility serving homeless and runaway youth in New York City, 5.3 per cent were found to be HIV positive (Stricof *et al.* 1991).

Among adolescents 13 to 19 years of age, the prevalence of HIV infection rises with increasing age. The distribution of both AIDS and HIV infection among adolescents differs from the distribution found in adults. Whereas the ratio of AIDS cases of adult men to adult women is 10:1, reported cases of AIDS among male adolescents outnumber those of female adolescents by 4:1. The ratio of male to female seroprevalence of HIV reported among adolescents varies depending on the population studied. However, the relative preponderance of male cases seen in adult populations is not characteristic of HIV prevalence among adolescents. The ratios of HIV prevalences in male compared to female adolescents in the various populations studied have been closer to unity, with a higher HIV seroprevalence rate among female adolescents in the Washington DC study.

School problems

School related problems represent a potential threat to adolescent cognitive development and future employment opportunities. The exact number of adolescents affected by educational deficits is not known. The US government does not maintain statistics reflecting the number of students who fail in high school or drop out before completing high school *per se*. However, the Center for Education Statistics monitors the number of students graduating from high school each year compared to the number which would be expected if all students who were in ninth grade four years earlier had completed high schools on schedule. Students who are required to repeat a grade, or those who entered private schools after the ninth grade, are included in the percentage of 'non-completers'.

In 1989, 29 per cent of students who were in the ninth grade (14–15 year olds) in 1985 did not complete the 12th grade (17–18-year-olds) (National Center for Education Statistics 1991). There is marked variation among the states with respect to the percentage of students who do not complete high school in a timely manner. Only 11 per cent of students in Minnesota did not complete high school by the expected date, compared to 42 per cent of students in the district of Columbia.

School failure has been cited as both a predictor and a consequence of substance use, early sexual activity, and delinquent behaviour (Dryfoos 1990). Jessor and Jessor (1975) found that a lower relative value placed on academic achievement than independence, as well as lower grade-point averages, predicted early sexual debut, initiation of marijuana use, and problem drinking in adolescents.

Conversely, increasing substance use has been associated with deteriorating school performance and truancy (Anglin 1987). In addition, among 12 to 16 year old adolescents, Orr (1991) and others found that sexually experienced males were almost seven times as likely to consider dropping out of school and seven times as likely to have been suspended from school in the past compared to sexually inexperienced males. Sexually experienced adolescent females in this study were four times as likely to consider dropping out of school and five times as likely to have been suspended from school in the past compared to sexually inexperienced females.

Substance use

The consequences of substance abuse are legion. As mentioned above, substance abuse is associated with behavioural problems at school and within the family, and with sexual activity. In addition, alcohol consumption has been linked to injury morbidity and mortality. In addition, adolescent females who consume alcohol during pregnancy risk giving birth to an infant with fetal alcohol syndrome (American Academy of Pediatrics 1987).

Short term consequences of smokeless tobacco use by adolescents include increased dental carries and periodontal disease. Cigarette smoking of less than two years' duration in adolescents is associated with a reduction of lung function, and with depression of high-density lipoprotein cholesterol (HDL-C) levels (Centers for Disease Control 1987). Lower HDL-C levels have been associated with an increased risk of developing heart disease. Long term tobacco use is associated with heart disease and cancer. Adolescent females who smoke cigarettes during pregnancy increase their risk of delivering low birth-weight infants.

Marijuana use has declined among adolescents since the late 1970s. However, the potency of the marijuana has increased substantially. The concentration of δ-9-tetrahydrocanabinol in marijuana currently available in the US has increased by 250 per cent over the past decade (Schwartz *et al.* 1989). The immediate pulmonary effect of smoking marijuana is bronchodilatation. With chronic use, the smoked particles cause irritation and bronchoconstriction and eventually airway obstruction (American Academy of Pediatrics 1991). Heavy marijuana use has been associated with decreased sperm motility, decreased sperm counts, and decreased circulating testosterone. Other consequences of chronic marijuana use include learning difficulties related to short term memory deficits that continue for at least six weeks after the last use of marijuana (Schwartz *et al.* 1989), and possibly increased risk of infection secondary to suppression of cell-mediated immunity and diminished circulating immunoglobulin.

Use of tobacco, alcohol, and particularly marijuana have been associated with progression to using other illicit substances with potentially grave consequences, including chemical dependence and death from complications or overdose of illicit drugs. Medical complications of acute cocaine use include convulsions, CNS heamorrhages, hyperthermia, respiratory paralysis, and potentially fatal cardiac arrhythmias and infarctions. Chronic cocaine use is associated with weight loss, lethargy, and impotence.

Youth at high risk

A disproportionate share of risk-related morbidity and mortality is contributed by a subset of youth who engage in high-risk behaviours at greater frequencies than the general adolescent population. As mentioned above, high school dropouts experience higher rates of substance use, earlier sexual debut, and higher rates of unintended pregnancy than those who complete high school (Dryfoos 1990).

In a study comparing imprisoned youth to a similarly aged high school sample in San Francisco, DiClemente and others (1991) found that knowledge of AIDS transmission was high in both groups. However, fewer imprisoned youth identified condom use, sexual abstinence, and not having intercourse with intravenous drug users as AIDS risk-reduction strategies. In addition, imprisoned youth were more likely to be sexually active, initiated intercourse at earlier ages, reported more sexual partners, and were less likely to use condoms consistently compared to adolescents from the high school.

Approximately 1.2 million adolescents leave home annually. Twenty-five per cent of these runaways will become homeless 'street youth' (Farrow et al. 1991). A third to half of runaway youth left home because of a history of physical or sexual abuse (Deisher and Rogers 1991). More than half of runaway youth in Seattle in 1985 had dropped out or had been suspended from school, 63 per cent had problems with alcohol or drugs, and 43 per cent had been involved with the juvenile justice system (Smart 1991).

In Los Angeles, the use of illicit substances other than marijuana was substantially higher among runaway youth compared to similarly aged adolescents attending outpatient clinics who were not runaways. Over a third of the runaway youth reported using intravenous drugs in the past, ten times the rate found among non-runaway youth (Yates et al. 1988).

In order to survive on the street, homeless youth may sell small goods or used clothing. However, more often, street youth beg, deal drugs, and steal (Luna 1991). More than half of street youth have been involved in prostitution (Deisher and Rogers 1991). Adolescents who engage in so-called 'survival sex' are at great risk of sexually transmitted diseases and physical harm from violence.

In a study comparing homeless and runaway youth in Los Angeles who were involved in prostitution to those who were not, Yates and others (1991) found that adolescents involved in prostitution were 14 times as likely to be diagnosed with PID and three times as likely to have a diagnosis of rape than homeless or runaway youth who were not involved in prostitution. A recent study in downtown Rio de Janeiro found that 69 per cent of males 11 to 23 years of age who engaged in sexual activity for money were infected with HIV (Luna 1991).

As many as 900 000 adolescents are involved in prostitution in the US (Yates et al. 1991). Street youth who are involved in prostitution have higher rates of substance use, sexually transmitted diseases, and serious mental illness (other than depression) than homeless and runaway youth who are not involved in prostitution. Adolescents who receive food, lodging, clothes, drugs, or money in exchange for sexual favours are among the highest risk youth for HIV infection and personal violence.

Prevention

The policies of the past 20 years in the US have failed to reduce the incidence of sexually transmitted diseases, unintended pregnancy, school drop-out, substance use, or unintentional injury among American youth. This may be due in part to the narrow focus on the prevention of separate social problems rather than the integrated promotion of improved overall adolescent well-being, including coping skills, self-esteem, and social supports (Scales 1990).

The US Preventive Services Task Force (1989) recently emphasized the critical role that health care providers plans in counselling patients on substance use, sexual practices, and injury prevention, both for the 13–18 as well as the 19–39 year age groups. Health-risk behaviours, often initiated in adolescence, are responsible for the majority of morbidity and mortality which occurs in the fourth decade. Therefore effective intervention with respect to adolescent risk-taking behaviours may result in long-term positive outcomes, well into adulthood.

Efforts to prevent risk-taking behaviours and their consequences include legal interventions, school and community based interventions, and public and private institution-based interventions. Prevention of risk-behaviour related morbidity and mortality may be primary, secondary, or tertiary. Although a multitude of interventions have been developed in the arena of risk-taking behaviour among adolescents, few have been critically evaluated.

Some empirically derived general principle of intervention with variable support in the literature include the following (Dryfoos 1991; Boyer 1990; Pentz et al. 1989).

1. Approaches grounded in established behavioral theory, such as social learning theory or problem behaviour theory, tend to be more effective.

2. The more successful interventions are multifaceted, targeting both groups and individuals, utilizing didactic and interactive approaches, peer and adult involvement, and print and audiovisual information.

3. Education may lead to attitude change but 'skill building' is necessary for behaviour change.

4. Programmes are initiated in the early adolescent years are more promising than those initiated later in adolescence.

Primary prevention, as it relates to risk-related morbidity and mortality among adolescents, involves intervention before risk behaviour becomes manifest. Examples of primary prevention include programmes discouraging or delaying the onset of sexual activity and substance use, or encouraging the safe operation of vehicles, including the use of safety belts and bicycle helmets.

A recent primary intervention programme in Canada involved physicians in a relatively affluent area providing patients with information and pamphlets about the dangers of riding bicycles without protective headgear (Cushman et al. 1991). The results showed no difference in the purchase or use of bicycle helmets between subjects and controls who did not receive the information. The investigators concluded that the intervention would have been more successful if it had been part of a multidisciplinary community-based campaign.

The 'Midwest prevention project', a multidisciplinary community-based intervention to prevent adolescent substance use, has shown promising early results (Pentz *et al.* 1989). The project includes mass-media programming, a school-based education programme for youth 10 to 14 years of age, parent education and organization, community organization, and health policy components that are introduced sequentially into communities during a six year period. Results from the one year follow-up showed that the net increase in drug use prevalence in the intervention schools was half that of the delayed intervention schools. Long-term effects of the intervention await evaluation.

Secondary prevention with regard to risk behaviours involves intervening after the behaviour has been established in order to prevent some of the potential negative consequences. Examples of secondary prevention include promoting the use of a 'designated' abstaining driver when adolescents with a history of substance use are participating in events in which alcohol is likely to be consumed, or encouraging 'safe' sexual practices among adolescents who are already sexually active.

A number of studies have shown that the knowledge of negative consequences of a behaviour does not necessarily translate into behaviour change. Kegeles and others (1988) found that knowledge of the protective effect of condoms with regard to STD and a high value placed on avoiding STD did not result in increased condom use among sexually active adolescents. Over a two year study period, however, from 1988 to 1990, runaway adolescents involved in an HIV risk-reduction programme increased their condom use compared to runaways who were not involved in the intervention (Rotheram-Borus *et al.* 1991).

The HIV risk-reduction programme involved high-risk adolescent living in a shelter. The programme's components included general knowledge through multi-media activities, training in coping skills, increasing access to resources, and addressing individual barriers to safer sex. The gains in condom use were modest but significant and the effect of the intervention increased with increasing number of sessions in which the runaways participated. The longevity of the behaviour change has not been evaluated.

The School/Community Program for Sexual Risk Reduction Among Teens, was a comprehensive intervention aimed at reducing the occurrence of unintended pregnancies among unmarried adolescent females in a western county in South Carolina, USA. The programme targeted parents, teachers, clergy, community leaders, and children in the public school system and emphasized development of decision-making and communication skills, self-esteem enhancement, and understanding human reproductive anatomy, physiology, and contraception. Among adolescent females aged 14 to 17 years in the intervention county, estimated pregnancy rates declined from 60 per 1000 to 25 per 1000 between 1982 and 1985. The reduction in adolescent pregnancy rates was not seen in neighbouring counties not participating in the intervention.

Tertiary prevention involves mitigating the consequences of risk behaviours. Examples include providing early recognition and treatment of lower genital tract infection to prevent the development of PID and its potential sequelae, and providing services to pregnant and parenting adolescents to ameliorate the negative consequences of early childbearing.

A recent five year follow-up evaluation of 'project redirection' (Polit 1989), a comprehensive programme for pregnant and parenting teens, found that programme participants had better employment records, higher average earnings, and lower rates of welfare dependency than similar young mothers who had not enrolled in 'project redirection'.

Legislative efforts to reduce risk-taking behaviours and their consequences have had limited success. Forty-four states and the district of Columbia have laws restricting minors' access to tobacco (Centers for Disease Control 1990*a*). These laws are not consistently enforced, however. In a study in Colorado, where the sale of tobacco to persons under the age of 18 was outlawed in 1987, minors successfully purchased cigarettes in 64 per cent of their attempts (Centers for Disease Control 1990*d*).

Legal intervention has been more successful in the arena of injury-risk reduction. By raising the legal driving age to 17 years, New Jersey has virtually eliminated fatal crashes involving 16-year-old drivers. A 13 per cent reduction in night time traffic fatalities involving adolescents was found in states that raised their minimum drinking age from 18 or 19 to 21, compared to states that did not raise their minimum drinking age (Agran *et al.* 1990).

Conclusion

Risk-taking behaviours represent the most serious threat to the lives and health of adolescents. Premature sexual activity may result in unintended pregnancy and sexually transmitted diseases including AIDS. Substance use is associated with school failure, early sexual debut, and increased rates of motor-vehicle and other injury-related fatalities. Finally, injury-related behaviours may result in disability or death. These major sources of morbidity and mortality, initiated in adolescence, persist through the fourth decade (Irwin 1990).

In order to achieve the developmental milestone of the second decade, including autonomy and identity formation, all young people need a safe context in which to explore their environments. Therefore intervention strategies addressing risk-taking behaviours must strive to increase adolescent safety while maintaining a perspective on their developmental needs for growth and exploration.

Acknowledgements

During the preparation of this manuscript, the authors were supported in part by grants from the Bureau of Maternal and Child Health, Department of Health and Human Services, grant No MCJ000978, and the William T. Grant Foundation.

References

Agran P., Castillo, D., and Winn, D. (1990). Childhood motor vehicle occupant injuries. *American Journal of Disease in Childhood* **144**, 653–62.

Amaro, H., Zuckerman, B., and Cabral, H. (1989). Drug use among adolescent mothers: profile of risk. *Pediatr.* **84**, 144–51.

American Academy of Pediatrics (1987). Committee on Adolescence, Alcohol use and abuse: a pediatric concern. *Pediatrics* **79**, 450–5.

American Academy of Pediatrics (1991). Committee on Adolescence, Committee on Substance Abuse. Marijuana: a continuing concern for pediatricians. *Pediatr.* **88**, 1070–72.

Anglin, T.M. (1987). Interviewing guidelines for the clinical evaluation of adolescent substance abuse. *The Pediatric Clinics of North America* **34**, 381–98.

Bachman, J.G., Wallace, J.M., O'Malley, P.M., Johnston, L.D., Kurth, C.L., and Neighbors, H.W. (1991). Racial/ethnic differences in smoking, drinking, and illicit drug use among American high school seniors, 1976–89. *Am. J. Public Health* **81**, 372–7.

Bagnall, G., Plant, M., and Warwick, W. (1990). Alcohol, drugs and AIDS-related risks: results from a prospective study. *AIDS Care* **2**, 310–17.

Baumrind, D. (1987). A developmental perspective on adolescent risk-taking in contemporary America. in Irwin CE Jr. (ed.) Adolescent social behavior and health. *New Directions for Child Development*.

Baumrind, D. (1991). The influence of parenting style on adolescent competence and substance abuse. *J. Early Adolescence* **11**, 56–95.

Biglan, A., Metzler, C.W., Wirt, R., Ary, D., Noell, J., Ochs, L., French, C., and Hood, D. (1990). Social and behavioral factors associated with high-risk sexual behavior among adolescents. *J. Behav. Med.* **13**, 24–61.

Blum, R.W. (1991). Global trends in adolescent health. *J. Am. Med. Assoc.* **265**, 2711–19.

Boyer, C.B. (1990). Psychosocial, behavioral, and educational factors in preventing sexually transmitted diseases. *Adolescent Medicine: State of the Art Reviews* **1**, 597-613.

Brooks-Gunn, J. and Chase-Lansdale, P.L. (1991). Children having children: effects on the family system. *Pediatr. Ann.* **20**, 467–81.

Brooks-Gunn, J. and Furstenberg, F.F. (1989). Adolescent sexual behavior. *Am. Psych.* **44**, 249–57.

Cates, W. (1990). The epidemiology and control of sexually transmitted diseases in adolescents. *Adolescent Medicine: State of the Art Reviews* **1**, 409–28.

Centers for Disease Control (1987). Psychosocial predictors of smoking among adolescents. *Mobility and Mortality Weekly Reports* **36**, 1S–47S.

Centers for Disease Control (1989). Results from the national adolescent student health survey. *Morbidity and Mortality Weekly Report* **39**, 147–50.

Centers for Disease Control, (1990*a*). State laws restricting minors' access to tobacco. *Morbidity and Mortality Weekly Report* **39**, 349–51.

Centers for Disease Control (1990*b*). Childhood injuries in the United States. *American Journal of Disease in Childhood* **144**, 627–46.

Centers for Disease Control (1990*c*). Fatal injuries to children—United States, 1986. *Morbidity and Mortality Weekly Report* **39**, 442–51.

Centers for Disease Control (1990d). Cigarette sales to minors—Colorado, 1989. *Morbidity and Mortality Weekly Report* **39**, 794–5, 802–3.
Centers for Disease Control (1990e). Abortion surveillance, United States, 1988. *Morbidity and Mortality Weekly Report*, **40**, 15–57.
Centers for Disease Control (1991a). Premarital sexual experience among adolescent women—United States, 1970–1988. *Morbidity and Mortality Weekly Report* **39**, 929–32.
Centers for Disease Control (1991b). Alcohol-related traffic fatalities among youth and young adults—United States, 1982–1989. *Morbidity and Mortality Weekly Report* **40**, 178–9.
Centers for Disease Control (1991c). AIDS-related knowledge and behaviors among teenagers—Italy, 1990. *Morbidity and Mortality Weekly Report* **40**, 214–15, 221.
Centers for Disease Control (1991d). Tobacco use among high school students—United States, 1990. *Morbidity and Mortality Weekly Report* **40**, 617–19.
Centers for Disease Control (1991e). *Sexually transmitted disease surveillance 1990*. US Department of Health and Human Services, Atlanta.
Chollet-Traquet, C. (1992). *Women and Tobacco*. WHO, Geneva.
Cloninger, C.R. (1987). Neurogenetic adaptive mechanisms in alcoholism. *Science* **236**, 410–16.
Covey, L.S., and Tam, D. (1990). Depressive mood, the single-parent home, and adolescent cigarette smoking. *Am. J. Public Health* **80**, 1330–1.
Cushman, R., James, W., and Waclawik, H. (1991). Physicians promoting bicycle helmets for children: a randomized trial. *Am. J. Public Health* **81**, 1044–5.
D'Angelo, L.J., Getson, P.R., Lubann, N.L.C. and Gayle H.D. (1991). Human immunodeficiency virus infection in urban adolescents: can we predict who is at risk? *Pediatr.* **88**, 982–6.
Deisher, R.W. and Rogers, W.M. (1991). The medical care of street youth. *J. Adolesc. Health* **12**, 500–3.
DiBlasio, F.A., and Benda, B.B. (1990). Adolescent sexual behavior: multivariate analysis of a social learning model. *J. Adolesc. Res.* **5**, 449–66.
DiClemente, R.L., Lanier, M.M., Horan, P.F., and Lodico, M. (1991). Comparison of AIDS knowledge, attitudes, and behaviors among incarcerated adolescents and a public school sample in San Francisco. *Am. J. Public Health*. **81**, 628–30.
Dielman, T.E., Campanelli, P.C., Shope, J.T., and Butchart, A.T. (1987). Susceptibility to peer pressure, self-esteem, and health locus of control as correlates of adolescent substance abuse. *Health Ed. Quart.* **47**, 207–21.
Donovan, J.E., Jessor, R., and Costa, F. (1991). Adolescent health behavior and conventionality–unconventionality: an extension of problem-behavior theory. *Health Psychol.* **10**, 52–61.
Dryfoos, J.G. (1990). *Adolescents at risk*. Oxford University Press.
Dryfoos, J.G. (1991). Adolescents at risk: a summation of work in the field—programs and policies. *J. Adolesc. Health* **12**, 630–7.
Farrow. J.A., Deisher, R.W., and Rogers, W.M. (1991). Introduction: Proc. West Coast Symp. of Health Care of Runaway Street Youth. *J. Adolesc. Health*. **12**, 497–9.
Fielding, J.E., and Williams, C.A. (1991). Unintended pregnancy among teenagers: important roles for primary care providers. *Ann. Int. Med.* **114**, 599–601.
Forrest, J.D. and Singh, S. (1990). The sexual and reproductive behavior of American women, 1982–1988. *Fam. Plann. Persp.* **22**, 206–14.

Friedman, I.M. (1985). Alcohol and unnatural deaths in San Francisco youths. *Pediatr.* **76**, 191–3.

Fullilove, M.T., and Fullilove R.E. (1989). Intersecting epidemics: black teen crack use and sexually transmitted disease. *Journal of the American Medical Womens Association* **44**, 146–53.

Fullilove, R.E., Fullilove, M.T., Bowser, B.P., and Gross, S.A. (1990). Risk of sexually transmitted disease among black adolescent crack users in Oakland and San Francisco, Calif. *J. Am. Med. Assoc.* **263**, 851–5.

Furstenberg, F.F., Brooks-Gunn, J., and Chase-Lansdale, L. (1989). Teenaged pregnancy and childbearing. *Am. Psych.* **44**, 313–20.

Guyer, B. and Ellers, B. (1990). Childhood injuries in the United States. *American Journal of Disease in Childhood*, **144**, 649–52.

Halebsky, M.A. (1987). Adolescent alcohol and substance abuse: parent and peer effects. *Adolescence*, **22**, 961–7.

Halperin, S.F., Bass, J.L., Mehta, K.A., and Betts, K.D. (1983). Unintentional injuries among adolescents and young adults: a review and analysis. *J. Adolesc. Health Care*, **4**, 275–81.

Hardy, J.B., and Duggan, A.K. (1988). Teenage fathers and the fathers of infants of urban, teenage mothers. *Am. J. Public Health* **78**, 919–22.

Haverkos, H.W. Bukowski, W.J., and Amsel, Z. (1989). The initiation of male homosexual behavior. *J. Am. Med. Assoc.* **262**, 501–5.

Hayes, C.D. (ed.) (1987). *Risking the future: adolescent sexuality, pregnancy and childbearing*. National Academy Press, Washington, D.C.

Hibbs, J.R., and Gunn, R.A. (1991). Public health intervention in a cocaine-related syphilis outbreak. *Am. J. Public Health* **81**, 1259–62.

Irwin, C.E. Jr, (1987). Adolescent social behavior and health (ed.) *New Directions for Child Development* **37**, 1–12.

Irwin, C.E. Jr (1990). The theoretical concept of at-risk adolescents. *Adolescent Medicine: State of the Art Reviews* **1**, 1–14.

Irwin, C.E. Jr (1993). Adolescents and risk taking: how are they related? In *Risk taking in the life cycle* (ed. N. Bell and R. Bell). Texas Tech University Press, Lubbock, Texas.

Irwin, C.E. Jr and Millstein, S.G. (1986). Biopsychosocial correlates of risk-taking behaviors during adolescence. *J. Adolesc. Health Care* **7**, 82S–96S.

Irwin, C.E. Jr and Shafer, M.A. (1992). Adolescent sexuality: the problem of negative outcomes of a normative behavior. In *Adolescent at risk medical and social perspectives* (ed. D. Rogers and E. Ginzberg), Ch. 4. Westville Press, Boulder, Colorado.

Jessor, R. (1982). Problem behavior and developmental transition in adolescence. *J. School Health* **May**, 295–300.

Jessor, R. (1991). Risk behavior in adolescence: a psychosocial framework for understanding and action. *J. Adolesc. Health Care* **12**, 597–605.

Jessor, S.L. and Jessor, R. (1975). Transition from virginity to non-virginity among youth: a social–psychological study over time. *Develop. Psycho.* **11**, 473–84.

Jessor, R. and Jessor, S.L. (1977). *Problem behavior and psychological development: a longitudinal study of youth*. Academic Press, New York.

Jessor, R., Costa F., Jessor L., and Donovan, J.E. (1983). Time of first intercourse: a prospective study. *J. Person. Social Psychol.* **44**, 608–26.

Jones, E.F., Forrest, J.D., Goldman, N., Henshaw, S.K., Lincoln, R., Rosoff, J.I., Westoff, C.F., and Wulf, D. (1985). Teenage pregnancy in developed countries: determinants and policy implications. *Fam. Plann. Persp.* **17**, 53–62.

Kandel, D.B., and Logan J.A. (1984). Patterns of drug use from adolescence to early adulthood: I. Periods of risk for initiation, continued use and discontinuation. *Am. J. Public Health* **74**, 660–6.

Kaplan, H.B., Martin, S.S., and Robbins, C. (1984). Pathways to adolescent drug use: self-derogation, peer influence, weakening of social controls, and early substance use. *J. Health Soc. Behav.* **25**, 270–89.

Kegeles, S.M., Adler, N.E., and Irwin, C.E. Jr (1988). Sexually active adolescents and condoms: changes over one year in knowledge, attitudes and use. *Am. J. Public Health* **78**, 460–61.

Kelly, K.B., Ehrver, M., Erneholm, T., Gundevall, C., Wennerberg, I., and Wettergren, L. Self-reported health status and use of medical care by 3500 adolescents in western Sweden, part I. *Acta Paediatr. Scand.* **80**, 837–43.

Kokkevi, A., and Stefanis, C. (1991). The epidemiology of elicit and illicit substance use among high school students in Greece. *Am. J. Public Health* **81**, 48–52.

Luna, G.C. (1991). Street youth: adaptation and survival in the AIDS decade. *J. Adolesc. Health*, **12**, 511–14.

Marlatt, G.A., Baer, J.S., Donovan, D.M., and Kivlahan, D.R. Addictive behaviors: etiology and treatment. *Ann. Rev. Psychol.* **39**, 223–52.

Marx, R., Aral, S.O., Rolfs, R.T., Sterk, C.E., and Kahn, J.G. (1991). Crack, sex, and STD. *Sex. Transm. Dis.* **18**, 92–101.

McAnarney, E.R. (1987). Young maternal age and adverse neonatal outcome. *American Journal of Disease in Childhood*, **141**, 1053–9.

Millstein, S.G., Irwin, C.E. Jr, Adler, N.E., Cohn, L.D., Kegeles, S.M., and Dolcini, M.M. (1992). High-risk behaviors and health concerns among young adolescents. *Pediatr.* **89**(3):422–8.

Mosher, W.D. and Horn, M.C. (1989). First family planning visits by young women. *Fam. Plann. Persp.* **21**, 33–40.

Mosher, W.D. and McNally, J.W. (1991). Contraceptive use at first premarital intercourse: United States, 1965-85. *Fam. Plann. Persp.* **23**, 108–28.

Mott, F.L. and Haurin, R.J. (1988). Linkages between sexual activity and alcohol and drug use among American adolescents. *Fam. Plann. Persp.* **20**, 128–36.

National Center for Education Statistics (1991). *Public high school graduates, 1988–89*, compared with *ninth grade enrolment in fall 1985, by state*. US Department of Education, Washington DC.

National Center for Health Statistics, CDC (1990*b*). Wanted and unwanted childbearing in the United States: 1973–88. *Advance Data* **189**, 1–8.

National Center for Health Statistics, CDC (1990*c*). Advance report of final natality statistics, 1988. *Monthly Vital Statistics Report* **39**, (Suppl., No. 4), 1–13.

National Center for Health Statistics, CDC (1991). Firearm mortality among children, youth, and young adults 1–34 years of age, trends and current status: United States, 1979–88. *Monthly Vital Statistics Report* **39**, (No. 11), 1–14.

National Center for Health Statistics, CDC (1992). Advance report of final mortality statistics, 1989. *Monthly Vital Statistics Report* **40**, (No. 8, Suppl. 2), 21–5.

Newcomb, M.D., and Bentler, P.M. (1986). Cocaine use among adolescents: longitudinal associates with social context, psychopathology and use of other substances. *Addictive Behaviors* **11**, 263–73.
Newcomb, M.D. and Bentler, P.M. (1989). Substance use and abuse among children and teenagers. *Am. Psych.* **44**, 242–8.
Newcomb, M.D., Maddahian, E., and Bentler, P.M. (1986). Risk factors for drug use among adolescents: concurrent and longitudinal analysis. *Am. J. Public Health* **76**, 525–31.
Newcomb, M.D., Maddahian, E., Skager, R., and Bentler, P.M. (1987). Substance abuse and psychosocial factors among teenagers: associations with age, sex, ethnicity, and type of school. *Am. J. Drug Alcohol Abuse*, **13**, 413–33.
Newcomer, S., and Udry, J.R. (1987). Parental marital status effects on adolescent sexual behavior. *J. Marriage Fam.* **49**, 235–40.
Orr, D.P., Wilbrandt, M.L., Brack, C.J., Rauch, S.P., and Ingersoll, G.M. (1989). Reported sexual behaviors and self-esteem among young adolescents. *American Journal of Disease in Childhood*, **143**, 86–90.
Orr, D.P., Beiter, M., and Ingersoll, G. (1991). Premature sexual activity as an indicator of psychosocial risk. *Pediatr.* **87**, 141–7.
Osgood, D.W., Johnston, L.D., O'Malley, P.M., and Bachman, J.G. (1988). The generality of deviance in late adolescence and early adulthood. *American Sociological Review* **53**, 81–93.
Paulson, J.A. (1988). The epidemiology of injuries in adolescents. *Pediatr. Ann.* **17**, 84–96.
Pentz, M.A., Dwyer, J.H., MacKinnon, D.P., Flay, D.R., Hansen, W.B., Wang, EYI, and Johnson, C.A. (1989). A multicommunity trial for primary prevention of adolescent drug abuse. *J. Am. Med. Assoc.* **261**, 3259–66.
Phinney, V.G., Jensen, L.C., Olsen, J.A., and Cundick, B. (1990). The relationship between early development and psychosexual behaviors in adolescent females. *Adolescence* **98**, 321–32.
Polit, D.F. (1989). Effects of a comprehensive program for teenage parents: five years after project redirection. *Fam. Plann. Persp.* **21**, 164–9, 187.
Reuben, N., Hein, K., Drucker, E., Bauman, L., and Lauby, J. (1988). Relationship of high risk behaviors to AIDS knowledge in adolescent high school students. *J. Adolesc. Health* **9**, 263.
Richardson, J.L., Dwyer, K., McGuigan, K., Hansen, W.B., Dent, C., Johnson, C.A., Sussman, S.Y., Brannon, B., and Flay, B. (1989). Substance use among eight-grade students who take care of themselves after school. *Pediatr.* **84**, 556–66.
Rockett, I.R.H and Smith, G.S. (1989). Homicide, suicide, motor vehicle crash, and fall mortality: United States' experience in comparative perspective. *Am. J. Public Health* **79**, 1396–1400.
Rosenbaum, E. and Kandel, D.B. (1990). Early onset of adolescent sexual behavior and drug involvement. *J. Marriage Fam.* **52**, 783–98.
Rotheram-Borus, M.J., Koopman, C., Haignere, C., and Davies, M. (1991). Reducing HIV sexual risk behaviors among runaway adolescents. *J. Am. Med. Assoc.* **266**, 1237–41.
Saucier, J.F. and Ambert, A.M. (1983). Parental marital status and adolescents' health-risk behavior. *Adolescence* **18**, 403–11.
Scales, P. (1990) Developing capable young people: an alternative strategy for prevention programs. *J. Early Adolesc.* **10**, 420–38.

Schwartz, R.H., Gruenewald, P.J., Klitzner, M., and Fedio, P. (1989). Short-term memory impairment in cannabis-dependent adolescents. *American Journal of Disease in Childhood*, **143**, 1214–19.
Schydlower, M., and Shafer, M.A. (1990). Chlamydia trachomatis infections in adolescents. *Adolescent Medicine: State of the Art Reviews* **1**, 615–28.
Selbst, S.M., Alexander, D., and Ruddy, R. (1987). Bicycle-related injuries. *American Journal of Disease in Childhood*, **141**, 140–4.
Shafer, M.A., Beck, A., Blain, B., Dole, P., Irwin, C.E., Sweet, R., and Schachter, J. (1984). Chlamydia trachomatis: important relationships to race, contraception, lower genital tract infection and Papanicolaou smear. *J. Pediatr.* **104**, 141–6.
Smart, D.H. (1991). Homeless youth in Seattle: planning and policy-making at the local-government level. *J. Adolesc. Health* **12**, 519–27.
Smith, T. (1993). Influence of socio-economic factors on attaining targets for reducing teenage pregnancies. *British Medical Journal*, **306**, 1232–5.
Sonenstein, F.L., Pleck, J.H., and Ku, L.C. (1989). Sexual activity, condom use and AIDS awareness among adolescent males. *Fam. Plann. Persp.* **21**, 152–8.
Sonenstein, F.L., Pleck, J.H., and Ku, L.C. (1991). Levels of sexual activity among adolescent males in the United States. *Fam. Plann. Persp.* **23**, 162–7
Stricof, R.L., Kennedy, J.T., Nattell, T.C., Weisfuse, I.B., and Novick, L.F. HIV seroprevalence in a facility for runaway and homeless adolescents. *Am. J. Public Health* **81**, (Suppl.), 50–3.
Studer, M., and Thornton, A. (1987). Adolescent religiosity and contraceptive usage. *J. Marriage Fam.* **49**,117–28.
Taket, A. (1986). Accident mortality in children, adolescents and young adults. *World Health Stat. Quart.* **39**, 232–56.
Turner, R.A., Irwin, C.E., and Millstein, S.G. (1991). Family structures, family processes, and experimenting with substances during adolescence. *J. Res. Adolesc.* **1**, 93–106.
Udry, J.R. (1988). Biological predispositions and social control in adolescent sexual behavior. *Am. Sociolog. Rev.* **53**, 709–22.
Udry, J.R., and Billy, J.O.G. (1987). Initiation of coitus in early adolescence. *Am. Sociolog. Rev.* **52**, 841–55.
US Preventive Services Task Force (1989). *Guide to clinical preventive services: an assessment of the effectiveness of 169 interventions*. Williams and Wilkins, Baltimore.
Wadhera, S., and Silins, J. (1990). Teenage pregnancy in Canada, 1975–1987. *Fam. Plann. Persp.* **22**, 27–30.
Washington, A.E., Sweet, R.L., and Shafer, M.A. (1985). Pelvic inflammatory disease and its sequelae in adolescents. *J. Adolesc. Health Care*, **6**, 298–310.
Werner, J.J. (1991). Adolescent substance abuse. *Maternal and child health technical information bulletin*. National Center for Education in Maternal and Child Health, Cincinnati.
Williams, A.F. and Carsten, O. (1989). Driver age and crash involvement. *Am. J. Public Health*, **79**, 326–7.
Williams, B.C., and Kotch, J.B. (1990). Excess injury mortality among children in the United States: comparison of recent international statistics. *Pediatr.*, **86**, 1067–73.
Wintemute, G.J. (1990). Childhood drowning and near-drowning in the United States. *American Journal of Disease in Children*, **144**, 663–9.
Wyatt, G.E., (1989). Re-examining factors predicting Afro-American and white women's ages of first coitus. *Arch. Sexual Behav.* **18**, 271–98.

Yamaguchi, K., and Kandel, D.B. (1984*a*). Patterns of drug use from adolescence to young adulthood: III. Predictors of progression. *Am. J. Public Health* **74**, 673–81.

Yamaguchi, K., and Kandel, D.B., (1984*b*). Patterns of drug use from adolescence to young adulthood: II. Sequences of progression. *Am. J. Public Health* **74**, 668–71.

Yates, G.L., MacKenzie, R., Pennbridge, J., and Cohen, E. (1988). A risk profile of runaway and non-runaway youth. *Am. J. Public Health* **78**, 820–1.

Yates, G.L., MacKenzie, R.G., Pennbridge, J., and Swofford, A. (1991). A risk profile comparison of homeless youth involved in prostitution and youth not involved. *J. Adolesc. Health* **12**, 545–8.

Zabin, L.S. (1984). The association between smoking and sexual behavior among teens in US contraceptive clinics. *Am. J. Public Health* **74**, 261–3.

PART VI

The new morbidity

Childhood morbidity in developed countries has changed during this century; iatrogenic, social, emotional, and chronic problems have replaced acute infections as the principal causes of child morbidity. The term 'new morbidity' has been coined to describe this change. The main manifestations of the 'new morbidity' are considered in this part.

16 The new iatrogenesis
Ulla Fasting

Life begins at conception

The creation of life has always appeared to be beyond man. Recent technological developments, however, challenge this assumption. Until only a few years ago it was impossible for a child to be conceived outside the body of its mother—today it is a routine procedure: a fertilized human ovum can develop under artificial conditions for a period of 3–4 weeks outside the womb. The subsequent 20 weeks of development are still dependent on the body of the mother but at a gestation age of 23–24 weeks, the fetus can survive outside the womb. Post-menopausal women can become pregnant by the use of eggs from fertile women; the same procedure can be used for women with ovarian dysgenesis (Turner's syndrome).

The early development of a child is no longer a mystery. The fortunate go through their early development undisturbed, only to leave their cosy environment to enter the hi-tech world of today—the younger and less mature the child, the greater the chances of an early introduction to technology. Little is known of how the child experiences this encounter and how it affects their development. We have gained some knowledge but are far from knowing enough; this creates difficult ethical problems as to the application of new technology to fetuses and small children. The prologue to the UN Convention on the rights of the child states the following.

Bearing in mind that, as indicated in the declaration of the rights of the child, 'the child, by reason of his physical and mental immaturity, needs special safeguards and care, including appropriate legal protection, before as well as after birth.'

This statement is important because it is the only one in which the Convention defends the right of the unborn child. The 'Declaration of the rights of the child' of 1959 included the same statement, but in practice, the legal rights of the fetus have been weakened over the past 30 years. In the last 20 years in Europe, the right to abortion on demand and the use of new technical innovations have impinged upon the rights of the fetus. At the same time, however, these technological advances have improved the chances of survival of a child or fetus, thereby supporting their rights in the periods before, during, and after birth.

This development is by no means surprising but that does not make it less serious. A fundamental element of the European way of thinking is the principle that the powerful rule the weak: Aristotle stated that 'those who have knowledge are entitled to rule over the ignorant'. From this standpoint, the child is usually evaluated in adult terms and has necessitated the principle that the weak need protection a principle which, perhaps, is an intrinsic part of human nature since children can trigger our instincts to nurture. So, perhaps we should look for solutions based on moral rather than legal principle, with the emphasis on needs rather than on rights.

The new technology has a strong impact on two areas: the development of the fetus in connection with *in vitro* fertilization (IVF), and the treatment of premature babies. These topics introduce ethical dilemmas in which the child's life is created and preserved at a cost.

This chapter discusses first, the ethics of infertility and the technical development created to overcome it, and second, the ethics of treating premature babies. The child's perspective is taken in the ethical analysis, which is supported by the *UN Convention on the rights of the child*, and where the main objective is to create happy, confident children who are ready to take on the responsibility of the future. Measures for the prevention of iatrogenic morbidity are also discussed.

In vitro fertilization

In vitro fertilization (IVF) exemplifies the many technical methods used to treat infertility. Some of the medical complications that affect the pregnant woman can also make an impact on the growing fetus, such as in extra-uterine pregnancies which are three times as common in IVF. Furthermore, caesarean sections and toxic reactions in pregnancy are more common. Another important risk related to the fetus or child is the risk of spontaneous abortion which terminates every fourth IVF pregnancy. The risks of malformation and chromosome defects are probably not increased, but perinatal deaths are more common, with three per cent compared to the 0.3 per cent for normal pregnancies. Thirty five per cent of children have a low birth-weight and 27 per cent are born prematurely, compared to five per cent for normal pregnancies. This partly explains the increased morbidity and mortality rates. A further explanation is the higher risk of a pregnancy with multiple fetuses, but these risks also affect single-fetus pregnancies, which represent 18 per cent of cases.[1] Multiple fetuses occur in about 30 per cent of cases, causing an increased risk of prematurity, which in turn increases the mortality and morbidity rates and the risk of neurological sequelae.[2]

IVF raises many ethical questions: the technology, as such, has been rejected by the Roman Catholic Church because it separates conception from intercourse and the love connected with it.[3] Is it always the responsibility of a society to satisfy the needs of its citizens, even when scarce resources may force a choice between the treatment of cancer and IVF? On a global perspective, overpopulation causes innumerable deaths among children each day, because of malnutrition in combination with bad health and lack of potential for children to develop physically and mentally. There is also the question of the fertilized eggs that are not implanted and used for research, or implanted in the womb of another woman.

Research

Some countries, such as the UK, have sanctioned research on fertilized human eggs up until 14 days of age. Peter Singer, an Australian philosopher, has suggested that research should be allowed up to five or six weeks of gestation because the fetus lacks sensory reactions until the seventh week.[4] A longer limit of 18 to 20 weeks has also been discussed. This longer limit is only possible if the concept of 'a higher order of brain death' is accepted, i.e. the loss of brain functions which steer consciousness and awareness.[5] If one could declare a person who has lost the higher brain functions as dead, there is a logical consequence that a fetus which has not yet gained these functions is declared as 'not being alive'. Acceptance of these criteria would solve some of the moral problems involved in transplantation, treatment, and research on fetuses and their organs. However, conceived eggs and fetuses have increasingly become dehumanized. This is illustrated in the vocabulary of research such as the term 'experimental substance', which represents an abortus; and unused *in vitro* fertilized eggs which are known as 'excessive products'.

Donation of human eggs

Sperm donation is not without problems but the donation of eggs is more complicated in relation to children. Who is the 'real' mother, the genetic, biological or social mother? And who does the child 'belong' to? These are new problems, and the long-term consequences to the child are unknown. How will the child react on finding out how he or she was 'created', and what happens if the child wants to contact the genetic parents and siblings? Will the child feel in any way 'rejected' by the 'real' parents and perhaps feel jealously towards the siblings? Many adopted children have strong urge to know their origins. It might not be easy for a child to accept that one or both parents are not, in fact, the 'real' (or genetic) parents. One of the basis principles of the UN Convention is the right to know your origin. Adoption is a special case, and as stated in article 21, 'State parties that recognize and/or permit the system of adoption shall ensure that the best interests of the child shall be the paramount consideration'. The 'Declaration of human rights' stresses the child's right to know its origins equally strongly: 'The first priority for a child is to be cared for by his or her own parents' and 'The need of a foster- or an adopted child to know about his or her background should be recognized by persons responsible for the child's care unless this is contrary to the child's best interests'.

Premature children

We do not have accurate knowledge about the long-term outcome for premature children: there have been no follow-up studies of extremely pre-term children into school age, and so we have no clear idea of the outcome of premature birth and its effect from the child's point of view. However, there are children now four or five years of age who spent their first months in hospital or under intensive care, who are often described as withdrawn and overprotected. They do not respond well to either positive or negative stimuli, have clumsy movements, and do not react to physical contact. Their drawings show few details and they lack colour. Drawings of the 'self' show a person with diffuse outlines, floating in the air. Some of these children are in long-term therapy because of a diagnosis of 'early frustration' and 'organic brain damage',[6] the symptoms of which are similar to Bowlby's classic observations of deprived children.[7]

Some basic facts on the premature child

Cerebral palsy (CP) increases with lower birth-weight and is about 50 per cent more common among very low birth-weight children (<1,500 g). Perinatal mortality among the premature has decreased in recent years but the number of children with CP has increased. Twenty years ago about 20 per cent of premature children survived; five per cent of those had cerebral palsy. Today 80 per cent survive with the same proportion having CP, which means that the total number of children disabled by CP has increased.

The disease pattern has changed from 'a slight to moderate form of diplegia in an otherwise healthy child having normal mental capacities', which was the clinical picture previously attributed to prematurity. Only half of the present day CP syndromes in very low birth-weight children have these clinical features; instead there is an increasing number of quadriplegic children, hydrocephalus, severe visual impairments, epilepsy, and mental retardation.[8] A similar pattern is seen if gestational age is used as the measure 50 per cent of infants born before 29 weeks' gestation survive, and of these, 23 per cent are severely disabled, 13 per cent are moderately disabled, 29 per cent have mild impairment and only 35% are normal at four years of age.[9]

Are the healthy children really healthy?

The causes of CP are important aetiological factors related to learning difficulties, but the follow-up period is at present too short to enable a full evaluation of cognitive skills, motor skills, or visual capacities. Also, social context influences the child's development, which was illustrated by a 1956 study showing an increase in hospital admissions related to poor housing conditions.[10] A 30 year follow-up to this study tried to clarify what conditions in childhood created problems later in adulthood: housing conditions had the greatest impact on somatic and psychiatric hospital admissions, and was also related to criminal behaviour.[11] The study proved that the basic causes of adverse health persisted in the welfare state in spite of an increase in resource allocation to the education, health, and social system. There are few children who have been able to break this social heritage.

Ethical standpoints

There are great uncertainties connected to the evaluation of premature children immediately after birth. Attitudes and practices differ between countries, centres, and individuals.

The following principles have been constituted by The Hastings Center, based on a project called '*The imperiled newborns*'.[12] The principles are intended to guide the treatment of the extremely premature child and the very ill child.

1. *The statistical approach.* According to this decision strategy, if a premature infant were to fall below a cut-off level for age and size, aggressive treatment would not be provided.

The opposing principle is called

2. *The 'wait until near-certainty' approach.* Here, treatment is provided for every infant that is even potentially viable, and to continue active treatment until it is certain that a particular baby will either die or will be so severely impaired that, under any substantive standard, parents could legitimately opt for termination of treatment.

The intermediate approach is called

3 *The individualized approach.* Treatment is begun for every infant, but parents are allowed the option of termination before it is absolutely certain that a particular infant will either die or be so devastingly disabled that he or she will be unable to relate to others or to the environment. Under this strategy doctors will periodically reassess the infant's probable prognosis, taking into account such factors as severe intraventricular haemorrhages or other indicators of probable neurological impairment, and will allow termination of treatment if there is a high chance (though not certainty) of severe disability.

The statistical approach uses a strictly objective view of the child where the understanding of the child is based on an understanding of statistical probabilities. The problem is reduced to a purely medical problem where ethical issues are neglected and the parents do not participate in the decision making.

The same applies to the 'near certainty' approach where attention is drawn towards all available technical possibilities, leaving aside the sufferings of the child in relation to the treatment. Ethical dilemmas are neglected and the parents are merely bystanders.

The 'individual' approach mainly concentrates on the child in conjunction with the parents. The difficult ethical problems related to each situation are considered. The objective is to deal with ethical decisions rather than with certainty.

Technology in relation to 'the needs of the child'

According to one of the persons involved in the preparation of the *UN Convention on the rights of the child*, Dr Lars H. Gustavsson, each child has seven basic needs:

(1) to have roots;

(2) to be seen;

(3) to have the devoted time of adults;

(4) to have two parents

(5) to be associated with several proud adults;

(6) the right to their own personal human rights;

(7) to have a future.

These seven basic needs are relevant from the start and it is the responsibility of adults to help the child fulfil these needs. It is not only a parental responsibility to achieve this but a moral and political responsibility. It is possible to constitute laws and take the necessary political initiatives which secure the best possible start for each child. The new technology has been available for such a long time that our moral decisions and actions no longer have to be steered by this uncontrolled machinery.

Remmen has classified the technological development from 1970 onwards into three categories.[13]

1. *Evaluation of consequences*: a reactive mode of decision making (i.e. to reduce harmful effects).

2. *A holistic evaluation*: proactive (i.e. to develop the technologies needed).

3. *A constructive evaluation*: interactive (i.e. to influence technical development).

In the early 70s the focus was on reducing the harmful effects of technology by developing new technology. Within neonatology this meant highly intensive, highly technological and invasive treatment of the premature with little consideration of the social or psychomotor consequences to the child. The reaction was a focus on alternative treatments, such as the 'kangaroo method'.

Both these attitudes still exist but gradually a third approach has developed—the constructive evaluation of technology. This means that one tries to anticipate the consequences, to the individual, of technical development at the stages of research, planning, and construction. The consequence is that the latest technical development in neonatal care is non-invasive and aims not to be harmful to the child; for instance, the incubators of today are constructed in a way which stimulates the sensorimotor development of the newborn.

The change in perspective on technological development is clear; from being an 'external decoy' where activities were limited by the possible negative consequences, the technology of today has a social construct where the human being and the environment are considered at the stages of research, planning, and design—this development enables a dialogue between the consumer and the expert.

If the seven points regarding the needs of the child are related to the development of the technology involved in early life it becomes possible to make clear what demands must be placed on technology.

- To have *roots* means that the child has sensory needs, that the child belongs to the family and a group of relatives which form a good basis for growth.

- To be *seen* can be interpreted as the need of the child to be seen as a human being with all potentials, resources, and possibilities which have to be respected in medical interventions.

- To have the *devoted time of the adults* means that people who love and care and devote time to the child are also able to listen, talk to, and represent the child and defend it against technical maltreatment, thus making the world less terrifying.

- Unless you have *two parents* it is difficult to know who you are, i.e. to know your origins.

- To have several *proud adults* gives emotional strength and self-respect.

- To have *human rights* means being respected as a human being.

- To have a *future* places a demand on adults not to hurt the child and to guarantee that all children are met by a loving and caring environment, enabling full development of the child's potential.

It is easier to understand the ethical problems when these seven basic needs of the child are kept in mind. Using them as a starting point it is possible to limit the negative technical consequences and decide how this development can be beneficial to the child. It can be helpful to evaluate whether it is a question of the adults' need of children or the child's need of responsible adults. Furthermore, the seven basic needs can have an impact at the child's point of entry into the world, when the relationship between the prematurely born and technology is encountered. They can guide research, development, treatment, and care.

The needs of the premature child in relation to technology: a coexistence determined by the child's needs

Premature children have first of all the same basic needs as full-term children, but they have been deprived of their optimal natural environment—the womb. This should therefore serve as a model for the artificial environment one has to design when essential new technology is developed for the premature child, which should support the sensorimotor development of the premature child. The child and its demands on the environment should guide the technical development.

Sensorimotor development

The sensorimotor development of a child follows a biological clock. In a sense it is preconditioned, and trigger mechanisms need to be stimulated at the right time in order to have optimal development. Any misinterpretations may lead to suboptimal sensorimotor and emotional development. An integration of the senses means to coordinate all sensory stimuli, and the principle of learning should be connected to desire because the child has a natural need to learn and integrate the impulses. For example, the first time hunger is experienced, the child starts to cry, the mother takes the child to her breast and the child experiences a success. A similar reaction is induced when the bladder is filled and emptied. The repetition of these patterns of 'stimulus and response' induces a sense of security and increases the sense of self-confidence. The child is able to imitate the behaviour of the parents from birth, which is an example of advanced sensory integration.

The tactile sense

Already in the seventh week of gestation the child is able to react to sensory stimuli. This early development is an indication that this sense is vital to survival. Jean Ayers, who has developed a method of stimulating sensory integration, thinks that the skin functions as an 'external central neutral system'.[14] She says that 'a constant bombardment of tactile stimuli to the brain is essential for the maintenance of a stable central neural system. If not stabilised, there is a risk of sensory deprivation which, later in life, may cause problems on the emotional and perceptual levels'. The skin of very small children is very thin and sensitive at a time when the brain is especially vulnerable. This intimate relationship may lead to brain damage if wrongly induced.

When the child is unable to float in the amniotic fluid it is especially important to consider other forms of stimuli. The skin of the parents is the next best choice, especially in the area between the breasts of the mother where it is moist and warm. This can serve as an alternative to the incubator and is the principle behind the so-called 'kangaroo method'. The child remains between the mother's breasts, close to the nipple where feeding is easily induced until sucking becomes independent. This guarantees optimal sensory integration and access to breast-milk whenever needed. Combined to this method the child is placed on a lamb skin—which induces faster weight gain.[15]

The vestibular sense

The sense of balance is developed at about 20 weeks of gestation. The vestibular stimuli are processed in the cerebellum which is in a stage of rapid development in the last three months of gestation. Almost full maturation is reached at the age of one year. This development is necessary to enable the child to sit and walk later. A premature child in an incubator easily loses this sensory stimulus; a child in the womb or a newborn which is kept in contact with the skin of the mother or father, or rocked in a chair or moved around in a cushioned pram has constant stimuli. The rocking movement as well as touch stimulates the respiratory centre and also reduces anxiety. Lack of these stimuli could be one explanation of spells of apnoea which can occur in the prematurely born. An alternative to the mother's body is an incubator incorporating a water-bed, or a cot which can be rocked manually.

The auditory sense

Auditory senses are developed simultaneously with the vestibular senses. They are intimately connected to perceptions of rhythm and sound. The sound of the mother's heartbeat, her breathing and voice, plus all the natural sounds of her daily activities are part of the child's development and sense of security. A child in an incubator loses all these stimuli and has only the monotonous mechanical sounds of the machines or sudden sounds in the environment such as phones ringing or alarms going off. This is being encountered today in the early life of the premature. It has also been shown that human voices, soft music, occasional periods of relative silence, or the beat of a heart increases the child's sucking intensity and also makes the child calm. This is one of the explanations of better weight gain than that seen in babies subjected to high levels of noise or total silence.

The visual sense

Rhythm is also relevant to light, as seen in the daily rhythms of light. It has been shown that children who are exposed to light constantly have a slower weight gain than children who have a variation of light and dark. Premature children who are stimulated by strong light around the clock show greater risks of developing retinopathy than prematures who have rhythmic lights.[16]

Sensory integration and technology

The senses are not only to be stimulated, they are also to be integrated and the child must not be over- or under-stimulated. It is of no use to give massage to all premature children even though we know that touch is an important part of development—it might be that the skin is too thin and could be damaged if stimulated too strongly. Too strong a stimulus can cause too strong a sensation, when just the touch of a hand may be appropriate to comfort the child.

Interaction with premature children demands an increased awareness, to understand and sense the needs of the child, and to be able to react to what is experienced and seen. The adult must be able to love the child as a fellow human being.

The development of technical equipment has to be based on the knowledge of the needs and development of the unborn and newly born child. Only through this knowledge it becomes possible to develop a technology which is supportive the child's development and does not cause injuries. The only demand which cannot be placed on technology is to love the child. On the other hand, it is possible to use technical equipment in such a way that prevents the child from becoming an object, failing which much energy has to be put into repairing the damage caused. The greater the vulnerability of the child, the greater the demand on technical compatibility and the more careful one has to be to initiate technical interventions. Technology is not there to disturb and break the relationship between the child and its parents, which can easily occur in this extremely sensitive stage of development, with possibly fatal consequences. When survival is beyond the reach of technology and the child's capabilities, treatment must be discontinued. It is then appropriate to create a respectful, loving atmosphere where the child is in immediate physical contact with the parents.

References

1. Konsensusuttalande (1990). Assisterad befruktning vid ofrivillig barnlöshet. *Medicinska forskningsrådet*. SPRI, Stockholm.
2. Lindemann, R. and Finne, P.H. (1988). Pediatriske aspekter ved in vitro fertilisering. *Tidskr. Nor Lægeforen* **108**, 405–6.
3. Lauritzen, P. (1990) *What price parenthood?* pp. 38–46. Hastings Center Report, March/April.
4. Singer, P. (1989). Embryo experimentation and the moral status of the embryo. Paper presented to the Aberdeen Conference, HELP, July 1989.
5. Wikler, D. and Weisbard, A.J. (1989). Appropriate confusion over 'brain death'. *J. Am. Med. Assoc.* **261**, Editorial.
6. Rygaard, N.P. (1991). *Tidlig frustration*. Socialpædagoisk Bibliotek, Munksgaard, Copenhagen.
7. Bowlby, J. (1988). *Clinical applications of attachment theory*. Routledge, London.

8. Konsensus-rapport (1990). *Ekstremt tidligt fødte børn.* Danish Medical Research Council and Danish Hospital Institute, Copenhagen.
9. Johnson, A., Townshend, P., Yudkin, P., Bull, D. and Wilkinson, A. (1993). Functional abilities at four years of children born before 29 weeks of gestation. *British Medical Journal*; **306**, 1715–8.
10. Christensen, V. (1956). *Boligforhold og børnesygelighed, en undersøgelse af hospitalsindlæggelsen under forskellige boligforhold.* Munksgaard, Copenhagen.
11. Andersen, T.F. (1984). Persistence of social and health problems in the welfare state: a Danish cohort experience from 1948 to 1979. *Soc. Sci. Med.* **18**, 555–60.
12. Caplan, A. and Cohen, C.B.(ed.) (1987). *Imperiled newborns.* pp. 5–32. Hastings Center Report, December.
13. Remmen, A. (1990). *Konstruktiv teknologivurdering—at komme bagklogskaben i forkøbet.* Institut for Samfundsøkonmi og Planlægning, Aalborg Universitetscenter.
14. Ayres, J. (1984). *Sensory integration and learning disorders* (7th edn.) Western Psychological Services Los Angeles, USA.
15. Scott S. Lucas, P., Cole, T., and Richards, M. *et al.* (1983). Weight gain and movement patterns of very low birth weight babies nursed on lambswool. *Lancet* 1014–16.
16. Glass, P., Avery, G., Subramaniam, K., Keys, M., Sostek, A., and Friendly, D. *et al.* (1985). Effect of bright light in the hospital nursery on the incidence of retinopathy prematurity. *New Eng. J. Med.*, 313, (7), 401–4.

17 Suboptimal nutrition
Ann Aukett and Brian Wharton

The Declaration of Alma-Ata at the WHO international conference on primary health care in 1978 (WHO, 1978) expressed the need for urgent action to protect and promote the health of all the people of the world. Section VII No 3 refers to the promotion of food supply and proper nutrition (WHO 1978). Article 24 of the *UN Convention on the rights of the child* also places emphasis on the combating of malnutrition and the provision of adequate, nutritious foods (United Nations 1991).

Whereas in many parts of the world frank malnutrition and prevention of death from it is a major concern of health professionals, in Europe such frank malnutrition is rare but under-nutrition and the problems relating to it are still common. This chapter will aim to cover aspects of nutrition in European children, concentrating mainly on experience in the UK but drawing generally applicable conclusions from that experience.

Against the perspective of malnutrition in the Third World, problems of under-nutrition in Europe may seem trivial and, since they rarely lead to death, statistics concerning them are hard to find. Data on what normal children actually eat even where available usually reflect national data and it is important to remember, in interpreting such data, that statistics vary quite markedly according to social class.

It is often impossible to single out the nutritional problems of the child completely, as their nutritional state may well depend on the nutrition of the mother during pregnancy and lactation. However, this suboptimal nutrition in pregnancy—affecting the newborn child and low birth-weight infants in particular—will not be dealt with in this chapter as these aspects are covered elsewhere in the text. However, just as the nutrition of the child *in utero* may affect his nutritional status and health in childhood, so may the nutritional state of the child affect the nutritional state and health of the adult, and patterns of eating established during childhood may continue into adulthood. The diets of free living, healthy children cannot be taken in isolation from the diet of the whole population in which they are growing up.

Normal physiological nutrition in Europe: what is optimal?

In order to discuss suboptimal nutrition, some baseline of what is optimal needs to be established. Many countries, including the UK, have tried to produce recommended daily intakes of nutrients. The most recent of these, published in the

UK in 1991 (DOH 1991), moves away from RDI (recommended daily intakes) and RDA (recommended daily amounts) to 'dietary reference values?. The RDA are defined as 'the average amount of the nutrient which should be provided per head in a *group* of people if the needs of partically all the members of the group are to be met'. They are not, therefore, indicators for the diets of individuals. The recommended levels are well above the physiological requirements in order to cover 'practically all members of the group'. The new dietary reference values draw a distinction between EAR (estimate of average requirement)—i.e. half the group will need more, half will need less, the RNI (reference nutrient intake)—the amount that is enough for about 97 per cent of people in a group, and the LRNI (lower reference nutrient intake)—the amount that is enough for only the few people in a group who have low needs.

The use of such tables for children poses particular problems as age is used as the basis for recommendations without regard to the considerable variations in body size which occur in children of the same age. As many countries have their own tables of recommended daily amounts, some more comprehensive than others, and showing considerable variation, it is quite possible for a child's diet to be 'adequate' in one country and 'deficient' in another, and indeed RDA should not be used in this way.

RDA are also used for food labelling, public health assessment of populations, agricultural planning, diets for institutions, as well at the diagnosis of under-nutrition and malnutrition. In order to place these in context it is worth noting that many would regard the scientific facts that have been used to derive the RDA to be inadequate (Whitehead 1991).

It is also important that health professionals are clear about the difference between RDA and dietary guidelines. The figures for RDA have frequently been set following metabolic balance studies or from observations of nutrient deficiency states. Each country will have only one set of RDA. Dietary guidelines are aimed at protecting the health of the general population by reducing the adult degenerative diseases believed to be wholly or partially attributed to diet. Some specifically exclude children below certain ages. These guidelines tend to address the quality of the dietary components rather than the quantity—the new 'healthy' diet being one which is lower in sugar and fat and higher in fibre. These diets may not always be appropriate for children.

Nutritional practice in Europe

In the UK there have now been three reports for the Committee on medical aspects of food policy on 'Present day practice in infant feeding' (DHSS 1974, 1980, 1988). The last of these also deals with the diet of the toddler and young child and subsequent health in later life. In 1988 a major report dealt with the diet of British schoolchildren (DOH 1989). Both of these reports were published at a time when public interest in the relationship between diet and health was increasing.

In the UK there have been several changes in nutritional practice over the past 20 years and these have been reflected in many other European countries, notably Scandinavia (Soderhjelm and Zetterstrom 1990). Some of these changes and the factors associated with them are considered below.

Breast-feeding

Breast-milk, with its correct balance of nutrients and chemical constituents, is the nutritionally ideal food for babies. The psychological, anti-infective, and other protective mechanisms that breast-feeding promotes are also well described. In spite of this the overall incidence of breast-feeding in many children is disappointingly low. In the early part of the twentieth century most babies were breast fed and there was then a decline to very low rates in the 1960s. Over the following 20 years there was a gradual increase from, in the UK, 51 per cent in 1975 to 67 per cent in 1980 and there has been little change since that time (DHSS 1988). The number of babies still being breast-fed at six to eight weeks has also increased but is still disappointingly low (40 per cent). In Holland it is slightly higher at 53 per cent (Geuns *et al.* 1985), and in Sweden even higher—80 per cent at two months. (Soderhjelm and Zetterstrom 1990; Hillervik-Lindquist 1991).

First or second born child, education of the mother, higher social class, living in more prosperous areas, and mother being over 25 years are all factors associated with the highest incidence of breast-feeding. In the UK in 1985, 87 per cent of social class I mothers (i.e those with husbands in professional occupations) breast-fed compared with 43 per cent of social class V (those with husbands in unskilled manual occupations) (DHSS 1988). The influence of social factors has been described also in the USA and Scandinavian countries (Stahlberg 1985). Clearly, education about the benefits of breast-feeding has to be targeted at poorer mothers from lower socio-economic classes but the issue may not be as simple as this and the changes probably reflect complicated and profound changes in society.

In response to concerns about the nutrition of babies worldwide, the WHO International code on the marketing of breast-milk substitutes was adopted in 1981 (WHO 1981) in order to protect and promote breast-feeding and to ensure the proper use of infant formulae. It has been up to individual Governments to ensure that infant formulae in their country are marketed in accordance with the WHO code. It is not clear how far this has been implemented in the whole of Europe but many would feel there is still room for improvement!

The reasons for the poor rates of initiation of breast-feeding in women from lower socio-economic groups warrants further investigation. One study in a socially disadvantaged area of London (Rajan and Oakley 1990) indicated that improved social support from health professionals and others in the postnatal period could increase breast-feeding success rates and a study in Poland indicated that the lack of knowledge, attitudes, and activities of health service workers could be obstructive to the initiation of breast-feeding (Mikiel-Kostyra and Galecki 1990 *a,b,c*). As approximately 30 per cent of mothers decide on the feeding method before they become pregnant and the rest decide early in pregnancy, attention should be directed perhaps to schoolgirls rather than pregnant women.

Much more research has been centred on the reasons for cessation of breast-feeding once started. In the UK, although in 1985 65 per cent of mothers started to breast-feed, this had fallen to 57 per cent by one week, 40 per cent by six weeks, and 26 per cent by four months. Only 12 per cent were still breast-feeding at nine months.

Mothers in the groups which were most likely to start breast-feeding were also those who continued the longest. The most common reason given for cessation is 'insufficient milk'. Studies in Sweden (Hillervik-Lindquist 1991) and Denmark (Weile *et al.* 1990) have looked at this phenomenon and what might influence it. Apart from purely physiological influences such as maternal diet, age, smoking habits, and contraceptive use, there are also indirect influences such as maternal time constraints, sociocultural factors, maternal comfort factors, and infant factors. The socio-cultural factors again seem to have the most influence (Hill and Humenick 1989). The complexity of the problem is illustrated by a study in the USA where an intensive programme of post-partum counselling did not affect the duration of breast-feeding in low income women (Grossman *et al.* 1990).

Infant formula and bottle feeding

Most infant formulae presently available in Europe are based on cow's milk. Some contain other proteins, e.g. soya, but in general, these more specialized formulae are used for babies with special requirements. Whilst nutritionally, bottle-feeding is a safe alternative to breast-feeding as long as an approved infant formula is used, it does not carry the immunological and other advantages of breast-feeding. In the UK in 1985, 36 per cent of mothers gave infant formula from the start and by four weeks the majority of babies were receiving some formula. At four months, 75 per cent of babies were bottle-fed (DHSS 1988). Comparative figures for Sweden indicate that 40–50 per cent are bottle-fed at four months (Soderhjelm and Zetterstrom 1990) and in Holland 30–50 per cent (Geuns *et al.* 1985).

In planning nutrition education programmes it is clearly important, therefore, that bottle-feeding is not ignored as most babies are fed in this way at some stage. Consequently, parents still need education about the use of infant formulae. Balance needs to be sought, however, so that the instruction in the correct use of bottle-feeds does not carry an implied support for artificial feeding over breast-feeding. In particular, samples of infant formulae should not be given to mothers and the WHO code on their marketing should be adhered to (WHO 1981). The choice of infant formula should be up to the mother. All formulae should meet acceptable compositional standards and governments should ensure that they do so.

The Scientific Committee for food of the European Economic Community have introduced specific definitions for infant formulae and follow-up milks.

- *Infant formulae* are 'products intended where necessary to replace human milk and to meet, by themselves, the normal nutritional needs of infants during the first four to six months of life' and 'which can satisfactorily be used for feeding infants aged over four to six months provided they are suitably enriched with iron'—to be labelled as *'infant formulae'* and 'suitable for infants from birth to one year'.

- *follow-up milks* are 'products intended to constitute the basic milk element in the progressively diversified diet of infants aged over four months'—to be labelled as 'follow-up milks' and 'suitable for infants over the age of four months and young children', accompanied by a statement to the effect that the product should form part of a diversified diet.

Follow-up milk are used extensively in Belgium, France, Greece, Italy, and Spain but to a much lesser extent elsewhere in Europe and North America. They have no particular advantage over continued use of an iron-fortified infant formula, but if a mother wishes strongly to change from an infant formula then a follow-up milk is preferable to whole cow's milk.

The Scientific Committee for food has also made recommendations concerning the composition of these products (Astier-Dumas *et al.* 1983) and these have been adopted as a directive of the European Commission. Numerous other expert bodies have issued recommendations and there are a number of differences (Wharton 1984). All recommend a lower concentration (per unit volume and per unit energy) of protein and the major minerals such as phosphorus, sodium, calcium, potassium, etc., than are found in cow's milk.

However, WHO/FAO and particularly the USA, are not as stringent as others in this and some formulae which would be allowed by those regulations would not be acceptable to current paediatric opinion. All except WHO/FAO and the USA insist on some lactose in the formula and in France, a formula described as 'maternise' must have lactose as the only carbohydrate. All except the UK insist on a minimum of 300 mg per 100 kcal of linoleic acid (UK suggests 100 mg). UK, France, and the EEC also define an upperlimit for linoleic acid. Other recommendations concerning fat composition are expressed only in general terms concerning fat absorption, but the EEC sets an upper limit on the amounts of lauric and myristic acid; the use of cotton oil, sesame oil, and fats containing more than eight per cent *trans* isomers of fatty acids is prohibited. France limits vegetable oils to a maximum of 40 per cent of the total fat, so that in practice most formulae in France contain some cow's milk fat. In the UK, no recommendations as to compositional guidelines are made regarding trace elements at present. WHO/FAO, USA, and France set minima for copper, iodine, manganese, and zinc; EEC does not set a lower limit for manganese. The UK suggests, and the EEC sets, maxima too for these trace elements. Fortification with iron is allowed by all, but France does not allow fortification with vitamin D.

The French and USA (American) limits are enforceable by law and the EEC limits will become enforceable shortly.

Weaning

Weaning begins when semi-solid food starts to be given in addition to milk. It is usually a gradual process. The introduction of cereals and other complex foods before four months is discouraged (DHSS 1988). The baby in the first six months of life is vulnerable, particularly to diarrhoeal diseases, because of the immaturity of the digestive, absorptive, and local defence systems (Milla 1986) and for this reason the time of weaning is a dangerous one for the child, particularly in the developing world where the malnutrition/diarrhoea complex is a major cause of mortality (Wharton 1986). However, the relationship between diarrhoea and diet are not merely 'tropical' considerations. Gastro-enteritis is a continuing problem to child health even in the UK, and deaths from this show a considerable social gradient with a nine-fold difference between social classes I and V. In addition to this, iron deficiency and rickets continue to be major problems in the weaning period, as do the lesser ones of zinc deficiency, allergy, and obesity.

Weaning practices in the UK have changed. As breast-feeding declined and cow's milk was consumed earlier, so solid foods were given earlier too. Then the trend reversed. (See Table 17.1.)

In all surveys there is a strong association between bottle-feeding and starting solid foods early. In interpreting national data it is important to remember the major social class differences, particularly in bottle- and breast-feeding. However, in the UK the indications are that there has been a relative improvement right across the social spectrum (Whitehead *et al.* 1986). In Scandinavia, weaning seems to occur somewhat later with four months being the earliest time solid foods are introduced (Soderhjelm and Zetterstrom 1990) with the mean age being nearer five months in successfully breast-fed babies (Hillervik-Lindquist 1991). Although early weaning can be problematic, if solids are intro-

Table 17.1 *Consumption of solid foods by age and year (DHSS 1988)*

Year	Age		
	Four weeks	Eight weeks	Three months
1975	18%	49%	85%
1980	4%	24%	55%

duced late, the child may experience difficulties in establishing a nutritionally adequate diet. This seems to be a particular problem with Asian children in the UK (Jivani 1978).

Not only the timing of weaning but the types of foods introduced needs to be considered. In the UK, mothers who started weaning early tended to choose rusks, cereals, and commercial baby foods. At four to five months only 35 per cent used home-made weaning foods (DHSS 1988). In Sweden and Finland, gruels made from oat or wheat flour or a manufactured mixture were given as first food, and in Norway porridge. Tinned baby foods have been used less and prepared fruit and vegetables are often used by six months (Soderhjelm and Zetterstrom 1990). Amongst the Swedish breast-feeding mothers quoted above (Hillervik-Lindquist 1991) mashed potatoes was the most common first food (64 per cent). Many cultures have a traditional first food so there is likely to be considerable variation across Europe. As babies get older a much wider variety of foods is eaten in all countries and the nutritional adequacy or otherwise of the diet may well depend on many socio-economic factors. A considerable body of opinion believes that the continuation of some sort of fortified food, either formula or fortified solid food, would produce a safety net, particularly of vitamins and minerals, that would help the child through this difficult period of weaning until the child is on 'sensible' family foods (Wharton 1986).

Traditionally the first weaning foods offered throughout most of Europe have been cereals; in some countries a cereal 'pap' (i.e. with milk or water) is offered for many months. Cereals are used as weaning foods in many ways, e.g. alone, mixed with milk or water, baked as biscuits and rusks, or combined with other foods. In addition the infant may consume some of the wide selection of cereal foods available for older children and adults, e.g. breakfast, cereal, bread, etc.

The exact uses of commercially available weaning foods containing meat, poultry, or fish also vary considerably from one country to the other within the European Community. Some mothers, particularly in Italy, use a meat-only preparation as the basis of a dish, adding vegetables, etc. themselves. Others, e.g. in UK, give their babies a 'complete dish' to start with, e.g. lamb and vegetables, and then a second dish or course—dessert, pudding, or fruit. Yet others, e.g. in Germany, use a 'complete meal' from one can or jar. Clearly, a meat-only dish would be relatively high in protein, a complete dish might rely on the second course for various nutrients and energy, while a 'complete meal' would contain reasonable amounts of many nutrients, reasonably balanced.

Fruit juices and nectars have traditionally been used as a vehicle for vitamin C supplementation in Europe, and this practice may have helped to eliminate, almost completely, infantile scurvy from Europe. Most mothers regard fruit and vegetables as a good source of vitamin C. If necessary, vitamin C should be added to commercially available fruit juices for children so that the final concentration is not less than that found in many fruits. Vegetable juices may be used instead of fruit juices and these should have a minimum vitamin C content too.

There have been a number of investigations describing the diet of the weanling in Europe (Stolley et al. 1972; Black et al. 1976; Van Steenbergen 1978; Lestradet et al. 1979; McKillop and Durnin 1982; Boggio et al., 1984) but no recent ones. In the early weanling months, formulae provided a substantial proportion of the total energy and nutrient intake. In later infancy and beyond, this role was taken over by cow's milk which provided about a quarter of the total energy and a third of protein intakes. Total energy intakes studied mostly met the recommended allowances. In general, boys ate more than girls, and energy intakes tended to be a little higher in less-favoured social groups. If the child was not taking vitamin preparations, the intake of vitamin D was frequently below 10 μg (400 International Units) per day. The intake of most other nutrients met the recommended dietary allowances (RDA) of the regions studied except for iron, and the UK report noted that children who drank little milk had intakes of calcium and riboflavin well below the average. The RDA for protein were at that time set to provide about a tenth of the energy intake, but the observed protein intake exceeds this in most countries, particularly in later infancy, reflecting the contribution of cow's milk to the total diet.

As cow's milk in the weanling's diet is replaced by continued use of an infant formula or a follow-up milk, there should be an overall reduction in the intake of protein, calcium, and sodium and there is some evidence that this is occuring.

The European Commission has introduced a draft directive based on a report of the Scientific Committee on food (Wharton et al. 1990) concerning the composition of commercially available weaning foods.

The pre-school child

There is little documented about the diets of toddlers and pre-school children nor indeed little advice as to what an optimal diet for them should be. Children under five were specifically excluded from the COMA report of 1984 (DHSS 1984) while recommended a lower fat, salt, and sugar, and higher fibre diet. Most young children are apparently offered a wide range of foods but the chosen diet of healthy normally growing toddlers varies widely in quality and quantity. The high-fat diet of the infant should be gradually shifted towards the lower fat diet currently recommended for adults, but this needs to be done without compromising the intakes of energy and other nutrients needed for growth. Studies in France (Boggio et al. 1984) and Sweden (Hagmen et al. 1986) suggest that some toddlers have excessive intakes of fat.

A study in a kindergarten in Spain (Farre-Rovira et al. 1990) indicated that children had a high protein (mainly dairy products) and low carbohydrate intake, and low intakes of iron, zinc, folic acid, and vitamin D were seen. This diet is clearly not optimal but may not reflect national trends. Other considerations should be gradual increase in fibre-rich foods and a restriction of salt intake.

Because of the dearth of information on the nutrition of pre-school children, the Department of Health in the UK has recently commissioned a separate report on this age group.

The school-age child

The diet of children from age five upwards should move towards our present concept of a healthy diet for adults. The adequacy of the diet should be measurable by the child's rate of growth, lack of obesity (or thinness), and the absence of any deficiency states such as iron deficiency.

Although the majority of school children in the UK are growing well, some from the lower socio-economic groups rely on free school meals to provide a significant proportion of their nutritional intake (DOH 1989). At weekends and during school holidays these children may receive a much poorer diet. In the 1950s and 60s most British school children received free school milk and a cheap school meal that had to conform to nutritional standards. In the late 1960s, free school milk was stopped for most children and in 1980 local authorities were free to decide the form, content, and price of school meals. Certain children from disadvantaged families were still eligible for free milk and meals. In order to monitor the effect of these changes a survey of the diets of schoolchildren was set up in 1983 and the final report published in 1989 (DOH). The main sources of energy in the diets of British school children were bread, chips, milk, biscuits, meat products, cake and puddings. There were regional variations an variations with social class and other socio-economic variables. Higher chip consumption was recorded among social classes IV and V and children with unemployed fathers and children from families receiving supplementary benefit. Milk consumption was low amongst most of these groups.

Although most children were above the 50th centile for both height and weight, children from families where the father was unemployed were considerably smaller than those from families in social classes I, II, and III. Energy intakes were adequate but three quarters of children had intakes of fat over the level of 35 per cent of energy recommended by COMA (DHSS 1984). Intakes of protein, thiamin, and vitamin C were adequate but girls' iron intake was below the RDA and 60 per cent of older girls had calcium intakes below the RDA. Some older children who ate their meals at 'cafes' had a diet which was the poorest of all the group.

These findings leave no room for complacency and, with the present emphasis on childhood diet and its relationship to adult morbidity/mortality, give considerable cause for concern. Further analysis of the data (Crawford et al. 1987) has confirmed that the diets leave much to be desired from the point of view of preventing cardiovascular disease and are also lacking in many of the nutrients known to be important for general health, growth, and development. Two studies from the former GDR and the USSR (Mior et al. 1988; Gobedzhishvili et al. 1990) would indicate that the UK school children are not unusual.

The adolescent

At adolescence, weight increases in both sexes; girls accumulate relatively more fat and boys more lean tissue. This adolescent growth spurt means that this is a time of increased nutritional requirement and therefore a time when suboptimal nutrition can become important. Most adolescents' appetites increase in proportion to their accelerating rate of growth. In the UK two nutritional problems can occur, iron deficiency and rickets, and these are dealt with below.

Many adolescents worry about their body and this can lead to abnormal eating and exercise problems. In a survey, at least five per cent of girls aged 14/15 years were dieting to lose weight (DOH 1989). Adolescence is also a time when some rebel against conventional foods, other become concerned about the environment, animal rights, and other issues. These young people need support so that a nutritionally adequate intake may be ensured.

Extensive nutritional surveillance takes place during the early period of rapid growth of a child but little attention is focused on the adolescent. We are unsure of the role of school meals or other food supplementation programmes (Wharton and Wharton 1987). As these young people may soon become parents themselves, perhaps some emphasis should be placed on them in the 1990s.

The primary nutritional disease in Europe: Rickets

Rickets is a disorder characterized by the deficient mineralization of bone. It particularly affects the growing epiphyseal ends of the metaphyses in children. The groups mainly affected are toddlers and adolescents and the disease is due to a deficiency of vitamin D (calciferol). About 25 per cent of circulating calciferol is of dietary origin, 75 per cent being synthesized in the skin by sunlight. Although originally known as the 'English Disease', the incidence in the UK has decreased, but it remains a worldwide phenomenon despite recent advances in knowledge of vitamin D metabolism (Belton 1986). There are reports of infantile and toddler rickets even in countries where there is abundant sunlight, e.g. Turkey (Ozsolu 1977) and Greece (Doxiadis *et al.* 1976). A recent study of Asian toddlers in Birmingham, UK showed 40 per cent to have low plasma concentrations of 2,5-hydroxy vitamin D (Grindulis *et al.* 1986). However, in the UK as a whole, the problem may be confirmed to certain susceptible groups (Brook 1983). There are many reasons why children may develop rickets, these are listed below.

1. Lack of exposure to sunlight. This applies particularly to the urban poor. The 43 per cent incidence reported in Glasgow in 1913 was probably due to this factor (Boyle 1991). The city was overcrowded, children played in narrow streets, and there was massive smoke and air pollution which, combined with the weak sunlight, virtually excluded all the ultraviolet light needed to allow the synthesis of vitamin D. Although cured by oral vitamin D supplementa-

tion, this was an air-pollution disease. Although in the UK air pollution has been reduced, this is not true of all European countries. When there has been little exposure to ultra-violet radiation (UVR) during the summer months, the vitamin D status of infants and young children may become low in winter, especially if dietary sources are also poor (DHSS 1988).

2. Poor vitamin D stores due to maternal vitamin D deficiency during pregnancy.
3. Prolonged breast-feeding.
4. Early introduction of unfortified cow's milk.
5. Use of unfortified weaning foods.
6. Vegetarian diets. Many Asian children with rickets (particularly adolescents) have a very low meat intake. It is possible that lean meat, as opposed to fatty meat, contains more vitamin D than had previously been thought.
7. Regulation of vitamin D metabolism may be different in black children compared to those who have fair skin (Belton 1986).
8. Prematurely born infants are especially prone to disturbances of vitamin D metabolism.

Various options have been put forward as methods of prevention, these are listed below.

1. Increasing exposure to sunlight. Reducing air pollution should be the major thrust here but cultural differences in the exposure of the skin to sunlight may play a part and traditional beliefs (e.g. purdah) are not easily overcome. Oral supplementation may provide just as much vitamin D as the UK summer (Grindulis et al. 1986).
2. Fortification of foods, e.g. margarine, chapati, flour, rusks, breakfast cereals.
3. Fortification of cow's milk. If this were done to the present level applied in the USA, the daily requirements of most children would be met.
4. Use of fortified formulae. If these were used up to one year and ideally beyond, this would provide a 'safety net'.
5. Encouraging use of vitamin supplements. The present recommendation in the UK (DHSS 1988) is for vitamin A, C. and D supplements to be given to all infants and children from six months up to at least two years and preferably five years. These should be supplied free to all at-risk groups.
6. Modifications to diet. Health education campaigns to modify diet, e.g. replacing 'ghee', with fortified margarine, must always remain culturally sensitive.
7. Supplementation of vitamin D to pregnant women.

There have been various attempts in the UK to reduce the incidence of rickets, particularly in the Asian community, by health promotion campaigns. The Scottish campaign (Dunnigan et al. 1985), based on the issue of vitamin D supplements, was successful. A health education campaign encouraging dietary change was not successful (Stephens et al. 1982). A 'stop rickets campaign' launched by the DHSS (Deparment of Health and Social Security) and the 'Save the Children Fund' in 1981 (Save the Children Fund 1983) showed an overall increase in the knowledge of rickets as the result of the campaign, but there are no data concerning the uptake of vitamin drops, nor of the effect on the incidence of rickets.

Iron deficiency

The incidence of iron deficiency worldwide is high and it remains so in many European countries (10–40 per cent). In the UK there have been several surveys of this and these are summarized in Table 17.2. Other countries, notably the USA (Dallman and Yip 1989) and some European countries (Haschke and Javaid 1991) have achieved success in prevention. Iron deficiency can develop for a variety of reasons and these are listed in Table 17.3.

Table 17.2 *Incidence of iron deficiency*

Study		Place	Age of children	Ethnic group	Prevalence (%)
Erhardt	(1986)	Bradford	6–48 months	European	12
				Asian	28
Grindulis et al.	(1986)	Birmingham	21–23	Asian	31
Aukett et al.	(1986)	Birmingham	17–19	European	18
				Asian	27
James et al.	(1988)	Bristol	12–48	European	4
				Caribbean	8
				Indian	17
				Vietnamese	20
Wright et al.	(1989)	Newcastle	9–15	Affluent	11
				Deprived	16
Earley et al.	(1990)	London	6–72	European	10
				Asian	27
Mills	(1990)	London	8–24	European	17
				Asian	26
				Caribbean	18
Mardar et al.	(1990)	Nottingham	15–24	European	16
				Asian	26
				Caribbean	20

Table 17.3 *Causes of iron deficiency*

Severe maternal iron deficiency

Prematurity, low birth-weight

Lack of breast-feeding

Prolonged *exclusive* breast-feeding

Early introduction of and excessive intake of cow's milk

Blood loss from GI tract due to cow's milk

Late introduction of suitable weaning foods

Poor utilization of suitable weaning foods (fortified foods and 'natural' foods)

Poor economic circumstance

Blood loss (hookworm)

Although the amount of iron in breast-milk is small, its bioavailability is high and the breast-fed baby does not become iron deficient in the first six months. However, if breast-feeding continues with no added source of iron, the baby will become iron deficient. Most modern infant formulae are fortified with iron and this has been a large factor in the decline of iron deficiency in many countries, but if whole cow's milk is introduced, this can become a major factor in iron deficiency as it contains very little iron which is poorly absorbed. There is also some evidence that cow's milk can induce blood-loss from the gastrointestinal tract (Ziegler *et al.* 1990; Walter *et al.* 1990). An added factor is that many children consume large amounts of milk and little else, hence other souces of iron are not available to them.

The child's solid food at weaning should contain either fortified infant foods or foods containing natural iron. Many do not receive such a diet either for cultural reasons, e.g. being strict vegetarians, Hindus, Moslems, or because of food fads. The bioavailability as well as the iron content of the food needs to be considered. There has always been concern that the iron in fortified cereals may not be in an easily absorbable form (Foman 1987). Recently, more emphasis has been placed on the addition of vitamin C to a child's diet as this increases the bioavailability of non-haem iron (Fairweather-Tait 1989).

Socio-economic circumstances play a major role as higher prevalences of iron deficiency are seen in areas of socio-economic deprivation (Wright *et al.* 1989). In Budapest, Hungary, where there is an incidence of 18–20 per cent overall, this rises to 40 per cent in poor areas (Schuler, personal communication).

Iron deficiency is important because it has consequences that go beyond the production of anaemia itself. These non-haemotological effects are listed in Table 17.4.

Table 17.4 *Non-haematological effects of iron deficiency*

Growth

Skin and mucous membranes

Exercise tolerance

Susceptibility to infection

?GI abnormalities

Ice eating (pagiophagia)

Behaviour

Psychomotor development

School performance

There is still debate about the effects of iron deficiency on susceptibility to infection (Oppenheimer 1989). A more definite and important link has been established between iron deficiency and cognitive development. In adolescence, poor scholatic performance and disruptiveness is described and iron-deficient schoolchildren have poorer educational achievement (Soemantri *et al.* 1985). Several studies have shown that anaemic pre-school children tend to be developmentally delayed, but they improve when given iron. In our own study (Aukett *et al.* 1986) anaemic children grew faster and developed at a faster rate when given iron than children who were not. A more recent worrying study in the USA (Walter *et al.* 1989) showed that some of the deficit was not reversible with iron therapy, hence a shift in emphasis away from screening alone towards prevention.

Prevention of iron deficiency does seem possible and several strategies are necessary (Dallman 1990):

(1) the improvement of infant nutrition in general, particularly around the time of weaning;

(2) the promotion of breast-feeding and its maintenance for at least six months;

(3) the use of iron-fortified formulae if formulae are used;

(4) the avoidance of the early introduction of cow's milk (before one year);

(5) the use of fortified weaning foods;

(6) utilization of vitamin C containing foods to promote absorption of iron;

(7) supplemental iron for low birth-weight babies.

Iodine deficiency

The WHO published data in 1989 (Delange and Burgi 1989) which indicated that iodine deficiency was still prevalent in many European countries in spite of attempted prohpylaxis in some of them. An adequate intake of iodine is said to be 40–120 μg per day for children up to 10 years. With an adequate intake, urinary excretion is more than 10 μg per day and deficiency can be detected in a urinary excretion of less than 50 μg/ per 100 ml.

There are marked regional differences. In northern Europe where seafood is part of the staple diet, cow's milk is rich in iodine due to iodinization of cattle-feed, and iodinated salt is used on a national basis, iodine intake is high and deficiency states are few. In central and southern Germany, virtually all babies were deficient in iodine (values < μ5 g/100 ml), and severe iodine deficiency exists in some parts of Italy—particularly Sicily. Moderate to severe deficiency exists in parts of Austria, Greece, Portugal, Romania, and Spain, and to lesser degrees in many other countries.

As iodine is an essential nutrient, gross deficiency causes clinically apparent problems. In adults, this consequence is usually goitre, but because of the high susceptibility of the developing brain, children under three years are particularly susceptible, this susceptibility starting around 20 weeks of gestation. A second period of high iodine requirement seems to occur in adolescence (Tajtakova *et al.* 1990).

Lack of iodine can cause short stature, mental deficiency, hearing loss, and other neurological impairments, but more recently defective neuromotor and cognitive ability have been reported in otherwise apparently 'normal' school-children with mild to moderate iodine deficiency (Vermiglio *et al.* 1990; Fenzi *et al.* 1990).

Preventive approaches have concentrated mainly on the iodinization of salt, but this approach has not been totally successful (WHO 1990). The daily salt intake has been overestimated and sources of salt from other foods ignored. In some countries not all salt is iodinated and the salt that is may be four to five times more expensive than non-iodinated, placing an additional financial burden particularly on poorer families. Some countries, e.g. Hungary (Delange and Burgi 1989), have successful iodine prophylaxis and in the former GDR an interdisciplinary approach involving both iodinization of salt and animal feeds was extremely successful (Bauch *et al.* 1989; Bauch *et al.* 1990). A similar approach appears to have worked, at least partially, in Sicily (Vermiglio *et al.* 1989). However, opposition to prophylaxis can be culturally determined as belief in hereditary causation has hampered dietary intervention (Lellep-Fernandez 1988). Any preventative approach, therefore, must also be accompanied by information to the community which addresses these beliefs.

Protein-energy deficiency (growth faltering)

Poor weight gain/growth can be caused by not getting enough of the right food, inability to suck or swallow, poor retention of food, malabsorption, or an inability to utilize food. Many of these are purely clinical problems and will not be discussed here.

Protein-energy malnutrition and infection are largely responsible for the very high post-neonatal and toddler mortality rates in developing countries (Wharton 1991). Availability of food is just one environmental factor in the aetiology. Many others such as the size at birth, infections, and culture play a role. Although frank malnutrition is rare in Europe, it is possible, with major changes in economic circumstances, wars, and social upheavals, that it will be seen in the next 10 years and we already have disturbing reports of severely malnourished children in some institutions. Apart from these severe forms, milder forms of protein-energy deficiency causing growth faltering are seen in many European countries, particularly in the poor inner cities.

Most studies suggest some permanent defect in stature if growth is arrested by malnutrition below the age two, but there are problems with control groups. Similarly the effects of malnutrition on the function of the developing brain have the same problems. Common sense dictates that these possible effects should not be ignored.

Malnutrition can be seen as the result of poor education, poor hygiene, poor earning capacity, poor agricultural practices, overpopulation, and inappropriate use of resources. It is clearly associated with poverty.

We have studied children living in the inner city of Birmingham (Leach *et al.* 1987 unpublished data); 36 per cent were one-parent families and 57 per cent on supplementary benefit. We found that only six per cent were receiving a nutritionally adequate diet, and only nine per cent had three meals per day. Although 86 per cent had one protein-rich food every day, only 26 per cent had two protein-rich foods every day. Sixteen per cent never had fruit or vegetables and only 17 per cent had fruit or fruit juice every day. What seems to characterize the poor diet of povery is not the lack of staple food, but a lack of variety of foods—monotony is the hallmark of poverty in this respect (Golden 1991).

As a family becomes poorer, first the luxury items are dropped from the diet, then the more expensive but common foods. Money is then not spent on foods that are perceived as not giving 'value for money' in terms of satisfying the appetite, e.g. fruits and vegetables, and with increasing poverty the diet becomes more and more restricted. This diet, which is adequate in quantity but not in quality, can also lead to malnutrition. It is almost certainly lacking in the nutrients essential for adequate growth.

Particular groups of children seem to be particularly vulnerable to this growth faltering, e.g. inner city Asian children (Jivani 1978; Harris *et al.* 1983). Another group working in London has found that almost 25 per cent of inner city socio-economically disadvantaged children with chronic growth retardation had some disorder of oral-motor functioning. These children tended to come from relatively disorganized homes and they had poor relationships with their mothers, particularly around meal times (Mathisen *et al.* 1989).

Prevention of this problem must occur on several levels. It will have to work at the level of the mother and child and the health professionals but must not ignore the environment outside the family itself, which is influenced by external policies affecting the choice and price of food. Governments and the food industry are the main players here.

Obesity

In adults, the 'body mass index' is used as an indicator of obesity (weight/height). In children this is not as helpful; because of the variation in size with age an alternative method using standard growth charts can be used (Poskitt 1987).

Obesity is a common problem in children of all ages. It has been highlighted as a cause for concern in child health because in adult life severe obesity is associated with reduced lifespan, hypertension, cardiovascular problems, and diabetes mellitus. One-third of obese adults were obese children and 50 per cent of obese adolescents were obese in infancy (Poskitt 1986). For this reason studies are underway to investigate the risk factors of obesity in children (Ladodo *et al.* 1988).

In the 1960s and 1970s obesity in infancy was common and often attributed to overfeeding with unmodified cow's milk formulae and the early introduction of solids. However, studies gave conflicting results. Low social class was an important determinant both for obesity and for not breast-feeding (thought to be protective). As feeding practices changed, obesity in infancy did seem to decrease.

Excess weight must be due to an excess of energy intake over expenditure on growth, exercise, and maintenance, but genetic and environmental influences are important factors which appear to modify both intake and expenditure (Poskitt 1986; Poskitt and Cole 1978).

Single child, single parent, large family, and low socio-economic class are all associated with obesity in young children (Jacoby *et al.* 1975; Wilkinson *et al.* 1977) and one can only speculate as to the reasons for this—possibly the quality of the food rather than the quantity, emotional conflicts, and so on.

Prevention of obesity on a population level is a difficult task. Concentration on high-risk groups is not feasible as the risk factors are so prevalent, but we do know that obesity becomes more prevalent as the population has reduced levels of activity—surely this is amenable to change. We know it becomes more prevalent when a population's diet contains more energy-dense foods—we could encourage the intake of 'wholefoods'. We know it also becomes more prevalent as the population is generally warmer and healthier—but we surely would not want to alter these aspects.

The changes in diet needed to reduce levels of childhood obesity require widespread changes in national diet. This requires intensive education, not only of the general public, but also of food manufacturers. Appropriate foods need to be available at affordable prices. It is salutory to note that the consumption of chips in UK schoolchildren showed a marked class gradient with a three-fold difference between social classes I and V (DOH 1989). The Department of Employment's 'family expenditure survey' at the same time showed that family expenditure on food varies with socio-economic status. Chips are a cheap source of calories.

Children fed on 'inappropriate diets'

A new term has been coined for children fed on one kind of inappropriate diet—'meusli belt malnutrition'. These children, usually from better off families, are fed on an adult 'healthy diet' regime of high-fibre, low-fat foods. This food tends to be bulky, low in energy density, and may also be low in nutrient availability. Although suitable for adults, this type of diet is not suitable for children who are still growing and parents often need careful explanation of the special nutritional needs of children in comparison to adults.

Separate from this are children fed on special diets because of the beliefs—religious or otherwise—of their parents. The diets adopted may exclude food of animal origin to a variable degree. Vegans are vegetarians whose diet totally excludes food derived from animals; other vegetarians eat some animal products but exclude red or all meats. Vegetarianism has been growing in popularity, not just on religious grounds but because of conservation and environmental issues. Well-informed vegetarians offer satisfactory diets to their children but less knowledgeable parents may be responsible for nutritional disorders in their children (DHSS 1988). Good sensible advice to these parents is essential.

Table 17.5 summarizes some religious and cult-food regimes. Some of these have been studied extensively (Jacobs and Dwyer 1988; Sanders 1988), particularly in Holland (Van Staveran and Dagnelie 1988; Dagnelie et al. 1989 a,b,c, 1991). The more liberal vegetarian diets (lacto-vegetarian, lacto-ovo-vegetarian, and semi-vegetarian), which include a wide variety of foods, can fulfil nutritional requirements throughout childhood (Jacobs and Dwyer 1988). Vegan diets, particularly in infancy and early childhood, pose problems because of bulk (reducing energy consumption) and low intakes of protein, calcium, vitamin D, riboflavin, and vitamin B_{12} (Sanders 1988). However, most parents were aware of the need for supplements of vitamin B_{12} and if sufficient care is taken, a vegan child can have normal growth and development.

Table 17.5 *Foods avoided by some religions and cults*

Food	Pork	Beef	Other meat	Non-scaly fish, shellfish	Eggs	Milk	Canned foods
Religion							
Buddhist	x	x	x	x	x	?	
Hare Krishna	x	x	x	x	x		x
Hindu	x	x			?		
Jain	x	x	x		x		
Jewish	X			x			
Macrobiotic (Zen)	x	x	x	x	x	x	x
Muslim	X						
Rastafarian	x	x	x	x	x	?	x
Seventh-day Adventist	x	x	x	x			
Sikh		x					

* Dietary restrictions may be greater if foods not prepared in acceptable way.
x Foods generally avoided.
? Denotes considerable variation within religion over consumption of these foods.

The Dutch studies showed that the children on macrobiotic diets were at most risk; their growth deviated from the Dutch standard curves after five months of age with no catch-up growth. The children seemed to be particularly vulnerable around the time of weaning with low dietary intakes of protein, energy, calcium, riboflavine, vitamin B_{12}, and vitamin D (Dagnelie *et al*. 1989*b*). Babies tended to be breast-fed beyond one year and solid food was introduced late. The authors report a 25 per cent incidence of rickets. Iron deficiency was seen in 15 per cent of the children and vitamin B_{12} deficiency (B_{12} concentration < 136 pmol/l) in 45 per cent (Dagnelie *et al*. 1989*a*), the latter raising serious concerns about long-term neurological development.

As well as the poor growth, both in terms of weight, height, and arm circumference, gross motor and language development were slower in macrobiotic infants (Dagnelie *et al*. 1989*c*). However, there was no reported abnormal mental development at age four to six years. They suggested that the macrobiotic diet should be supplemented with fat, fatty fish, and dairy products (Dagnelie *et al*. 1991).

Parents adopting very restrictive dietary practices may be alienated from the rest of society by their beliefs and the widely media-reported cases of malnutrition can perpetuate this. There is need for a balance between more tolerance on the part of the health professionals and sensible dietary advice from the vegetarian and vegan organizations.

Special problems of ethnic minority groups

A wealth of information has been published on the medical and cultural problems of ethnic minority children, particularly in the UK. This is dealt with by another author in this text (Chapter 25), and by ourselves (Aukett and Wharton 1989) elsewhere. It is often very difficult to decide how much of the nutritional problems of these groups are due to their ethnicity and cultural practices and how much to other social and economic factors such as poverty. In general the majority of investigators find that the ethnic group they reviewed have nutrition and health problems greater than those of the population at large, but the judgement that ethnic group membership places children at greater risk than the general population, of which other groups are a part, is often impossible to make because of this interrelationship with poverty (Pelto 1991). However, there do seem to be some particular nutritional problems which are worth highlighting.

Asians

There are many sub-ethnic differences in the diet of children of mothers who come from the Indian subcontinent (Wharton 1991); these are undoubtedly influenced by religion. The patterns of infant feeding show some differences from the non-Asian children living in the same areas (Aukett and Wharton 1989). Many studies indicate that the majority of babies are breast-fed for a very short time or not at all. The introduction of solids tend to be late and the first foods tend to be sweet. Cow's milk is introduced early and remains the major constituent of the child's diet for very much longer than their non-Asian counterparts. The use of vitamin supplements varies. Specific nutritional problems include growth faltering, rickets, and iron deficiency anaemia.

Afro-Caribbean

Normally Afro-Caribbean and African children living in the UK are well nourished although mild iron deficiency is common. A high percentage of Afro-Caribbean mothers start to breast-feed but the percentage falls quickly. In Birmingham 35 per cent of babies were breast-fed for less than one month. Traditional weaning foods are often used but there is no evidence that these cause nutritional problems. These mothers took more advice from their mothers and mothers-in-law than from health professionals (Douglas 1989). The particular problems of Rastafarian children are dealt with above.

Chinese/Vietnamese

Cultural food traditions can be very strong in this group, but in Birmingham, the nutritional problems we have seen have been similar to those for the Indian subcontinent, e.g. lack of breast-feeding, iron deficiency, and rickets. An inherited lactose deficiency may lead to avoidance of milk, and alternative sources of calcium may need to be sought.

To intervene in the nutritional problems of ethnic minority children, a team approach is required which is both nutritionally sound and culturally sensitive. This must involve the child's parents and ethnic minority communities as well as the health professionals.

Intervention and potential for change

Just as the physical growth of an individual child reflects its health and nutrition, so the growth pattern of a population reflects the collective well-being. As infant mortality decreases, physical growth and development assume increasingly greater importance as a monitor of children's health. Although the last 30 years have seen major advances in the nutrition and subsequent health of children in Europe, there is still potential for change and intervention that can bring about that change.

There has been intensive research in child nutrition throughout this century but still uncertainties remain in many areas, not least whether or not suboptimal nutrition in infancy and childhood can affect future health and performance (Lucas 1990). Studies on the effect of malnutrition are fraught with confounding factors such as poverty, poor social circumstances, and lack of stimulation. Good evidence seems now to exist on the effect of iron deficiency, but relatively few countries have managed to prevent the problem. Recently, research has centred on the effect of early nutrition on adult cardiovascular disease (Viikari *et al*. 1990; Lloyd 1991). Even this is not straigthforward as socio-economic conditions in childhood are significantly associated with adult ischaemic heart disease, but nutrition is not the only facet of poor socio-economic conditions that exerts an effect.

To alter levels of suboptimal nutrition in Europe, interventions can clearly occur on several levels. In as much as suboptimal nutrition is related to poverty, only major social and political changes can have effect and paediatricians can, in this respect, act as advocates for children.

At a pan-European level, the EEC Commission has produced directives which will have effects on child nutrition. The Directive on infant formulae and follow-on formulae was adopted in May 1991 (EEC 1991) and a directive on processed cereal-based foods and baby foods for infants and young children is in preparation. At an individual country level, nutritional feeding guidelines such as 'present day practice in infant feeding' (DHSS 1988) can not only provide a framework so that consistent advice is given, but also make recommendations to government departments which can have far-reaching effects on child nutrition. For instance, in the most recent of these reports there is a recommendation that infant feeding should be included as part of the education in child care taught to both girls and boys at school. They recommend that the 'welfare food scheme' should be continued and that regular assessment of nutritional status should be an essential part of health surveillance of all infants.

In setting up national nutrition policies, account needs to be taken of the social-economic context. Although it is said that a 'healthy' diet can cost no more than an 'unhealthy' diet, many would disagree. The London food commission estimated that the basic cost of a 'healthy' diet was 35 per cent more than a 'normal' diet, and this did not take into account additional hidden costs of preparation time and difficulty of cooking. The traditions and cultural view of different ethnic groups within the community as a whole also need to be considered, as advice which does not heed such beliefs will not be taken.

Experience in other countries needs to be drawn upon, such as the Special Supplemental Food Programme for Women, Infants and Children (WIC) in the USA (Miller *et al.* 1985). We can also draw lessons from developing countries where 'road to health' style parent-held records have long been used to help parents understand the nutritional status of their children. The implementation of a national parent-held record which not only incorporates growth charts but also nutritional advice which gets into *every* home should be a major advance.

Our own experience (Leach *et al.* 1987) has been that it is possible not only to increase parents' awareness of what they *should* feed their children, but also to affect what they *actually* feed them. In an inner city area the dietary diaries of a group of children improved significantly following a period of nutrition education given by a health visitor. The advice given was tailored to the culture of the family, took into account the level of income of the family, and was delivered in an easily understandable form.

Parents get advice on how to feed their children from a variety of sources—the extended family, friends, their own education, food advertising, the media, as well as from health professionals. Much of this advice is conflicting.

As we move towards the end of the twentieth century, there are clearly several priorities to be defined. First, we need effective continuing measurements of the state of the nutritional health of European children. Second, if health/nutrition education is to be effective, health professionals need to deliver the same, not conflicting, messages; and third, we must recognize that nutrition is only one aspect of child health and is closely related to other aspects. If health professionals, the food industry, and Governments all worked together to improve child nutrition, major improvements could be made.

References

Astier-Dumas initials, Fernandes, J., Marquardt, P., Nordio, S., Oppe, T.E., Rey, J., *et al.* (1983). First report of the Scientific Committee for food on the essential requirements of infant formulae and follow up milks based on cows milk proteins in food—Science and Techniques. *Report of the Scientific Committee for Food*, 14th Series, EUR 8752 EN, pp. 9–32. Commission of the European Communities, Luxembourg.

Aukett, M.A., Parks, Y.A., Scott, P.H. and Wharton, B.A. (1986). Treatment with iron increases weight gain and psychomotor development. *Archives of Disease in Childhood*, **61**, 849–57.

Aukett, M.A. and Wharton, B. (1989). Nutrition of Asian children: infants and toddlers. In *Ethnic factors in health and disease* (ed. J.K. Cruickshank and D.G. Beevers), pp. 241–8. Butterworth, London.

Bauch, K., Anke M., Gurtler H., Hesse V., Knappe, G., Korber, R., et al. (1989). Interdisciplinary aspects of iodine prophylaxis in German Democratic Republic. *Endocrinol. Exp.* **23**, 77–84.

Bauch, K., Seitz, W., Forster, S., and Keil, V. (1990). Dietary iodine-deficiency in East Germany following introduction of interdisciplinary preventive use of iodine. *Zeitschrift für gesamte Innere Medizin*, **45**, 8–11.

Belton, N.R. (1986). Rickets—not only the 'english disease'. *Acta Paediatrica Scandinavica* (Supplement) **323**, 68–75.

Black, A.E., Billewicz, W.Z., and Thomson, A.M., (1976). The diets of preschool children in Newcastle-upon-Tyne 1968–71. *British Journal of Nutrition*, **35**, 105–13.

Boggio, V., Lestradet, H., Astier-Dumas, S., Machinot, M., Suquet, J., and Klepping J. (1984). Characteristiques de la ration alimentaire des enfants francais de 3 a 24 mois. Alimentation des Nourissons francais. *Archives Francaises de Pediatrie* **41**, 499–505.

Boyle, I.T. (1991). Bones for the future *Acta Paediatrica Scandinavica* (Supplement) **373**, 58–65.

Brook, O.G., (1983). Supplementary vitamin D in infancy and childhood. *Archives of Disease in Childhood*, **58**, 573–4.

Crawford, M.A., Doyle, W, Drury, P.J., Meadows N. (1987). Food intakes of children, the DHSS, and the prevention of heart disease. *Nutrition and Health* **5**, 65–77.

Bagnelie P.C., Van Stavern W.A., Vergota, F.J.V.R.A., Dingjam P.G., Vander Berg H., and Hauvast J.G.A.J., (1989a). Increased risk of vitamin B_{12} and iron deficiency in infants on macrobiotic diets. *American Journal of Clinical Nutrition* **50**, 818–24.

Dagnelie P.C., Van Staveren W.A., Verschuren S.A.J.N., and Hautvast J.G.A.G., (1989b). Nutritional status of infants aged 4 to 18 months on macrobiotic diets and matched omnivorous control infants. A population-based mixed longitudinal Study. I: Weaning pattern/energy and nutrient intake. *European Journal of Clinical Nutrition* **43**, 311–23.

Dagnelie PC, Van Staveren WA, Vergote FJVRA, Burema J, Van't Hof MA, Van-Klaveren JD, et al. (1989c) Nutritional & status of infants aged 4 to 18 months on macrobiotic diets and matched omnivorous control infants : a population-based mixed longitudinal study. II: Growth and psychomotor development. *European Journal of Clinical Nutrition* **43**, 325–38.

Dagnelie, P.C., Van Staveren WA, and Hautvast JGJA, (1991). Stunting and nutrient deficiencies in children on alternative diets. *Acta Paediatrica Scandinavica* (Supplement) **374**, 111–18.

Dallman PR, and Yip R, (1989). Changing characteristics of childhood anaemia. *Journal of Paediatrics* **114**, 161–4.

Dallman PR, (1990). Progress in prevention of iron deficiency in infants. *Acta Paediatrica Scandinavica* (Supplement) **365**, 28–37.

Delange F, and Burgi H, (1989). Iodine deficiency disorders in Europe. *Bulletin of the World Health Organization* **67**, 317–25.

DHSS (Department of Health and Social Security) (1974). Present-day practice in infant feeding. *Reports on health and social subjects, No 9*. HMSO, London.

DHSS (Department of Health and Social Security) (1980). Present-day practice in infant feeding: 1980. *Reports on health and social subjects, No 20.* HMSO, London.
DHSS (Department of Health and Social Security) (1984). Diet and cardiovascular disease (COMA Report). *Reports on health and social subjects, No 28.* HMSO, London.
DHSS (Department of Health and Social Security) (1988). Present-day practice in infant feeding: third report. *Reports on health and social subjects, No 32.* HMSO, London.
DOH (Department of Health) (1989). The diets of British schoolchildren. *Reports on health and social subjects. No 36.* HMSO, London.
DOH (Department of Health) (1991). Dietary-reference valves for food energy and nutrients for the United Kingdom. *Reports on health and social subjects. No 41.* HMSO, London.
Douglas, J. (1989). Food type preferences and trends among Afro-Caribbeans in Britain. In *Ethnic factors in health and disease*, (ed. J.K. Cruickshank and D.G. Beevers)., pp. 249–54. Butterworth, London.
Doxiadis S, Angelis C, Karatzas P, Vrettos C, and Lapatsanis P, (1976). Genetic aspects of nutritional rickets. *Archives of Disease in Childhood* **51**, 83–90.
Dunnigan MG, Glekin BM, Henderson JB, McIntosh WB, Summer D, and Sutherland GR, (1985). Prevention of rickets in Asian children: assessement of the Glasgow campaign. *British Medical Journal* **291**, 239–42.
Earley A, Valman HB, Altman DG, and Pippard MJ, (1990). Microcytosis iron deficiency and thalassaemia in pre-school children. *Archives of Disease in Childhood* **65**, 610–14.
Erhardt, P. (1986). Iron deficiency in young Bradford children from different ethnic groups. *British Medical Journal* **292**, 90–3.
EEC (European Economic Community) (1991). Commission directive on infant formulae and follow-on formulae. *Official Journal of the European Communities*, L **175**, 35–49.
Fairweather-Tait, S.J. (1989). Iron in food and its availability. *Acta Paediatrica Scandinavica* (Supplement) **361**, 12–20.
Farre-Rovira R, Perez-Salvador A, Rodriogo Ramon S, Frasquet Pons M, and Frasquet Pons I (1990). Dietary survey at the nursery of the polytechnic university of Valencia. *Annals Espana Pediatrie* **32**, 122–8.
Fenzi G.F, Guisti LF, Aghini LF, Bartalena L, Marcocci C, Santini F, *et al.* (1990). Neuropsychological assessment in school-children from an area of moderate iodine deficiency. *Journal of Endocrinological Investigation* **13**, 427–31.
Foman SJ (1987). Bioavailability of supplemental iron in commercially prepared dry infant cereals. *Journal of Paediatrics* **110**, 660–1.
Geuns M, Huisinga C, Van Staveren WA, Deurenberg P and Hautvast JGAJ (1985). *Tijdschr Kindergeneeskd* **53**, 50–6.
Gobedzhishvili MS, Kondrateva II, and Abdushelishvili GV, (1990). Daily energy consumption, physiological standards of energy requirement and energy value of food rations for children in boarding schools of the Georgian SSR. *Vopr-Pitar* **4**, 37–9.
Golden MHN (1991). The nature of nutritional deficiency in relation to growth failure and poverty. *Acta Paediatrica Scandinavica* (Supplement) **374**, 95–110.
Grindulis H, Scott PH, Belton NR, and Wharton B (1986). Combined deficiency of iron and vitamin D in Asian toddlers. *Archives of Disease in Childhood* **61**, 843–48.
Grossman LK, Harter C, Sachs L, and Kay A (1990). The effect of post partum lactation counselling on the duration of breast feeding in low income women. *American Journal of Diseases in Childhood* **144**, 471–4.

Hagman V, Bruce A, Persson L, Samuelson G, and Sjolin S (1986). Food habits and nutrient intake in childhood in relation to health and socio-economic conditions. A Swedish multicentre study 1980–81. *Acta Paediatrica Scandinavica* (Supplement) **328**, 4–56.

Harris RJ, Armstrong D. Al R and Laynes A (1983). Nutritional survey of Bangladeshi children aged under 5 in the London borough of Tower Hamlets. *Archives of Disease in Childhood* **58**, 428–32.

Haschke F and Javaid N (1991). Nutritional anaemias. *Acta Paedictrica Scandinavica* (Supplement) **374**, 38–44.

Hill PD and Humenick SS (1989). Insufficient milk supply. *Image* **21**, 145–8.

Hillervik-Lindquist C (1991). Studies on perceived breast milk insufficiency. Doctoral Thesis, Uppsala University. *Acta Paediatrica Scandinavica* (Supplement) **376**, 1–27.

Jacobs C and Dwyer JT (1988). Vegetarian children: appropriate and inappropriate diets. *American Journal of Clinical Nutrition* **48**, 811–18.

Jacoby A, Altman DG, Cook J, Holland WW, and Elliot A (1975). Influences of some social and environmental factors on the nutrient intake and nutritional studies of school-children. *British Journal of Preventive Social Medicine* **29**, 116–20.

James J, Evans J, Male P, Pallister C, Hendrikz JK, and Oakhill A (1988). *Journal of the Royal College of General Practitioners* **28**, 250–2.

Jivani SKM (1978). The practice of infant feeding among Asian immigrants. *Archives of Disease in Childhood* **53**, 69–73.

Ladodo KS, Kopylova NV, Kulinskaia EV, Beider AI, and Tomberg EE (1988). Characteristics of the actual nutrition of Estonian and Finnish children. *Vopr-Pitan* **6**, 17–21.

Leach K, Alexander E, and Aukett A (1987). A Study of the dietary patterns of children aged 1–5 years in an inner city health district. ICP Project. (Unpublished data.)

Lellep-Fernandez R (1988). Biocultural belief and iodine prophylaxis.*Soc.Sci.Med.* **27**, 578–96.

Lestradet H, Machinot S, Greneche MO, Dufour C, *et al.* (1979). L'alimentation des nourissons francais de 2 a 9 mois. *Rev. Pédiatr.* **15**, 11–19.

Lloyd JK (1991). Cholesterol: should we screen all children or change the diet of all children? *Acta Paedictrica Scaninavica* (Supplement) **373**, 66–72.

Lucas A (1990). Does early diet program future outcome? *Acta Paediatrica Sandinavica* (Supplement) **365**, 58–67.

McKillip FM and Durnin JVGA (1982). The energy and nutrient intake of a random sample (305) of infants. *Human Nutrition: Applied Nutrition* **36 A**, 405–21.

Mardar A, Nicoll A, Polnay L, and Shillman CE (1990). Discovering anaemia at child health clinics. *Archives of Disease in Childhood* **65**, 892–4.

Mathisen B, Skuse D, Wolke D, and Reilly S (1989). Oral-motor dysfunction and failure to thrive among inner city infants. *Developmental Medicine and Child Neurology* **31**, 293–302.

Mikiel-Kostyra K and Galecki A (1990*a*). Education of health personnel for promotion of breast-feeding—a pilot study (Part I–the level of knowledge). *Wiad-Lek* **43**, 57.

Mikiel-Kostyra K and Galecki A (1990*b*), Education of health personnel for promotion of breast-feeding—pilot study. II: Attitudes. *Wiad-Lek* **43**, 658–61.

Mikiel-Kostyra K and Galecki A (1990*c*). Preparation of health service personnel for widespread use of breast-feeding—a pilot study. Part III: Practice and declared contraindications to breast-feeding. Wiad-Lek **43**, 718–23.

Milla PJ (1986). The weanling's gut. *Acta Paediatrica Scandinavica* (Supplement) **323**, 5–13.
Miller V, Swaney S, and Deinard A (1985). Impact of the WIC program on the iron status of infants. *Paediatrics* **75**, 100–5.
Mills AF (1990). Surveillance of anaemia-risk factors in patterns of milk intake. *Archives of Disease in Childhood* **65**, 428 31.
Mior M, Poze G, Korman M, Mikalauskaite D, and Valatkaite A (1988). The food behaviour of school-children in the GDR and the Lithuanian SSR. *Vopr-Pitan* **5**, 43–6.
Oppenheimer SJ (1989). Iron and infection: the clinical evidence. *Acta Paediacrica Scandinavica* (Supplement) **361**, 53–62.
Ozsolu (1977). Breast feeding and rickets. *Lancet* **ii**, 560.
Pelto GH (1991). Ethnic minorities, migration and risk of undernutrition in children. *Acta Paediatrica Scandinavica* (Supplement) **374**, 51–7.
Poskitt EME (1986). Obesity in the young child. Whither and whence. *Acta Paediacrica Scandinavica* (Supplement) **323**, 24–32.
Poskitt EM.E (1987). Management of obesity. *Archives of Disease in Childhood* **62**, 305–10.
Poskitt EME and Cole TJ (1978). Nature, nuture and childhood overweight. *British Medical Journal* **1**, 603–5.
Rajan L and Oakley A (1990). Infant feeding practice in mothers at risk of low birth weight delivery. *Midwifery* **6**, 18–27.
Sanders TAB (1988). Growth and development of British vegan children. *American Journal of Clinical Nutrition* **48**, 822–5.
Save the Children Fund (1983). *Stop rickets campaign.* Save the Children Fund, London.
Soderhjelm L and Zetterstrom R (1990). Trends in infant feeding in Sweden during the 20th Century. *Acta Paediatrica Scandinavica* (Supplement) **365**, 5–6.
Soemantri AG, Pollitt E, and Kim I (1985). Iron deficiency anaemia and educational achievement. *American Journal of Clinical Nutrition* **42**, 1221–8.
Stahlberg MR (1985). Breast feeding and social factors. *Acta Paediatrica Scandinavica* **74**, 36–39.
Stephens WP, Klimivk PS, Warrington S and Taylor JL (1982). Observations on the dietary practices of Asians in the UK. *Nutrition and Applied Nutrition* **36A**, 438–44.
Stolley H, (1982). Zeitpunkt und Zusammensetzung der 'Beikost' für Säuglinge im ersten Lebensjahr. In: *Säuglingsernährung Heute*, (ed. R. Gruttner), p. 17. Springer, Berlin.
Tajtakova M, Hancinova D, Langer P, Tajtak J, Foldes O, Malinovsky E *et al.* (1990). Thyroid volume by ultrasound in boys and girls 6–16 years of age under marginal deficiency as related to age at puberty. *Klein-Wochenschrift* **68**, 503–6.
United Nations (1991) Convention on Rights of the Child.
Van Staveren WA and Dagnelie PC (1988). Food consumption, growth and development of Dutch children fed on alternative diets. *American Journal of Clinical Nutrition* **48**, 819–21.
Van Steenbergen WM, (1978). De voeding van Surinaamse, Antiliaanse en Nederlandse zuigelingen in de Bijlmermeer. *Voeding*, **39**, 2–8.
Vermiglio F, Finocchiaro MD, Lo-Presti VP, La Torre N, Nucifora M, and Trimarchi F, (1989). Partial beneficial effects of the so called 'silent iodine prophylaxis' on iodine deficiency disorders (IDD) in North Eastern Sicily endenia. *Journal of Endocrinological Investigation* **12**, 5–14.

Vermiglio F, Sidoti M, Finocchiaro MD, Battiato S, Lo Presti VP, Benvenga S, *et al.* (1990). Defective neuromotor and cognitive ability in iodine-deficient schoolchildren of an endemic goiter region in Sicily. *Journal of Clinical Endocrinology and Metabolism* **70**, 379–84.

Viikari J, Akerblom HK, Rasanen L, Kalavainen M, and Pietarinen O, (1990). Cardiovascular risk in young Finns. *Acta Paediatrica Scandinavica* (Supplement) **365**, 9.

Walter T, de Andraca I, Chaducl P, and Perales CG, (1989). Iron deficiency anaemia: adverse effects on infant psychomotor development. *Paediatrics* **84**, 7–17.

Walter T, Hertrampf E, Arredano M, and Vega V, (1990). Effect of different milk diets on gastrointestinal blood loss in infancy. *Paediatric Research* **28**, 296.

Weile B, Rubin DH, Krasilnikoff PA, Kuo HS, and Jekel JF, (1990). Infant feeding patterns during the first year of life in Denmark: factors associated with the discontinuation of breast-feeding. *Journal of Clinical Epidemiology* **43**, 1305–11.

Wharton B.A (1984). Infant formulae. *Bulletin of the British Nutrition* Foundation **9**, 83–93.

Wharton BA (1986). Food for the weaning: the next priority in infant nutrition. *Acta Paediatrica Scandinavica* (Supplement) **323**, 96–102.

Wharton B (1991). Protein-energy malnutrition: problems and priorities. *Acta Paediatrica Scandinavica* (Supplement) **374**, 5–14.

Wharton B and Wharton P (1987). Nutrition in adolescence. *Nutrition and Health* 4, 195–203.

Wharton BA, Oppe TE, Astier-Dumas M, Fernandes J, Ferro-Luzzi A, Rey J, *et al.* (1992). *First report of the Scientific Committee for food on the essential requirements for weaning foods.* 24 Series, EUR 131140 EN, 9–38. Food-Science and Techniques Commission of the European Communities, Luxembourg.

Whitehead RG (1991). Dietary allowances: what to recommend. *Acta Paediatrica Scandinavica* (Supplement) **373**, 25–32.

Whitehead RG, Paul AA, and Ahmed EA (1986). Weaning practices in the United Kingdom and variations in Anthropometric development. *Acta Paediatrica Scandinavica* (Supplement) **323**, 14–23.

Wilkinson PW, Parkin JM, Pearlson J, Phillips, and Sykes P (1977). Obesity in childhood: a community study in Newcastle-upon-Tyne. *Lancet* **i**, 350–3.

WHO (1978). *Declaration of Alma-Ata*, (International Conference on Primary Health Care). WHO, Geneva.

WHO (1981). *International code of marketing of breast milk substitutes.* WHO, Geneva.

WHO (1990). Nutrition: iodine deficiency and its effects in Europe. *Weekly Epidemiological Record* **44**, 339–41.

Wright CM Reading RF, Halse PC, and Watson JG (1989). Iron deficiency in adolescents. *British Medical Journal* **298**, 1035–6.

Ziegler EE, Foman SJ, Nelson SE, Rebouche CJ, Edwards BB, Rogers RR *et al.* (1990). Cows milk feeding in infancy: further observations on blood loss from the gastrointestinal tract. *Journal of Paediatrics* **116**, 11–18.

18 Unexpected death in infancy
Elizabeth Taylor

Introduction

The death of a child from any cause is a major tragedy in the life of the family concerned, but, when the death is unexpected and unexplained, feelings of shock, grief, anger, and guilt may be overwhelming.

In Europe, approximately 1–2 per thousand apparently normal babies die unexpectedly. All these deaths are described as 'cot deaths'. A small proportion of cot deaths are found at necropsy to have either an undiagnosed, potentially lethal, congenital abnormality or an overwhelming infection such as meningococcal septicaemia. The remainder fulfil the criteria for registration as 'sudden infant death syndrome' or 'sudden unexpected death in infancy'.

There is considerable variation in the incidence of unexpected death in infancy between different countries in Europe and between different geographical areas within individual countries. Rates appear to be lowest in the Scandinavian countries, The Netherlands, and in Italy, although the incidence in the Scandinavian countries has risen slightly and may be associated with changing child care patterns (Norvenius *et al.* 1991). The incidence of unexpected infant death tends to be higher in large urban areas compared with small towns and rural areas, and is higher in areas of socio-economic deprivation. In the early 1990s some, but not all, European countries have experienced a marked decline in their rates.

The definition of the sudden infant death syndrome as 'The sudden death of an infant or young child which is unexpected by history and in which a full post-mortem examination fails to show an adequate cause of death' was accepted at the second International Conference on sudden infant death in Seattle in 1969. This rather vague definition resulted in considerable discrepancy in reporting and, more recently, an attempt has been made to tighten up the definition by restricting the age group to infants dying between the ages of one month and one year and by insisting on an investigation of the death. However, it is still the case that in several European countries deaths are registered as 'SIDS' without either a post-mortem examination or a full investigation of the death having been carried out.

Until this century, most unexpected infant deaths were thought to be due to infanticide or accidental suffocation by the mother's body during sleep (overlying). In the distant past, infanticide was tacitly accepted as a means of regulating family size, but is now viewed with horror, and it seems probable that only a small proportion of deaths currently registered as unexpected death in infancy

(SIDS) are associated with infanticide (Taylor and Emery 1990). References to overlying as a cause of infant death occur in the Old Testament and in Roman records. The compulsory use of wooden cradles was introduced in Florence in the seventeenth century and subsequently also in Germany. Studies of infant death in the nineteenth century blamed overlying as a major cause, particularly as these deaths were often associated with poverty, overcrowding, and drunkenness (Templeman 1892).

As early as 1855, a *Lancet* editorial called for routine pathological investigation of infant deaths (Lancet 1855). Enlargement of the thymus was suggested as a cause in 1889 (Paltauf 1889) and this theory held sway for many years. In the 1930s many infants with a normal thymus received unnecessary and potentially damaging irradiation. The first suggestion of a cardio-respiratory cause was made in 1923 (Still 1923). The search for 'a cause' for these unexplained deaths then gathered pace. In 1971 Froggatt (Froggatt *et al.* 1971) postulated a critical combination of extrinsic (e.g. infection) and intrinsic factors and it is now generally accepted that the sudden infant death syndrome is both multicausal and multifactoral.

Epidemiology

The epidemiological study of unexpected death in infancy is beset by problems of identification. Comparison of data may be made difficult by the lack of standardization of age limits, by variation in interpretation of pathological findings, and by the presence or absence of an adequate enquiry into the death. More accurate comparisons can be made by including deaths registered as due to infection, accident, or non-accidental injury (possibly preventable mortality) (Carpenter 1983). It is hoped that a standardized database will be established by the middle of the 1990s to record early childhood mortality in most European countries. However, much careful epidemiological work has been done on sudden infant deaths and an epidemiological profile has emerged.

Sudden unexpected infant deaths appear to be uncommon (but not unknown) in the neonate. The peak age incidence is two to four months and between 80 and 85 per cent of deaths occur before the age of six months. They then become progressively less common. There is some evidence that children dying in the presence of respiratory infection are older than those who were apparently completely well at the time of death. (Knowelden *et al.* 1984). Deaths occur more commonly during the winter months or following episodes of bad weather (Kraus *et al.* 1967). Sudden infant deaths are more common in males, in low birth-weight babies, and in multiple births (whether or not they were low birth-weight). They can occur in any part of the community, but are more common in areas of socio-economic deprivation. Deaths are more common in bottle-fed babies, but can occur in breast-fed infants. Babies of mothers who are both young and parous appear to be particularly vulnerable (Froggatt *et al.* 1971).

The risk appears to be increased by excessive alcohol consumption or drug-taking by mothers during pregnancy or the child's life. All studies show a positive relationship with maternal smoking in pregnancy. Recent European studies have shown a higher incidence in gypsies (Schuler *et al.* 1991).

Recent studies in Sheffield (Taylor and Emery 1990) appear to indicate that the epidemiology of unexpected infant death does not apply equally to all these deaths. Infants registered as unexpected death in infancy who died during the course of potentially treatable or minor infection were found to have more adverse family and social factors, their parents were less likely to own their own homes, a car, or a telephone, and their mothers were more likely to be young, to smoke, and to present late in pregnancy. Babies who died with no evidence of terminal illness were younger at the time of death and were more likely to be male. Their families were demographically similar to the control group and to the general population.

Causes of unexpected death in infancy

Occasional unexpected infant deaths may have a single overwhelming cause. More probably, causal factors may be associated with increased vulnerability or with trigger factors which precipitate death in an already vulnerable infant. Causal factors may be genetic (for example, inheritable metabolic defect) or may have their origin in an adverse intrauterine or postnatal environment.

Many hypotheses have been produced and many lines of research followed. Much has been learned of the profound physiological changes that take place in the early months of life, but the multicausal and multifactorial nature of unexpected infant death militates against the validation of any individual causal hypothesis.

Research methods may be divided into four areas: (1) physiological—experiments on newborn animals and studies of living babies; (2) pathological and biochemical studies of babies who have died; (3) studies on babies who have suffered a so called 'near miss' or 'apparent life-threatening event' (ALTE); and (4) studies of the siblings of babies who have died. Fields of study include the cardiorespiratory systems, allergy, metabolic defects, and pathology. It is only possible here to touch on some of the major and exciting fields of research which have particular significance for the social paediatrician.

Respiration

The 'apnoea' theory of unexpected infant death was first postulated in the 1920s. Because some infants suffer episodes of apnoea, usually described as 'near miss' or 'apparent life-threatening events' (ALTE) from which they recover and are, therefore, available for investigation, and because low birth-weight babies are prone to respiratory disorders and are also known to be at increased risk of unexpected infant death, this is one of the most thoroughly investigated hypotheses of cause. The maturation of respiratory mechanisms and reflexes in the first months of life is a complex process. Non-physiological apnoea may be associated with sleep (Haidmayer et al. 1991) or with respiratory infection (Devlieger et al. 1991). Infants who die tend to have longer periods of central apnoea, although these remained within the normal range (Kahn et al. 1990a). Further evidence of the importance of hypoxia in the aetiology of some unexpected deaths comes from studies in Oslo (Rognum et al. 1988) which found raised levels of hypoxanthine in eye fluids indicating the presence of hypoxia. However, the relationship between ALTE and SIDS is uncertain (Wennergren et al. 1987) and the majority of babies who die unexpectedly do not have a history of apnoea. Studies on functional testing to identify infants at risk have been inconclusive and do not improve on epidemiological identification of high risk infants (Bentele and Albani 1988).

The use of apnoea monitors in the 'prevention' of unexpected infant death has escalated and many are now issued with little or no guidance or supervision (Kahn et al. 1990b). The few controlled studies that have been undertaken (Emery et al. 1985) do not show a significant reduction in the number of deaths. Newer, more sophisticated monitors are cumbersome and invasive. They may prove effective in some vulnerable infants in that a threatening situation may be identified before the onset of apnoea (Southall, personal communication), but have yet to be fully evaluated. However, many paediatricians believe that apnoea monitors have an important role to play, particularly for subsequent siblings, in enabling anxious parents to live a more normal life, knowing the alarm will sound if their baby stops breathing. The effectiveness of resuscitation following cessation of breathing is likely to depend on the underlying cause, and is only likely to be effective in cases of cardiorespiratory origin.

Infection

Both intrauterine and postnatal infection have a role in the complex aetiology of SIDS. The Oxford record linkage study (Golding et al. 1985) showed a clear association between maternal infection in pregnancy (particularly respiratory and urinary tract infection) and increased risk of SIDS. Variend and Pearse (1986) reported on four infants with post-mortem evidence of cytomegalovirus inclusion disease who had been apparently thriving.

Infection may act as a trigger. More than a third of infants dying unexpectedly have evidence of infection in the pre-terminal period (Knowelden et al. 1984) and there may be an underestimation of the presence of respiratory viruses at necropsy (Van Velsen and Peters 1988). Although the presence of respiratory infection in a normal baby is a poor predictor of death (Gilbert et al. 1990), it seems sensible to encourage early and energetic response to illness in vulnerable infants in the first six months of life. Morley et al. (1991) have developed a system called 'Babycheck' designed to encourage parents and professionals to

Immunization

Because of the age distribution of the incidence of unexpected infant death, it is inevitable that infants will sometimes die unexpectedly shortly after routine immunization. A large American epidemiological study (Hoffman *et al.* 1987) of 757 pathologically verified cases of SIDS compared with living controls found that SIDS victims were less likely to have received diptheria, pertussis and tetanus (DPT) immunization and provides convincing evidence that DPT immunization is not a cause of unexpected death in infancy. No parent should be deterred from immunizing their child because of fear of cot death.

Pathology

Studies by pathologists (Vawter and Kozakewich 1982; Hinchliffe *et al.* 19930 have found an increased incidence of dysplastic and dysmorphic lesions and of minor congenital anomalies in infant dying unexpectedly compared with deaths from other causes. Post-mortem examination and investigation may explain some deaths and is necessary for further epidemiological studies and to indicate future lines of research (Cheron *et al.* 1990). Full post-mortem examination should form an integral part of the investigation which should follow all unexpected infant deaths.

Sleeping position and temperature regulation

The apparent association of SIDS with babies sleeping in the prone position was highlighted by work in The Netherlands (De Jonge *et al.* 1989) and confirmed by other studies (Nicholl and O'Cathain 1988). Some areas have experienced a marked and encouraging decline in the incidence of SIDS after changing to the supine position (Taylor *et al.* 1991). Prone sleeping has been identified as a major causal factor in some studies (Wigfield *et al.* 1992). Although it now seems sensible to encourage parents to place small babies on their sides or in the supine position, these results should still be treated with caution as the incidence of unexpected infant deaths in all communities is known to fluctuate widely and the relationship between statistically associated factors and cause is complicated and difficult to elucidate.

Emphasis on prevention of overheating both during warm weather and during cold weather, when parents may overcompensate by using more clothes and bedding, also could be of importance (Stanton *et al.* 1980). Small babies appear to be able to lose heat even when grossly overclothed, but at some metabolic cost to themselves (Wailoo *et al.* 1989). Other studies have shown an association between SIDS and the use of excessive clothing and bedding, with a higher room temperature, with the use of duvets (quilts), and with the practice of infants sleeping in the parents' bed (Bacon et al. 1991). Prone sleeping and overheating appear to be independent risk factors (Fleming et al. 1990) and there is no evidence that prone sleeping reduces the infant's ability to lose heat (Petersen et al. 1991).

Only a small proportion of the fields of research into the causes of unexpected infant death have been briefly discussed here, but the cumulative view of the mechanisms involved is that many infants destined to die unexpectedly have minor abnormalities or have been damaged by prenatal influences which result in increased vulnerability to trigger factors such as infection, hypoglycaemia, or thermal stress.

Risk scoring and intervention programmes

A number of 'scoring systems' have been developed, aimed at identifying infants at increased risk of unexpected infant death. A scoring system for risk can be constructed for any condition or groups of conditions which have a known epidemiological profile, for example, it would be possible to score young adults for risk of heart disease in later life. Such scoring systems for increased risk of unexpected death in infancy utilize information available at birth or shortly after to identify factors which occur more frequently in infants who die compared with survivors. On the results of a retrospective study, each factor is assigned a value using one of several appropriate statistical methods. The factors used in this way are statistically associated with increased risk and do not necessarily have a direct causal relationship and the resulting curve, Fig. 18.1, shows that, although the majority of infants are at medium risk, babies at lower than average or higher than average risk can be identified. For the purpose of intervention, the 'cut off' can be taken at a point which gives a population of manageable size in relations to the availability of resources for intervention. Risk scoring is, therefore, quite distinct from screening procedures which aim to identify a condition which is already present but not clinically apparent.

Risk scoring systems appear to work best for the populations from which they were derived (Peters and Golding 1986), but certain factors (Table 18.1) occur in all or most systems and knowledge of these and of other factors (Table 18.2) which have been found in some studies to be statistically associated with increased risk, enable the individual practitioner to assess the risk status of children with whom they work.

Population-based education programmes aimed at altering practices that are associated with increased risk at birth (e.g. smoking, drinking and drug-taking in pregnancy) or child care practices associated with increased risk (e.g. overwrapping) have been associated with a reduction in the mortality rate (Taylor et al. 1991). Specific intervention programmes aimed at infants assessed at birth as being at increased risk usually involve a programme of increased health visitor,

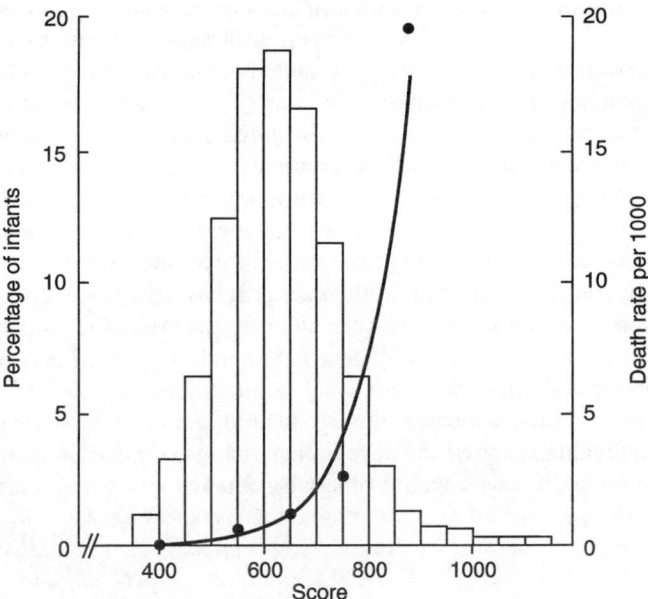

Fig. 18.1 The distribution of month scores and the observed and fitted relation of 'possibly preventable' infant mortality to score (Carpenter *et al.* 1988).

Table 18.1 *Risk factors in all or most scoring systems*

Low birth-weight
Low maternal age
High maternal parity
Multiple births
Short birth interval
Bottle-feeding
Maternal smoking

Table 18.2 *Risk factors occurring in some scoring systems*

Alcohol or drug abuse	Low APGAR score
Late antenatal booking	Small for dates
History of maternal depression	Low social class
Short second stage of labour	Black race
Unemployed or absent partner	Month of delivery
Maternal infection in pregnancy	Social problems
Poor weight gain in pregnancy	

nurse, or family doctor contacts with emphasis on education, and identification of and response to illness. These have been difficult to evaluate because of the problem of control data (most areas that undertake scoring do so with the stated aim of introducing an intervention programme). However, a recent assessment of comparative mortality trends in areas using risk related intervention and comparable areas in the same regions shows a consistent reduction in the mortality rates in the areas using intervention (Limerick 1992). In addition, a recent Sheffield study (Taylor et al.1993) shows that energetic intervention can reduce the number of deaths in very high risk infants who otherwise appear to have fewer than average contacts with health care professionals.

These scoring systems have also been shown to be predictive of later morbidity and child abuse (Golding and Peters 1985) and of poor achievement in the early school years (Maddocks, personal communication). Use of these and similar scoring systems, or the intelligent application of knowledge of risk factors by individuals, allows the development of positive discrimination in care to vulnerable children who would otherwise receive less health care than the average child.

Recurrence

All parents who have suffered a cot death worry about the risk of recurrence. Early studies of recurrence rates depended on parental recall and showed a very variable incidence, but a competent prospective assessment (Irgens and Skjaerven 1984) puts the statistical likelihood of recurrence encouragingly low at 4.8 per thousand (only approximately twice the incidence of first deaths). However, counselling of individual families should only take place following a full investigation of the death, as, theoretically, the risk of recurrence for any individual family may vary from 1 in 4, if the death was due to an undiagnosed familial condition, to the normal population risk of 1 in 500–1000 if the death was associated with the effects of one specific factor, e.g. low birth-weight, which is absent from the subsequent child. A study of 12 families who have suffered more than one cot death (Emery 1986) reported that three deaths were probably due to a familial disorder, two were associated with poor child care practices, five were probably due to an action by one of the parents, and only two were completely unexplained.

Effect on the family

The immediate needs of the family are for support and reassurance. These needs are best met by the professionals routinely involved with the family and already well known to them. Help may be needed with the suppression of lactation and with the practical problems of coping with a death. This immediate support may be difficult for professionals to provide as they may have little experience of cot death and may find themselves emotionally affected by the episode. However, most parents appreciate the early support of professionals with whom they are already familiar. Many parents are young, this may be their first experience of death, and they may need practical guidance in making arrangements for the disposal of the body.

Later the parents may need to talk through the episode, perhaps several times, with a professional who has specialized knowledge of the problem of cot death. This can be undertaken as part of a confidential enquiry or by a paediatrician with a particular interest in unexpected death in infancy. The period of shock following the death may be more prolonged than following an expected death and feelings of anger and guilt may last for many years. Parents may channel their feelings of anger against their own professional advisers, against other agencies such as housing authorities, or more generally against fate or their God. They may blame quite obviously unrelated factors such as fetal monitoring during labour. Parents' own feelings of guilt are usually related to their concept of total responsibility for the child's welfare. Regrets may centre on quite obviously unrelated incidents or on the minor failures in parenting which occur in all families. Occasionally guilt or anger may be associated with more significant failures in parenting or of health care, and counselling in these circumstances is more difficult. In addition to help from professionals, parents may obtain great comfort from parents' groups or from non-professional befrienders or just by developing friendship with another parent who has lost a child.

Grandparents may also need help. They are doubly bereaved, mourning the loss of a grandchild and affected by their own child's unhappiness. They often react by pressing the parents to have another baby quickly, in the hope that this will ameliorate their son or daughter's grief.

Siblings are always affected. The nature of the reaction depends on age and maturity of understanding. Babies react to disturbance in their environment and young children have fears that other members of the family or they themselves will disappear. Children may believe themselves responsible for the death because of the inevitable anger and jealously felt towards a younger sibling. Younger children will react with regression and behaviour disturbances, and all children may become very protective towards their parents and towards any subsequent baby. Sometimes grief reactions recur as the child develops intellectually and is able to experience a more mature reaction to the death. This is particularly the case for the survivor of twins who may, even as an adult, grieve for and feel responsibility for the other twin's death.

Subsequent pregnancies

The majority of families who experience a cot death go on to have another child. Many will embark on another pregnancy as quickly as possible, but others will seek advice. Most professionals advise parents to delay pregnancy to allow themselves time to mourn their lost child. My own practice is not to advise a specific period of time, but to advise parents to wait until they feel they are their normal selves again with normal energy and enthusiasm for life. In general, it is advisable to avoid anniversaries, for example a new baby born on or near the birthday or anniversary of the death of the child who died.

Parents having a subsequent child will inevitably feel increased anxiety until the age at which their previous child died is well past. All families should be offered support with a subsequent child. This may take the form of an apnoea monitor with appropriate paediatric back up, and should always include an increased level of professional involvement with the family and emphasis on restoring parents' confidence and improving parenting skills (Emery et al. 1985; l'Hoir et al. 1991). It is important that local areas should develop a system of identification so that all parents are offered a service, because the younger, less articulate parents who would most benefit from increased professional involvement are the least likely to request it. In England and Wales, the CONI (care of next infant) programme is promoted by the Foundation for the Study of Infant Death, and each health authority involved identifies a paediatrician and a nursing coordinator to take local responsibility for the programme.

Conclusion

Unexpected infant death is not a single entity. Although it has a clear, epidemiological profile, it is multicausal, and individual deaths may be multifactoral, the infant being vulnerable because of genetic predisposition or intrauterine disadvantage to one or more trigger factors such as infection or overheating. There is continuing need for high quality research and the European Society for the Study and Prevention of Infant Death (ESPID) has been formed to promote research within Europe. However, a reduction in the incidence of unexpected infant death may be achieved by changing child care practices and by positive discrimination in care. In the early eighties Guntheroth (1982) stated that 'the single most effective remedy for SIDS would appear to be a general improvement of maternal and infant health' and this remains true today.

References

Bacon, C.J., Bell, S.A., Clulow, E.E., and Beattie, A.B. (1991). How mothers keep their babies warm. *Archives of Disease in Childhood* **66**, 627–32.

Bentele, K.H.P. and Albani, M. (1988). Are there tests predictive for prolonged apnoea and SIDS? *Acta Paediatrica Scandinavica* (Supplement) **342**, 1–21.

Carpenter, R.G. (1983). Scoring to provide risk related primary health care; evaluation and updating during use. *Journal of the Royal Statistical Society* (Series A) **146**, 1–32.

Carpenter, R.G., Gardner, A., Harris, J., Judd, M., Lowry, J., Maddock, C.R., et al. (1988). Prevention of unexpected infant death. A review of risk related intervention in six centres. *Annals of the New York Academy of Sciences* **533**, 96–103.

Cheron, G., Rambaud, C., and Rey, C. (1990). La mort subite du nourrisson, interet du bilan post mortem. *Progrès en Néonatologie, 10, XXes Journee Nationales de Neonatologie*, 111–22. Karger, Paris.

De Jonge, G.A., Engelberts, A.C., Koomen-Lieftung, A.J.M., Kostense, P.J. (1989). Cot death and prone sleeping position in the Netherlands. *British Medical Journal* **298**, 722.

Devlieger, H., Daniels, H., de Zegher, F. and Eggermont, E. (1991). RSV infection presenting as life threatening event in young infants. *European Society for the Study and Prevention of Infant Death, Founding Congress June 1991*. Workshop abstract 50 C.R.A.M. Normandie

Emery, J.L. (1986). Families in which two or more cot deaths have occurred. *Lancet*, **1**, 313–15.

Emery, J.L., Waite, A.M., Carpenter, R.G., Limerick, S.R., and Blake, D. (1985). Apnoea monitors compared with weighing scales for siblings after cot death. *Archives of Disease in Childhood* **60**, 1055–60.

Fleming, P.J., Gilbert, R., Azaz, Y., Berry, P.J., Rudd, P.T., Stewart, A., and Hall, E. (1990). Interaction between bedding and sleeping position in the sudden infant death syndrome: a population based case-control study. *British Medical Journal* **301**, 85–9.

Froggatt, P., Lynas, M.A., and Mackenzie, G. (1971). Epidemiology of sudden deaths in infants (cot deaths) in Northern Ireland. *British Journal of Preventive Social Medicine* **25**, 119–34.

Gilbert, R.E., Fleming, P.J., Azaz, Y., and Rudd, P.T. (1990). Signs of illness preceding sudden unexpected infant death. *British Medical Journal*, **300**, 1237–9.

Golding, J. and Peters, R.J. (1985). What else do SIDS risk prediction scores predict? *Early Human Development* **12**, 247–60.

Golding, J., Limerick, S., and Macfarlane, A. (1985). In *Sudden infant death. Patterns, puzzles and problems*, pp. 58–9. Open Books, Somerset, UK.

Guntheroth, W.G. (1982). Management and prevention of SIDS. In *Crib death, the sudden infant death syndrome*, pp. 161–202. Futura, New York.

Haidmayer, R., Loscher, W.N., Einspieler, C., and Kerbl, R. (1991). Cardiorespiratory control mechanisms in infants during sleep. *European Society for the Study and Prevention of Infant Death, Founding Congress* June 1991. Workshop abstract 58 C.R.A.M. Normandie.

Hinchliffe, S.A., Howard, C.V., Lynch, N.R.J., Sargent, P.H., Judd, B.A., and van Velsen, D. (1993). Renal developmental aspect in sudden infant death syndrome. *Paediatric Pathology* **13**, 333–43.

Hoffman, H.J., Hunter, J.C., Damus, K., Pakter, J., Peterson, D.R., van Belle, G. et al. (1987). Diphtheria–tetanus–pertussis immunisation and sudden infant death: results of the National Institute of Child Health and Human Development (NICHD) co-operative epidemiologic study of sudden infant death syndrome risk factors. *Journal of Pediatrics* **79**, 598–611.

Irgens, L.M. and Skjaerven, R. (1984). Prospective assessment of recurrence risk in sudden infant death syndrome siblings. *Journal of Paediatrics* **104**, 349–51.

Kahn, A., Rebuffat, E., Sottiaux, M., Muller, M.F., Bochner, A., and Grosswasser, J. (1990a). Brief airway obstructions during sleep in infants with breath holding spells. *Journal of Pediatrics* **117**, 188–93.

Kahn, A., Blum, D., Rebuffat, E., Sottiaux, M., Levit, J., Bochner, A. et al. (1990b). Home monitors for infants: use, misuse and 'over the counter' use. *European Journal of Paediatrics* **149**, 356–8.

Knowelden, J., Keeling, J., and Nicholl, J.P. (1984). *A multicenre study of postneonatal mortality*. Medical Care Research Unit, University of Sheffield, pp. 20–1, 26, HMSO, London.

Kraus, A.S., Steel, R., and Langworth, J.T. (1967). Sudden unexpected death in infancy in Ontario Part II. Findings regarding season, clustering of deaths on specific days and weather. *Canadian Journal of Public Health* **58**, 364–71.

Lancet (1855). Infants found dead in bed. Medical jurisprudence. *Lancet* **i**, 103.

L'Hoir, M.P., Horstink, J., Neeleman, C., and Huber, J. (1991). Managing subsequent siblings of cot death victims. *European Society for the Study and Prevention of Infant Death, Founding Congress June 1991*. Workshop abstract 128 C.R.A.M. Normandie.

Limerick, S.R. (1992). Sudden infant death in historical perspective. *Journal of Clinical Pathology* (Suppl.) **45**, 3–6.

Morley, C.J., Thornton, A.J., Cole, T.J., Hewson, P.H., and Fowler, M.A. (1991). Baby check: a scoring system to grade the severity of acute systematic illness in babies under six months old. *Archives of Disease in Childhood* **66**, 100–6.

Nicholl, J.P. and O'Cathain, A. (1988). Sleeping position and SIDS. *Lancet* **ii**, 106.

Norvenius, G., Milerad, J., Wennergren, G., Lagercrantz, H., Rammer, L., Dahlberg, K. et al. (1991). The development of SIDS in Sweden. *European Society for the Study and Prevention of Infant Death, Founding Congress June 1991*. Workshop abstract 23. C.R.A.M. Normandie.

Paltauf, A. (1889). Ueber die Beziehungen der Thymus zum Plotzlichen Tod. *Wiener klinische Wochenschrift* **2**, 877.

Peters, T.J. and Golding, J. (1986). Prediction of SIDS. An independent evaluation of four scoring methods. *Statistics in Medicine* **5**, 113–26.

Petersen, S.A., Anderson, E.S., Lodemore, M., Rawson, D., and Wailoo, M.P. (1991). Sleeping position and rectal temperature. *Archives of Disease in Childhood* **66**, 976–9.

Rognum, T.O., Saugstad, O.D., Oyasaeter, S., and Olaisen, B. (1988). Elevated levels of hypoxanthine in vitreous humor indicate prolonged cerebral hypoxia in victims of sudden infant death syndrome. *Pediatrics* **82**, 615–17.

Schuler, D., Klinger, A., Agfalvi, R., and Barko, E. (1991). The effect of social-cultural and ethnic factors on infant mortality in Hungary. *European Society for the Study and Prevention of Infant Death, Founding Congress June 1991*. Workshop abstract 29. C.R.A.M. Normandie.

Stanton, A.W., Scott, D.J., and Downham, M.A.P.S. (1980). Is overheating a factor in some unexpected deaths? *Lancet* **i**, 1054–7.

Still, G.F. (1923). Attacks of arrested respiration in the newborn. *Lancet* **i**, 431.

Taylor, E.M. and Emery, J.L. (1990). Categories of preventable unexpected infant deaths. *Archives of Disease in Childhood* **65**, 535–9.

Taylor, B.J., Nelson, E.A.S., and Mackay, S. (1991). Changing childcare practice in an area with a high postneonatal mortality. *European Society for the Study and Prevention of Infant Death, Founding Congress June 1991*. Workshop abstract 30. C.R.A.M. Normandie.

Taylor, E.M., Spencer, N.J., and Carpenter, R.G. (1993). Evaluation of attempted prevention of unexpected infant death in very high risk infants by planned health care. *Acta Paediatrica Scandinavica* **82**, 83–6.

Templeman, C. (1892). Two hundred and fifty eight cases of suffocation of infants. *Edinburgh Medical Journal* **38**, 322.

Van Velsen, D and Peters, P.W.J. (1988). Underestimation of viral infection in sudden infant death. *Pediatric Pathology Abstracts* **8**, 350.

Variend, S and Pearse, R.G. (1986). Sudden infant death syndrome and cytomegalovirus inclusion disease. *Journal of Clinical Pathology* **39**, 383–6.

Vawter, G.F. and Kozakewich, H.P.W. (1983). Aspects of morphologic variation amongst SIDS victims. In *Proceedings of 1982 International Research Conference on the sudden infant death syndrome* (ed. J. Tyson *et al.*). Academic Press.

Wailoo, M.P., Petersen, S.A., Whittaker, H., and Goodenough, P. (1989). The thermal environment in which 3–4 month old infants sleep at home. *Archives of Disease in Childhood* **64**, 600–4.

Wennergren, G., Milerad, J., Laercrantz, H., Karlberg, P., Svenningsen, N.W., Sedin, G. *et al.* (1987). The epidemiology of sudden infant death syndrome and attacks of lifelessness in Sweden. *Acta Paediatrica Scandinavica* **76**, 898–906.

Wigfield, R.E., Fleming, P.J., Berry, P.J., Rudd, P.T., and Golding J. (1992). Can the fall in Avon's sudden infant death rate be explained by changes in sleeping position? *British Medical Journal* **304**, 282–3.

19 Child abuse and neglect
Stella Tsitoura

The problem of child abuse

Child abuse and neglect refers to a wide variety of damaging care-taker omissions and commissions. Endangering a child includes creating substantial risk to a child's health or safety, by violating duty of care, support, or protection. This includes torture or cruel abuse and excessive punishment, or restraint that creates substantial risk of physical harm to the child. Child abuse is also repeated unjustified discipline that poses substantial risk to the child's mental health or development, or death, that is not caused by allowable physical discipline. Abuse of children does not only occur in families. Abuse of children can also take place in schools, children's homes, children's courts, child care centres, hospitals, and mental health establishments.

The physically abused infant or child is deprived of the precious state of safety, predictability, and love which is so crucial for development. With each physical attack comes a message of 'badness', worthlessness, and 'unlovability'.

The abuse of children has been a feature of society for many centuries. Many cultures used infanticide as an accepted method of family planning and for the disposal of weak, premature, or deformed infants. At times children were killed for superstitious reasons. It was believe that slain infants would benefit the sterile woman, kill disease, and confer health, vigour, and youthfulness. To ensure durability of important buildings, children were buried under the foundations (Radbill 1974).

The repeated experience of nations first denying the existence of child maltreatment only to 'discover' it later (Kempe 1978a) stimulated interest in the broader cross-cultural record. At international congresses and regional meetings sponsored by the International Society for the Prevention of Child Abuse and Neglect (ISPCAN), more and more nations participated, indicating that child maltreatment is a concern within their boundaries.

The history of child abuse can be grouped into four periods (Oates 1985). In the first period prior to 1946 child abuse was professionally unrecognized, even though the medical features of child abuse were first described in 1860 by Ambrose Tardieu, a specialist in forensic medicine working in Paris. This long period was followed by the early scientific phase when scientists from the field of medicine, such as radiologists, paediatricians, and psychiatrists, reported a number of unidentified syndromes of broken bones, bleeding, and bruising in journal articles between 1946 and 1962 (Caffey 1946; Astley 1953; Silverman

1953). The third period started in 1962 when the classic paper by Henry Kempe's group (Kempe et al. 1962) ushered in a period of professional awareness and concern. These authors coined the phrase 'the battered child syndrome' and concluded that physical abuse was a significant cause of death and injury among children and suggested that psychiatric factors were likely to be of importance in understanding the disorder. Early approaches were focused on diagnosis, pathogenesis, and aetiology and their primary concern was on saving lives of the victims of this 'disease'. In the fourth period which dates from the mid-1970s it was recognized that to save the child, one had to diagnose the syndrome, and that traditional medical examination alone was not sufficient. Hence, professionals in the behavioural field were drawn in to help with identification and diagnosis. This pathway led to understanding the dynamics of the abusing adults. Emphasis was placed on protection and therapy. To ensure the survival of children, alternatives to living with abusing parents were developed which involved child protection agencies and legal systems, courts, and police. At the same period child abuse legislation was widely introduced and rewriting of laws took place to deal optimally with this syndrome, a process that is still going on. Despite this progress, child abuse remains a major problem. Further efforts have to be made before a fifth phase, encompassing the widespread prevention of child abuse, can be said to have occurred.

Epidemiology and comparative statistics

Physical abuse

Incidence and prevalence statistics of child abuse are unreliable even in nations with legally mandatory reporting systems. One must consider whether the figure given is based on the actual reported incidents of child abuse to an official agency or whether the figure was an estimate to include cases thought to have occurred but not reported. Varying definitions of child abuse used by different authorities compound the difficulties in the interpretation of data, and whilst many cases go unreported, there is also a considerable amount of over-reporting.

Methods of obtaining data on child abuse incidents can be from surveys within a defined community or by making estimates from the number of cases presented to medical services.

Using a strict definition of severe physical abuse, Baldwin and Oliver (1975) carried out a retrospective study in north-east Wiltshire, England. They found a rate of one case per thousand children in their prospective survey, a rate that was 2.6 times that found in their retrospective study.

Child abuse and neglect remain a significant problem in the USA. Results of a recent national study (US Department of Health and Human Services 1988) indicates that countable cases of child maltreatment increased 66 per cent over the rate found in the previous (1980) national incidence study. Under 1986 definitions, there were an estimated one and a half million children nationwide who experienced abuse or neglect. Approximately 10 per cent of the incidents were classified as serious and 0.1 per cent were fatal (US DHHS 1988). Experts in the field suspect that the true incidence of fatalities is far higher, with estimates ranging from 2000–5000 per year (Massachusetts Legislative Commission 1988). Children who are left in severely mistreating homes have a 40–70 per cent chance of being re-injured (Ferleger et al. 1988) and as much as five per cent chance of being killed (Schmitt and Kempe 1975).

About 10 per cent of injuries to children under five years of age seen in hospital emergency rooms are due to abuse. The ages of victims of physical abuse are estimated to be one-third under one year, one-third between one and six years of age, and one-third over six years old. Premature infants are at a threefold greater risk of abuse. The abuser is a related care-taker in 90 per cent of cases, a male friend (boyfriend) of the mother in five per cent, an unrelated babysitter in four per cent, and a sibling in one per cent.

Data from the UK reported 16 000 severely abused children in 1986. There was a 70 per cent increase between 1979 and 1986. The death rate was nine per cent in 1986. A study of the Committee on Violence in the Family considered child abuse as the fourth cause of death in pre-school children. In the rest of Europe only Portugal and Sweden presented national data based on national epidemiological studies and on representative samples. Research in Sweden of families with children 3–17 years old proved that 30 per cent of parents used more severe abuse than a 'simple strike or slap' and four per cent described the abuse as severe. Statistics in Portugal show that only 0.58 per cent of children are abused (Council of Europe 1987), a percentage which is considered low and inaccurate by the researchers. France reports 300 000 cases of abused children of ages 0–6 each year and approximately 90 000 at-risk children per year whose protection is taken care of by social services.

Although there is a lack of clarity about the definition of child abuse and its true incidence, the important conclusion that should be drawn from all studies is that child abuse is a relatively common problem. It is far more prevalent than many other diseases to which considerable paediatric time and resources are devoted; as such it is worthy of a greater share of resources as well as further studies for appropriate treatment and prevention.

Sexual abuse of children

According to incidence figures during a single year (1984), 200 000 new cases of child abuse were reported to child protection services in 19 states of the USA. However, only 100 000 of these cases were substantiated, 22 per cent involving a male child and 78 per cent involving a female child (American Humane Association 1984). It is unlikely, however, that the confirmed cases were the only victims of sexual abuse. A sizeable portion of victims never come to the attention of the child welfare system. Included among this group are those whose abuse is investigated but does not stand up to the rigours of the court. And finally, there are unknown numbers of children who remain silent and never tell. Victims below the age of 18 years are often subjected to physical and psychological coercion to ensure their participation and silence in abusive relationships (Finkelhor 1979). If and when they disclose their abuse they are often not believed, ignored, punished, and not supported by non-abusive adults and professionals (Russels 1983).

Current prevalence or lifetime rates for at least one incident having occurred before the age of 18 years range from 6 per cent to 62 per cent for females and from 3 per cent to 31 per cent for males (Peters *et al*. 1986). There is a substantial range in reported rates, due to methodological variations, especially in data collection and sampling techniques and to differences in how child sexual abuse is defined. As far as the UK is concerned, and accepting all the problems, an estimate of one in ten children (7000 per year) being sexually abuse is widely accepted by professionals as a 'true' rate (La Fontaine 1988).

Austria reports to 10 000 children per year, Switzerland between 40 000 and 50 000 children per year, while during a survey in Sweden using random sample of adults (18–70 years of age) it was discovered that nine per cent of women and three per cent of men had experienced sexual abuse at least once by the time they reached 18 years of age.

Childhood victims of sexual misuse have a median age of 11 years, but significant numbers of episodes occur as early as the first year of life. Girls are abused more often, but it is estimated that one out of four girls and one out of five boys will be molested by the age of 18 years. Family members, close relatives, neighbours, and friends account for 30–50 per cent of all incidents and 80 per cent of children know their attackers. Incestuous relationships in particular frequently involve stepfathers.

At least 0.2–0.3 per cent of children have been involved in persistent incestuous relationships for an average period of five years. Brief sexual encounters occur more frequently. Victims of incest are 90 per cent female and 10 per cent male. In cases of third party molestation in child care centres, which are being recognized with increasing frequency, the sex ration is more nearly equal. No age of child is exempt. Approximately one-third are less than six years old, one-third 6–12 years, and one-third 12–18 years old. Incest is often repeated with successive daughters. The offenders are 99 per cent male. The incidence among stepfathers is about five times higher than among natural fathers. Incest cuts across socio-economic boundaries to a greater degree than physical abuse.

Substance abuse and child abuse

Estimates of the number of children living in drug-dependent families can be obtained only indirectly by dependent families of adult substance abuse. There are approximately 10 million adult alcoholics, 500 000 heroin addicts, and between five and eight million regular cocaine users in the USA. Most drug users are in their child-bearing years. More than 300 000 infants are born annually to American women who use opiates. From these figures the NCPCA estimates that 10 million children in the USA are being raised by addicted parents and at least 675 000 children are seriously mistreated by an alcoholic or drug-abusing care-taker (Bays 1990).

Changing patterns of abuse

Socio-economic and sociocultural changes have been linked in the literature with an increase in child maltreatment. Most often this is attributed to a breakdown in traditional patterns and practices. The above changes have an impact on parent–child relationships and integration. In the change from an agrarian to an urban economy, children become consumers rather than producers and an economic liability rather than an asset. Through formal schooling, immigrant children acquire more knowledge of the new environment and society than their parents possess. They become less obedient and compliant, providing greater opportunity for parent–child conflict. Children's behaviour in urban areas is more aggressive and disruptive while mothers who move to urbanized areas and come into situations of new culture contact are less confident about their efficacy in child rearing and uncertain which of the conflicting models of child care to adopt. These problems are compounded by increased social isolation of families from traditional kin and social networks and thus diminished availability of others in child care (Korbin 1991).

Although battered children as described by Kempe are now not often seen, children suffering from physical abuse, sexual abuse, emotional abuse, physical neglect, emotional neglect, medical care neglect, and educational neglect are regularly encountered. Munchausen's syndrome by proxy, in which the child's carer invents fictitious illness or induces illness, has been discovered and many professionals become overwhelmed by babies born to drug-addicted mothers.

Types of abuse

Physical abuse

A child maltreatment situation is one in which through purposive acts or marked inattention to the child's basic needs, behaviour of a parent/substitute or other adult care-taker causes foreseeable and avoidable injury or impairment to a child or materially contributes to unreasonable prolongation or worsening of an existing injury or impairment (National Center on Child Abuse and Neglect 1981).

The essential first step in diagnosis is a knowledgeable evaluation of physical injuries by the physician. Injuries of the skin in various stages of healing, lacerations, scars, bruises (especially when confined to the buttocks and lower back), finger and thumb prints, human bite marks, lash marking, choke marks, and traumatic alopecia may be found.

Bone trauma is found in 10–20 per cent of physically abused children. Fractures of the long bones and skull, metaphyseal 'chip' or 'corner' fractures, subperiosteal haematoma, or later bone remodelling may be apparent.

Approximately 10 per cent of cases of physical abuse involve burns. The most severe inflicted injuries, in terms of morbidity and mortality, are head injuries leading to subdural haematomas. Over 95 per cent of serious intracranial injuries during the first year of life are the result of abuse. Intra-abdominal injuries are the second most common cause of death in battered children. A tentative diagnosis of physical abuse should be made if an injury is inadequately explained. Inconsistencies are common between the history offered and the child's development level. Delay in seeking medical attention for inflicted injuries and use of multiple health providers are common. Families in distress will often make medical visits that are inappropriate superficially but can precede incidents of physical abuse.

Sexual abuse

Sexual abuse can be defined as the engaging of dependent, developmentally immature children and adolescents in sexual activities that they do not fully comprehend, to which they are unable to give informed consent, or which violate the social taboos of family roles (Kempe 1978*b*). This definition is broad and includes intrafamilial and extrafamilial forms and all types of sexual activities (e.g. exhibition, fondling, child pornography, oral, anal, and genital sexual contact).

Incest refers to any sexual activity between persons too closely related to marry; most legal codes include adopted and/or stepchildren in the definition. Incest in the most common type of sexual mistreatment, followed by sexual abuse by a person closely involved with the family. Least common is sexual abuse by strangers.

It is common in all classes of society, both urban and rural, and often occurs in subsequent generations. The abuser is an adult or adolescent who uses a child for a sexual act to satisfy his need for power, bravado, tenderness, and contact as well as his erotic desires.

Because secrecy is generally enforced many children exhibit symptoms for some time before disclosure and someone needs to be attentive so the child can be given permission 'to tell'. Early warning may take various forms. Some children make broad general statements. More often there are numerous behavioral changes. Sleep and appetite disorders, phobias, withdrawal, depression, guilt, temper tantrums, excessive anger, excessive masturbation, runaway behaviour, suicide attempts, neurotic and conduct disorders, hysterical conversion reactions may all be the first recognized symptom. We may notice sexual awareness inappropriate to the child's age, constant preoccupation with sexual identity, repressive behaviour, withdrawal from friends, poor school performance, and truancy. Promiscuity and prostitution are late presenting signs of sexually abused adolescents. Substance abuse provides an escape from the sexual abuse experience. Perpetration to others is seen predominantly in boys (Krugman 1986).

Medical conditions may be overt or 'masked' (Hunter et al. 1985). Genital trauma or infection are most common, followed by non-specific abdominal pain. Recurrent urinary tract infections, enuresis, and encopresis may also be presentations of sexual abuse. Sexually transmitted disease in children, such as gonorrhoea and syphilis, are highly correlated with sexual transmission and herpes simplex, chlamydia, trichomonas, *Gardnerella vaginalis*, and *Lymphogranuloma venereum* are often found in sexually abused children. Adolescent pregnancy, especially in the 12 to 15 years age group, may be another presentation.

The diagnosis of child molestation and most instances of sexual intercourse is the most uncomfortable task of paediatricians and rests on the history offered by the victim. Children do not generally tell lies about abuse. Physical findings are usually absent because of the long delay before disclosure. In pre-pubertal girls, a hymenal opening of 5mm or greater is probably abnormal.

The presence of hymenal changes suggests penetration. Interpretation of these findings is difficult and readers are returned to more comprehensive texts (see references). If sexual intercourse has occurred within the previous 72 hours laboratory evidence of acid phosphatase or sperm helps to confirm the diagnosis. Normal physical and laboratory examinations, however, are compatible with most types of sexual abuse.

Non-organic failure to thrive (FTT)

This is a substained subnormal weight velocity, usually identified in children under three years of age, and significant whether the weight has gone below the third percentile or not. Clinically we define FTT as a decreased weight velocity resulting in a weight curve that has crossed at least two major percentiles. Linear growth may also be affected although usually to a lesser extent, and there may be evidence of delay in psychomotor development (Oates 1984).

Investigation of these children fails to reveal an organic cause for the growth disorder and the history is suggestive of emotional or nutritional deprivation, or both. The implication is that the child's social, emotional, or nutritional environment is disturbed to the point where it interferes with normal growth and development.

This is accompanied by signs such as apathy, poor hygiene, withdrawal behaviour, and disorders of oral intake, which may be manifested as anorexia, voracious appetite, or pica. Vomiting, regurgitation, diarrhoea, and general neuromuscular spasticity or hypotonia may be concurrent.

Sills (1978) studied the degree of usefulness of laboratory investigations in non-organic failure to thrive and found only 1.4 per cent of the tests to be of positive diagnostic assistance.

Hospitalization frequently leads to dramatic improvement in weight gain and in social responses and thus provides evidence that environmental factors are causative.

Munchausen's syndrome by proxy (MSBP)

This is a form of child abuse wherein the mother falsifies illness in her child through simulation and/or production of illness, and presents the child for medical care, disclaiming knowledge as to aetiology of the problem.

In 117 cases of MSBP that were reviewed from the literature (Rosenberg 1987), the most common presentations of MSBP were bleeding (44 per cent), seizures (42 per cent), central nervous system depression (19 per cent), apnoea (10 per cent), diarrhoea (11 per cent), vomiting (10 per cent), fever (10 per cent), and rash (9 per cent).

The short-term morbidity rate, defined as pain and/or illness which resolved and did not leave permanent disfigurement or permanent impairment of function, was 100 per cent. Morbidity caused by medical staff was related to investigations and procedures. At least eight per cent had long-term morbidity, including multiple surgeries for laparotomy, colectomy, or ileostomy, predisposing to future medical problems, serious psychiatric problems, destructive joint changes, and a mental retardation with cerebral palsy and cortical blindness. The mortality rate was nine per cent (all children were less than three years). Failure to thrive was associated with MSBP in 14 per cent of cases.

All perpetrators were mothers frequently complaining of either somatic or depressive symptoms, none of which have responded well to a variety of treatment. If a psychiatric referral was made, the usual diagnosis was 'reactive depression' or 'personality problems'.

The mothers tried to attract attention to themselves and receive sympathy and support that might otherwise not be forthcoming, either from inside or outside the family. The mothers differed greatly in some aspects but loneliness and isolation in these women's lives were unusually prominent.

Emotional and psychological abuse

This involves the continual rejection or scapegoating of a child by care-takers and is generally synonymous with verbal abuse. For a young child, reality is the world portrayed by his or her parents. The verbally abused child will accept that he is bad, stupid, or worthless, and may be burdened by his low self-esteem and sense of incompetence. Emotional abuse is difficult to prove. Psychological terrorism (e.g. locking a child in a dark cellar or threats of mutilation) may also occur.

Emotional neglect

This refers to a lack of loving interaction between parent and child. For the preschool child both affective and cognitive needs are often unmet.

Physical neglect

This is the inability to provide adequate food, shelter, clothing, and hygiene and is the form of maltreatment most closely related to poverty. We should bear in mind, however, that in indigent populations, many children with inadequate clothing and hygiene are loved and safe in their homes.

Neglect of medical care

Non-compliance for immunizations and dental and illness follow-up is a common problem for many paediatricians. Occasionally the magnitude of neglect is extreme, especially for a child with chronic disease, and may lead to deterioration in the condition. This calls for aggressive intervention with court-enforced supervision, or placement in foster care or out-reach health systems.

Educational neglect

This refers to either passive collusion with a child's truancy or actual active prevention of a child's school attendance.

Unusual presentations of child maltreatment

These include fatal pepper aspiration, internal microwave oven burns, thirsting and hypernatremic dehydration, 'tin ear syndrome'—a clinical triad consisting of ear bruising, retinal haemorrhages, and cerebral oedema, deprivational dwarfism and kwashiorkor due to cult diets, and ritual abuse in childhood by satanic cults. Satanic cults are intrafamilial, transgenerational groups that engage in explicit satanic worship which includes the following criminal practices: ritual torture, sacrificial murder, deviant sexual activity, and ceremonial cannibalism (Young *et al.* 1991).

As drug use has escalated in the past decade, a new category of children at risk has emerged—drug-affected infants. The effects of drugs may be compounded by factors such as poor nutrition, exposure to infectious diseases, lack of medical care, inadequate child-bearing practices, criminal lifestyle, and parental mental illness.

Societal and institutional child abuse

The issue of the state as a parent cannot be studied in isolation but should be approached through a broad analysis of existing political, economic, and social systems while considering historical developments and respecting cross-cultural variations.

History has provided us with ample examples of the state assuming a destructive parenting role in the name of political ideologies (disguised under scientific initiatives). A recent sad example is Romania. An entire generation is now paying for a dictator's ambition to increase the country's population from 22 million to 30 million by the end of the century (Dobbs 1990). His obsessive campaign resulted in increasing numbers of orphans, an infant mortality rate higher than anywhere else in Europe, and the deaths of thousands of women who attempted illegal or self administered abortions (Marie Claire 1990). The list of examples of the state's exploitation and even extermination of children is endless. Should we overlook the recent killing by the Brazilian police of more than 400 street children who were bothering shop-keepers on the Cabacabane (Copacabana) beach?

The traditional care for children provided by the extended and nuclear family systems had been steadily decreasing over the years under the pressure of various historical, social, and economic vicissitudes. As a result, the state has been gradually assuming a parental role either with or without statutory power.

The question naturally emerging is 'can the state parent?'. The characteristics of parental love are that it is unconditional, continuous, does not have cut-off points, is long-suffering, and does not evaluate. The state cannot replicate this, it delegates parenting to subsidiaries such as foster parents, adoptive parents and residential care workers, only some of whom can offer a satisfactory service. The state then reacts with dismay when things go wrong (Parker and Millham 1989). Such dismay may result in children being shifted from setting to setting, from one foster family to another, or back to their natural families, without any family evaluation or support.

A close look at child protection systems reveals systems overwhelmed by reports often impossible to substantiate, inadequate staffing of services, inadequate finance, over-reporting, professional 'burn-out', staff turn-over, and inadequate professional 'parenting'.

In most countries, traditional institutional care shares characteristics parallel with intrafamilial child abuse and neglect: there is a special parent, a special child, and a crisis situation (Agathonos 1983). Institutions and their staff assume the role of the special parent: poorly educated and poorly paid staff, with low professional status and often brought up in care themselves, assume the role of the special parent; but children in residential care have lived mostly in multi-problem families, in emotional deprivation, and in antecedent conditions of family breakdown. Their personality has been formed with poor attachment experiences while few enjoy any corrective experiences while in residential care. They may well be described as 'special' children, as children with special needs. Lastly, most residential care settings are in a state of chronic crisis. Buildings are housing children rather than offering them a home. All types of abuse can be found (Grenleese and Henderson 1987):

(a) programme abuse: institutional procedures which operate below normally accepted standards, or which rely on inhumane techniques to control behaviour;

(b) system abuse: when the whole system is stretched beyond its limits and is incapable of adequately caring for children in its custody;

(c) abuse akin to familial child abuse and neglect: when the abusive act—be it physical, psychological, or sexual—is committed by a member of staff.

The paradigm of residential care for children depicts quite clearly the role of the state as 'a needy parent' and as the bigger consumer of public expenditure and resources for children in care. If safety valves such as research and programme evaluation do not exist, the needs of the system assume greater priority over the needs of the consumer, thus the system perpetuates itself by recycling its own needs rather than meeting those of the population it should serve (Agathonos 1988).

Consequences of child abuse

There is sufficient empirical evidence to support the widely held assumption that child abuse and neglect have deleterious effects on the physical, neurological, intellectual, and emotional development of the child. A significant number of abused children have demonstrated failure to thrive at the time of abuse identification and some of them continued to show signs of growth retardation at follow-up. There is sufficient evidence to suggest that there is a substantial proportion of children mentally handicapped as a direct consequence of physical abuse (baby battering or shaking) and neglect. Not only is brain damage a very real consequence of child abuse, but so too is death (Martin et al. 1974). Intellectual development has also been found to be delayed among neglected children. Learning disabilities and significant deficiencies in speech and language are greatly increased in these children. Poor self-concept, lack of joy and play ability, poor sense of self, and deviant object-relations are common findings (Martin 1976; Lynch and Roberts 1982).

Common emotional traits of abused children are fearfulness, aggression, and hyperactivity. These children may also become the juvenile delinquents and violent members of our society and the next generation of child abusers. Concerning non-organic failure to thrive, approximately 5–10 per cent of these infants sustain superimposed physical abuse. Weight loss and understature from malnutrition are reversible, but normal head circumference and brain growth may not be achieved if the infant has had marasmus persisting beyond six months of age. Emotional and educational problems occur in over half of these children (Schmitt and Krugman 1987). Lynch and Roberts (1982) identified various common characteristics of the abused children whose outcome was good at follow-up. These children tended to lack neurological deficits and were likely to have experienced perinatal problems or developmental and behavioural abnormalities before the onset of intervention. If they had been subject to legal proceedings, then these were usually resolved quickly with few placement changes. The possession of above-average intelligence appears to have been a possible protective factor. The children who did well demonstrated an ability to enjoy themselves, possessed self-confidence, spontaneity, and an ability to form good relationships.

The impact of sexual abuse on a child may vary from minimal, acute, and reversible—as is often the case with a single, non-violent, heterosexual, extra-familial episode—to catastrophic developmental and psychological damage wrought by long-term incest. There are four traumatic dynamics that account for the impact of sexual abuse: traumatic dynamics alter a child's cognitive or emotional orientation to the world and cause trauma by distorting the child's self-concept, world view, or affective capacities. Later on there are sexual problems–including aversion to sex, and difficulty with arousal and orgasm. Some of the victims inappropriately sexualize their own children in ways that lead to sexual or physical abuse. Depression is noted as a result of the disillusion and loss of a trusted figure. Sometimes extreme dependency and clinging behaviour is seen; victims are often observed to be hostile and angry, to distrust men or intimate relationships in general, and to have a history of failed relationships or marriages. Victims often feel isolated and gravitate towards stigmatized groups of society—for example among drug abusers, into criminal subcultures, or into prostitution. Low self-esteem, self-destructive behaviour, and suicide attempts appear. Fear and anxiety reflect the experience of having been unable to control their own life. The post-traumatic stress disorder symptoms include nightmares, phobias, hypervigilance, dissociations, somatic complaints, sleep problems, and deadness of affect (Finkelhor 1988). Girls who had no symptoms in adult life had had support from friends and family during childhood and had not been blamed for the events: they had also found several partners in adulthood who were sympathetic and understanding.

Concerning alcohol and drug use there are many deleterious effects when parents use them during pregnancy (i.e. teratogenesis, mental retardation, growth failure, facial anomalies, symptoms of withdrawal in neonates). Long-term effects include persisting psychosocial problems, learning disabilities, hyperactivity, impulsivity, and antisocial behaviour. Neurobehavioural deficits, abnormalities in T-cell functions, and a 10-fold increased risk of acute non-lymphoblastic leukaemia is reported in children whose mothers used marijuana just before and during pregnancy (Robinson *et al.* 1989).

Cultural attitudes to abuse

Child maltreatment has occurred throughout history and is known across cultures, in developing and developed countries, in the East as well as in the West. Repeated experience with nations that first denied the existence of child abuse only to 'discover' it later has promoted scepticism that severely abused and neglected children look sadly similar across cultural boundaries. A definition of child abuse that can be used internationally is that given by Finkelhor and Korbin (1988): 'child abuse is the portion of harm to children that results from human action that is proscribed, proximate, and preventable'. Cross-cultural variability in child rearing beliefs and behaviours makes it clear that there is not a universal standard for optimal care for child abuse and neglect. Conceptions of 'badness' are culturally bound. Behaviours that are considered acceptable in one culture may be viewed as detrimental to children in another. Some helpful guidelines for understanding child rearing practices from other countries have been produced by Korbin (1980, 1981). She suggests that in trying to decide whether a practice is harmful to the child one should consider the cultural acceptance of the act, the intent of the adult who performs it, the way the child perceives the incident, and what it means to the development of the child as a member of his culture, and proposes three levels for culturally appropriate definitions of child maltreatment.

1. *Cultural differences in child rearing practices and beliefs.* Some practices that are viewed as acceptable in the culture in which they occur may be considered as abusive or neglectful by outsiders. Many Euro-American child care practices, even those as seemingly benign as sleeping arrangements in which infants have separate beds and rooms, are seen as ill-informed at best, uncaring and abusive at worst, by many of the world's societies (Korbin 1981). The same parental behaviour may have different meanings and interpretations in different cultural contexts. For example, continual physical contact with an infant increases chances of survival in societies with high infant mortality, while the same behaviour in societies with low infant mortality carries a meaning of indulgence. Similarly, child outcomes may have different meanings. It does not make sense to equate bruises inflicted on a child by angry parents in Western societies with a child who is bruised in the process of the Vietnamese curing practice of 'coin rubbing' (Yeatman 1976). Even normal child rearing practices differ markedly between cultures and the possibility of conflict in defining child maltreatment increases.

2. *Idiosyncratic departure from one's cultural continuum of acceptable behaviour.* All cultures have criteria for behaviours that fall outside the range of acceptability and some individuals in all cultures exceed the boundaries of their society's standards (Agathonos *et al.* 1982). Virtually all societies have

proscriptions of sexual behaviour, some societies permit fondling of the genitalia of infants and very young children to soothe them or get them to sleep. However, such fondling of older children, or for the sexual gratification of adults, would fall outside of the acceptable cultural continuum (Korbin 1987). Also, cultural practices have been documented in which incest occurs openly, in exempted situations (religious and ceremonial occasions or prior to battle) and for exempted individuals (from specific classes such as royalty or nobility). These cultural exceptions and exemptions do not diminish, but rather underline the rules (Schneider 1976).

3. *Societal harm of children that is beyond the control of individual parents and care-takers.* This level refers to the degree of poverty, unemployment, homelessness, and hunger that nations are willing to tolerate for children and families. The cross-cultural literature suggests that child maltreatment is less likely in cultures in which children are highly valued for their economic utility, for perpetuating family lines and the cultural heritage, or as sources of emotional pleasure and satisfaction (Korbin 1987). However, inflicting these cultural values on children may place them in jeopardy, for example, if the welfare of orphans who are taken as economic helpers is dependent on their continued utility. If children are valued for the perpetuation of family lines and cultural traditions, in societies that require males to perform ceremonies, females are less valued and at greater risk of maltreatment. Furthermore, if children are expected to be sources of psychological and emotional satisfaction, they may fail parental expectations, making them vulnerable to abuse. Even in cultures that place high value on children in general, some children are less valued than others. Such children may be subjected to deliberate infanticide, physical abuse and neglect, sexual misuse, psychological maltreatment, or economic exploitation (Korbin 1991).

Early detection

What causes abuse?

It is necessary to know the factors which constitute abuse. Helfer and Kempe (1972) pointed out the following three factors:

(1) a certain type of adult, the abusogenic parent;

(2) stress, both chronic and in acute crises;

(3) a special child, i.e. a child who has some qualities making him different or special to the parent.

There are some characteristics common to abusive parents (Steele 1975) such as immaturity and dependency, social isolation, poor self-esteem, difficulty in seeking or obtaining pleasure, distorted perceptions of the child (often role reversal), fear of spoiling the child, belief in the value of punishment, and impaired ability to empathize with the child's needs and respond appropriately. Abusive parents were often themselves abused or neglected, physically or emotionally, as children. They share common misunderstanding with regard to the nature of their own parenting emotional needs. Only a few of the parents show severe psychotic tendencies (Spinetta and Rigler 1972). The child is being raised in a home where there is mistrust of strangers, minimal contact with people outside the nuclear family, and without modelling for the child in how to find enjoyment and gratification from social contact with others (Martin 1976).

Unlike the frequently chaotic, unstable, physical abuse families, incestuous families are generally very 'tight', locked in a perpetual conspiracy of secrecy, with the child's silence and compliance crucial for maintaining a pathologic balance. The mothers are generally withdrawn. In many cases they are aware of the sexual activity occurring between the father or boyfriend and the child and they collude in it, to maintain the family unit. The perpetrators also tend to be passive and dependent people. They have weak and generally asexual relationships with the mothers. They turn to the daughters out of loneliness and dependency, finding this refuge much less threatening than independence or an extramarital affair.

Abusive parents are often under chronic or acute stress. Gil (1970, 1975) has emphasized the social stresses which are believed to be the primary aetiological factors in abuse. Gil reports that he found most abusive families to come from low income, poorly educated urban communities. Fifty-five per cent of the parents had not finished high school, 48 per cent of the fathers had a history of deviancy in social and behavioural functioning, and 29 per cent of the families had no man in the home.

Low social class, poverty, and overcrowding have been described as prominent factors in the occurrence of child sexual abuse but these findings have mainly been derived from court or prison settings. Other studies (Finkelhor 1986) have shown that child sexual abuse occurs in families from all socio-economic backgrounds.

Franklin (1977) suggests that all parents should be considered capacity to attack their children physically. This potential for abusing children varies in intensity. Given a parent with a higher than usual potential to abuse a child, and given certain life stresses which might increase that potential, some characteristics or attribute of the child may be just enough to tip the scale.

Premature, mentally retarded, and physically handicapped children are at greater risk of abuse. Any factor which interrupts the early attachment process places the child at greater risk of abuse (Klaus and Kennel 1976). Medical illness is a contributing factor (Lynch 1975). Mild neurologic immaturity in child increases the difficulty of establishing parenting patterns. All this suggests that the following factors increase the chances of physical abuse given a parent with high potential for becoming an abusive parent (Franklin 1977):

(1) any factors which intrude into the early bonding and attachment of mother and child, such as prematurity, or separation of mother and newborn;

(2) characteristics of a child which make him a less gratifying child: a child for whom it is more difficult to care and who gives less reinforcement for good parenting;

(3) any child who does not meet the expectations of the parents. This may be a child of the 'wrong' sex, or a normal child who does not measure up because the parents' expectations are so unrealistic and distorted;

(4) the development level of the child may represent special stresses to a specific parent. Almost all parents find some developmental stages more stressful than others. Some do not find the dependencies of infancy easy to meet, while others deal poorly with the tempestuous teenager;

(5) the child who invites abuse. We have seen abused children who seem to invite or provoke abuse. This may be the child's only way of obtaining attention from the parent, as if equating punishment with love.

Knowing all the factors that cause abuse our efforts must be directed at identifying families at risk for abuse. These families are in need of help and we should provide help. Based on a framework of blame where abusive parents are considered guilty of crime, it is not easy to maintain a constructive outlook. A broadened preventive framework with a lowered threshold for helping and less emphasis on blaming might be more acceptable and effective.

Prevention

During the past decade, there has been growing recognition that some families are unable to offer a protective, nurturing environment to their children, despite the most rigorous attempts at treatment and that it might be more effective to intervene earlier in high-risk situations to prevent abuse or neglect. Prevention can occur at different levels.

The earlier support can be provided the better, but we must not forget that families need support at many different times. Thus, there must be programme directed towards each phase of the life cycle, beginning with the prenatal period and continuing through a child's school years. A comprehensive approach to *primary prevention* (Cohn 1991) includes the following:

- perinatal support programme—to prepare individuals for parenting and to enhance parent–child bonding;
- education for parents—to provide parents with information about child development and with skills in child care;

- early and periodic childhood screening and treatment—to identify and deal with physical and developmental problems in children at an early age;

- programme for abused children—to minimize the longer term effects on children who have been abused and to reduce the likelihood of their becoming abusive parents;

- life-skills training for children and young adults;

- self-help groups and other neighbourhood supports—to reduce the social isolations so often associated with abuse;

- family support services, including health care, family planning, child care, crisis care, marriage counselling—to provide families with the range of supports they need to survive the stresses of life and to stay together;

- public education on child abuse prevention;

- community organization activities—to increase local opportunities for job training, employment, access to social and health services, and other supports that reduce family stress.

Others (Chamberlin 1988; Schorr 1988) argue that the main emphasis of primary prevention should be on community-wide approaches which raise the level of support to *all* families caring for young children, and avoid the 'labelling' and 'ruin-blaming' (Parton 1985) associated with risk-based programmes.

Primary prevention of sexual abuse includes encouraging children to 'not keep secrets', 'say no', and to 'tell someone'. The new preventive strategies focus on development of self-esteem, conflict-resolution skills, and adult–child and peer–peer relations as tools in self-protection.

If resources are limited, it has been suggested that the maximum gain is via *secondary prevention*, and that significant benefit occurs in the highest risk group: poor, single, teenaged mothers having their first baby. Abuse and serious neglect may be prevented when such families receive an intensive form of well-baby care, contact between mother and baby in the delivery room, 'rooming in', more frequent visits, a variety of one-to-one prevention services tailored to their needs, ongoing counselling regarding discipline, nurseries to which their children can be admitted for short-term respite care at the times of family crises, telephone lifelines, arrangements for day care, and assistance in family planning.

In addition there must be efforts to change the environment in which we are trying to prevent abuse with changes in legislation, policy, social conditions, public participation and values.

Tertiary prevention, or treatment of child abuse, depends on the accurate identification of cases. For that purpose a need exists for a collaborative effort between the members of a multidisciplinary child protection team (CPT).

Multidisciplinary child protection teams (CPT)

No single professional, regardless of his or her sophistication in his or her own field, is going to be able to satisfactorily carry out the complex diagnostic and dispositional processes that cases of child abuse and neglect demand. To meet these needs, multi-agency, multidisciplinary protection teams have been developed. Some of them are hospital based, some are community based, and some are an integral part of each country's protective services agencies. Child protection teams in large communities will generally have the following core membership: a paediatrician (who is knowledgeable and interested in the management of these cases), a social worker, a psychologist or psychiatrist, a health visitor, a legal advisor, and a protective services representative. The primary goals of CPT case management are the safety of the child, an acceptable developmental environment for the child, family unity (where the child's safety and development are not compromised), and the provision of services to prevent the recurrence of abusive or neglectful behaviour. A comprehensive treatment plane for the family must be implemented. The specific medical, psychiatric, developmental, and socio-economic needs of each family will determine the particular combination of services offered. This approach would emphasize the following:

(1) a reinstitution of the helping approach to families, with certain professionals clearly helping rather than assuming an investigatory role;

(2) a focus on prevention;

(3) the rebuilding of the infrastructure for children and families.

References

Agathonos, H. (1983). Institutional child abuse in Greece: some preliminary findings. *Child Abuse and Neglect* **7**, 1.
Agathonos, H. (1988). Some concepts on issues of child welfare. Children at risk, future developments. Child welfare and family policy. European Centre for Social Welfare Training and Research, RChP/Paper No1.
Agathonos, H. Stathakopoulou, N., Adam, H., and Nakou, S. (1982). Child abuse and neglect in Greece: Sociomedical aspects. *Child Abuse and Neglect* **6**, 307–11.
American Humane Association (1984) Denver, CO.
Astley, R. (1953). Multiple metaphyseal fractures in small children (metaphyseal fragility of bone). *British Journal of Radiology* **26**, 577–83.
Baldwin, J.A. and Oliver, J.E. (1975). Epidemiology and family characteristics of severely abused children. *British Journal of Preventive and Social Medicine* **29**, 205–21.
Bays, J. (1990). Substance abuse and child abuse. Impact of addiction on the child. *Pediatric Clinics of North America* **37**, 881–904.
Caffey, J. (1946). Multiple fractures in the long bones of infants suffering from chronic subdural hematoma. *American Journal of Roentgenology* **56**, 163–73.

Chamberlin, R (ed) (1988). *Beyond individual risk assessment: Community-wide approaches in promoting the health and development of families and children*. The National Center for Education in Material and Child Health Washington DC.

Cohn, H.A. (1991). What we have learned about prevention: what we should do about it. *Child Abuse and Neglect* **15**, 99–106.

Council of Europe (1987). *Colloquy on violence within the family measures in the social field*, 25–27 November; CDPS-VF. 14. Revised. Council of Europe, Strasbourg.

Dobbs, M. (1990). Romania: the biological degradation of a Nation. *The Guardian*, January 14.

Ferleger, N., Glenwick, D.S., Gaines, R.W., and Green A.H. (1988). Identifying correlates of reabuse in maltreatment parents. *Child Abuse and Neglect* **12**, 41–9.

Finkelhor, D. (1979). *Sexually victimized children*. Free Press, New York.

Finkelhor, D. (1986). *A source book on child sexual abuse*, pp. 115–16. Sage, Beverly Hills.

Finkelhor, D. (1988). The trauma of child sexual abuse. In *Lasting effects of child sexual abuse*, pp. 61–82. Sage, Beverly Hills.

Finkelhor, D. and Korbin, J. (1988). Child abuse as an international issue. *Child Abuse and Neglect* **12**, 3–23.

Franklin, A.W. (1977). *Child abuse: prediction, prevention and follow-up*, pp. 13–14. Churchill Livingstone, Edinburgh.

Gil, D. (1970). *Violence against children*. Harvard University Press, Cambridge, MA.

Gil, D. (1975). Unraveling child abuse. *American Journal of Orthopsychiatry* **45**, 346–56.

Granleese, J. and Henderson, P. (1987). Prevention institutional child abuse: a review. Paper presented at the *London Conference of the British Psychological Society*, University of London, 17-18 December.

Hunter, R.S., Kilstorm, N., and Loda, F.A. (1985). Sexually abused children: identifying masked presentations in a medical setting. *Child Abuse and Neglect* **9**, 17–26.

Kempe, C.H. (1972). *Helping the battered child and his family*. J.B. Lippincott, Philadelphia.

Kempe, C.H. (1978a). Recent developments in the field of child abuse. *Child Abuse and Neglect* **2**, 261–7.

Kempe, C.H. (1978b). Sexual abuse: another hidden pediatric problem. *Pediatrics* **62**, 382–9.

Kempe, C.H., Silverman, F.N., Steele, B.F., Droegmueller, W., and Silver, H.K. (1962). The battered child syndrome. *Journal of the American Medical Association* **181**, 17–24.

Klaus, M.H. and Kennel, J.H. (1976). *Maternal infant bonding: the impact of early separation or loss on family development*. Mosby, St. Louis.

Korbin, J. (1980). Cultural context of child abuse and neglect. *Child Abuse and Neglect* **4**, 3–13.

Korbin, J. (1981). *Child abuse and neglect: cross-cultural perspectives*. University of California Press, Berkeley, CA.

Korbin, J. (1987). Child maltreatment in cross-cultural perspectives: vulnerable children and circumstances. In *Child abuse and neglect: biosocial dimensions*, (ed. R. Geles and J. Lancaster). Aldine, Chicago.

Korbin, J. (1991). Cross-cultural perspectives and research directions for the 21st century. *Child Abuse and Neglect* **15** (Supplement I), 67–77.

Krugman, R.D. (1986). Recognition of sexual abuse in children. *Pediatrics in Review* **8**, 25–30.
La Fontaine, J. (1988). *Child sexual abuse* (An ESRC Research Briefing). ESRC, London.
Lynch, M. (1975). Ill health and child abuse. *Lancet* **ii**, 317–19.
Lynch, M.A. and Roberts, J. (1982). *Consequences of child abuse.* Academic Press, London.
Marie Claire (1990). Roumanie: la vie maintenant. F. quipe Medivale du Secours Populaire Francais, July.
Martin, H.P. (1976). The environment of the abused child. In *The abused child: a multi-disciplinary approach to developmental issues and treatment*, Ch. 2, pp. 11–26. Ballinger, Cambridge, MA.
Martin, H.P. and Miller, T. (1976). Treatment of specific delays and deficits. In *The abused child*, (ed. H.P. Martin), Ch. 14. Ballinger, Cambridge, MA.
Martin, H.P., Beezley, P., Conway, E.F., and Kempe, C.H. (1974). The development of abused children. *Advanced Pediatrics* **21**, 25–73.
National Center on Child Abuse and Neglect (1981). *Study findings: national study of incidence and severity of child abuse and neglect.* Department of Health, Education and Welfare, Washington DC.
Oates, R.K. (1984). Nonorganic failure to thrive. *Australian Paediatric Journal* **20**, 95–100.
Oates, R.K. (ed.) (1985). The problem of child abuse. Historical aspects. In *Child abuse and neglect*, Ch. 4, pp. 41–4. Butterworths, London.
Parker, R. and Millham, S. (1989). Introduction: Research on organization and accountability for state intervention. In *The state as parent—international research perspectives on interventions with young persons*, J. Hudson and B. Galaway. Kluwer Academic Publishers, Lancaster.
Parton, N. (1985). *The politics of child abuse.* Macmillan, London.
Peters, S.D., Wyatt, G.E., and Finkelhor, D. 91986). Prevalence. In *A sourcebook of child sexual abuse*, (ed. D. Finkelhor). Sage, Beverley Hills, CA.
Radbill, S.X. (1974). This history of child abuse and infanticide. In *The battered child* (2nd edn) (ed. R.E. Helfer and C.H. Kempe). University of Chicago Press, Chicago.
Robinson, L.L., Buckley, J.D., Daigle, A.E. Wells, R. Benjamin, D. Arthur, D.L. *et al.* (1989). Maternal drug use and risk of childhood nonlymphoblastic leukaemia among offspring. *Cancer* **63**, 1904.
Rosenberg, D.A. (1987). Web of deceit: a literature review of Munchausen syndrome by proxy. *Child Abuse and Neglect* **11**, 547–63.
Russels, D.E.H. (1983). The incidence and prevalence of intrafamilial and extrafamilial sexual abuse of female children. *Child Abuse and Neglect* **7**, 133–46.
Schmitt, B. and Kempe C. (1975). Neglect and abuse of children. In *Nelson textbook of pediatrics* (10th edn) (ed. V. Vaughn and R. McKay). Saunders, Philadelphia.
Schmitt, B.D. and Krugman, R.D. (1987). Nonorganinc failure to thrive. In *Nelson textbook of pediatrics* (13th edn) pp. 83–4. Saunders, Philadelphia.
Schneider, D. (1976). The meaning of incest. *Journal of the Polynesian Society* **85**, 149–69.
Schorr, L. (1988). *Within our reach: breaking the cycle of disadvantage.* Anchor Doubleday, New York.
Sills, R.H. (1978). Failure to thrive the role of clinical and laboratory evaluation. *American Journal of Diseases of Childhood* **132**, 967–9.

Silverman, F.N. (1953). The Roentgen manifestations of unrecognized skeletal trauma in infants. *American Journal of Roentgenology* **69**, 413–27.

Spinetta, J.J. and Rigler D. (1972). The child abusing parent. A psychological review. *Psychological Bulletin* **77**, 296–304.

Steele, B. (1975). *Working with abuse parents: from a psychiatric point of view*. Office of Child Development, US Dept. of Health, Education and Welfare, Washington, DC.

US Department of Health and Human Services (1988). *Study findings: study of national incidence and prevalence of child abuse and neglect*. Washington, DC.

Yeatman, G.W. (1976). Pseudobattering in Vietnamese children. *Pediatrics* **58**, 617–18.

Young, W.C., Sachs, R.G., Braun, B.G., and Watkins, R.T. (1991). Patients reporting ritual abuse in childhood: a clinical syndrome. *Child Abuse and Neglect* **15**, 181–9.

20 Young children with special needs
Agnes Lànyi Engelmayer

Definition of the population

The concept of 'children with special needs' or 'special needs children' has replaced such former notions as 'impaired', 'disabled', or 'handicapped' children, in the vocabulary of remedial education. Scientific revisions, along with the introduction of new terminology, are usually due to several reasons, one of which is that the terms mentioned above have become loaded with negative connotations. By introducing euphemistic, yet understandable alternatives, the group of people (including parents) involved with such children were attempting to erase such negative meanings. Introducing the term 'person with a disability' instead of 'disabled person' is based on real anthropological thought, not hairsplitting. The underlying meaningful message is that these people are, above all, persons with expectations, desires, and rights common to all human beings, and their disability is only a secondary peculiarity of theirs, in the same way as nationality, race, or religion is secondary to humanity.

The necessary renewal of the professional terminology reflects changing attitudes to 'people with disabilities'. Phrases like 'impairment disability' or 'handicap' were recommended by the WHO in the 1970s in order to replace the formerly frequented notions of 'defect', 'deficiency', and 'abnormality'.[1] However, 'mental deficiency/retardation' or 'intellectual impairment' had, in turn, replaced the even earlier term 'oligophrenia'.[2] However, the alterations have more significant reasons as well. In our case it represents a paradigmatic change within the philosophy of special education—which, in our context, means the complex, interdisciplinary field of research, which, besides teaching methodology and strategy, involves the sciences examining the causes and outcomes of the handicapping condition.

The impact of psychology and sociology is reflected above all in the fact that the so-called medical–clinical model is gradually being replaced by explanatory principles. The representatives of the medical–clinical model maintain that most of the problems are rooted in the individual, and the keynote of the assessment is to diagnose the aetiology and the causally related symptoms. Special educational psychologists stressed the same idea when psychodiagnosing disabled children. The sociological attitude, pointing out the errors of the diagnostic process, has managed to turn the tide, focusing attention on the weaknesses of the labelling approach.[3] It was realized that early labelling may function as a self-fulfilling prophecy. As a consequence, more and more researchers admitted the correlation between the diagnosis, the person making the diagnosis, and the degree of his/her competence.

Simultaneously, the effect of harmful environmental impacts on the development of the child were paid more attention. In extreme cases of social deprivation the symptoms resemble mental deficiency, although it is not actually the case. A multitude of studies were made on institutionalized children after Spitz, in which the effects of lacking or dysfunctioning early interpersonal relationships on the somatic development, weight gain, emotional life, and verbal and cognitive development were thoroughly studied.[4,5]

In the first period following the description of institutionalized children special educational professionals assumed that the main diagnostic task was to separate the children retarded only as a result of social harm from the 'real' mentally deficient cases. According to their theories, the long-term prospects of the former group were better. Under primarily North American influence, the 'enrichment programmes' were favoured as they were believed to accelerate the child's cognitive and social development. The problems of the socially disadvantaged and of the various ethnic groups were especially dramatized. Some authors doubted whether the children's failure to acquire academic skills was due to a disability. They also criticized the traditional assessment procedures that tried to measure the output of children raised in other cultures/socializational experience relative to white middle-class standards.[6]

The core of the debate was about defining the difference between the socially backward and the disabled/handicapped children. Does the different aetiology represent a different direction of development and long-term effects? How are the four Ds—delay, deficit, difference, deviance—represented in a child's development? These questions can only be answered by such experimental follow-up studies in which the psychology of handicapped children and developmental psychology find common ground. This interdisciplinary encounter is reflected in the emergence of 'developmental psychopathology' and the spreading of its research methods and practice.

According to Rutter[8]

'Developmental psychopathology as a research approach draws on both developmental and psychopathologic perspectives to tackle questions about causal mechanisms. Developmental perspectives are discussed in terms of the implications that flow from age differences in prevalence, age trends in remission of disorders, developmental appropriateness of psychiatric conditions, continuities and discontinuities in psychopathology between childhood and adult life, and age differences in the effects of psychiatric risk factors. Psychopathologic perspectives are considered in terms of continuities and discontinuities between normality and pathology and the contrasts between pervasive and situation-specific disorders, and by the differences between single variables and behavioural composites.'

Since the 1980s experts have become less concerned about the reliable differentiation of the endogenic versus the exogenic, the biological versus the environmental aetiology. The nature–nurture debate was also re-evaluated, as the interrelation of the causes became more and more obvious. It is virtually impossible to distinguish cause from effect. For example, poverty is associated with intellectually impaired underfed children. However, the expectant mother's under-nourishment leads to the biological injury of the embryo's developing brain. Socially neglected children are exposed to several diseases, and their development is thus influenced by biological as well as social risk factors.

Surveying epidemiological research in an attempt to separate the effects of experience from genetic influences, Rutter,[9] referring to Cadoret,[10] concludes that 'the quasi-experimental separation of genetic and environmental effects does not mean that either can operate in the absence of the other; nor does it mean that gene–environment interactions are unimportant'.

Simultaneously, the experts interest turned from the deficit and aetiology-oriented framework to the intervention-oriented approach. What special needs must be satisfied by a child- and parent-centred service? This is how the new concept of 'special need' comes to the fore, but in what sense is it special? The Warnock Report,[11] which analyses the overall situation of special education in the late 70s, introduces the notion of special educational need. The 'children with special educational need' are only partially the same as the disabled–handicapped ones who were educated in traditional, segregated special schools.

In the mean time, the practise of integrating normal and disabled children has gained pace, and many children with specific learning disabilities have attended regular elementary schools. However, the demand of 'satisfying their special educational needs' applies to them as well. The size of this population is significantly larger than the group of students learning in special schools for the disabled. In the European countries there are various schooling systems, and the proportion of the school-aged population in special schools varies widely. Therefore, because there is no clear definition of the population, obtaining international size/incidence and prevalence data is understandably difficult.

Prevalence the incidence rates

We have comparative data, based on UNESCO records taken in past decades, on the percentage of the school-age population enrolled in special educational provision.[12,13] In the European countries the percentage of students learning in special schools ranges between 2.5 and 4.5 per cent. Wherever the differentiated system of special schooling was highly developed, with each category and level of disability having its own appropriate school, (e.g, in West Germany or the Netherlands), this figure was relatively high. In these countries not even the severely, multiply, and profoundly handicapped children were excluded from schooling. In those countries where integration has taken place rapidly and across a wide range, it is not possible to say how many pupils are enrolled in special educational provision since there are no strict boundaries between regular and special education.

According to UNESCO estimates, 10–15 per cent of the school-age population is in educational need. This figure includes defects of speech, major behavioural problems, and the various forms of learning disability. In most cases, the special need is temporary (e.g. for the first one or two years of schooling). The problem may disappear as a result of the correctional, re-educational, or other therapeutic and training programmes. However, in many cases the disappearance of certain symptoms is related to development and maturing and not to the therapy applied (14). According to the clinical experience of child psychotherapists, certain learning disabilities may be influenced effectively by mere psychotherapeutic intervention, without applying specific learning therapy. This underlines the fact that in the background of learning problems, besides perceptual and cognitive disabilities, there are non-specific emotional and/or affective factors as well.[15]

It has been proved that children, 'problematic' for any reason in the first period of their lives, appear over-represented among the teenage and young adult persons with behavioural and socializational problems. These appear to be late negative psychical consequences of early developmental disabilities.

These facts explain why it is virtually impossible to gain reliable incidence and prevalence parameters. This is especially so with the notion of 'special educational needs children', which is difficult to interpret as the appearance of these needs are highly dependent on the level of the given country's educational system. Education in the ex-communist countries is characterized by strong centralization, achievement-orientedness, didactic teaching methods, overcrowded classrooms, and a lack of individualization, as well as teachers' inability to handle problem children. In such conditions, problems, regarded as regular elsewhere, appear as a special educational need.[16]

Several epidemiological surveys have attempted to present an overall picture of the prevalence of certain classical development impairments, disabilities, and handicaps. The experimental data are contradictory.[17] This is not due to the different frequency of certain disabilities in the various countries, but rather to the different research conditions. The studies differ in terms of

(a) the size and representativeness of the sample;

(b) whether they are based on multidisciplinary examinations involving the whole population or on screening of the risk-factor groups; and

(c) the quality and extend of 'special needs' registration.

In certain European countries, such as the former Federal Republic of Germany, there was, and still is, no unified system of registration of disabled person. During Nazi rule, the disabled were regarded as eliminable, worthless persons, and even decades later, strong moral resistance makes registering handicapped persons impossible. In Hungary the monitoring system of persons suffering from hereditary diseases and congenital anomalies operates efficiently. This allows tracing of the geographical and gender distribution of these diseases and the temporal changes which occur in congenital anomalies.[18] Strangely enough, in the course of planning special educational services, this rich database is barely utilized. It is well known that there is a gender difference within the disabled population: in almost every group, boys form the majority; yet the new Hungarian boarding schools for the deaf and mentally and multiply disabled are being built with equal numbers of rooms for both sexes.

The prevalence of disabilities alters at different stages of childhood. Inherited anomalies may be diagnosed late, disabilities may be acquired through illness or trauma and genetically determined conditions may become manifest later in childhood.[9] Only a longitudinal research design can explore all these factors. From among such studies, that by Becker and his colleagues[19] following up 600 children between the ages of three and nine is worthy of note. The main purpose of their multidisciplinary research was to examine the children's developmental dynamics and to establish the frequency of developmental disorders.

Early childhood special education

Historical background, present situation, changing outlook

In the first half of the twentieth century 'special education' referred only to the education and training of school-aged disabled children. Including children younger than school age in the scope of special education primarily meant developing special kindergartens. However, it became obvious in the 1960s that early special education is necessary before the nursery school age.

In the mean time a multitude of studies have been made on the subject. Periodicals and significant handbooks have been published on it, early developmental training centres and associations have been established, international conferences arranged, and, in different ways in the various countries, the services of early intervention took shape. Many studies examined the myths about early intervention, observing a tendency to make exaggerated promises and the potential hazards of early intervention, and analysing the efficiency of early intervention. With emancipated, active parents and by integrating special needs children into regular pre-school settings, educational philosophy and practice in early childhood special education has changed significantly.[20-25]

The conditions of early intervention

Interdisciplinarity

Early childhood special education turned into an overall early interventional strategy when the various fields involved began to cooperate in finding common ground. Developmental neurology, social paediatrics, infant psychiatry, medical rehabilitation (providing prostheses, orthoses, and technical aids), motor rehabilitation, physiotherapy, speech therapy, special education, special and developmental psychology, theory of counselling, and legislation philosophy were all necessary to create really comprehensive, helpful intervention programmes.

Early detection, early diagnosis, and assessment

Every therapeutic and developing intervention is based on a thorough check-up, with the exact mapping of the initial status, i.e. the diagnosis. As well as medical check-ups, it is essential, to follow up the child's psychological development. This is especially so in the case of biological and sociological risk factors where the symptoms do not inevitably manifest, while in the case of other clinical diagnoses certain disabilities are predictable. Several debates have been concerned with the use of developmental tests or the so-called 'infant test'. The growing criticism questioned the usefulness of these tests for predicting later intelligence functions. The use of the developmental quotient (DQ) to categorize children was criticized; yet these tests, given high quality analysis, allow some insight into a few of the functions of early development. The assessment of motor and essential cognitive functions, the way of social maturing and preverbal communication, vocalization, and speech development may help significantly in exploring potential delays and disabilities. Some of these tests serve as screening and developmental check-up purposes. If developmental disorder is suspected, a thorough psychological examination is always necessary.

Following decades of testing, development researchers are gradually turning their attention towards targeted methodical observation. These observations involve the child's social interactions, self-conducted activity, playful initiations, his/her level of awareness, concentration, interests, communicational initiations, and the displaying of emotional needs and wishes. The norm-orientated, standardized tests pin-point the lack of certain functions, i.e. the negative aspects of development, whereas observation explores the child's existing positive abilities and functions in order to build the developing therapy on to them. The observation can be supported by various check-lists.[26]

Involving parents and other family members in early education

Special educational professionals realized that their intervention is only effective if they can convince parents of the efficacy of treatment and teach them the therapeutic exercises. In the beginning of the early educational movement, it was thought that the parents should be trained as co-therapists. During this period, 'helping intervention' primarily meant expert-controlled functional training. However, a significant change of attitude occurred and the 'early' experts of the 80s maintained that parents should be kept in their traditional roles. They suggested that instead of teaching them functional training, the parents should be made sensitive to the signals and needs of their disabled child, who communicates and develops unusually. Psychologists pay special attention to the initial 'telling of the news'. In maternity wards, departments of neonatology, and childrens' hospitals, mother are often traumatized by the information heard from doctors. Initial telling should never be a 'one-off' announcement but the first step towards the acceptance of a child with special needs, which requires tact, empathy, and therapeutic skill.

The parents—primarily the mother—and the brother/sister of the handicapped child might need to participate in therapeutic groups (or in personal psychotherapy), where the distress and guilt caused by the disability can be discussed freely.[27]

Access to counselling services

Since the 1970s and 80s, a self-supportive movement created by disabled children's parents has become more significant. The growth of their solidarity and self-responsibility has resulted in the deprofessionalization of the 'early movement'. Parents were frequently upset that some expert had inflicted the psychic harm of disability on them. They demanded information—about the origin of the child's status, the risk of recurrence in subsequent children, the developmental prognosis, the various services available (e.g. baby sitters, respite care, and vacation and leisure-time programmes, etc.). It is also important that parents find out about the social benefits available for families with a child in need (e.g. increased family benefit, extended infant-care aid, longer vacations, etc.). They want to know their rights, and the degree of their responsibility when considering issues like sending their children to a special school or some other institution. They expect information about the various non-professional, voluntary, and non-governmental associations helping the disabled.

For the experts it was difficult to understand and to accept the process of parental emancipation and frequent subsidiary resistance. New cooperational methods had to be learned in forming a partnership in which each participant has their own competence and responsibility. In the mean while, counselling practice has developed into a self-contained discipline.[28]

Establishing the institutional framework of the early services

In the 1960s, in Europe and especially in West Germany, so-called 'social-paediatric centres', operating under medical control, were established rapidly. Hellbrügge[27] played an eminent role in organizing these centres and creating a model in his Munich institute for multidisciplinary work. According to his proposal, for each one million citizens, one social-paediatric centre should be established.[30,31]

In Germany, so-called 'early training centres' (Frühförderungszentren) came into existence in another organizational framework, operating under psychological and special educational control, often in cooperation with universities teaching the theory of early education. At the end of the 1970s the Education Commission, set up by the Federal Government of the Federal German

Republic, proposed the erection of one early training centre for every 200 000 citizens. According to the original concept these services should be easily available, so that the parents involved do not have to take on the additional burden of extensive travelling with a handicapped child, which makes keeping regular contact problematic.[32] In many countries a home-visitor system for special education has been introduced with special regard to the early detectable sensory failures. This system had significant consequences for the training of experts, since working with infants in a family setting requires an attitude entirely different from that of the traditional schoolteacher.

The system of the services mentioned above took different shapes in the various European countries. UNESCO's publications on special education also offer rich information on this subject.[33,34] In the post-communist Eastern and Central- European countries the variety of services is more limited than in the West. At present, social security payments do not cover these services. It usually takes diligent search and financial sacrifice for the parents to gain access to these institutions. In these countries, experiments modelling the various forms of early intervention have been performed in order to convince policy-makers about the importance of this form of education. Reform of the schooling system is under way there, and early special education will hopefully find its lace in it.[35]

Conclusion

The twentieth century has seen a major change in attitude towards children with special needs. In Europe and North America, they have to come to be seen primarily as children with expectations, desires, and rights common to all children. As part of this change in attitude, educational approaches have developed with the result that integrated education with active parental participation is now the universally accepted goal.

The continuing progress of education and health services for children with special needs will depend on adequate registration, the success of partnership with parents (see Chapter 33), and the provision of adequate financial resources, despite financial constraints imposed by government in response to economic recession.

References

1. Secretariat of the Council of Europe (1989). *The use of the International Classification of Impairments, Disabilities and Handicaps (ICIDH) in rehabilitation.* Council of Europe Publishing and Documentation Service, Strasbourg.
2. Secretariat of the Council of Europe (1985). *Glossary and list of principal terms used in the rehabilitation of disabled people,* (3rd edn). Council of Europe Publishing and Documentation Services, Strasbourg.

3. Mercer, J. (1873). *Labeling the mentally retarded.* University of California Press, Berkeley, CA.
4. Singer, T.L., Drotar, D., Fagan, F.J., Devost, L., and Lake, R. (1983). The cognitive development of failure to thrive infants: methodological issues and new approaches. In *Infants born at risk: physiological, perceptual and cognitive processes,* (ed. T. Field and A. Sostek), pp. 221–420 Grune & Stratton, New York.
5. Wolf, H., Karte, H., Otten, A, and Turski, J. (1989). Der Einfluss von Deprivation und Vernachlässigung auf Wachstum and Entwicklung. *Sozialpädiatrie in Praxis and Klinik* **11**, 333–40.
6. Swanson, H.L. and Watson, B.L. (1982). *Educational and psychological assessment of exceptional children. Theories, strategies and application.* St. Louis, Toronto.
7. Rauh, H. (1987). Kognitive Entwicklung von Risikokindern und von behinderten Kindern: Entwicklungspsychologische Sichtweise. *Frühförderung Interdisziplinär* **1**, 1–4.
8. Rutter, M. (1988). Epidemiological approaches to developmental psychopathology. *Archives of General Psychiatry* **45**, 486–95.
9. Rutter, M. (1989). Age as an ambiguous variable in developmental research: some epidemiological considerations from developmental psychopathology. *International Journal of Behavioral Development* **12**, 1–34.
10. Cadoret, R.J. (1985). Genes, environment and their interactions in the development of psychopathology. In *Genetic aspects of human behavior,* (ed. T. Sakai and T. Tsuboi). Igaku-Shoin Tokyo, New York.
11. Warnock Committee (1978). *Report of the Warnock committee of enquiry into the education of handicapped children and young people.* HMSO, London.
12. UNESCO (1988). *Review of the present situation of special education.* UNESCO, Paris.
13. UNESCO (1988). *Consultation on special education. Final Report.* UNESCO, Paris.
14. Barnett, W.D., Macmann, M.G., and Carey, T.K. (1992). Early intervention and the assessment of developmental skills: challenges and directions. *Topics in Early Childhood Special Education* **12**, 21–43.
15. Canino, F.J. (1981). Learned helplessness theory: implications for research in learning disabilities. *Journal of Special Education* **15**, 471–484.
16. Lányi-Engelmayer, A. (1987). Diagnostische und schulpolitische Kriterien in Entscheidungsprozess einen adäquaten Beschulung Behinderter. *Behinderten-pädagogik* **26**, 370–5.
17. Speck, O. (1991). Die Verbreitungshäufigkeit von Behinderungen (Schädigungen). In *System Heilpädagogik. Eine ökologisch reflexive Grundlegung,* pp. 149–55. Ernst Reinhardt, München.
18. Czeisel, A.E. (1988). The activities of the Hungarian Centre for Congenital Anomaly Control. *World Health Statistics Quarterly* **41**, 219–227.
19. Becker, K.P. (ed.) (1991). Entwicklungsdynamik drei bis neunjäriger Kinder. Ergebnisse einer interdisziplinären Längsschnittstudie über die biopsychosoziale Entwicklung. Gesundheit, Berlin.
20. Walthes, R. and Trost, R. (1991). Frühe Hilfen für entwicklungsgefährdete Kinder. Wege und Möglichkeiten der Frühforderung aus interdisziplinärer Sicht. Campus, Frankfurt.

21. Bricker, D.D. (1986). *Early education of at-risk and handicapped infants, toddlers, and pre-school children.* Little Brown, Glenview, IL.
22. Vereinigung für Interdisziplinäre Frühförderung, (gg). Familienorientierte Frühförderung. Dokumentation des 6. Symposiums Frühförderung. Hannover. Ernst Reinhardt, München.
23. Neuhäuser, G. (1987). Frühe Hilfen für Kinder mit Entwicklungsstörung und Hirnschädigung im europäischen Vergleich. *Gynäkologe* **20**, 70–76.
24. Davis, H. and Rushton, R. (1991). Counselling and supporting parents of children with developmental delay: a research evaluation. *Journal of Mental Deficiency Research*, **35**, 89–112.
25. LeLaurin, K. (1992). Infant and toddler models of service delivery: are they detrimental for some children and families? *Topics in Early Childhood Special Education* **12**, 82–104.
26. Schonkoff, J.P. (1983). The limitations of normative assessments of high-risk infants. *Topics in Early Childhood Special Education* **3**, 29–43.
27. Hornby, M. (1983). Group programmes for parents of children with various handicaps. *Child care, Health and Development* **9**, 185–98.
28. Gladding, S.T. (1992). *Counselling. A comprehensive profession.* Maxwell Macmillan International, New York.
29. Hellbrügge, Th. (ed.) (1981). *Klinische Sozialpädiatrie. Ein Lehrbuch der Entwicklungsrehabilitation im Kindesalter.* Spinger, Berlin.
30. Masur, R. (1989). Sozialpädiatrie und Sozialarbeit—Ergänzung und Chance. *Sozialpädiatrie in Praxis und Klinik* **11**, 779–85.
31. Hellbrügge, Th., Blüm, N., and Schlack, H.G. (1989). Zur Leistungsfinanzierung in Sozialpädiatrischen Zentren. *Sozialpädiatrie in Praxis und Klinik* **11**, 754–8.
32. Speck, O. (1991). Fröhförderung. In *System Heilpädagogik. Eine ökologische reflexive Grundlegung,* pp. 349–59. Ernst Reinhardt, München.
33. Council of Europe (1991). Ad hoc *conference of ministers responsible for policies on people with disabilities. Council of Europe, Paris.* Strasbourg.
34. Secretariat of the Council of Europe (1990). *Activities in favour of disabled people. Activity Report 1989–1990.* Council of Europe Publishing and Documentation Service, Strasbourg.
35. Illyés, S. (1990). Kontinuität und Diskontinuität in der Theoriebildung der Heilpädagogik. In *Trends und Perspektiven der gegenwärtigen ungarischen Heilpädagogik,* (ed. W. Bachmann and Zs. Mesterházi), pp. 13–4. Giessener Dokumentationsreihe Heil- und Sonderpädagogik Band 11.

21 Adolescents and young people with special needs

Robert Wm Blum, Joan-Carles Suris, and Joan Patterson

Introduction: the demographic picture

While reliable international data are scarce, the World Health Organization has suggested that as many as one in five children in the world have handicaps in the sense of 'serious obstacles to a child's development' (Kohler and Jakobsson 1991). Of these, perhaps three quarters are in the developing world (Noble 1981). In industrialized countries such as the United States, prevalence of childhood chronic illnesses and disabilities has been estimated at 10 per cent (Blum and Geber 1992). As Kohler and Jakobsson (1991) note, part of the variability among prevalence data can be explained by differences in the definitions used (e.g. conditions under treatment vs. diagnosed conditions vs. self-defined health problems). In addition, cross-national variations in disability rates are the result of differences in survey design, the statistical concepts and definitions used, and the survey and screening devices employed (Chamie 1989). Despite these methodologic variations, there appears to be a positive correlation ($r=0.6851$) between rates of disabilities and Gross National Product, indicating that cultural, political, and economic factors may also influence these rates. The following age-specific (15–24-year-olds) prevalence data are from United Nations' statistics (1990).

Prevalence of disabling conditions

In Africa, disability prevalence rates for the 10–19 year age group vary from 469 per 100 000 in Cape Verde to 3396 per 100 000 in rural Ethiopia (United Nations 1990). Rates for rural populations in Mali are double those in urban settings, while urban rates in Tunisia are 33 per cent higher than in rural areas.

In the Americas, rates vary widely from 540 per 100 000 15–19 years old in Trinidad and Tobago to 6726 per 100 000 10–14 years old in Canada. In South America, only data for Guyana (733 per 100 000) and Venezuela (1085 per 100 000) are available. In Venezuela, rates in urban areas are lower than in semi-urban settings and those rates are lower than in urban areas.

The same variability is found in Europe, where Austria has a disability rate of 4708 per 100 000 for 15–19 year olds, while Ireland's rate is only 591 per 100 000. In Oceania, rates for the 15–24 year age group vary from 326 per 100 000 in Kiribati to 1361 per 100 000 in Fiji and 5770 per 100 000 in Australia.

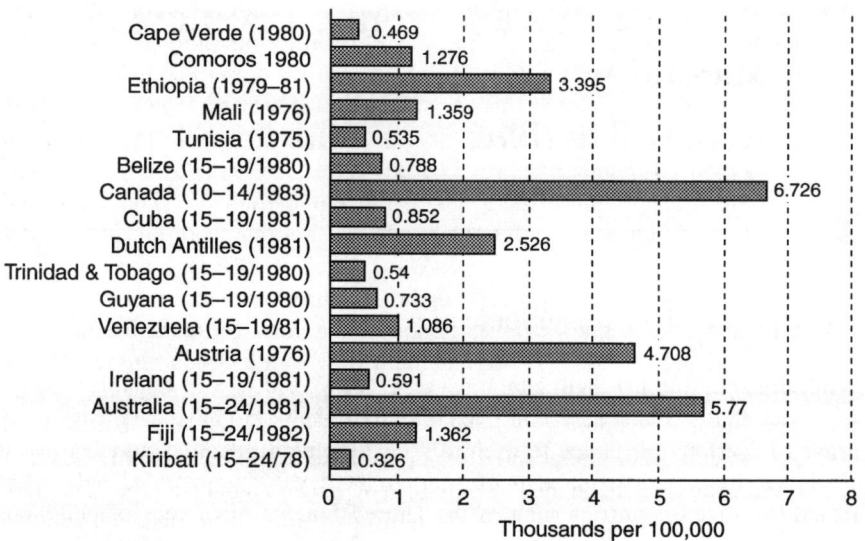

Fig. 21.1 Disability rates for young people in selected countries.

In Asia, rates range from 143 per 100 000 in Myanmar to 2780 per 100 000 in the Philippines. When comparisons between urban and rural areas are available, the latter have higher rates, with a ratio of approximately 1.5:1.

Rates for motor impairments in developing countries range from 240 per 100 000 for males and 146 per 100 000 for females in Tunisia to 718 per 100 000 and 357 per 100 000, respectively, in Netherlands Antilles. Rates for total visual impairment also vary widely, and for Mali, Netherlands Antilles, and Pakistan, are higher among females (United Nations 1990).

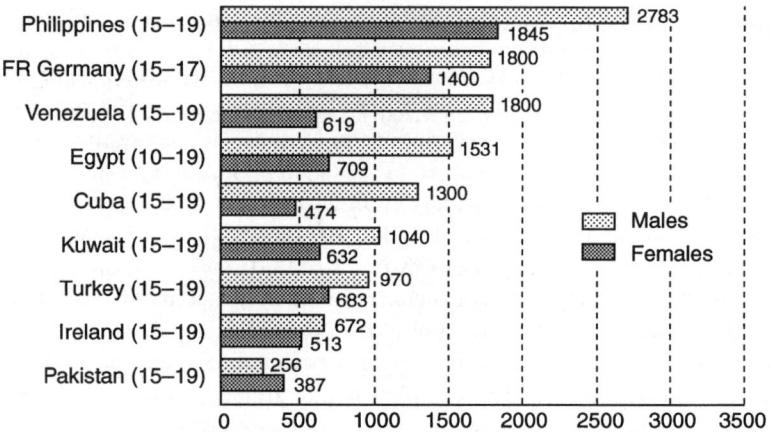

Fig. 21.2 Disability rates by gender in selected countries.

Overall, with the exception of Pakistan, rates are higher for males (United Nations 1990) which may reflect actual variations or cultural attention to males. In the United States, prevalence is higher among individuals living below the poverty level. At the same time, prevalence diminishes as the years of education of the head of household increase (Newacheck 1989).

Chronic illness prevalence

Prevalence data for chronic disease among adolescents are scarce, and usually based on small samples. In addition, uniform age groupings are seldom used.

The 1981 US health interview survey reported a prevalence of chronic condition for the 12–17 age group of 9.4 per cent (Blum and Geber 1992). Data from the National health interview survey indicate that the prevalence of *activity-limiting* chronic conditions among children under 17 years of age doubled from 1960 to 1981, from 1.8 per cent to 3.8 per cent (Newacheck *et al.* 1986). In 1984 the US prevalence of disability for 10–18 year old youths was estimated to be 6.2 per cent, the leading causes being mental disorders, diseases of the respiratory system, followed by diseases of the musculoskeletal system and connective tissue, the nervous system, and the ear and mastoid process (Newacheck 1989).

A survey of 19 year old male draftees in Finland found that 1.8 per cent of them had asthma. While this figure is low compared with other countries, it represents a six-fold increase from 1966 (Haahtela *et al.* 1990). Asthma prevalence in a rural New Zealand adolescent population (12–18 years of age) increased from 26.2 per cent in 1975 to 34 per cent in 1989 (Shaw *et al.* 1990). In the United States (1984), chronic respiratory conditions represented 21 per cent of all adolescent disabilities (Offord *et al.* 1989).

The child health study in Ontario, Canada (Cadman *et al.* 1986) found that 18.8 per cent of males and 21.8 per cent of females of 12–16 years of age had one or more of four psychiatric disorders: conduct disorder, hyperactivity, emotional disorder, somatization. The same study found that for the 12–16 year age group, 146 per 1000 boys and 138 per 1000 girls had a chronic illness or condition. The figures were 231 per 1000 and 218 per 1000, respectively, for chronic health problems (Cadman *et al.* 1986). Mental disorders represent one third of all adolescent disabilities in the US (Newacheck 1989). Prevalence rates for mentally disabled/handicapped children in developing countries vary widely, with males consistently outnumbering females (United Nations 1990).

A study among mentally retarded young people in a Swedish county found that the prevalence of epilepsy for the 10–19 year age group was 1.6 per 1000 for females and 1.4 per 1000 for males (Forsgren *et al.* 1990). A survey among male draftees in Lombardy (Italy) found a prevalence of active epilepsy at 4.73 per 1000 (Cornaggia *et al.* 1990). In England (Southampton and south west Hamphsire), the prevalence of multiple sclerosis for 15 to 29-year-olds was 35 per 100 000. Females had higher rates than males (58 per 100 000 vs. 14

per 100 000) (Roberts et al. 1991). Diseases of the nervous system affect six per cent of all disabled adolescents in the United States (Newacheck 1989).

A survey in Copenhagen in 1978–79 found a prevalence of diabetes for the 10–19 year age group of 2.1 per 1000 males and 1.8 per 1000 females (Snorgaard et al. 1989). For the 10–19 year age group in a Nigerian population, the prevalence of diabetes was 0.58 per cent (Erasmus et al. 1989)

Despite the wide variability in the quality of the data, this sampling of reported global data suggests that chronic illnesses and disabilities affect young people in significant numbers. Whether one chooses the more conservative figure of 10 per cent or the WHO estimates of nearly 20 per cent, it would appear that improvements in public health and improvements in medical and surgical technologies have increased the number of youths who are faced with chronic illnesses and disabling conditions.

Pubertal maturation

Chronic illnesses and disabling conditions can make an impact on the physiologic process of puberty in a variety of ways. This impact can be mediated through a range of mechanisms: centrally (e.g. central nervous system involvement), nutritionally (e.g. malnutrition), medically (e.g. through medications), and socially (e.g. through physical exertion). Conditions associated with pubertal delay and precocity are reported in Table 21.1.

Table 21.1 *Pubertal dyssynchrony associated with chronic conditions*

Conditions associated with pubertal delay	Conditions associated with pubertal precocity
Chronic illnesses	Central nervous system tumors
Cystic fibrosis	Optic gliomas
Chronic renal failure	Hypothalamic gliomas and teratomas
Protein-losing enteropathies	Astrocytomas
Central nervous system tumors	Ependymomas
Craniopharyngiomas	Germinomas in males
Germinomas in females	Hormone-secreting hamartomes
Astrocytomas	McCune–Albright syndrome
Hypothalamic and optic gliomas	Neurofibromatosis
Chromophobe adenomas (rarely)	Neural tube defects
Central nervous system lesions	Spina bifida
Septo-optic dysplasia	Encephalocele
Holoprosencephaly	
Cleft lip and palate	
Down syndrome	

Early pubertal development is associated with a host of acute and chronic conditions. Central nervous system (CNS) tumours, such as optic and hypothalmic gliomas, both of which are associated with neurofibromatosis (Fineman and Yakovak 1970); astrocytomas, ependymomas, and germinomas in males (in females, these tumours are associated with delayed puberty); hypothalmic teratomas; and hormone-secreting hamartomas are all associated with true sexual precocity. So, too, McCune–Albright syndrome (polyostotic fibrous dysplasia), which is associated with irregularly edged 'café-au-lait' spots, fibrous dysplasia, and bone cysts (Benedict 1966); and neurofibromatosis, which has associated smooth-bordered 'café-au-lait' spots, axillary freckles, and subcutaneous and internal masses (neurofibromas) are associated with early pubertal development. Seizures, visual defect, and mental retardation may be associated with alterations of pubertal development as well. Neural tube defects are associated with precocious puberty; females with spina bifida, for example, experience menarche on average more than a year prior to their able-bodied peers.

Delayed pubertal development is associated with at least as extensive a list of chronic and disabling conditions as is precocious development. Gonadatrophin deficiency from a variety of aetiologies is the primary cause of pubertal delay. The most common type of CNS mass leading to sexual infantilism is craniopharyngioma, which has its peak incidence between six and 15 years of age. Other extracellular masses encroaching on the hypothalamus can also result in delayed sexual development: germinomas, hypothalamic and optic gliomas, astrocytomas, and, rarely, chromophobe adenomas. Congenital CNS lesions ranging from ceptooptic dysplasia and holoprosencephaly to cleft lip or palate may be associated with hypothalamic dysfunction (Yen and Jaffe 1978). Syndromes and chronic illnesses with concomitant pubertal delays are numerous. Girls with Down syndrome, for example, on average menarche behind their healthy peers (Salerno *et al.* 1975). There are also some data to support the observation of later onset of menstruation and irregular cycling in mentally retarded girls whose deficiencies are prenatal and organic in nature (Rundle and Sylvester 1970).

Body image and disability in adolescence

We know that while the tempo of puberty may be altered by disease, the process is rarely affected. When puberty is dyssynchronous from their peers, research suggests concurrent concerns. The young adolescent who does not enter puberty with his peers has persistent questions of adequacy. For example, Perrin (1984) has found that such teens have more concern about height and weight than peers without disabilities. Carroll *et al.* (1983) in Montreal compared a group of teens with chronic illness to a population-based sample of adolescents and found that in relationship to the comparison group, those with disabilities reported twice the anxiety (50.0 per cent vs. 29.2 per cent), nearly seven times the weight concerns (40.0 per cent vs. 5.9 per cent), double the acne problems (37.3 per cent vs. 18.3 per cent), almost four times the health worries (35.0 per cent vs. 9.0 per cent), and three times the headaches (26.7 per cent vs. 8.9 per cent).

In a series of studies on youth with asthma, cancer, or cystic fibrosis, Offer *et al.* (1984) reported that their self-perceived body image compared favourably with healthy peers. They found that girls with either asthma or cancer did not report significantly different perceptions from their peers, but the same did not hold for cystic fibrosis, where major differences were found in perceived body image (more negative for those with cystic fibrosis).

The interrelationship between self and chronic illness has been well described on a personal level by Robert Massie: 'Chronic illness is the constant and sometimes overwhelming companion, a shadow both inseparable and internal…"having a chronic illness" is sometimes an elusive concept because one's illness becomes melded into one's identity. To ask what I would be like without hemophilia is an impossible question to answer' (Massie 1985).

While the literature suggests that youths with special health care needs have more somatic concerns and emotional problems than their peers, it is also clear that chronic illness does not have a uniformly negative emotional impact on body image. Rather, there are a whole set of factors that determine the impact of chronic illness.

- *Degree and type of incapacitation*: contrary to expectations, those with *mild* gait disturbance seem to have more emotional difficulties than those with *more severe* mobility limitations.

- *Degree of visibility*: contrary to common belief, those who have *invisible* conditions have consistently been found to have more emotional problems than those with *more visible* limitations or deformities.

- *Prognosis*: the stress of an uncertain prognosis is greater than when the course is known, even when the clinical trajectory leads to death.

- *Course of illness*: rather than chronic persistent conditions, those which are remitting and relenting are most burdensome.

- *Costs*: as one would anticipate, those conditions with treatments that are most costly in terms of pain, home care, time, and money are also those that have the highest emotional costs.

Beyond the factors associated with the condition are other individual and family factors that greatly determine the extent of body image disturbance, altered self-esteem, and depression experienced by youths with disabilities. For example, while in the general population girls have more somatic concerns than boys, the converse is true among those with disabilities. Age is another important variable, for it is the early adolescent going through puberty who appears to be most vulnerable. Because differences from peers are most extreme during puberty, it may be that the psychological sequelae are greatest, or perhaps developmentally, it is during early adolescence that the individual begins to become aware of differences from peers.

To observe self-image alterations, however, is not to say that such adolescents have more psychopathology than the general population. While those with chronic illnesses and disabilities report more depression than peers, it is frequently associated with reporting more social isolation. If youth with disabilities are more socially and developmentally delayed than their peers, it may be because they have not had equal access to those socializing experiences that enhance maturation. To most, *psychopathology* implies that the problem is within the individual. This is less likely to be the case for those with chronic and disabling condition; rather, the problem lies more within society, which limits access and which stereotypes. A *disability* is a restriction in functional capability imposed by physiology; a *handica*p, on the other hand, is determined by the social context coupled with the restriction in functional capability.

Sexual maturation

One of the major consequences of pubertal development is the establishment of sexual dimorphism: the acquisition of secondary sex characteristics and with it the development of adult reproductive capabilities. Yet sexuality goes beyond the boundaries of pubertal maturation to include sexual socialization, physical maturation and body image, social relationships with the same and opposite sex, and future plans, including the possibilities of childbearing, child rearing, and marriage (Blum 1984).

Among the barriers to the development of healthy sexuality are the prevailing *myths* that permeate society regarding the sexuality of those with disabilities. These include the beliefs that people with disabilities

- are asexual while also having uncontrolled urges;
- are vulnerable and need protection;
- wish to socialize with others who have disabilities;
- will have children who have disabilities;
- cannot have orgasm.

What, in fact, is known is that the social desires of youths with disabilities parallel the rest of society. For example, in a comparative study of youths with spina bifida and cerebral palsy, Blum *et al.* (1991) found that nearly 75 per cent of both groups wished to marry when they were older. In addition, 63.7 per cent of those with spina bifida and 76.7 per cent of youths with cerebral palsy wished eventually to have children.

On the other hand, the majority of youths in the Blum (1991) study reported far more restricted social contacts than peers without disabilities. Limited social contacts with peers has a number of significant consequences including: delay in gender appropriate behaviour, delay in socially appropriate behaviour, and limited knowledge about sexuality. Due to lack of information, those with disabilities tend to have greater difficulty than peers in sorting fact from fiction. In addition, sexual behaviour is learned, shaped, and reinforced by the environments within which one lives. Mainstream environments are more likely to reinforce mainstream behaviours. Thus, the lack of sexual experiences as well as inappropriate expressiveness is learned. As has been observed: 'It is not the sex act but the inability to locate a partner that is the major problem'. Finding a partner and establishing social relationships are the first stages of sexual relations.

Chronic illnesses and disabilities may affect one's sexual capabilities in a variety of ways. In Table 21.2, examples of the consequences of four prevalent conditions of youth are presented.

Table 21.2 *The impact of four chronic conditions on sexual functioning*

Condition	Consequences	
	Female	Male
Spinal cord injury	Diminished or absent sensation	Erection possible in up to 50 per cent
	Post-traumatic amenorrhea Fertility usually normal	Fertility markedly reduced
Diabetes mellitus	Dyspareunia	Impotence Retrograde ejaculation
Cancers	Nitrogen mustard may cause amenorrhea Pelvic radiation may cause dyspareunia	Vincristine may cause neuropathy-based impotence Cyclophosphamide may cause zoospermia Pelvic irradiation may cause erectile dysfunction, painful ejaculation, and reduced ejaculatory volume
Cystic fibrosis	Endocercival glandular hyperplasia Viscous leukorrhea Dyspareunia due to diminished lubrication	Sterility may exist secondary to anatomical abnormalities No organic erectoejaculatory dysfunction

Coping and adjustment to disability

Most early research took a psychopathological approach to understanding the emotional sequelae of chronic illness. Epidemiologic studies such as that of the Isle of Wight (Rutter 1975) substantiated that perspective. Simply stated, the psychopathological model posited that a stressor (e.g. chronic illness, physical disability) that is unrelenting (e.g. chronic) would push otherwise emotionally stable people (both parents and children) beyond their ability to cope, with the manifestation of maladaptation being symptoms of psychopathology.

Drotar (1981) notes that 'research in chronic illness has been dominated by a personality-focused paradigm focused on differences between chronically ill and physically healthy children'. The consequences, in part, of this perspective were both to 'overpathologize' chronically ill children (Offer *et al.* 1984) and to neglect factors associated with successful coping (Pless 1984).

The literature is filled with studies which indicate greater emotional and/or behavioural problems of many children with chronic illnesses and disabilities. However, this research provides few cues to interventions which may improve adjustment and outcome. Over the past decade there has been a growing body of research which explored the role of stress as a key factor in psychological well-being *within* specific conditions such as sickle cell disease, chronic renal failure and transplantation, and cystic fibrosis rather than comparing them solely with able-bodied controls.

Pless and Pinkerton (1975) argue that the processes of maturation and emotional development are complex; to understand adjustment to chronic illness in children, there is a need for a model that takes into consideration a number of variables. Their model implies that psychosocial functioning is affected by a number of characteristics, only some of which are related to the condition. Interrelated factors include personality, temperament, past experiences with illnesses and/or disability, family characteristics, and disease/disability related factors (e.g. nature of the condition, age of onset, severity). Pless and Pinkerton (1975) believe that it is functioning in early childhood (either premorbid or early morbid functioning) which is predictive of adolescent and adult outcomes.

Abrahamson *et al.* (1979) offered a model that emphasized potentially positive outcomes across diverse social environments and was facilitated by positive attitudes leading to acceptance, self-esteem, independence, high expectation, high performance, heterosexual relationships, and a vocational future.

In contrast to these individual-focused models, Rolland (1987) has presented a model for understanding chronic illness within a family context. Specifically, Rolland proposed that the family, faced with chronic illness (or physical, sensory, or intellectual impairment) in one of its members, forms an interactive system with the illness. One interaction is between the developmental phase of the individual, the developmental phases of the family, and the different phases of the condition. The time phases of a condition are important both because of the differing physiologic impact at different stages and the different meanings ascribed to the condition at different ages by the individual, the family, and the broader social environments. In the absence of longitudinal studies, these interactions of family development and illness evolution are poorly understood.

Rolland (1987) also emphasized the interactions between the instrumental and affective style of the family and the demands of the illness. Prior research has not adequately accounted for variability in illness demands. Historically, research on the psychosocial consequences of chronic illnesses has tended either to have: (1) a specific illness orientation—where findings are believed to be non-generalizable, or (2) a generic orientation—where findings with one condition are almost indiscriminately applied to others. What is generic and what is condition-specific remains poorly understood. Rolland proposed a typology of chronic conditions, based on differences in course, cause, prognosis, and incapacitation which produce differential impacts on the family system.

Family issues

There is no question but that chronic illness or disability places an increased set of demands on the family. Numerous studies have emphasized that poor family functioning interacts with the stress of managing chronic illness or disability and leads to poorer psychosocial outcomes in the child. (Newbrough *et al.* 1985; Seidel *et al.* 1975; White *et al.* 1984). Children and families who experience an accumulation of other life events and strains concurrent to managing the chronic condition are reportedly more at risk. Rutter (1979) has observed that 'the stresses potentiated each other so that the combination of chronic stresses pro-

Table 21.3 *Rolland's model of impact of chronic illness on family*

Five elements of the conditions				
Progression	*Time phase*	*Expectations*	*Incapacitation*	*Treatments*
Static	Crisis (e.g.	Initial	Degree	Complexity
Progressive	early phase)	Change over	Nature	Requirements
Slow	Chronic (time	time	Sensory	Additive
Rapid	between early	Degree of	Motoric	Restrictive
Relapsing/remitting	readjustment	certainty or		Ending old
	and death	predictability	Disfigurement	behaviour
Uncertain	Death	re. aetiology	Energy	Inviting
		re. course	production	new
			Social	behaviour
			stigma	Efficacy

vided very much more than a summation of the effects of the separate stresses considered singly.'

The patterns of interaction between different dyads (e.g. parent–child) and the total family system may be protective or may be strained and increase the risk. The 'goodness of fit' between the child and parent in terms of temperament and personality (Thomas and Chess 1980) will influence how well a child's developmental needs are met. The child's condition has an impact on these interaction patterns.

At the family level, Minuchin et al. (1978) have identified interaction patterns characterized by rigidity, avoidance of conflict resolution, enmeshment, and overprotectiveness as predictive of psychosomatic symptoms in children with asthma, diabetes, or anorexia nervosa.

Over the past decade, a greater effort has been made to identify positive characteristics of families which protect the child and contribute to better outcomes. Family organization including clarity of rules and expectations, family routines, clear role allocation, and clear generational boundaries, with a parental hierarchy that works together to make decisions and establish and maintain child discipline lead to better child outcomes. This is particularly apparent when the condition calls for compliance with a home treatment regimen.

In addition, family emotional and communication patterns are also related to child outcomes. Cohesion, or bonds of family unity and emotional support, has been repeatedly identified as a critical protective factor for managing the stress of chronic illness or disability. This support needs to be coupled with firm parental control. The importance of father's support (in addition to mother's) has been emphasized. Sibling support is also helpful. Balancing high levels of support with appropriate challenges to the child's independence also has been reported to facilitate better outcomes (Steinhausen et al. 1977).

A clear, direct, and open family communication style where positive and negative feelings are expressed has been reported as adaptive for families of children with disabilities (Patterson 1985). In addition to expression of affect, communication directed at problem-solving and conflict resolution is also protective.

The way in which families cope with the chronic demands of caring for a child with a disability has received considerable attention in the literature. Paying attention to and managing multiple family needs (including the special needs child) has been related to better child outcomes. This includes efforts to maintain normal family functioning. Developing social support among relatives and friends is an identified buffer to this chronic stress.

Coping strategies that alter the meaning of the chronic illness situation have received considerable attention in more recent studies. An attitude of 'we can beat this', believing things could be worse, living day to day, and endowing the situation with meaning are examples of what is reported to help families (Hauser et al. 1986). Cowen et al. (1985) found that parents of chronically ill children minimized normal developmental stresses more than parents of non-sick children as a way of reducing demands. A form of denial (especially about long-term consequences) appears to help many of these families. It allows them to maintain hope that their child will get better or a cure will be found so that the family can continue to attach to and invest in the child's care.

We tend to view the relationships between children with chronic illness and families as linear (e.g. the impact of chronic illness on family). There is continuous interchange between the individuals and their families such that the functioning of one directly influences the functioning of the other. It is the continuous, recursive pattern of interaction which is critical to understanding child and family adaptation to chronic illness and disability over time. While we can artificially punctuate the cycle at any one point in time and speak of a linear direction of effects (e.g. family functioning predicts child outcome), it is important to always keep in mind the circular nature of these processes of individual family and adaptation.

Patterson (1991) has described an interactive model linking condition, the child, and the family. This interactive model acknowledges that any change in the system affects everyone. Conversely, the failure to acknowledge these interactive relationships can predispose to treatment failures. Take, for example, the adolescent with diabetes who is admitted to hospital with ketoacidosis—failure to understand that his problems with poor glycaemic regulation may stem from the social environment will limit treatment efficacy. To re-establish glycaemic control then, and return him to the social environment that predisposed him to the problem originally, does little to improve the long-term outcome.

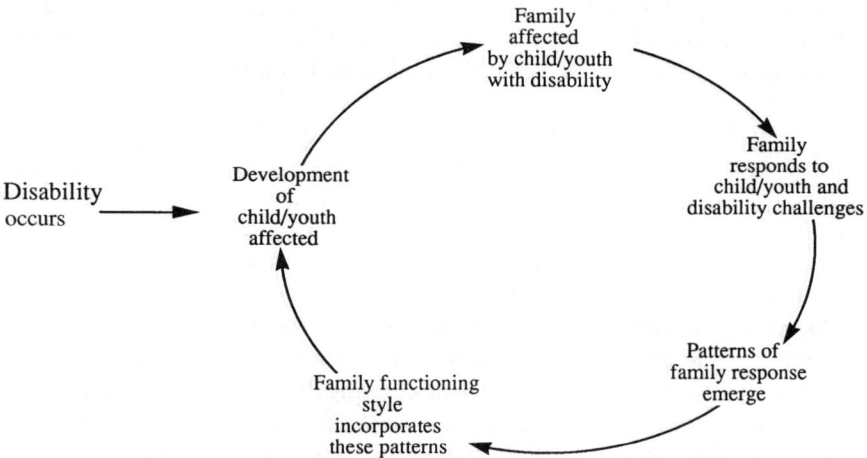

Fig. 21.3 Patterson's interactive model of condition–child–family impact.

Conclusion

Two major forces are occurring worldwide which raise our consciousness about issues related to youth with disabilities. First of all, improved health care coupled with new medical and surgical interventions means that today more children with disabling conditions will survive into adolescence and adulthood than ever before. These young people bring with them a host of questions and issues for which we have little experience. Concurrently, in most industrialized and many developing countries of the world, there is a growing awareness that the segregation of those with disabling conditions is both bad public policy and a costly destruction of human potential.

What becomes evident when speaking to young people who have disabilities is that their general health needs are not only parallel with those of their non-disabled peers, but, in addition, the common health worries and concerns of adolescence are more frequent and more persistent in these populations of teenagers.

We know that to be clinically effective with adolescents who have disabling conditions and chronic illnesses, we must understand their perceptions of the condition. We must learn about their lifestyle, their family functioning, their cognitive and social development. We must reorient our clinical style from being prescriptive to negotiative, modifying the regiment, when appropriate, so that physical health and social development can be maximized, so that the teenager does not feel more 'different' from his or her peers than is absolutely necessary and so compliance can be enhanced.

We must also be willing to acknowledge that we are at a new frontier in relation to teenagers and young adults with many chronic conditions which were previously fatal in childhood. We know regrettably little about the maturational and long-term consequences of some conditions; likewise, we know relatively little of what it means to grow up dependent on life-sustaining medical technologies.

As we have learned much about management of chronic conditions over the past 30 years, so too have we learned much about family functioning during adolescence. We have come to understand that the notion of the peer group replacing the family during adolescence as the primary reference group is simply not valid. It is not valid for adolescents in general; and it does not apply for those with disabling conditions. Rather, while peer groups are of increasing importance as the teenager matures, for better or worse the family is the central point of reference and the primary environment in which that young person matures. Families' attitudes, beliefs and behaviours have a dramatic impact on the young person with a chronic condition while concurrently the chronic condition has a dramatic impact on the family. Puberty is a very difficult period for many families as they come to realize that their children will not always remain young. It is a period when they begin to wrestle with the future and many of the complex issues which the future holds: (1) what are the genetic risks which my child has for transmitting the condition? (2) what are his or her sexual and reproductive capabilities? (3) what is his or her life expectancy? (4) what are his or her vocational capabilities? To be effective, we need not only to support families but also provide them with the information and the skills necessary to help their adolescents achieve independence. We need to help them separate and shift their focus from being solely on the child to broader social interests throughout, of home employment, volunteer work, and greater involvement with other children in the household.

The issues which face young people with chronic conditions and their families are both multi-faceted and complex, but research clearly shows that with appropriate care, the issues with which they are confronted can be the basis for building strength and resilience rather than defeat and psychopathology. The challenge for clinicians is to help them and their families access the appropriate supports.

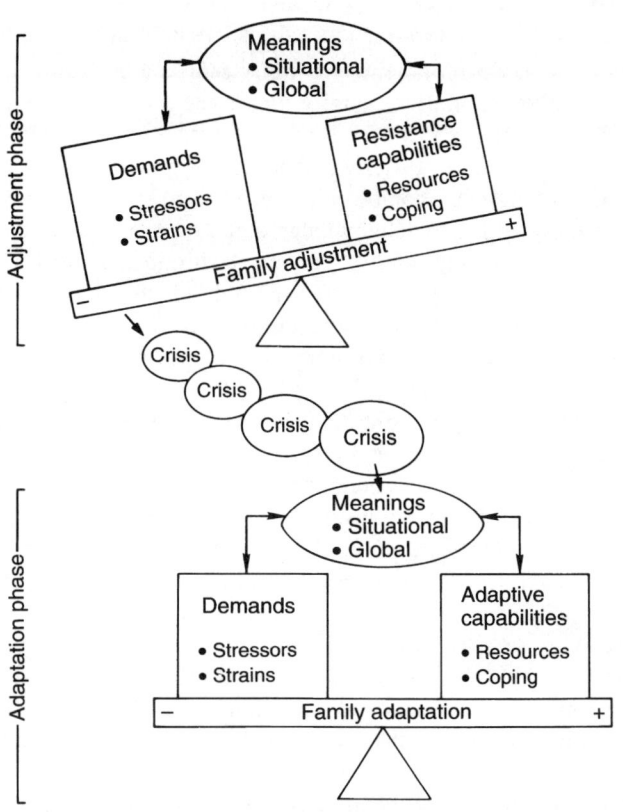

Fig. 21.4 The 'family adjustment and adaptation response' (FAAR) model.

Acknowledgements

The research for this chapter was supported in part by grant #MCJ-2736 (National Center for Youth with Disabilities) Maternal and Child Health Bureau, Department of Health and Human Services; and grant #H133B90012 (The Center for Children with Chronic Illness and Disability), National Institute on Disability and Rehabilitation Research, Department of Education.

References

Abrahamson, M., Ash, M., and Nash, W. (1979). Handicapped adolescents—a time for reflection. *Adolescence* **14**, 557–65.

Benedict, P.H. (1966). Sexual precosity and polyostotic fibrous dysplasia. *American Journal of Diseases in Children* **3**, 429–32.

Blum, R.W. (ed.) (1984). Sexual health needs of physically and intellectually impaired adolescents. In *Chronic illness and disabilities in childhood and adolescence*, pp. 127–42. Grune and Stratton, New York.

Blum, R. and Geber, G. (1992). Chronic illness in adolescence. In *Textbook of adolescent medicine*, (ed. E. McAnarney, R. Kreipe, and D. Orr). W.B. Saunders, Philadelphia.

Blum, R., Resnick, M.D., Nelson, R., and St. Germaine, A. (1991). Family and peer issues among adolescents with spina bifida and cerebral palsy. *Pediatrics* **145**, 994–8.

Cadman, D., Boyle, M., Offord, D., Szatmari, P., Rae-Grant, N., Crawford, J. et al. (1986). Chronic illness and functional limitations in Ontario children: findings of the Ontario child health study. *Canadian Medical Association Journal* **135**, 761–7.

Carroll, G., Massarelli, E., Opzoomer, A., Pekeles, G., Pedneault, M., Frappier, J. et al. (1983). Adolescent with chronic disease. Are they receiving comprehensive health care? *Journal of Adolescent Health Care* **4**, 261–5.

Chamie, M. (1989). Survey design strategies, the study of disability. *World Health Statistics Quarterly* **42**, 122–40.

Cornaggia, C., Canevini, M., Christe, W., Giuccioli, D., Facheris, M., Sabbadini, M., and Canger, R. (1990). Epidemiologic survey of epilepsy among army draftees in Lombardy, Italy. *Epilepsia* **31**, 27–32.

Cowen, L., Corey, M., Keenan, N, Simmons, R., Arndt, E., and Levison, H. (1985). Family adaptation and psychosocial adjustment to cystic fibrosis in the preschool child. *Social Science and Medicine* **20**, 553–60.

Drotar, D. (1981). Psychological perspectives in chronic childhood illness. *Journal of Pediatric Psychology* **6**, 211–28.

Erasmus, R., Fakeye, T., Olukoga, O., Okesina, A., Ebomoyi, E., Adeleye, M., and Arije, A. (1989). Prevalence of diabetes mellitus in a Nigerian population. *Trans. Royal Society Tropical Medicine and Hygiene* **83**, 417–18.

Fineman, N., and Yakovak, W. (1970). Neurofibromatosis in childhood. *Journal of Adolescent Health Care* **76**, 339–47.

Forsgren, L., Edvinsson, S., Blomquist, H., Heijbel, J., and Sidenvall, R. (1990). Epilepsy in a population of mentally retarded children and adults. *Epilepsy Research* **6**, 234–48.

Haahtela, T., Lindholm, H., Bjorksten, F., Koskenvuo, K., and Latinen, L. (1990). Prevalence of asthma in Finnish young men. *British Medical Journal* **301**, 266–8.

Hauser, S.T., Jacobsen, A.M., Wertlieb, D., Weiss-Perry, B., Follansbee, D., Wolfsdorf, J. *et al.* (1986). Children with recently diagnosed diabetes: interactions within their families. *Health Psychology* **5**, 273–96.

Kohler, L., and Jakobsson, G. (1991). *Children's health in Sweden*, p. 75. The National Board of Health and Welfare, Stockholm.

Massie, R.K., Jr (1985). The constant shadow: reflections on the life of a chronically ill child. In *Issues in the care of children with chronic illness*, (ed. N. Hobbs and J. Perrin), pp. 13–23. Jossey-Bass, San Francisco.

McCubbin, H., McCubbin, M., Patterson, J., Cauble, A., Wilson, L., and Warwick, W. (1983). CHIP—coping health inventory for parents: an assessment of parental coping patterns in the care of the chronically ill child. *Journal of Marriage and the Family* **45**, 359–70.

Minuchin, S., Rosman, B., and Baker, L. (1978). *Psychosomatic families*. Harvard University Press, Cambridge, MA.

Newacheck, P. (1989). Adolescents with special health care needs: prevalence, severity and access to health care services. *Pediatrics* **84**, 872–81.

Newacheck, P., Budetti, P., and Halfon, N. (1986). Trends in activity-limiting chronic conditions among children. *American Journal of Public Health* **76**, 178–84.

Newbrough, J.R., Simplins, C.G., and Maurer, M.A. (1985). A family development approach to studying factors in the management and control of childhood diabetes. *Diabetes Care* **81**, 83–92.

Noble, I.H. (1981). *Social inequity and the prevalence of disability. Projections for the Year 2000*. UNICEF, Assignment Children 53–54, Geneva. The National Board of Health and Welfare, Stockholm.

Offer, D., Ostrov, E., and Howard, K. (1984). Body image, self-perception and chronic illness in adolescence. In *Chronic illness and disabilities in childhood and adolescence*, (ed. R.W. Blum), pp. 59–74. Grune and Stratton, New York.

Offord, D., Boyle, M., Fleming, J., Blum, H., and Grant, N. (1989). Ontario health study: summary of selected results. *Canadian Journal of Psychiatry* **34**, 483–91.

Patterson, J. (1985). Critical factors affecting family compliance with home treatment for children with cystic fibrosis. *Family Relations* **34**, 79–89.

Patterson, J.M. (1988*a*). Families experiencing stress: The family adjustment and adaptation response model. *Family Systems Medicine* **5**, 202–37.

Patterson, J.M. (1988*b*). Chronic illness in children and the impact on families. In *Chronic illness and disability*, (ed. C. Chilman, E. Nunnally, and F. Cox), pp. 69–107.

Patterson, J. (1991). A family system perspective for working with youth with disability. *Pediatrician* **18**, 129–41.

Perrin, J. (1984). The organization of services for chronically ill children and their families. *Pediatric Clinics of North America* **31**, 235–57.

Pless, I. (1984). Clinical assessment: Physical and psychological functioning. *Pediatric Clinics of North America* **31**, 33–46.

Pless, I., and Pinkerton, P. (1975). *Chronic childhood disorder—promoting patterns of adjustment*, pp. 21–3. Yearbook Medical Publishers, Chicago.

Roberts, M., Martin, J., McLellan, D., McIntosh-Michaelis, S., and Spackman, A. (1991). The prevalence of multiple sclerosis in the Southampton and Southwest Hampshire health authority. *Journal of Neurology and Neurosurgical Psychiatry* **54**, 55–9.

Rolland, J. (1987). Chronic illness and the life cycle: a conceptual framework. *Family Process* **26**, 203–21.
Rundle, A.T. and Sylvester, P.E. (1970). The influence of retarded maturation on growth abnormalities in the mentally defective girl. *Journal of Mental Deficiency Research* **14**, 196–204.
Rutter, M. (1979). Protective factors in children's responses to stress and disadvantage. In *Primary prevention of psychopathology*, (Vol. 3) (ed. M.W. Kent and J.E. Rolf). University Press of New England, Arundale, NSW, Australia.
Rutter, M. (1975). *Helping troubled children*. Plenum New York.
Salerno, L.J., Park, J.K., and Giannini, M.J. (1975). Reproductive capacity of the mentally retarded. *Journal of Reproductive Medicine* **14**, 123–9.
Seidel, V.P., Chadwick, O., and Rutter, M. (1975). Psychological disorders in crippled children: a comparative study of children with and without brain damage. *Developmental Medicine and Child Neurology* **17**, 553–63.
Shaw, R., Crane, J., O'Donnell, T., Portous, L., and Coleman, E. (1990). Increasing asthma prevalence in a rural New Zealand adolescent population: 1975–1989. *Archives of Disease in Childhood* **65**, 1319–23.
Snorgaard, O., Eskildsen, P., Vadstrup, S., and Nerup, J. (1989). Diabetic ketoacidosis in Denmark: epidemiology, incidence rates, precipitating factors and mortality rates. *Journal of Internal Medicine* **226**, 223–8.
Steinhausen, H., Borner, S., and Koepp, P. (1977). The personality of juvenile diabetics. In *Pediatric adolescent endocrinology*, (Vol. 2) (ed. Z. Laron), pp. 1–7. Karger, Basel.
Thomas, A. and Chess, S. (1980). *The dynamics of psychological development*. Brunner/Mazel, New York.
United Nations (1990). *Disabilities statistics compendium*. (ST/ESA/STAT/SER. Y/4), United Nations, New York.
White, K., Kolman, M., Polin, G., and Winter, R.J. (1984). Unstable diabetes and unstable families: a psychosocial evaluation of diabetic children with recurrent ketoacidosis. *Pediatrics* **73**, 749–55.
Yen, S. and Jaffe, R.B. (1978). *Reproductive endocrinology*. W.B. Saunders, Philadelphia.

PART VII

Vulnerable children

The concept of vulnerable children, sometimes expressed as children 'at risk', is a useful tool in social paediatric practice in identifying groups of children within a population requiring special attention. This part deals with a range of factors leading to vulnerability, including poverty and family breakdown. The final chapter of this part considers the factors which protect children from the worst effects of factors which render them vulnerable.

22 Children in poverty
Nick Spencer and Hilary Graham

Introduction

The link between poverty and adverse social environments and child morbidity and mortality has long been recognized; social paediatrics and, to a large extent, paediatrics as a subspecialty of medicine arose from this recognition as outlined by Professor Manciaux in Chapter 1. In developing countries these links remain starkly obvious (see Chapter 5); in developed countries the links are less clear. Controversy has centred on the definition of poverty and the relative weight of poverty itself, and on the lifestyles of the poor in the causal pathways to poor health. This chapter considers the definition of poverty, the evidence for links between poverty and child mortality and morbidity in Europe, and the causal controversy in order to inform strategies for the reduction of poverty and its adverse effects on child health.

Definition of poverty

Early attempts to define poverty centred on the level of income below which the minimum requirements for physical efficiency could not be obtained. This is known as 'absolute' or 'primary' poverty and would apply to many children living in developing countries. Difficulties arise in defining physical efficiency and the concept is not useful in studying health inequalities in developed countries with social welfare systems which maintain people above a mere subsistence level. 'Relative' poverty, defined by Townsend (1979) as 'lack of the resources to obtain the types of diets, participate in the activities and have the living conditions and amenities which are customary in the society to which they (individuals, families, groups) belong', has been advanced as a means of accounting for the relative disadvantage experienced by those below a certain income level who, however, are manifestly not suffering from 'absolute' poverty. 'Relative' poverty is necessarily a changing and dynamic concept which is difficult to use over time as a reproducible measure of poverty. It is specific to particular societies, rendering comparisons between countries difficult, though innovative approaches to developing cross-national measures are being developed. Because measures of 'relative' poverty are usually based on household income, it does not take account of 'hidden' poverty suffered by women and children as a result of maldistribution of income within the family. Equally, 'relative' poverty measures do not take account of how poverty is mediated and created by racial discrimination.

None the less, relative poverty remains a useful concept and has been adopted by many European governments in order to define a level of income below which people are regarded as significantly disadvantaged. In EC countries this is now accepted as being less than 50 per cent of national average income, though some EC publications use a definition based on percentage of average expenditure. A 'poverty line' is not accepted by the UK government. Official statistics, until 1985 based on low income families (LIF) figures giving the number of families living at or below the level of supplementary benefit (the welfare safety net), now record households below average income (HBAI). Numbers of families with children living on incomes less than 50 per cent of the average income can be derived from these figures.

The inherent difficulties of defining relative poverty and the inclination of governments to use the statistics which seem most favourable to them is reflected in the variety of ways official statistics on low income households are presented. These problems will be addressed below in attempting to define the extend of child poverty in Europe and the trends in recent years.

An interesting recent attempt to define the level of relative poverty was made by a group of researchers for a television programme in the UK, 'Breadline Britain' (London Weekend Television 1991), in which opinion poll techniques were used to ascertain a consensus view of a representative sample of the population of the necessities required for life in modern Britain. Twenty-six necessities were identified by more than 50 per cent of the sample and data were analysed to obtain a proportion of the sample without one or more of these necessities as a result of lack of resources rather than choice (Mack and Lansley 1984). A follow-up study has been published recently (London Weekend Television 1991) which indicates, using comparable measures of poverty (lack of three or more of the items considered as necessities by the majority of respondents), an increase in child poverty from two million in 1983 to three million in 1991.

Health for all targets, the UN Convention, and poverty

The World Health Organization, through the *Health for all 2000* initiatives, and the United Nations, through the *Convention of the rights of the child*, explicitly recognize the importance of poverty as a determinant of childhood ill-health. Target 1 of *HFA 2000* states

'By the year 2000, the actual differences in health status between countries and between groups within countries should be reduced by at least 25 per cent, by improving the level of health of disadvantaged nations and groups.'

The reduction of differences among social groups and geographical areas within countries is seen as essential to the achievement of targets 6 and 7, concerned with increasing life expectancy at birth and reducing infant mortality, and the eradication or reduction of health inequalities underpins the whole initiative. Article 27 of the *UN Convention on the rights of the child* recognizes the right of every child to a standard of living adequate for the child's physical, mental, spiritual, moral, and social development. The Convention charges State Parties with providing material assistance and social security for children and specifically stresses the importance of nutrition, clothing, and housing (Articles 26 and 27).

In 1986, WHO (Europe) initiated a 'healthy cities' programme (see Chapter 2). Specific problems associated with living in cities can be identified and the programme is based on the reduction of inequalities and strategies to reduce the effects of inner city poverty and social disadvantage. The European Society for Social Paediatrics (ESSOP) has translated some of the *HFA* and *Healthy city* targets into child health targets, and the eradication of poverty and unemployment are seen as major steps to achieving improvements in health for city children.

In the UK, the Faculty of Community Medicine, in its response to the *HFA 2000* initiative, argues that it is the responsibility of central government to pursue policies designed to eliminate absolute and relative poverty and to ensure that available resources within the health services are used in the interests of raising health standards and reducing health inequalities. The recently enacted 1989 Children Act specifically recognizes the need for additional services and attention to 'children in need' and gives local government in the UK responsibility for offering a range of services to reduce disadvantage.

The international recognition of the importance of poverty as a determinant of child ill-health provides a valuable support to practitioners, service planners, and researchers engaged in formulating strategies for the reduction of health inequalities. However, controversy persists amongst social policy makers and child health workers in developed countries related to the extent of the effects of poverty on child health and the causal pathways by which these effects are mediated. Further analysis, research, and experience is required in order to inform intervention strategies based on the broad aims of reduction of child health inequality.

The extent of child poverty in Europe

As indicated above, variable definitions of poverty and absence of reliable data make it difficult to construct a comprehensive picture of the extent of child poverty in Europe. Identifying clear trends is even more difficult. However, using available data, a partial picture can be constructed from which some conclusions can be drawn.

Recent European data

Data for the 12 countries of the EC indicate that in 1985 43.9 million people were living in households with equivalent disposable incomes less than 50 per cent of the average equivalent disposal income (O'Higgins and Jenkins 1988). These people living in relative poverty represent 13.9 per cent of the EC population. Using a measure of 50 per cent of the average national income, 49.6 million people in 16.1 million households in EC countries (excluding Luxembourg) were estimated to be living in poverty (EC Commission 1991). Almost 20 per cent of children (12.2 million) in the EC (excluding Luxembourg) were living in households with less than 50 per cent of the national average equivalent expenditure in 1985.

Within these figures there were wide variations between countries; only 6.7 per cent of Belgian and 9.1 per cent of Danish children were living in poverty compared with 36.6 per cent in Portugal, 27 per cent in Ireland, and 24 per cent in the UK. Forty per cent of the poor children in the EC live in the UK and France.

Data for the rest of Europe are patchy and comparison is difficult as a result of different measures of poverty. Swedish figures based on less than 58 per cent of the average equivalent disposable income indicated that 11.5 per cent of families were poor in 1985 (Gustafsson 1989); Stjerno (1985) reports Norwegian figures for the early 1980s and, using 50 per cent of average income, five per cent of the Norwegian people were poor. Little data are available from Eastern Europe. In Czechoslovakia in 1985, 8.2 per cent of families with children were living below a 'minimum social level of consumption' (Cornia 1990). In Poland, 23 per cent of families were below the poverty line in 1987 and in Hungary in 1987, 12.7 per cent of the population and 20 per cent were defined as poor (Cornia 1990).

Trends in child poverty

Though direct comparisons across Europe are difficult and data on children are not universally available, comparisons and trends over time using the same national measures of poverty can be made. Table 22.1 is constructed from a number of sources; comparison between countries cannot be safely from these data but trends over time within countries can be discerned.

Trends are not consistent across Europe; in one group of countries, Spain, Greece, Belgium, Sweden, Italy, and Czechoslovakia, there was a decreasing trend in child poverty up to 1985 compared with countries such as the UK, Ireland, Germany (Federal Republic), The Netherlands, Poland, and Hungary in which child poverty increased in the early 1980s. Cornia (1990) summarizes the trends as follows:

'After more than two decades of steady progress involving all industrialised countries, poverty started to rise again in the mid-1970s in about two-thirds of the countries for which data are available—although with different characteristics and among different social groups. In the other third of the countries, poverty appears to have continued to decline although at a slower rate than before.' (p. 29)

Table 22.1 *Trends in child poverty for selected European countries and years*

Country	Around 1970 (%)	Around 1975 (%)	Around 1980 (%)	Around 1985 (%)
Czechoslovakia	–	11.4	9.3	8.2
Germany (FR)	14.0	7.4	8.7	8.9
Hungary	–	17.1	–	20.0
Ireland	–	15.7	18.5	26.0
Sweden	7.5	–	6.8	–
UK	–	–	9.0	18.1

Sources: Cornia (1990), p. 29.

Recent data from the Luxembourg income study (Mitchell 1990) suggests that the situation for families in industrialized countries may have deteriorated more than Cornia records. Using post-transfer incomes (after tax and benefits) below 50 per cent of the median, the trend between 1979 and 1986 (Fig. 22.1) for all the countries studies (including the USA, Canada, and Australia) is either no change or a sharp increase as in the UK and the USA.

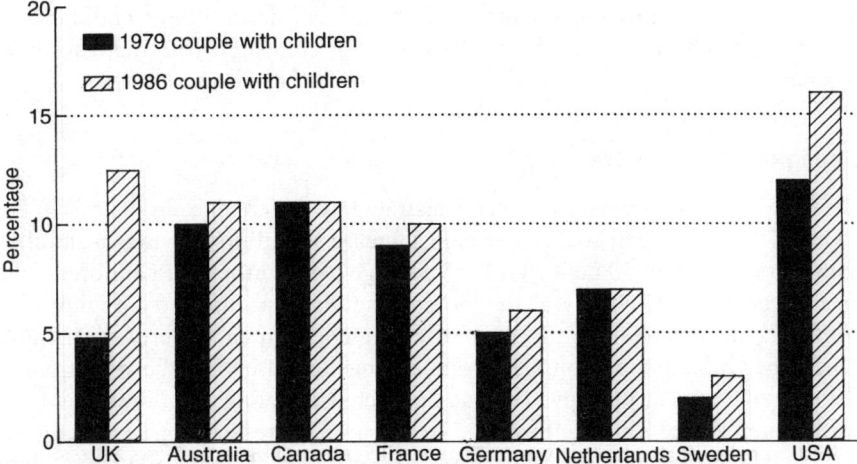

Fig. 22.1 Proportion of two-parent families with post-transfer incomes below 50 per cent of the median. (Source: Mitchell 1990.)

Table 22.2 *Comparison of trends in child and elderly poverty in three European countries*

Country	Around 1970 (%)	Around 1975 (%)	Around 1980 (%)	Around 1985 (%)
Germany (FR)				
Elderly	11.9	9.0	8.6	6.5
Children	14.0	7.4	8.7	8.9
Ireland				
Elderly	–	34.8	25.0	10.0
Children	–	15.7	18.5	26.0
Sweden				
Elderly	9.0	–	1.5	–
Children	7.5	–	6.8	–

From Cornia (1990).

Poverty affects some age groups in society more than others. Children and the elderly are most vulnerable to poverty and the elderly were the most affected group until recently. Table 22.2 compares the poverty trends for children and the elderly in three European countries between 1975 and 1985. All three countries show a consistent downward trend in poverty amongst the elderly; Germany (former West Germany) and Ireland show a clear upward trend in child poverty whilst in Sweden the trend is downward but considerably slower than for the elderly. Overall, despite the reduction in actual children in poverty in some European countries, the trend appears to be for children and families with children to become relatively poor compared with the rest of the population.

Child poverty in the UK

The trends in child poverty are well illustrated by the changes in the UK in the 1980s. There has been a 25.7 per cent increase in children living in families with incomes below 50 per cent of the average and families with children have taken over from the elderly as the largest single group in poverty. Figure 22.2 compares the changes in the proportion of children in poverty with those across the whole population. The trend amongst children and the whole population has been sharply upwards but the increase amongst children has been particularly sharp. This confirms the trends noted across Europe but suggests that the UK experience may have been worse for children than in some other countries.

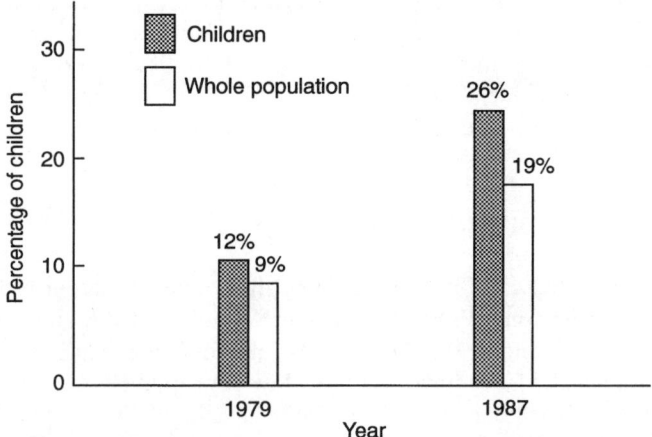

Fig. 22.2 Children and whole population living below 50 per cent income level after housing costs.

Groups of children vulnerable to poverty

National figures do not reflect the wide differences within countries in the experience of poverty. Regional differences are marked; in the UK in 1983–85, seven per cent of the population in the south-east had an income under 50 per cent of the national average compared with 26 per cent in Northern Ireland and in Italy in 1985, the average income of families in the north and central regions was 24.7 per cent higher than that of families in the south and Islands. Even within cities, marked differences are evident; in Sheffield in 1985, the unemployment rate varied between three per cent in the most prosperous areas to 30 per cent in the most deprived, and in Valencia in the early 80s a range between 15 and 30 per cent unemployment was noted.

Poverty increasingly affects children of the long-term unemployed, of single-parent families, of adults in precarious or low-paid jobs, and children of immigrants and ethnic minority groups (Cornia 1990). The recession which has affected all industrial countries in the eighties has led to a sharp increase in unemployment, and in parts of Europe the levels of long-term unemployment are high and increasing. Evidence from the UK suggests that tax and benefit changes have resulted in an actual fall in disposable income in real terms for the lowest decile income group in the last decade and that lone parents with one child have suffered disproportionately with an income loss of more than 25 per cent (Townsend 1991).

The doubling of lone-parent families over the last 25 years in the UK, a trend reflected in other European countries even those where divorce is uncommon, and the increasing disadvantage of this group may explain a significant part of the relative increase in child poverty. Data related to child poverty amongst immigrant and ethnic minority families is limited but available evidence from the UK (Blackburn 1991) indicates that ethnic minority and immigrant groups are more likely to be unemployed or in low-paid jobs, live in poor housing, and live in areas that lack social and educational resources. As with the rest of the population, children in these groups are most vulnerable.

The effects of poverty on child health

Broadly, international child health measures show a clear relationship between increasing Gross National Product (GNP) and national wealth and better child health outcomes (Grant 1991). There are some notable exceptions; countries such as Sri Lanka and Cuba have relatively low per capita GNPs and low infant mortality rates whilst Brazil and Saudi Arabia have high GNPs/capita with high infant mortality rates. These exceptions support the connection between poverty and child health as they indicate that income distribution within a country is important in determining the child health outcomes.

Health inequalities are marked within developing countries. The post-neonatal mortality rate (deaths at ages between one month and one year of age per 1000 live births) for children of agricultural workers in the 1970s for Senegal was 87 compared with 22 of those of professional workers; even in Jamaica where rates are closer to those of European countries the differential rates for the same occupational groups were 22 and 7 (Hobcraft *et al.* 1984). The 50th centile for height of low income Nigerian children is equivalent to the 10th centile on the growth charts devised by Tanner and Whitehouse, whereas the 50th centile for the children of professional Nigerians is just above that for the London children on whom the charts were based (Eveleth and Tanner 1976).

The focus in this chapter is on poverty and child health in present-day Europe but it is important to bear in mind the striking evidence from developing countries (see Chapter 5) and the historical importance of poverty in relation to health in nineteenth-century Europe (see Chapter 1).

Traditionally, health has been measured in terms of mortality and morbidity; measures of 'positive' health and quality of life (see Chapter 35) are underdeveloped and not widely available. The evidence for inequalities in child health presented here is in terms of mortality, growth and birth-weight, and various measures of morbidity. Where possible data from across Europe are used. However, much of the information is from the UK where a tradition of measuring social differences in mortality, and to a lesser extent morbidity, is well established.

Mortality

The 1988 perinatal, neonatal, and post-neonatal mortality rates (PNMR, NNMR, and PNNMR) by social class for England and Wales are shown in Figs. 22.3 and 22.4. It is important to note that these figures only include those infants born within marriage and the social class groups are based on the Registrar General's classification of the occupation of the head of the household and do not include a large group unclassified because of unemployment or single-parent status. As a consequence, the differential between those living in the most and the least favourable socio-economic circumstances in underestimated. Pamuk (1988) shows that the inclusion of births outside marriage significantly widens the differential for PNNMR. Comparison of the north-east of Italy with the south and Islands for PNMR and IMR in 1985 shows a marked differential between the prosperous north and the poorer south; rates of 12.6 (PNMR) and 8.4 (IMR)

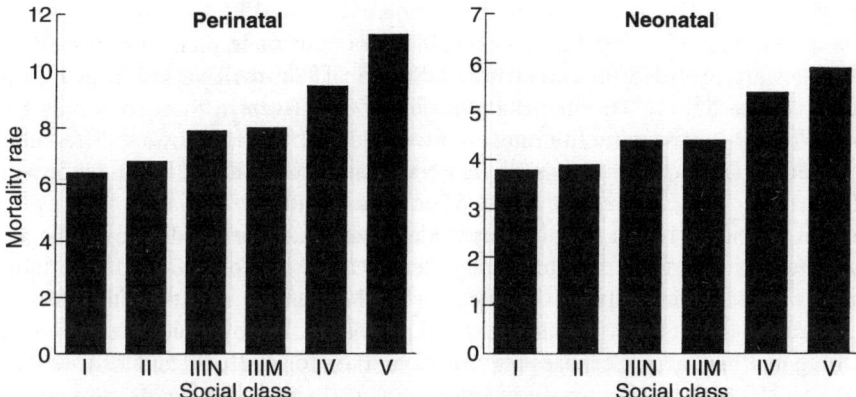

Fig. 22.3 Perinatal and neonatal mortality rates by social class, England and Wales 1988.

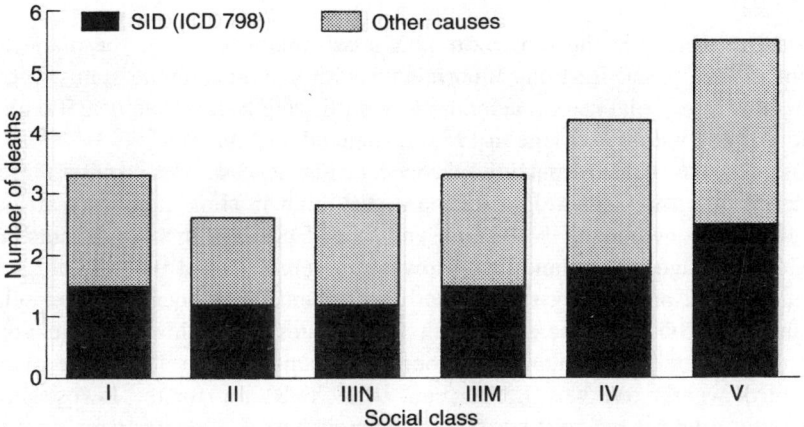

Fig. 22.4 Post-neonatal deaths per 1000 live births by social class, England and Wales 1988.

Table 22.3 *Perinatal and infant mortality rates and low birth-weight by socio-economic group in Sweden, 1976–81*

Socio-economic group	PNMR (per 1000)	IMR (per 1000)	LBW (%)
A (privileged)	7.7	5.9	3.5
B (middle)	8.9	7.4	4.5
C (underprivileged)	9.2	7.6	6.0

From Zetterstrom and Eriksson 1987, in Kohler and Jakobsson 1991, p. 28.

compared with 15.7 and 12.4 (Saraceno 1990). The same marked regional differences are recorded for parts of the USSR; in 1988, IMR varied from 11.0 in Lithuania to 53.0 in Turkmenistan (Cornia 1990). Even in Sweden, which has some of the lowest mortality rates in the world, Table 22.3 shows a differential between socio-economic groups in PNMR and IMR (Kohler and Jakobsson 1991).

Inequalities between social groups in mortality rates of children over the age of one year tend to be less than for infants. However, specific-cause mortality shows marked social class differences in England and Wales; the 'standardized mortality rates' (SMR) from injuries and poisoning for boys calculated from the Office of Population Censuses and Surveys' data for 1979–80 and 1982–83 are 50 and 150 respectively for social classes I and II and social class V. An almost identical pattern emerges for mortality due to traffic accidents in children aged 1–14.

Low birth-weight

Low birth-weight is the most common predisposing factor of perinatal and infant mortality and is strongly correlated with socio-economic status. Figure 22.5 shows the social class gradient in low birth-weight 'less than' (<2500 g) for children born within marriage in 1988 in England and Wales.

The absence of births outside marriage in Fig. 22.3 is important as there is evidence that low birth-weight rates are very high in some inner city areas in which many lone parents live (Townsend *et al.* 1988) and in 1978, infants born outside marriage in Scotland had a low birth-weight rate of 9.5 per cent compared with 4.2 per cent for social class I and II and 8.2 per cent for social class IV and V. In Sweden, where low birth-weight rates are the lowest in the world, differences persist between socio-economic groups (Kohler 1988); the overall low birth-weight rate was 4.5 per cent in 1976–81 but for the lowest socio-economic group it was 6.0 per cent compared with 3.5 per cent for the most advantaged group.

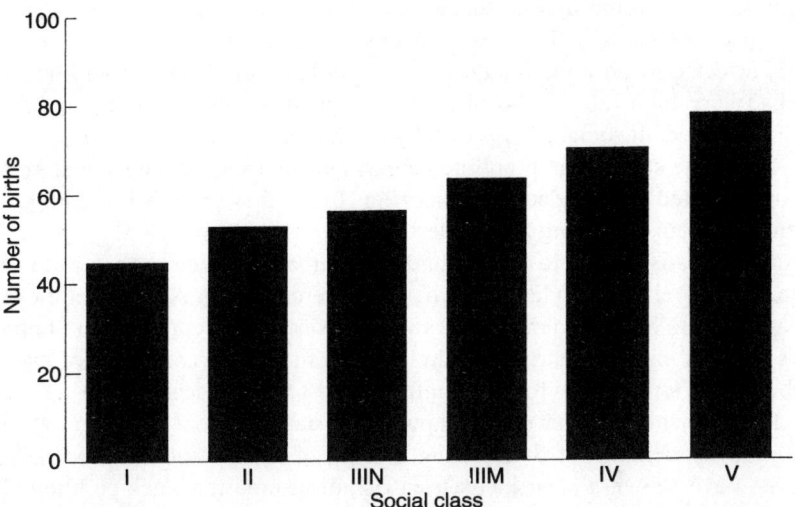

Fig. 22.5 Births under 2500 g per 1000 live births by social class, England and Wales, 1988.

Growth

Socio-economic differences in growth are well recognized; in the Newcastle 'Thousand families' study carried out in the 1940s and 50s, children in social class I and II were on average 4.5 cm taller than children from social class IV and V. In his fascinating analysis of inter-generational and longitudinal trends in a group of children born in the UK in 1946 (The National Survey of Health and Development), Wadsworth (1991) demonstrates that adult height differentials between social groups are already established by the age of four years. Using data from the 1958 cohort study (The National Childhood Development Study), Davie et al. (1972) conclude that the difference in height between the most and the least advantaged children in the sample was 13.8 cm. More recent UK surveys have shown persistent social class differences (Gulliford et al. 1991) though the authors conclude that social class differences are accounted for by 'biological' factors.

Morbidity

Morbidity data related to socio-economic status are difficult to obtain partly because of data collection problems and partly because of inconsistencies in definition. However, in countries where mortality rates are low, measures of morbidity are important in monitoring health inequalities.

In the 1946 UK national cohort study (Wadsworth 1991), a social class gradient was noted in pre-school children experiencing measles and whooping cough and for serious chronic illness, social class differences were noted for boys but not for girls. Respiratory illness was closely related to air pollution and in areas heavily affected by air pollution due to coal smoke and industrial pollution, children had very high rates of hospital admission for bronchitis and pneumonia, and this affected all social groups equally. However, many more children of low socio-economic status live in polluted areas. Differences between social groups have been noted for headaches, wheezing, bronchitis, mouth breathing, and repeated accidents (Golding and Butler 1986).

Bronchiolitis is known to affect children in urban areas more than rural children and is associated with large families and overcrowding. Analysis of the children admitted to hospital during the 1989–90 bronchiolitis epidemic in Sheffield shows a highly significant trend to admission from the deprived areas of the city which remains strong even for those infants with serious disease requiring active medical treatment (Spencer *et al.*, unpublished data). Recent work on bacterial meningitis has demonstrated clustering in areas of deprivation and studies from the USA have shown a clear increase in risk of asthma for black children. The authors conclude that poverty and associated factors account for part of this increased risk. A study in Ireland showed a clear social class gradient in hemiplegic and diplegic forms of cerebral palsy (Dowding and Barry 1990).

Cumulative evidence suggests that as with mortality, morbidity experience, particularly with respiratory illness, is greater in poor children than their more privileged peers. Causal mechanisms are unclear and some authors attribute the differences more to lifestyle and health behaviours of parents than to factors directly related to relative material deprivation. For example, Golding and Butler (1986) conclude that the class differences in childhood morbidity are mainly explained by parental smoking and other 'behavioural' factors. We will consider these issues in the next section.

Explanations for the effect of poverty on child health

As indicated above, there has been a long-running debate in developed countries, and particularly in the UK in the last 13 years since the publication of a government-initiated report on health inequalities (Townsend and Davidson 1982), on the explanation for differences in health outcome between socio-economic groups. Two major schools have emerged: the behavioural school who argue that differences in health outcome between social groups are explained by differences in health-related behaviour, which in the case of children usually refers to maternal behaviour, and the structural school who argue that differences in income and access to resources are the most causal explanation for inequalities.

WHO's *HFA 2000* encompasses both approaches and targets are concerned with structural as well as behavioural change. In the UK, the behavioural approach has dominated official publications related to health and a government publication *'Prevention and health: everybody's business'* (Department of Health and Social Security 1976) states 'the greatest potential, and perhaps the greatest problem for preventative medicine, now lies in changing behaviour and attitudes to health'. One important source of this orientation to the behavioural interpretation of health inequalities has been the conclusions drawn from various research studies. Brooke *et al.* (1989), from a major study of pregnancy in London, concluded that the most important factor accounting for a five per cent reduction in what they call 'corrected birth-weight' was maternal smoking, and socio-economic factors became non-significant after controlling for smoking. Gulliford *et al.* (1991) reach a similar conclusion related to height in cohort of children, arguing that the association with social class disappears when 'biological' factors, particularly parental height, are taken into account.

Golding and Butler (1984), reporting the results of the UK cohort studies, conclude that maternal smoking history is the major determinant of the differences in death rates and, for this reason, political action to equalize the wealth or housing of the lower socio-economic groups is unlikely to result in any reduction in health inequalities. They predict 'give the family more money and it is possible that their consumption of tobacco (and alcohol) would increase'.

There are some methodological problems with these conclusions. Smoking and 'biological' factors are assumed to be independent of socio-economic status. In the UK, smoking amongst women with young children has become increasingly associated with deprivation, and controlling for social class, in fact, means controlling for intra-class differences in income. Parental height is not independent of social class and, in the same way as for smoking, maternal short stature selects the most deprived within each class group.

Further evidence from the UK indicates that smoking is used by mothers in low-income families as a coping mechanism and that in the budgets of the poor, smoking takes on the characteristics of a 'fixed' payment behaving like rent and fuel payments rather than as a 'flexible' item such as luxuries and to some extent food (Graham 1989). Thus, at least in the UK, smoking amongst women with children is increasingly associated with disadvantage and is a mechanism through which health inequalities are expressed (Graham 1992). It appears to be part of an overall pattern of coping for the poor and one of their few pleasures which now behaves as an essential rather than a luxury item.

In addition, maternal smoking as the main explanation for socio-economic differences in child health outcomes is implausible. The marked social class gradient in women smoking in the UK is a recent phenomenon, with women smoking equally across the social classes in the 1950s. Before the Second World War, a negligible number of women were smokers and in some European countries, such as Spain and Greece, there is evidence that the social class gradient is reversed with women in higher social class groups smoking more. Health inequalities in mortality rates and low birth-weight rates have persisted throughout all these changes in maternal smoking patterns and exist in all European countries independent of maternal smoking habits.

Lack of clean water, inadequate housing, environmental dangers, and nutrition are some of the recognized mechanisms by which health inequalities are expressed in poor children in the developing countries. Damp and inadequate housing, dangerous living conditions, and pollution (Chapter 11) affect poor families in developed countries disproportionately, with adverse effects on their children's health. These mechanisms, through which health inequalities are expressed, have not figured greatly in the causal debate; in contrast, nutrition has joined smoking as one of the foci of this debate in the UK.

Table 22.4 shows a summary of the results of a survey of poor families carried out by the National Children's Homes (NCH) (National Children Homes

Table 22.4 *NCH poverty and nutrition survey, 1991*

The survey
The Food Commission were engaged to work with NCH Policy Unit in conducting the first nationwide study of nutrition for children and their families on low incomes.
In order to assess how families fare on low incomes, NCH gathered information from a total of 354 families with children under five in January 1991. In order to establish a complete picture four separate surveys were undertaken. These were:

- *Information on food expenditure, food consumption, and goods bought.* Detailed questionnaire parents and children under five were completed by 354 families using 52 NCH centres.

- *Detailed nutrition information on diet.* In-depth interviews on nutrition and diet were undertaken with 19 families by a community nutritionist in three NCH Family Centres near Nottingham, Oxford, and Newcastle.

- *Shopping basket survey.* Detailed questionnaire of food costs that identified the differences in costs between buying a 'healthy' basket of food—representing those foods which made up a nutritionally healthy diet—contrasted with the cost of an 'unhealthy' basket. Information was collected on the cost of shopping from the food shops most regularly used by the families using 43 NCH Family Centres in locations ranging from inner city estates to rural areas.

- *The role of NCH in providing advice and supplementing diet.* Information on the nutritional health advice and the food provided by 47 NCH projects.

Key findings

- 1 in 5 parents (73) said they had gone hungry in the last month, December 1990, because they did 'not have enough money' to buy food. 44 per cent (151) of the parents said they had gone short of food in the past year in order to ensure other members of the family had enough.

- 1 in 10 children under five (33) had gone without food in the last month because of lack of money. Nearly 1 in 4 had gone without food during the month because they did not like the food on offer. When money is tight, if a child does not like what is on offer, it may not be possible to offer an alternative.

Table 22.4 *(cont.)*

- No parent or child in the detailed nutritional study was eating a healthy diet—the diet recommended by nutritionists for a healthy life. Two-thirds of the children and over half of the parents were eating nutritionally poor diets. Of these, a third of parents and a quarter of children were eating very poor diets.

- The cost difference for a family of three on a healthy and unhealthy shopping basket was on average £5 per week. This was one fifth of the total weekly expenditure on food of families living on Income Support. The cost of food was highest and the differences in cost between healthy and unhealthy shopping baskets greatest, in rural areas.

- The average amount of money spent on food per person per week in the sample was under £10.00. The national average expenditure on food is over £13.00 comprising only 12.4 per cent of household expenditure. For the families surveyed, food comprised over 35 per cent of total household expenditure. Differences in the costs of healthy and unhealthy foods mean that at this level of expenditure it is virtually impossible for low income families to have a healthy diet.

- Poor diet was directly correlated with food expenditure. The survey showed that there was no evidence to suggest that parents are ignorant about what constitutes a healthy diet. They were unable to provide themselves or their families with an adequate diet because of their income.

1991) which is a charitable organization originally established to provide for abandoned and orphaned children and now providing a national network of family centres serving deprived areas. The publication of these results prompted a junior minister in the UK government to comment that the findings arose because of the unhealthy eating habits of the poor and their failure to 'shop around' for the cheapest food. The results of this survey and a growing number of others suggest that poor families are not only aware of healthy foods but within their limited resources purchase a greater percentage of healthy foods than high-income families (Blackburn 1991). However, what they buy is directly related to the resources available to spend on food, and healthy foods, at least in the UK, are more expensive than unhealthy foods (Lobstein 1988). A study in Valencia, Spain, comparing supermarket prices in two neighbourhoods, shows that within the same supermarket chain prices are higher for 'healthier' foods in the poorer area (Vaandrager 1990). Equally, in the UK, there is evidence that food in the shops to which the poor have easy access is more expensive and of poorer quality than in the supermarkets which are often difficult to reach without a car (Cole-Hamilton and Lang 1986).

It is interesting to note that the proportion of income spent on food by the poor families in the NCH Survey is 35 per cent compared with the average of 12 per cent for the whole population; 35 per cent is the median proportion of income spent on food by families in the group of countries, identified in the UNICEF publication *The state of the world's children*, with a middle level of rates of under-five mortality. It suggests that in nutritional terms, the experience of the poor in the UK is closer to that of families in much poorer countries than that of the 'average' UK family.

Available evidence suggests that far from having a 'free choice' of diet, the poor in developed countries are limited directly by their resources and not by ignorance or unhealthy eating habits. Health-related behaviours are intimately related to social circumstances and social environment and in some cases are a direct marker of disadvantage. Though alteration of lifestyle is an important component of the reduction in health inequalities, if it becomes an alternative to improvements in living conditions and the reduction in relative poverty, then health promotion is in danger of 'victim blaming' and can become an obstruction to necessary preventive approaches to health inequalities created by poverty and disadvantage.

Approaches to reducing health inequalities

Health services alone have a marginal effect on health inequalities. These are primarily determined by structural differences in society and by governmental social policy. However, health services can contribute positively to reduction of inequality in conjunction with other sectors and by instituting changes within their own structures.

On a simple level, practitioners can modify the services they offer by ensuring that they are accessible and acceptable to poor families. The simple expedient of taking services to isolated and deprived areas and ensuring a high quality primary care service has been evaluated in developing countries and its value confirmed. Accessibility also implies low or no cost to the family. Acceptability requires consideration of the perceptions of poor families of their own needs. Community participation and diagnosis (Chapter 34) are the most developed forms of this approach and a move by the child health services towards this model would constitute a major contribution to reducing inequalities. Even where this model is not fully established, child health practitioners can enhance service acceptability by deliberately setting out to reduce the barriers to service use which the poor currently experience as a result of their overall lack of power within society. Child health practitioners should attempt to empower rather than disempower parents. Genuine partnership in the care of their children is one means of achieving this aim (Chapter 33).

Though important for individual families using the services, the approach of individual practitioners cannot compensate for the effects of poor housing, suboptimal nutrition, and the other factors which contribute to health inequalities. Intersectoral plans and targets based on *HFA 2000* need to be set and enacted to improve living and playing conditions for children and to reduce accidents. Examples of the potential of such approaches for reducing environmental dangers to children in disadvantaged areas are outline in Chapter 12. Societies and their governments have a responsibility equal to that of parents to provide children with healthy contexts for living. This does not imply the absence of risk but the reduction of unnecessary risk.

Intersectoral plans and programmes are a political as well as a health responsibility. Financial resources and political will are required to underpin local initiatives. Child health practitioners need to become active advocates for children, especially those disempowered by the effects of poverty and deprivation. Advocacy does not imply 'speaking for the poor' but enabling the poor to speak for themselves and lending expert authority to their voice. Local and national professional organizations representing child health workers should highlight the situation of poor children and advocate social policy solutions which benefit children from poor families and which are acceptable to poor families themselves.

On a European level, child health workers through organizations such as the European Society for Social Paediatrics can exert a powerful influence on political and social policy to support and enhance local and national initiatives designed to reduce health inequalities. Child health inequalities, though resistant, are not inevitable; experience from Sweden (Kohler and Jakobsson 1991) and Japan (Wilkinson 1986) amongst other countries confirms that social policy designed to reduce relative poverty is effective in reducing health inequalities.

Preparation of this chapter has been hampered by lack of comparable data on both the extent and the effects of child poverty. Standardized European data as well as good quality local data are essential. National and European organizations urgently need to address this issue if progress towards reducing health inequalities is to be adequately monitored.

Conclusion

This chapter has outlined the evidence for poverty amongst European children and its effect on their health. We have drawn attention to the causal debate which has influenced, at least in the UK, the measures taken to overcome inequalities in child health and have indicated some of the strategies available to individual practitioners and services wishing to reduce the effects of poverty on child health. Poverty remains one of the most powerful determinants of poor health outcomes for children and its reduction is the legitimate concern of all child health workers. Information is vital in persuading politicians of the importance of poverty as a health determinant; systematic data collection across Europe is an urgent priority if the extent of and trends in child poverty are to be monitored and if strategies for reductions in health inequalities are to be evaluated.

References

Blackburn, C. (1991). *Poverty and health: working with families.* Open University Press, Milton Keynes, UK.

Brooke, O.G., Ross Anderson, H., Bland, J.M., Peacock, J.L., and Stewart, C.M. (1989). Effects on birth weight of smoking, alcohol, caffeine, socioeconomic factors and psychosocial stress. *British Medical Journal*, **298**, 795–801.

Cole-Hamilton, I. and Lang, T. (1986). *Tightening belts: a report on the impact of poverty on food.* London Food Commission, London.

Cornia, G.A. (1990). Child poverty and deprivation in industrialised countries: recent trends and policy options. *Innocenti Occasional Papers, Number 2.* UNICEF and International Child Development Centre, Florence, Italy.

Davie, R., Butler N., and Golding J. (1992). *From birth to seven.* Longmans, London.

Department of Health and Social Security (1976). *Prevention and health: everybody's business.* HMSO, London.

Dowding, W.M. and Barry, C. (1990). Cerebral palsy: social class differences in prevalence in relation to birthweight and severity of disability. *Journal of Epidemiology and Community Health*, **44**, 191–5.

EC Commission (1991). *Final report on the second European poverty programme 1985–89.* EC Commission, Brussels.

Eveleth, P.B. and Tanner, J.M. (1976). *Worldwide variations in human growth (International Biological Programme, 8).* Cambridge University Press, Cambridge.

Golding, J. and Butler, N. (1984). The socio-economic factor. *Child Health*, **3**, 31–46.

Golding, J. and Butler, N. (1986). *From birth to five.* Pergamon, Oxford.

Graham, H. (1989). Women and smoking in the United Kingdom: the implication for health promotion. *Health Promotion*, **3**, 4 No. 4, 371–82.

Graham, H. (1992). *Smoking amongst working class mothers with children: final report of project funded by the Department of Health.* Department of Applied Social Studies, University of Warwick, UK.

Grand, J. (1991). *The state of the world's children 1991.* UNICEF and Oxford University Press, Oxford.

Gulliford, M.C., Chinn, S., Rona, R.J. (1991). Social environment and height: England and Scotland 1987 and 1988. *Archives of Disease in Childhood*, **66**, 235–41.

Gustafsson, B. (1989). Poverty in Sweden 1975–1985. In *Welfare trends in Scandinavia*, (ed. E.S. Hansen, S. Ringen, H. Usiralo, and R. Erikson).

Hobcraft, J.N., McDonald J.W., Rutstein S.O. (1984). Socio-economic factors in infant and child mortality: a cross-national comparison. *Population Studies*, **38**, 193–223.

Kohler, L., Jakobsson, G. (1991). *Children's health in Sweden.* Swedish National Board of Health and Welfare, Stockholm.

Lobstein, T. (1988). *Poor children and cheap calories.* (Community Paediatric Group Newsletter, Autumn 1988, No. 4) British Paediatric Association, London.

London Weekend Television (1991). *Breadline Britain 1990s: the findings of a television survey.* LWT, London.

Mack, J., Lansley, S. (1984). *Poor Britain.* George Allen and Unwin, London.

Mitchell, D. (1990). *The efficiency and effectiveness of income transfer programmes in ten OECD countries.* (Luxembourg Income Study Working Paper, No. 64.) Centre for population, poverty and policy studies, Walfendange, Luxembourg.

National Children's Homes (1991). *NCH poverty and nutrition survey, 1991.* NCH, London.
O'Higgins, M., Jenkins, S. (1988). *Poverty in Europe.* European Programme to Combat Poverty, Centre for the Analysis of Social Policy, University of Bath, UK.
Pamuk, E.R. (1988). Social class inequality in infant mortality in England and Wales from 1921–1980. *European Journal of Population Studies,* **4**, 1–21.
Saraceno, C. (1990). Child poverty and deprivation in Italy: 1950 to present. *Innocenti Papers, Number 6.* UNICEF and International Child Development Centre, Florence.
Stjerno, S. (1985). *Den moderna fattigdommen.* Universitetsforlaget, Oslo.
Townsend, P. (1979). *Poverty in the United Kingdom.* Pelican, London.
Townsend, P. (1991). *The poor are poorer: a statistical report on changes in the living standards of rich and poor in the UK 1979–89.* University of Bristol, Department of Social Policy and Social Planning, UK.
Townsend, P., Davidson, N. (1982). *Inequalities in health: the Black report.* Penguin, London.
Townsend, P., Phillimore, P., Beattie, A. (1988). *Health and deprivation.* Croom Helm, Beckenham, UK.
Vaandrager, L. (1990). *The nutrition and supermarket research in two different social class areas of Valencia.* School of Public Health (IVESP), Valencia, Spain.
Wadsworth, M. (1991). *The imprint of time.* Clarendon, Oxford.
Wilkinson, R.G. (ed.) (1986). Income and mortality. In *Class and health: research and longitudinal data.* Tavistock, London.

23 Low birth-weight infants
S. Pauline Verloove-Vanhorick

All newborn infants are vulnerable: without extensive caretaking they cannot possibly survive. Their health and well-being depends on the amount and quality of the care provided by their parents or others: nutrition, protection, love, and attention are the main needs of all newborn babies.

Most infants are born after a gestational period of 37–42 weeks from the first day of the last menstrual period, with a birth-weight that varies between 2500 and 4500 g. Around 8 to 10 per cent of babies, however, are born too soon (preterm) and/or too small (with low birth-weight). These infants are more vulnerable, especially during their first few weeks of life, but later on as well.

Definition of the problem

The aetiology of preterm delivery and low birth-weight is still largely unknown. Demographic, socio-economic, and cultural–behavioural factors have been shown to be associated with preterm birth, as have maternal health, age, and lifestyle (Kliegman *et al.* 1990). In most cases, however, the cause of preterm delivery remains unknown. Whatever the cause, preterm infants are more vulnerable than full-term infants. Their organ systems are immature, resulting in disturbances in breathing, circulation, feeding, and temperature control. Special care is required to meet these infants' needs. The less mature the infant, the less capable it is of even the most basic vital functions. Artificial support of respiration and nutrition is required for such very preterm babies. Low birth-weight in newborn infants may be the result of one or more of several aetiological pathways: they may be either born at term but growth-retarded, genetically small, or congenitally malformed, or they may be born preterm with an appropriate weight for their gestational age.

Due to this mixture of very different types of low birth-weight, studies on epidemiology, treatment, and outcome may show large differences depending on the composition of the group studied. A relatively low weight at birth due to placental dysfunction in an otherwise mature infant seldom causes a need for artificial support systems. It does imply, however, that nutritional deficiency existed during fetal life, which, in turn, may carry other risks.

Gestational age used to be difficult to assess with certainty. Many mother-to-be were uncertain of the exact date of their last menstrual period. In addition, many young couples tampered intentionally with this date in order to create a period of nine months between their date of marriage and the expected date of delivery. These *so-called* 7-months' infants were very healthy indeed. Such uncertainties about gestational age caused paediatricians to depend on birth-weight rather than on gestational age when estimating the risks that newborn infants incurred. However, in developed countries gestational age can nowadays be estimated quite reliably during pregnancy with early pregnancy testing and ultrasound measurements of the fetus. The need for tampering with dates has also disappeared since 10 to 50 per cent of all births happen to unmarried couples (Yearbook of Nordic Statistics 1985; CBS 1991). When gestational age remains uncertain, the paediatrician's scoring of physical and neurological characteristics of the newborn infant can help to provide an estimate (Dubowitz *et al.* 1970; Ballard *et al.* 1979). Therefore, gestational age is now the more logical parameter to use as indicator for vulnerability. For the sake of historical comparisons, though, birth-weight has to be used as well.

Incidence

The incidence of **preterm birth** (for definitions see Table 23.1) in European countries has been estimated to be around six per cent (Alberman 1977; Kloosterman 1977; Piekkala *et al.* 1986; Rantakallio *et al.* 1991). In the USA it ranges from seven to nine per cent (NCHS 1983; van den Berg and Oechsli 1984). Very preterm birth at less than 32 weeks gestation is reported to occur in 0.6 to 1.5 per cent of live births in Europe (Hoffman and Bakketeig 1984; Verloove and Verwey 1987), whereas in the USA an incidence of 1.8 per cent has been found (NCHS 1985). Births before 28 weeks account for approximately 0.2 per cent of live births (Macfarlane *et al.* 1988).

In many countries in Europe as well as elsewhere attempts have been made to achieve significant reduction in the (very) preterm and low birth-weight rate, and, hence, in infant mortality. These attempts have been only partially successful. In a part of France, for instance, the preterm birth rate fell from 5.4 per cent in 1974 to 3.7 per cent in 1982 during an intervention study with a programme for prevention of preterm deliveries (Papiernik *et al.* 1985). During the same time, the rate in France as a whole fell from 8.2 to 5.2 per cent (Rumeau-Rouquette *et al.* 1984). In Finland, the incidence decreased from 9.5 to 5.3 per cent in the period between 1966 and 1985. Most countries, however, have shown little or no recent change (Lumley 1987*a*). This is possibly due to successful preventive strategies on the one hand, but also increased recording of very preterm birth occurring simultaneously.

During the past decades, gradual changes in prognosis have developed concurrently with and closely connected to technological development of obstetric and neonatal intensive care. Consequently, infants who used to be considered abortions or late fetal deaths are nowadays treated with intensive neonatal care and, thus, appear in the live-born statistics. This development does not happen at

Table 23.1 *Definitions*

The following definitions and recommendations have been given by the World Health Organization (WHO 1977) and have been adapted by FIGO (1976, 1982).

Live birth
Live birth is the complete expulsion or extraction from its mother of a product of conception, irrespective of the duration of the pregnancy, which, after such separation, breathes or shows any other evidence of life, such as beating of the heart, pulsation of the umbilical cord, or definite movement of voluntary muscles, whether or not the umbilical cord has been cut or the placenta is attached; each product of such a birth is considered live born.

Gestational age
The duration of gestation is measured from the first day of the last normal menstrual period. Gestational age is expressed in completed days or completed weeks (e.g. events occurring 280 to 286 days after the onset of the last normal menstrual period are considered to have occurred at 40 weeks of gestation)

Birth-weight
The first weight of the newborn obtained after birth. This weight should be measured preferably within the first hour of life before significant postnatal weight loss has occurred.

Preterm
Less than 37 completed weeks (less than 259 days).

Low birth-weight (LBW)
Less than 2500 g (up to and including 2499 g).

Early neonatal death
Death of a live-born infant during the first seven completed days (168 hours) of life.

Late neonatal death
Death of a live-born infant after seven completed days but before 28 completed days of life. (WHO, approved by FIGO, with the modification of 'completed days'.)

Neonatal death
Death of a live-born infant before 28 completed days of life.

In addition to these, FIGO (1976, 1986) issued the following recommendations.

Low birth-weight (LBW)
500 g to less than 2500 g (up to and including 2499 g).

Very low birth-weight (VLBW)
500 g to less than 1500 g (up to and including 1499 g).

Table 23.1 (*cont.*)

Extremely low birth-weight (ELBW)
500 g to less than 1000 g (up to and including 999 g).

The definitions mentioned above do not adequately cover all circumstances. In the absence of recommendations by WHO or FIGO, we use the following additional definitions.

Post-neonatal death
Death from 28 completed days to less than one year from birth (i.e. up to and including 364 days) (Pharoah 1976; Hack *et al.* 1980; Chiswick 1986).

In-hospital death
Death of a live-born infant during the hospital stay following birth and before discharge home, irrespective of transferral between hospitals within this period.

Very preterm
Less than 32 completed weeks of gestation (less than 224 days).

Extremely preterm
Less than 28 completed weeks of gestation (less than 196 days).

---

the same pace in various countries, or even regions, which puts some restrictions on (inter)national comparisons of incidence and outcome (Working group on the very low birth-weight infant 1990).

Low birth-weight incidence may vary considerably according to different ethnic factors and socio-economic conditions (Rooth 1980; Macfarlane 1980; Priolisi 1980). In Europe, low birth-weight rates are reported to be around six to seven per cent (Public Health 1987).

In the USA, the proportion of babies of low birth-weight was 6.8 per cent in 1982 (5.6 per cent of white infants and 12.4 per cent of black infants) (Wegman 1985). No recent changes have been found, the percentages in 1988 being 5.6 and 13.0 respectively (Wegman 1990). Besides ethnic differences in low birth-weight rates, there are large differences in rates between states within the USA (Kliegman *et al.* 1990).

The incidence of very low birth-weight in live-born infants has been described to be 0.5 per cent in France (Papiernik *et al.* 1985), 0.7 per cent in the Netherlands (Verloove and Verwey 1987), 1.0 per cent in England and Wales (Public Health 1987), 2.0 per cent in Hungary (Lee *et al.* 1980), and 1.1 in the USA (McCormick 1985; Kliegman *et al.* 1990).

Health care provisions

In 1922, a 'premature infant station' was opened in Chicago (Hess 1953), the objective being 'to provide care for premature infants born in homes or hospitals not equipped with the necessities for their complete care'. Stewart et al. (1981) described this as 'phase I': in the absence of special treatment, few very low birth-weight infants survived and almost none weighing less than 1000 g; most of the survivors were said to be healthy (Douglas and Gear 1976).

In 1951, a new unit was opened in Chicago (Hess 1953). Now, a permanent, well trained nursing staff, aseptic nursing techniques, maintenance of body temperature, careful and minimal handling, oxygen therapy, use of breast-milk, and careful feeding regulation were seen as significant factors in neonatal care. This was refered to as 'phase II' and took place during the 1950s and early 1960s (Rider et al. 1957; Stewart et al. 1981). It led to a gradual decrease in mortality, initially accompanied by an increase in the number of handicapped survivors. Technical progress was provided by introduction of the incubator, the humidifier, skin temperature monitoring, glucose infusion, and tube feeding.

After 1965 (Reynolds 1978), intensive care was introduced successively in centres all over the world (Stahlman 1984). 'Phase III' had begun, characterized by a falling mortality rate achieved 'by more rational use of modern knowledge and increasing sophistication of obstetric and neonatal care', without an increase in the proportion of handicapped infants (Stewart et al. 1981). In the years since then, the care has gradually been intensified: the initial cardiorespiratory monitoring, intermittent positive pressure ventilation, intravascular oxygen monitoring, exchange transfusion, orogastric feeding, and servo-controlled incubators were followed by continuous positive pressure ventilation, transcutaneous oxygen monitoring, phototherapy, transpyloric tube feeding, total parenteral nutrition, radiant heating, and diagnostic use of ultrasound. The most recent advance in the treatment of lung immaturity by preventive surfactant administration shows promising results (Merritt and Hallman 1988; Collaborative European Multicentre Study Group 1988; Kendig et al. 1991).

Simultaneously with these medical and nursing developments, the understanding has grown that the natural process of infant–parent bonding should be aided as much as possible. Because the circumstances in a neonatal intensive care ward put a severe strain on both the infant and the parents, special measures are required to promote their interaction. The role of the parents has therefore changed during the past decades. They used to be allowed a glimpse only now and then from behind a viewing glass. In contrast, nowadays in many units parents take part in the daily care for their baby however tiny it is and even during artificial ventilation. Breast-feeding is encouraged, for nutritional and immunological reasons as well as for the psychosocial benefits for mother and child. Even if expressing and tube feeding the breast-milk is necessary during the first weeks, many mothers nowadays breast-feed their preterm babies for many months thereafter.

Prognosis of preterm birth and low birth-weight

In the first half of this century, survival of premature infants was the exception rather than the rule (Ylppö 1919; Duyzings 1935; Blegen 1953). Especially in the very preterm or very low birth-weight category, mortality was reported to be between 70 and 95 per cent (Looft 1928; Baedorf 1937; Tyson 1946). A proportion of the surviving children was described as handicapped, varying from one per cent (Wall 1913) to the majority (Capper 1928a,b). Neonatal intensive care as described above has changed the prognosis of these infants enormously (Stahlman 1984). At a gestational age of 32 weeks or more, mortality is nowadays only slightly higher than in term births (Yu 1987), and the same holds true for newborn infants with a birth-weight over 1500 g (ICE 1992). For very preterm and very low birth-weight infants, the risk of death or disability is still considerably increased compared to more mature infants with appropriate weight.

Studies from neonatal intensive care units show a decline in very low birth-weight mortality from around 50 per cent in the sixties to 20 per cent in the late eighties (Verloove and Verwey 1987; van Zeben 1989). The greatest progress in reducing mortality, from 46 per cent to 28 per cent, was achieved in the 750–1000 g category (Ehrenhaft et al. 1989), while in the 1000–1500 g group a decline from 18 to 10 per cent occurred.

Very preterm birth is still the major cause of infant mortality in developed countries. Pooled data from three population-based studies performed during the past decade in England (Mersey region), The Netherlands, and Scotland, indicate mortality to be 95 per cent in the less-than-24 weeks category, 86 per cent in the 24–25 weeks category, 59 per cent in the 26–27 weeks category, 35 per cent at 28–29 weeks, and 20 per cent at 30–31 weeks (Powell et al. 1986; Verloove et al. 1986; Macfarlane et al. 1988). Similar data for the category below 29 weeks were established by the European Community collaborative study of outcome of pregnancy between 22 and 28 weeks' gestation (Working group on the very low birth-weight infant 1990).

Mortality after discharge from hospital is higher as well in these infants compared with full-term, normal birth-weight infants (Hack et al. 1980; Yu et al. 1984). These deaths may be caused by sequelae of preterm birth, of neonatal treatment, or of genetic factors (e.g. bronchopulmonary dysplasia, congenital malformation, or severe neurological dysfunction with epilepsy) (van Zeben et al. 1989). Cot death has been found to be an important component of late mortality in preterm infants. The cot death rate in infants born very preterm or with a very low birth-weight was 11.2 per 1000 live births and 15.0 per 1000 discharged infants, compared with one to two per 1000 infants in the general population (Wierenga et al. 1990). It is estimated to account for 15–20 per cent of all cot deaths.

Sequelae in surviving children

The greatest concern of those engaged in the care of high-risk babies and of the majority of their parents is the risk of survival with severe defects (Alberman *et al.* 1985; McCormick 1985; Aylward *et al.* 1989). Population-based studies, however, have shown that the clear increase in birth-weight-specific survival did not result in an increase of the percentage of major morbidity in survivors. Long term follow-up studies demonstrated that minor degrees of morbidity as well as developmental problems often arise at school or pre-school age. Morbidity can be caused by adverse factors in the pre-, peri-, or postnatal period or by any combination of them; over time, shifts in severity can originate from socio-economic, cultural, as well as biological developments. 'Major' morbidity is generally reported in terms of cerebral palsy, mental retardation, and abnormalities of vision and hearing, while 'minor' degrees of morbidity usually include minor neurological dysfunction, respiratory problems, behavioural disturbances and delay in school achievement. Although understandable, such categorization is not very helpful when estimating the impact of morbidity on the daily life of a developing child.

The World Health Organization (WHO 1980) has issued a classification according to the following definitions.

- An impairment is any loss or abnormality of psychological, physiological, or anatomical structure or function.

- A disability is any restriction or lack (resulting from an impairment) of ability to perform an activity in the manner or within the range considered normal for a human being.

- A handicap is a disadvantage for a given individual, resulting from an impairment or a disability, that limits or prevents the fulfilment of a role that is normal (depending on age, sex, and social and cultural factors) for that individual.

Thus, impairment represents disturbance at organ level, disability the consequences of impairment for function and activity, and handicap the social disadvantage experienced by the individual as a result of the disability.

In the Dutch follow-up study of very preterm, very low birth-weight infants, a child was considered impaired, if it was diagnosed in any of the ten areas that were examined with impairment(s) not causing any disability. A child was considered disabled if it was diagnosed with either a disability or if a multiplicity of impairments (in several areas) caused loss of function or activity. A child was considered handicapped, if it was diagnosed with a handicap or if multiplicity of disabilities caused a social disadvantage. All children needing special education were considered handicapped. A handicap was considered minor if it did not seriously interfere with daily life and did not require extensive care-taking;

major when it did interfere with daily life and when it caused a life of dependency or institutionalization. In case of doubt, the child was allocated to the more severe group to avoid underestimation. Thus, the WHO classification has proved to be a useful tool in reporting the follow-up of surviving very preterm or very low birth-weight infants (Veen *et al.* 1991).

Table 23.2 provides an overview of the prevalence of morbidity in several areas, as stated in the literature. Most researchers describe specific

Table 23.2 *Prevalence of morbidity in populations of children, surviving very preterm or very low birth-weight birth*

Morbidity	Percentage	Group	Reference
Cerebral palsy	5–8	VLBW	Saigal *et al.* 1984; Kitchen *et al.* 1984; Johnson *et al.* 1987; Stanley and Watson 1988; van Zeben *et al.* 1989; Hagberg *et al.* 1989; Riikonen *et al.* 1989
Minor neurological dysfunction	30–40	preterm	Hadders-Algra and Touwen 1990
Blindness (nearly)	2–13	VLBW	Avery and Glass 1988; Cats 1990; Gibson *et al.* 1990
Squint	20–30	preterm	Cats 1990
Loss of stereoscopy	2–21	preterm	Peckham 1986; Cats 1990
Deafness (sensorineural)	0.3–4	VLBW	Saigal *et al.* 1982; Lloyd 1984; Saigal *et al.* 1989; van Zeben *et al.* 1989
Bronchopulmonary dysplasia (oxygen-dependent)	0.5–19	VLBW	Avery *et al.* 1987; Horbar *et al.* 1988
School failure	22–54	VLBW	Hunt *et al.* 1982; Vohr and Garcia 1985; Calame *et al.* 1986; Lindahl *et al.* 1988; Lloyd *et al.* 1988; Portnoy *et al.* 1988; Marlow *et al.* 1989; Abel-Smith and Knight-Jones 1990; Largo *et al.* 1990
Handicaps (major and minor)	22	<1500 g	Saigal *et al.* 1982
	12	<1500 g	Powell *et al.* 1986
	21	<1500 g	Johnson *et al.* 1987
	12	<1500 g	Piekkala *et al.* 1988
	15	<32 weeks	Veen *et al.* 1991
	15	<1500 g	Veen *et al.* 1991
Disabilities (including handicaps)	27	<32 weeks	Veen *et al.* 1991
	29	<1500 g	Veen *et al.* 1991
Impairments (including disabilities and handicaps)	76	<32 weeks	Veen *et al.* 1991
	79	<1500 g	Veen *et al.* 1991

disease entities. Veen *et al.* (1991) used the functioning of the child as a whole in the terms of WHO. From these data it becomes clear that the majority of very preterm and very low birth-weight infants survive without handicap. Data on disabilities in the Dutch population at large (data from the Dutch continuous health enquiry; CBS 1990) show that 17 per cent of all children aged 5 to 14 have some 'physical' disability (i.e. including four per cent severe disabilities causing handicap, but without mental disorders and without institutionalized children). Adjusting for the same criteria, 23 per cent of 'physically' disabled children (including 13 per cent handicaps) were found in the very preterm, very low birth-weight population (Veen *et al.* 1991). Although considerably higher, this is not an overwhelming difference. In relation to the small number of cases involved, the contribution of very preterm and very low birth-weight infants to the absolute number of disabled and handicapped children is very low.

Impairments were found in another 50 per cent of the Dutch very preterm very low birth-weight cohort, according to the WHO definition. Since these impairments do not cause disabilities or handicaps, and since in a small control group the impairment rate was 52 per cents as well, they seem to be of limited importance as an outcome measure for follow-up studies of very preterm or very low birth weight studies.

As shown in Table 23.2, neurological abnormalities (cerebral palsy and minor neurological dysfunction) are an important component of disabilities and handicaps. However, in infants and toddlers it is difficult to predict the neurological outcome at pre-school age (den Ouden 1991). The same holds true for behaviour and school achievement. Therefore, a specialized follow-up programme at least well into school age is needed for all these high-risk infants (Veen *et al.* 1991; den Ouden 1991). Such a programme should include close medical supervision, ongoing developmental assessment, and screening, thereby addressing emerging vulnerabilities or deficits as early as possible, and impeding developmental progress minimally (Desmond *et al.* 1980).

The parents need additional support in the upbringing of these children. Due to the perinatal problems they have experienced, their confidence in their child and in themselves is affected and the rearing of such a child is not straightforward. The advice and support that is routinely available in many countries in the operative child health care systems is usually insufficient to meet the parents' needs, even if the child appears quite normal. Moreover, many of these children do have some slight abnormalities in neurological function, speech development, or behaviour for which the parents want guidance, and the children frequently require hospital readmissions and other use of health services (Mutch *et al.* 1986; Skeoch *et al.* 1987; van Zeben *et al.* 1991). Since parental education, lifestyle, and social-economic status play an important role as well, some families may need more help in order to prevent further inequities in the outcome of their children (Masi 1979). This requires intervention and support programmes for parents or guardians in the performance of their child-rearing responsibilities. A 'parents' society' may play an important role in reaching such goals.

Prevention

In order to prevent adverse outcomes associated with preterm and low birth-weight birth, several options are open for **primary prevention** depending on the presumed aetiology.

First, when biological or hereditary factors are assumed to be the cause of both the untimely birth and death or disability, prevention should be aimed at the period before (genetic counselling) or shortly after conception (induced abortion). In the future, gene therapy may play an important role in the primary prevention of some disorders associated with preterm birth, low birth-weight and adverse outcome.

Second, a fetus may be damaged during pregnancy, with an increased risk of preterm birth, low birth-weight, and later sequelae. At least some of the cases of brain damage resulting in cerebral palsy are thought to have an antenatal origin (Stanley and Alberman 1984; Nelson and Ellenberg 1985, 1986). Parental lifestyle, especially smoking, drinking, socio-economic status, occupation, and maternal age, is known to influence fetal growth as well as length of gestation (Kliegman *et al.* 1990; Verkerk and van Noord 1991). Programmes aiming at the prevention of low birth-weight and preterm birth are reported to have some success (Lumley 1987*b*). In the future, provision of material assistance and support programmes with respect to antenatal care and lifestyle may further reduce preterm birth and fetal growth retardation as well as fetal damage.

Third, death or disabilities may be caused by diseases due to immaturity of the newborn infant. Neonatal morbidity, such as respiratory distress causing hypoxaemia, or disturbances of cerebral circulation causing periventricular leucomalacia and cerebral haemorrhage, are associated with increased mortality and later disabilities. Such neonatal disorders should, therefore, be prevented whenever possible, by intensive treatment starting well before birth (obstetrical intensive care) and immediately after birth (neonatal intensive care).

Sufficient facilities should be available to provide adequate care for all infants in need of such care (Dunn 1985). At present, this situation has not yet been reached in many countries (Health Council of The Netherlands 1991). Because of the high immediate costs involved in employing neonatal intensive care facilities, continuing shortage of neonatal intensive care cots is expected in many countries in as well as outside Europe, resulting in suboptimal care and unnecessary deaths and disabilities. Ironically, cost-effectiveness of neonatal intensive care has been demonstrated repeatedly (Boyle *et al.* 1983; Walker *et al.* 1985; Pharoah *et al.* 1988). At the same time, however, there must be scope for withholding or withdrawing neonatal intensive care whenever the prognosis is clearly unfavourable.

Secondary prevention, mainly involving early recognition of disorders threatening to hamper a child's development, is very important in children born preterm or with low birth-weight. Either in the context of a special systematic follow-up programme by developmental paediatricians including neurological, visual, hearing, psychological and educational components or within the framework of community child health care, wherever this offers the mentioned above facilities, surviving preterm and low birth-weight children should be followed closely.

For impaired, disabled, and handicapped children special treatment facilities as well as extra support for their families should be available. Even profound impairment or disability need not necessarily result in handicap. It is, therefore, imperative that such **tertiairy prevention** be given greater prominence in both teaching and research (Pharoah 1990). As a prerequisite, health information systems should be operative to monitor incidence, mortality, and various sequelae of preterm birth and low birth-weight. An essential regional or national indicator of child health is the infant mortality rate according to gestational age or birth-weight. In some European countries, even these basic parameters are currently not available (NCHS 1992).

Future developments

Presently, the reported incidence of preterm and low birth-weight live births is influenced by several factors that partly have an opposing effect. Thus, although prevention programmes are at least partly effective, the incidence remains stable due to increased reporting of tiny live-born infants that in the past were regarded pre-viable. Similarly, the decrease in total perinatal and infant mortality seems only to be modest in many countries in Europe (Public Health 1987; ICE 1992), probably due to the very high death rate in the extremely preterm category that formerly did not enter the statistics on live-born infants.

There is some reason for caution. While on the one hand the public supports antenatal prevention programmes and neonatal intensive care facilities, demographic and social developments may take the opposite direction.

The currently older maternal age at which child-bearing is started carries an increased risk of twinning and preterm birth. It also is accompanied by lower fecundity (van Noord *et al.* 1991), resulting in an increased demand for assisted reproduction including gamete intrafallopian transfer (GIFT) and *in vitro* fertilization (IVF). Such procedures again increase the risk of (grand) multiple births and preterm births and, thereby, the need of medical and social services (van Duivenboden *et al.* 1991). In view of the limited resources available even in developed countries, the time may have come to emphasize the advantages of child-bearing at an age that is biologically optimal, that is between 20 and 30 years. By enabling women to combine work with a family, the need to postpone child-bearing may lessen and resources may be used more adequately. There is still room for the improvement of antenatal care, of postnatal (intensive) care, and of socio-medical care, surveillance and support of the surviving preterm and low birth-weight children. Continuing efforts shall be needed to effectuate such improvements and to achieve equal opportunities in life for these vulnerable children.

Acknowledgements

The author wishes to thank Dr S. Buitendijk, Dr R. Hirasing, and Professor J.H. Ruys for their comments on an earlier draft of the manuscript, and Mrs R. Huls for typing it.

References

Abel-Smith, A.E., and Knight-Jones, E.B. (1990). The abilities of very low-birthweight children and their classroom controls. *Developmental Medicine and Child Neurology* **32**, 590–601.

Alberman, E. (1977). Sociologic factors and birthweight in Great Britain. In *The epidemiology of prematurity*, (ed. D.M. Reed, and F.J. Stanley), pp. 146–56. Urban and Schwarzenberg, Baltimore, MA.

Alberman, E., Benson, J., and Kani, W. (1985). Disabilities in survivors of low birthweight. *Archives of Disease in Childhood*, **60**, 913–19.

Avery, G.B. and Glass, P. (1988). Retinopathy of prematurity: what causes it? *Clinics in Perinatology* **15**, 917–28.

Avery, M.E., Tooley, W.H., Keller, J.B., Hurd, S.S., Bryan, M.H., Cotton, R.B. *et al.* (1987). Is chronic lung disease in low birth weight infants preventable? A survey of eight centers. *Pediatrics* **79**, 26–30.

Aylward, G.P., Pfeiffer, S.I., Wright, A., and Verhulst, S.J. (1989). Outcome studies of low birth weight infants published in the last decade: a metaanalysis. *Journal of Pediatrics* **115**, 515–20.

Baedorf, K. (1937). Zur Frase des 'Aufzuchtwertes', besonders der geistigen Entwicklung Unreifgeborener unter 1700 g Geburtsgewicht. *Zeitschrift für Kinderheilkunde* **59**, 218–35.

Ballard, J.L., Kazmaier Novak, K., and Driver, M. (1979). A simplified score for assessment of fetal maturation of newly born infants. *Journal of Pediatrics* **95**, 769–74.

Blegen, S.D. (1953). The premature child. The incidence, aetiology, mortality and the fate of the survivors. *Acta Paediatrica* **42** (Suppl.), 88.

Boyle, M.H., Torrance, G.W., Sinclair, J.C., and Horwood S.P. (1983). Economic evaluation of neonatal intensive care of very-low-birth-weight infants. *The New England Journal of Medicine* **308**, 1330–7.

Calame, A., Fawer, C.L., Claeys, V., Arrazola, L., Ducret, S., and Jaunin, L. (1986). Neurodevelopmental outcome and school performance of very-low-birth-weight infants at 8 years of age. *European Journal of Pediatrics* **145**, 461–6.

Capper, A. (1928*a*). Progress in Pediatrics. The fate and development of the immature and of the premature child. Review of the literature and study of cerebral hemorrhage in the new-born infant. Part I. *American Journal of Diseases of Children* **35**, 262–88.

Capper, A. (1928*b*). Progress in Pediatrics. The fate and development of the immature and of the premature child. Review of the literature and study of cerebral hemorrhage in the new-born infant. Part II. *American Journal of Diseases of Children* **35**, 443–91.

Cats, B.P. (1990). Retinopathy of prematurity: what causes it? *Clinics in Perinatology* **15**, 917–28.

CBS (Centraal Bureau voor de Statistiek) (1990). *Physical disabilities in the Dutch population, 1986/1988*, p. 67. 's-Gravenhage, SDU-uitgeverij,

CBS (Centraal Bureau voor de Statistiek) (1991). Buitenechtelijke geboorte blijft stijgen. *Maandstatistiek Bevolking CBS*, **2**, 5.
Chiswick, M.L. (1986). Commentary on current World Health Organization definitions used in perinatal statistics. *Archives of Disease in Childhood* **61**, 708–10.
Collaborative European Multicenter Study Group (1988). Surfactant replacement therapy for severe neonatal respiratory distress syndrome: an international randomized clinical trial. *Pediatrics* **82**, 683–91.
den Ouden, A.L. (1991). Early recognition of neurodevelopmental disturbances in very preterm infants. Ph.D. Thesis, State University Leiden.
Desmond, M.M., Wilson, G.S., Alt, E.J., and Fisher, E.S. (1980). The very low birth weight infant after discharge from intensive care: anticipatory health care and developmental course. In *Current problems in pediatrics*, (ed. L. Gluck), pp. 3–59. Year Book Medical Publishers, Chicago.
Douglas, J.W.B. and Gear, R. (1976). Children of low birthweight in the 1946 national cohort. Behaviour and educational achievement in adolescence. *Archives of Disease in Childhood* **51**, 820–7.
Dubowitz, L.S.M., Dubowitz, V., and Goldberg, C. (1970). Clinical assessment of gestational age in the newborn infant. *Journal of Pediatrics* **77**, 1–10.
Dunn, P.M. (1985). Medical and nursing staff in the neonatal care unit. *Lancet* **ii**, 616.
Duyzings, A.J.M. (1935). Ueber die Frühgeburt und das zu frühgeborene Kind. *Archiven für Gynaecology* **159**, 524–36.
Ehrenhaft, P.M., Wagner, J.L., and Herdman, R.C. (1989). Changing prognosis for very low birth weight infants. *Obstetrics and Gynecology* **64**, 528–35.
FIGO (Federation Internationale de Gynécologie et Obstetrie) (1976). List of gynaecologic and obstetrical terms and definitions. *International Journal of Gynaecology and Obstetrics* **14**, 570–6.
FIGO (Fédération Internationale de Gynécologie et Obstetrie) (1982). *Report of the FIGO committee on perinatal mortality and morbidity* (Workshop on monitoring and reporting perinatal mortality and morbidity). FIGO, Geneva.
FIGO (Fédération Internationale de Gynécologie et Obstetrie) (1986). *Report of the FIGO sub-committee on perinatal epidemiology and health statistics* (Workshop in Cairo, November 11–18, 1984, on the methodology of measurement and recording of infant growth in the perinatal period). FIGO, London.
Gibson, D.L., Sheps, S.B., Hong Uh, S., Schechter, M.T., and McCormick, A.Q. (1990). Retinopathy of prematurity-induced blindness: birth weight-specific survival and the new epidemic. *Pediatrics* **86**, 405–12.
Hack, M., Merkatz, I.R., Jones, P.K., and Fanaroff, A.A. (1980). Changing trends of neonatal and postneonatal deaths in very-low-birthweight infants. *American Journal of Obstetrics and Gynecology* **137**, 797–800.
Hadders-Algra, M. and Touwen, B.C.L. (1990). Body measurements, neurological and behavioural development in six-year-old children born preterm and/or small-for-gestational age. *Early Human Development* **22**, 1–13.
Hagberg, B., Hagberg, G., Olow, I., von Wendt, L. (1989). The changing panorama of cerebral palsy in Sweden. V. The birth year period 1979–1982. *Acta Paediatrica Scandinavica* **78**, 283–90.
Health Council of the Netherlands (1991). *Neonatal intensive care: an estimate of needs*. Gezondheidsraad, The Hague. (Summary in English).
Hess, J.H. (1953). Experiences gained in a thirty year study of prematurely born infants. *Pediatrics* **11**, 425–34.

Hoffman, H.J. and Bakketeig, L.S. (1984). Risk factors associated with the occurrence of preterm birth. *Clinical Obstetrics and Gynecology* **27**, 539–52.

Horbar, J.D., McAuliffe, T.L., Adler, S.M., Albersheim, S., Cassady, G. *et al.* (1988). Variability in 28-day outcomes for very low birth weight infants: an analysis of 11 neonatal intensive care units. *Pediatrics* **82**, 554–9.

Hunt, J.V., Tooley, W.H., and Harvin, D. (1982). Learning disabilities in children with birth weights < 1500 grams. *Seminars in Perinatology* **6**, 280–7.

ICE (International Collaborative Effort on Perinatal and Infant Mortality (1992). *Conference Report 30 April–2 May 1990, Bethesda, USA*. NCHS, Hyattsville.

Johnson, M.A., Cox, M., and McKim, E. (1987). Outcome of infants of very low birthweight: a geographically based study. *Canadian Medical Association Journal* **136**, 1157–65.

Kendig, J.W., Notter, R.H., Cox, C., Reubens, L.J., Davis, J.M., Maniscalco, W.M. *et al.* (1991). A comparison of surfactant as immediate prophylaxis and as rescue therapy in newborns of less than 30 weeks' gestation. *The New England Journal of Medicine* **324**, 865–71.

Kitchen, W., Ford, G., Orgill, A., Rickards, A., Astbury, J., Lissenden, J. *et al.* (1984). Outcome in infants with birth weight 500 to 999 gm; a regional study of 1979 and 1980 births. *Journal of Pediatrics* **104**, 921–7.

Kliegman, R.M., Rottman C.J., and Behrman, R.E. (1990). Strategies for the prevention of low birth weight. *American Journal of Obstetrics and Gynecology* **162**, 1073–83.

Kloosterman, G.J. (1977). *De voorplanting van de mens*. Uitgeversmaat schappij Centen, Haarlem.

Largo, R.H., Molinari, L., Kundu, S., Lipp, A., and Duc, G. (1990). Intellectual outcome, speech and school performance in high risk preterm children with birth weight appropriate for gestational age. *European Journal of Pediatrics* **149**, 845–50.

Lee, K.S., Paneth, N., Gartner, L.M., and Pearlman, M. (1980). The very low-birthweight rate: principal predictor of neonatal mortality in industrialized populations. *Journal of Pediatrics* **97**, 759–64.

Lindahl, E., Michelsson, K., Helenius, M., and Parre, M. (1988). Neonatal risk factors and later neurodevelopmental disturbances. *Developmental Medicine and Child Neurology* **30**, 571–89.

Lloyd, B.W. (1984). Outcome of very-low-birthweight babies from Wolverhampton. *Lancet* **ii**, 739–41.

Lloyd, B.W., Wheldall, K., and Perks, D. (1988). Controlled study of intelligence and school performance of very-low-birthweight children from a defined geographical area. *Developmental Medicine and Child Neurology* **30**, 36–42.

Looft, C. (1928). Importance de la naissance avant terme dans l'étiologie des troubles de l'intelligence et du système nerveux chez l'enfant. *Acta Paediatrica* **VII**, 15–59.

Lumley, J. (1987*a*). Epidemiology of prematurity. In *Prematurity*, (ed. V.Y.H. Yu and E.C. Wood), pp. 1–24. Churchill Livingstone, Edinburgh.

Lumley, J. (1987*b*). Prevention of preterm birth. In *Prematurity*, (ed. V.Y.H. Yu and E.C. Wood), pp. 54–75. Churchill Livingstone, Edinburgh.

Macfarlane, A. (1980). Low birthweight revised. *Lancet* **i**, 930–1.

Macfarlane, A., Cole, S., Johnson, A., and Botting, B. (1988). Epidemiology of birth before 28 weeks of gestation. *British Medical Bulletin* **44**, 861–93.

Marlow, N., Roberts, B.L., and Cooke, R.W.I. (1989). Motor skills in extremely low birthweight children at the age of 6 years. *Archives of Disease in Childhood* **64**, 839–47.

Masi, W. (1979). Supplemental stimulation of the premature infant. In *Infants born at risk*, (ed. T.M. Field). SP Medical and Scientific Books, New York.
McCormick, M.C. (1985). The contribution of low birth weight to infant mortality and childhood morbidity. *The New England Journal of Medicine* **312**, 82–90.
Merritt, T.A. and Hallman, M. (1988). Surfactant replacement. *American Journal of Diseases of Children* **142** 1333–9.
Mutch, L., Newdick, M., Lodwick, A., and Chalmers, I. (1986). Secular changes in rehospitalization of very low birthweight infants. *Pediatrics* **78**, 164–71.
NCHS (National Center for Health Statistics) (1983). *Advance report of final natality statistics*. NCHS.
NCHS (National Center for Health Statistics) (1991). *Monthly vital statistics report* Vol. 34, No 6 (suppl.) NCHS, Hyattsville, Maryland.
NCHS (National Center for Health Statistics) (1992). *International health data reference guide*. NCHS, Hyattsville, Maryland.
Nelson, K.B. and Ellenberg, J.H. (1985). Predictors of low and very low birthweight and the relation of these to cerebral palsy. *Journal of the American Medical Association*, **254**, 1473–79.
Nelson, K.B. and Ellenberg, J.H. (1986). Antecedents of cerebral palsy. Multivariate analysis of risk. *New England Journal of Medicine* **315**, 81–6.
Papiernik, E., Bouyer, J., Dreyfus, J., Collin, D., Winisdorffer, G., Guegen, S., et al. (1985). Prevention of preterm births: a perinatal study in Haguenau, France. *Pediatrics* **76**, 154–8.
Peckham, C.S. (1986). Vision in childhood. *British Medical Bulletin* **42**, 150–4.
Pharoah, P.O.D. (1976). International comparisons of perinatal and infant mortality rates. *Proceedings of the Royal Society of Medicine* **69**, 335–8.
Pharoah, P.O.D. (1990). Impairment, disability, and handicap. *Archives of Disease in Childhood* **65**, 819.
Pharoah, P.O.D., Stevenson, R.C., Cooke, R.W.I., and Sandu B. (1988). Costs and benefits of neonatal intensive care. *Archives of Disease in Childhood*, **63**, 715–18.
Piekkala, P., Kero, P., Erkkola, R., and Sillanpää, M. (1986). Perinatal events and neonatal morbidity:an analysis of 5380 cases. *Early Human Development* **13**, 249–68.
Piekkala, P., Kero, P., Sillanpää, M., and Erkkola, R. (1988). The developmental profile and outcome of 325 unselected preterm infants up to two years of age. *Neuropediatrics* **19**, 33–40.
Portnoy, S., Callias, M., Wolke, D., and Gamsu, H. (1988). Five-year follow-up study of extremely low-birthweight infants. *Developmental Medicine and Child Neurology* **30**, 590–8.
Powell, T.G., Pharoah, P.O.D., and Cooke, R.W.I. (1986). Survival and morbidity in a geographically defined population of low birthweight infants. *Lancet* **i**: 539–43.
Priolisi, A. (1980). Low birthweight revised. *Lancet* **i**, 930–1.
Public Health (1987). Low birth weight 1975–85 and perinatal mortality. *Public Health* **101**, 1–2.
Rantakallio, P., Oja, H., and Koiranen, M. (1991). Has the intrauterine weight-gain curve changed in shape? *Paediatric and Perinatal Epidemiology*, **5**, 201–10.
Reynolds, E.O.R. (1978). Neonatal intensive care and the prevention of major handicap. *Ciba Foundation Symposia*, Vol. 59, pp. 77–106. Elsevier, Amsterdam.
Rider, R.V., Harper, P.A., Knobloch, H., and Fetter, S.E. (1957). An evaluation of standards for the hospital care of premature infants. *Journal of the American Medical Association*, **165**, 1233–6.

Riikonen, R., Raumavirta, S., Sinivouori, E., and Seppälä, T. (1989). Changing pattern of cerebral palsy in the Southwest region of Finland. *Acta Paediatrica Scandinavia* **78**, 581–7.
Rooth, G. (1980). Low birthweight revised. *Lancet* **i**, 639–41.
Rumeau-Rouquette, C., du Mazaubrun, C., and Rabarison, Y. (1984). *Naître en France. 10 ans d'évolution*. Editions INSERM, Paris.
Saigal, S., Rosenbaum, P., Stoskopf, B., and Milner, R. (1982). Follow-up of infants 501 to 1500 g birthweight delivered to residents of a geographically defined region with perinatal intensive care facilities. *Journal of Pediatrics* **100**, 606–13.
Saigal, S., Rosenbaum, P., Stoskopf, B., and Sinclair, J.C. (1984). Outcome in infants 501 to 1000 g birth weight delivered to residents of the McMaster Health Region. *Journal of Pediatrics* **105**, 969–76.
Saigal, S., Rosenbaum, P., Hattersley, B., and Milner R. (1989). Decreased disability rate among 3-year-old survivors weighing 501 to 1000 grams at birth and born to residents of a geographically defined region from 1981 to 1984 compared with 1977 to 1980. *Journal of Pediatrics*, **114**, 839–46.
Skeoch, H., Rosenberg, K., Turner, T., Skeoch, C., and McIlwaine, G. (1987). Very low birthweight survivors:illness and readmission to hospital in the first 15 months of life. *British Medical Journal* **295**, 579–80.
Stahlman, M.T. (1984). Newborn intensive care:success or failure? *Journal of Pediatrics* **105**, 162–7.
Stanley, F. and Alberman, E. (1984). Birthweight, gestational age and the cerebral palsies. In *The epidemiology of the cerebral palsies* (ed. F. Stanley and E. Alberman), pp. 57–68. Blackwell Scientific, Oxford.
Stanley, F.J. and Watson, L. (1988). The cerebral palsies in Western Australia:trends, 1968 to 1981. *American Journal of Obstetrics and Gynecology* **158**, 89–93.
Stewart, A.L., Reynolds, E.O.R., and Lipscomb, A.P. (1981). Outcome for infants of very low birthweight:survey of world literature. *Lancet* **i**, 1038–41.
Tyson, R.M. (1946). A fifteen-year study of prematurity. From the standpoint of incidence, mortality and survival. *Journal of Pediatrics* **28**, 648–64.
Van den Berg, B.J. and Oechsli, F.W. (1984). Prematurity. In *Perinatal epidemiology*, (ed. M.B. Bracken). Oxford University Press.
Van Duivenboden *et al.* (1991). Infertility treatment: implications for perinatology. *European Journal of Obstetrics and Gynecology and Reproductive Biology*, **42**, 201–4.
Van Noord *et al.* (1991). Delaying childbearing: effect of age on fecundity and outcome of pregnancy. *British Medical Journal* **302**, 1361–5.
Van Zeben-van der Aa, T.M. (1989) Outcome at two years of age in very preterm and very low birthweight infants in the Netherlands. Ph.D. Thesis. State University, Leiden.
Van Zeben-van der Aa, T.M., Verloove-Vanhorick, S.P., Brand, R., and Ruys, J.H. (1989). Morbidity of very low birthweight infants at corrected age of two years in a geographically defined population. *Lancet* **i**, 253–5.
Van Zeben-van der Aa, T.M., Verloove-Vanhorick, S.P., Brand, R., and Ruys, J.H. (1991). The use of health services in the first 2 years of life in a nationwide cohort of very preterm and/or very low birthweight infants in the Netherlands: rehospitalisation and outpatient care. *Paediatric and Perinatal Epidemiology* **5**, 11–26.
Veen, S., Ens-Dokkum, M.H., Schreuder, A.M., Verloove-Vanhorick, S.P., Brand, R., and Ruys, J.H. (1991). Impairments, disabilities, and handicaps of very preterm and very low birthweight infants at five years of age in Netherlands. *Lancet*, **338**, 33–36.

Verkerk, P.H. and van Noord- B.M. (1991). *Lifestyle, environmental factors, outcome of pregnancy and neonatal health*. TNO Institute for Preventive Health Care, Leiden.

Verloove-Vanhorick, S.P., Verwey, R.A., Brand, R., Bennebroek Gravenhorst J., Keirse, M.J.N.C., and Ruys J.H. (1986). Neonatal mortality risk in relation to gestational age and birthweight. Results of a national survey of preterm and very-low-birthweight infants in the Netherlands. *Lancet* **i**, 55–7.

Verloove-Vanhorick, S.P. and Verwey, R.A. (1987). Project on preterm and small for gestational age infants in the Netherlands 1983. Ph.D. Thesis. State University, Leiden.

Vohr, B.R. and Garcia Coll, C.T. (1985). Neurodevelopmental and school performance of very low-birth-weight infants:a seven-year longitudinal study. *Pediatrics* **76**, 345–50.

Walker, D.J.B., Vohr, B.R., and Oh, W. (1985). Economic analysis of regionalized neonatal car for very-low-birth-weight infants in the State of Rhode Island. *Pediatrics* **76**, 69–74.

Wall, M. (1913). Ueber die Weiterentwicklung fruehgeborener Kinder mit besonderer Beruecksichtigung spaeterer nervoeser, psychischer und intellektueller Stoerungen. *Monatsschrift fuer Geburtschuelfe und Gynaekologie* **XXXVII**, 456–86.

Wegman, M.E. (1985). Annual summary of vital statistics—1984. *Pediatrics* **76**, 861–71.

Wegman, M.E. (1990). Annual summary of vital statistics—1989. *Pediatrics* **86**, 835–47.

WHO (World Health Organization) (1977). Recommended definitions, terminology and format for statistical tables related to the perinatal period and use of a new certificate for cause of perinatal deaths. *Acta Obstetricia et Gynecologica Scandinavica* **56**, 247–53.

WHO (World Health Organization) (1980). *International classification of impairments, disabilities, and handicaps*. World Health Organization, Geneva.

Wierenga, H., Brand, R., Geudeke, T., van Geyn, H.P., van der Harten, H., and Verloove-Vanhorick, S.P. (1990). Prenatal risk factors for cot death in very preterm and small for gestational age infants. *Early Human Development* **23**, 15–26.

Working group on the very low birthweight infant. (1990). European Community collaborative study of outcome of pregnancy between 22 and 28 weeks' gestation. *Lancet* **336**, 782–84.

Yearbook of Nordic Statistics (1985). (ed. Nordic Statistical Secretariat). Vol. 24. Nordic Statistical Secretariat, Copenhagen.

Ylppö, A. (1919). Pathologisch-anatomische Studien bei Fruehgeborenen. Makroskopische und mikroskopische Untersuchungen mit Hinweisen auf die Klinik und mit besonderer Beruecksichtigung der Haemorrhagien. *Zeitschrift Kinderheilkunde* **20**, 213–381.

Yu, V.Y.H., Watkins, A., and Bajuk, B. (1984). Neonatal and postneonatal mortality in very low birthweight infants. *Archives of Disease in Childhood* **59**, 987–99.

Yu. V.Y.H. (1987). Survival and neurodevelopmental outcome of preterm infants. In *Prematurity*, (ed. V.Y.H. Yu and E.C. Wood), pp. 223–45. Churchill Livingstone, Edinburgh.

24 Children and families in distress: the case of family breakdown

Bengt Lindström and Lennart Köhler

This chapter will exemplify children in disharmonious family situations by analysing one of the most common causes of distress, i.e. children in families at risk of breakdown. First the epidemiology of divorce is explained whereafter a general strategy for protection and enhancement of the child in these situations is explained using a salutogenic approach. These strategies can be used in a much wider context. The changes in the world and on the European continent in the last decade have increased the number of refugee and migrating children separated from one or two parents. A new pattern of family formation, i.e. families formed without official recognition, has become more common and there is a need to look at the situation of these children. So far, little research interest has been focused on this issue. As these patterns have been more common in the Nordic countries the research reports from this area are collected here as an example.

Introduction

Over the past decades there has been an increase in divorces or family breakdowns all over the world. Officially, in Europe alone, at least 5.5 million women, children, and men annually face the loss of their intimate relationships, discounting other types of separations and unofficial marriages. In order to be able to manage the situation there is a need to analyse and understand the family breakdown process and its health consequences. For public health workers this situation should encourage us to use the tools available for a salutogenic and health promotive approach, as recommended in the new directions of the WHO *Health for all* target. The ultimate target is to create healthy social settings for the coming generations, our children.

The global WHO *Health for all* strategy is changing focus towards the development of health resources and promotion of health. Some of the key elements in this reorientation deal with the creation of healthy environments, also in a social context, and more directly trying to improve social settings thus enabling the formation of healthy patterns of living and avoiding health damaging behaviour. One such setting is the family, where the potential for the future lies in the conditions that can be created for the child. In the past decades, families all over the world have increasingly been facing breakdowns or what is generally called divorce, which also has had an impact on children.

This text will approach family breakdown first from a theoretical and epidemiological point of view, whereafter the possibility of preserving and enhancing the health of children in divorce is discussed in order to develop strategies for professionals dealing with this rather common phenomenon. The suggested strategies can also be used in the wider context of promoting health in social settings. The focus is deliberately centred on the conditions of children since they are often most vulnerable in family breakdowns.

Social support networks are considered to be one of the strongest health enhancing factors for human beings, as has been proved in many health studies (Berkman 1984; Bergström and Tengvall 1985). The loss of a supporting network can be devastating to any individual. To witness the disruption of one's closest supporting network without being able to understand what is happening, without being able to control the process, sometimes not even being aware of what is going on or even wanting it to happen describes, in short, the situation of a child in a divorce.

The epidemiology of divorce

According to the 1982 *UN Demographic yearbook*, the annual number of individuals in Europe that officially are involved in a divorce amount to over 5.5 million people, out of which at least 2 million are children under the age of 18 (Table 24.1). Furthermore, there has been rapid increase in the number of divorces over the last decades, which has decelerated in the last few years (Fig. 24.1). Globally, the highest figures are found in the USA, while countries having strong religious traditions linked to the Catholic or Orthodox church tend to have the lowest figures. One curiosity is the rapid increase and then decrease in divorce rates in the mid 1970s in Sweden, which was caused simply by a change in legislation which made it easier to have a divorce. Similar changes have been seen in other countries for the same reason. Statistically, there is at least one child involved per official divorce (Lindström 1989).

The data presented in the figure only represent official statistics. Family formation patterns have changed as people also increasingly form 'unofficial' rela-

Table 24.1 *Population annually affected by divorces in Europe (UN Demographic Yearbook 1982)*

Number of divorces in Europe	1 833 500
Number of adults affected	3 667 000
Number of children affected	2 016 850
Total population affected	5 683 850

Since 1982 collective data to estimate the number of children involved in divorce has not been published.

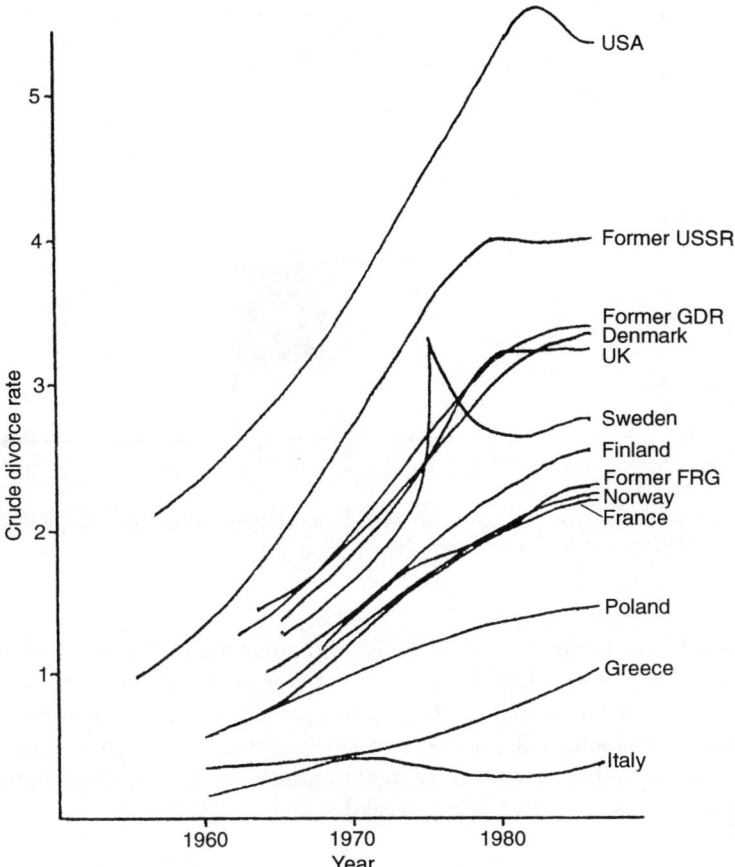

Fig. 24.1 Crude divorce rate in selected European countries and USA, 1955–1988. (Source: *UN Demographic yearbook* 1955–1988.)

tionships (so-called consensual unions) which in some parts of the world, as in some of the Nordic countries, have become the dominating form of intimate couple formation (Fig. 24.2). This figure describes two similar age cohorts (15–30 years) in 1968 and 1981. In 1968 40.3 per cent of the population had formed couples out of which only 0.3 per cent were not officially married. In 1981 the proportion living as couples was 40 per cent but only 17 per cent were in official marriages, which means that most couples were 'unofficial'. There are few reliable data about these relationships but they tend to last for a shorter period of time and produce fewer children (Köhler *et al.* 1986). In 1980, 84 per cent of all newly formed couples in Sweden were consensual unions; this percentage increased to 88 per cent in 1985 and the number of children living with unmarried parents had simultaneously increased by 30 per cent although they

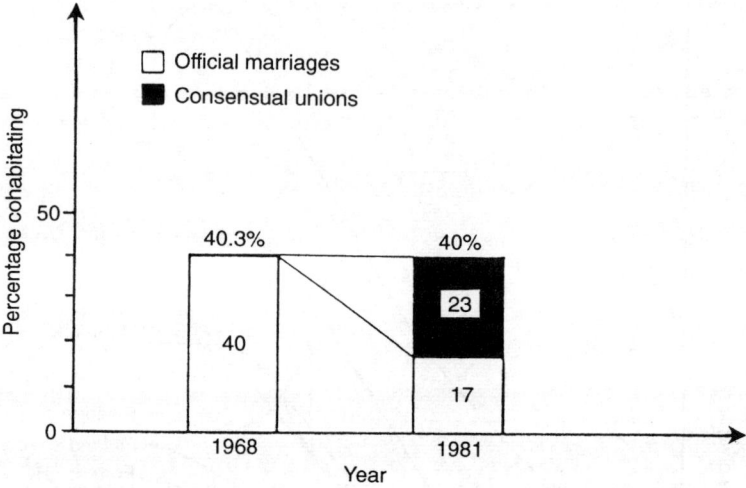

Fig. 24.2 Percentage of population in Sweden cohabiting and mode of cohabitation. Age group 15–30 years, calendar years 1968, 1981.

comprised only 15 per cent of the total child population (*Statistical yearbook of Sweden* 1991). The group of children that were most likely to face a family breakdown were under the age of three, had parents of low socio-economic class in consensual unions and who lived in small households in urban areas. These were also the children who were at the greatest risk of losing contact with non-custodial parents after family breakdown (Bing 1991).

Table 24.2 *Number of deaths per 100 000 inhabitants in Sweden by sex, age, and marital status, 1974–1978*

	Age (years)					
	20–24	30–34	40–44	50–54	60–64	70–74
Men						
Unmarried	118	232	579	1074	1292	5468
Married	60	78	187	546	1573	4446
Divorced	357	303	736	1519	3054	6440
Widowed	–	216	632	1025	2353	5783
Women						
Unmarried	47	115	289	589	1093	2932
Married	29	51	133	326	801	2463
Divorced	98	117	291	591	1082	2463
Widowed	–	112	244	436	989	2756

Also the length of marriages is decreasing. A marriage formed 40 years ago had only half the risk of ending in divorce after 10 years compared to a marriage formed 20 years ago and this tendency seems to be continuing (Fig. 24.3). The peak divorce frequency for Northern Europe (after the year of marriage) is between two and four years, while the peak divorce rate in the USA occurs after the first year of marriage. The time trends in Europe approach those of the USA (*UN Demographic yearbook*). There is no simple explanation of the global increase in divorce rates. Societies have changed, as have the functions of families. Historically, having been the primary group for production, reproduction, and socialization, families now face a divergence of functions:

- working life (production) has moved outside the family;
- socialization of children largely happens within institutions;
- the meaning of reproduction has changed—today sexuality and reproduction can be separated because of modern contraceptive methods;
- attitudes towards the creation of relationships between men and women have changed; issues of equity, economic independence, and the quality of the relationship have become more important.

Most of these changes started long before the rapid increase in divorce rates occurred, which makes it difficult to relate the causes and effects directly. Other

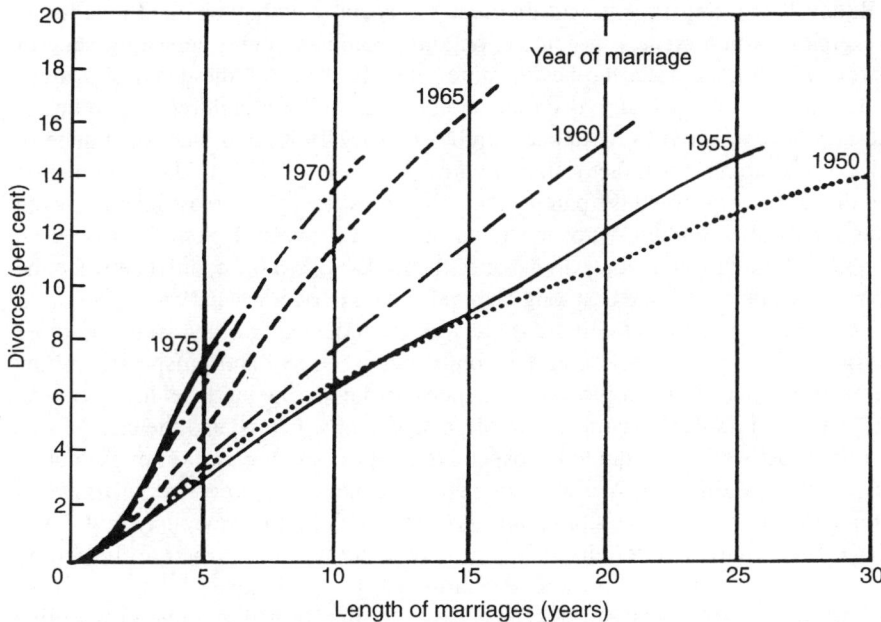

Fig. 24.3 Divorces in original cohorts of marriage.

important changes are, for instance, the mobility of the population, causing an increasing urbanization which has disrupted traditional networks. The secularization of societies has decreased the importance of religious constraints and also changed norms, causing an increased independence which for many, has been experienced as increased insecurity. The traditional sex roles have changed and demands on partners have increased, with individual interests becoming more important than family values. Finally, people tend to live longer, which allows more time for divorce.

The health consequences of divorce

The direct and negative health consequences of divorcing are unquestioned and well documented for the adult population. There is almost no disease that is less frequent among divorced persons compared with married (Nyström 1979). Men seem to run greater risk for unwanted health consequences (Jacobs 1982), which has been explained as being that men lose their only intimate friend when separating. Women tend to have better support networks which are utilized in a crisis (Pearson and Hendrix 1979).

When computing groups of married, single, and widowed with the divorced or newly separated, there is a pattern of a general increase in morbidity and mortality among the divorced and separated. The explanation for these differences is considered to be that social support functions as a protective factor in a crisis situation (Rutter 1985). Separations and divorces are socially ambiguous and potentially reversible which creates insecurity, ongoing conflicts, and a persisting state of stress which may affect the health more severely than, say the death of a loved one. The risk of psychiatric disorders are twice as high for children in families of discord as compared to harmonic families (Emery 1982) and a constant state of discord is a higher risk factor than divorce (Power et al. 1974). The combination of discordance between the parents and other stress factors increases the risk even further for the children, with or without a divorce involved.(Schwarzberg et al. 1983). Children who manage to distance themselves from the conflict between the parents seem to have the best long-term prognosis (Bridgewater 1984).

Children's reactions to divorces are well documented but the results are more difficult to interpret. Earlier studies, both cross-sectional and prospective, show clear evidence of negative consequences to behaviour and health (Douglas 1970). The population samples are often selected, which is also the case of one of the most frequently quoted prospective studies which based on middle-class families in California (Wallerstein 1984). Today there are some prospective studies which show that behavioural patterns in children, previously thought to have been caused by the divorce itself, were in fact present before the family disruption occurred (Elliot and Richards 1991). Boys tend to have a worse health outcome than girls, a fact that has been questioned in some prospective studies (Allison and Furstenberg 1989).

When reviewing the literature on the outcome for children after a divorce, several factors are said to be important:

- age;
- sex;
- personality traits;
- development;
- social support (siblings);
- the process of divorce;
- the relationship of the parents before, during, and after divorcing;
- societal values and attitudes.

There are no specific general outcomes of divorces because each divorce has unique features. Some ages are considered to be more sensitive to separations: young children because of cognitive reasons and parents having been the foundation for their basic trust, while teenagers are threatened because they are in the process of forming their first personal intimate relationships.

Family breakdown—a process system

A divorce is not a single phenomenon caused by the same underlying reasons and creating the same patterns of reactions. It should rather be seen as a process occurring over time and caused by several factors which also create different outcomes. The process has been described as follows (Ahrons 1984):

1. *Individual cognition.* One partner as an individual reflects on a separation without informing the rest of the family.

2. *Metacognition.* The rest of the family is informed, often creating the most chaotic, unstable, and uncertain phase in the process of divorce as earlier roles and structures are disrupted and the future is completely unknown.

3. *Physical separation.* This phase, when the partners separate, is called divorce in everyday talk. If the future structures and roles have been discussed in the previous phase the physical separation may be less chaotic than generally considered.

4. *Reorganization.* The new constellations are established and recognized internally.

5. *Reorientation.* The family members, social networks, and society accept and recognize the new roles and structures of the original family.

The above process has also been called family transformation from nuclear to binuclear family (Fig. 24.4). Each phase is reversible and can vary with respect to time. The last phase takes the longest and in cultures or societies where divorce is not socially or legally accepted it tends never to end.

If this process model were used when calculating divorce rates, thus more accurately reflecting that part of the population which is actively involved in a family breakdown process, one could easily multiply by five or tenfold the figures given in official statistics. Also, the number of separations of consensual unions could be added.

Each phase in the process is reversible, which means that the crisis can be resolved without a 'divorce'. However, the process often occurs unnoticed, protected by the intimacy and privacy of the family, making a professional intervention almost impossible even when the skills are available. Children are often forgotten and made invisible in the process of family breakdown as the crisis of the adults dominates the scene. Even well trained and skilled professional helpers find it difficult to understand and even recognize the crisis of the child. A ten year old child who manages the family breakdown brilliantly, not causing the family or helpers any problems, not showing any external signs of crisis, may easily be misinterpreted and given an adult responsibility, while in reality the child is lacking the means of expressing grief and pain. The long-term consequences for the child may be devastating. Time perception is often misunder-

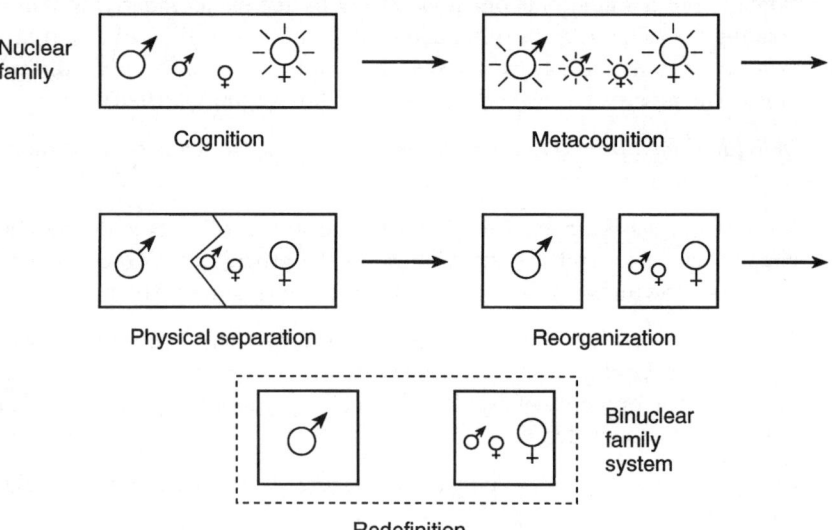

Fig. 24.4 Stages of transformation in the breakdown process from nuclear family to a binuclear family system.

stood in legal processes; losing a parent for three months may be an eternity to a young child, while an adult can easily overlook such a time interval.

Pathogenic mechanisms in family breakdown

Several studies have shown that divorces are among the least desired life events for children (Coddington 1972; Rutter 1985). Only the death of a parent is considered to be less desired. If the general theory of major life events is used (Rahe and Arthur 1978) there are three phenomena that have to be avoided in a divorce if the outcome is to be improved: lack of control, clustering of events, and the occurrence of undesired events (Kaplan 1983). These will be considered in the perspective of children and family breakdown.

1. *Lack of control.* Children seldom have the potential to control the situation. On the contrary, though feeling guilty, and responsible for the separation, children have no power to stop it.

2. *Clustering.* A family disruption often includes many events: loss of parent, change of housing, change of school, loss of friends and siblings. If these events are clustered in a short period of time their health-damaging potential increases dramatically.

3. *Desirability.* Children and young people often experience the loss of a family member by separation or death as being the least-desired life event.

In the light of life–event theory, family breakdowns for children include many of the negative possibilities considered above.

Another theoretical framework that could be used in health promotive activities has been developed by Antonovsky (1979, 1987), when describing what makes human beings able not only to survive but maintain their health in life-threatening situations. Antonovsky's original study was made on women who had survived the horrors of concentration camps in the Second World War. Much to his surprise there was a group of women who were able to lead a normal life, form good and lasting relationships with other people, maintain their jobs, and raise children successfully. In the pursuit of factors that enhance health, or have a salutogenic effect, Antonovsky later discovered that these women had developed a sense of coherence, which enabled them to make the world comprehensible, gave them a sense of mastering life, and finally gave them a meaning in life. From this framework Antonovsky formed a general theory of salutogenesis in which the sense of coherence is one of the central concepts. Applied to the scene of children in divorce it is easy to understand why the health consequences are so negative since children are seldom given the chance to understand, lack the means of mastering the situation and are rarely able to comprehend the reasons for a family breakdown.

Promoting health, the salutogenic approach

The elements of life events and salutogenesis described above can be used in a health promotive strategy for children in family breakdown situation.

1. *Control and mastering*. Children need a stable position in the chaotic situation, when the energy of the parents is used to manage their own situation and their parenting role is lost. Other persons need to step in and form substitutes or act as mediators to the parents. Such persons can be siblings, relatives, neighbours, teachers, or even health professionals. Furthermore, children can be given a sense of mastering the situation if they are given adequate information about the family breakdown and the possible outcomes. This information has to be given in a way that it is comprehended by the child where factors such as age, sex, and development play a major role. This will give the child a means to act and participate, thereby acquiring the active skills of mastering.

2. *Clustering of events*. The chain of events (losing parents, siblings, home, friends, school) should be based on the child's conceptual capabilities, with the possibility of also slowing the process being important for the child's health. Strategically, parents also find it easier to accept conditions based on the needs of the child rather than the needs of the partner.

3. *Desirability*. In the eyes of the child a separation of the parents is hardly ever desired, not even when the child suffers physically or mentally in a family. There is no appropriate age for a child in a family breakdown, although theoretically one may argue that children who are unable to cognitively understand the family breakdown suffer more from family breakdown. The right to maintain contact with both parents after the separation should be given priority. This fact is stated in the *UN Convention on the rights of the child*.

4. *Meaning*. According to Antonovsky (1987) the motivational factor, or meaning, has the strongest salutogenic effect. It is difficult to find a meaning for a family breakdown for a child in both the short and long-term perspective. Is it meaningful for children to realize that nothing is permanent in this world, that our existence is fragmented and that it is meaningful to survive in spite of hardships?

The above factors could be considered when trying to make the best of the situation for the children. Antonovsky (1979) also discusses factor that enhance health, or so-called general resistance resources (GRR). These are of a general character, such as personality traits, intelligence, social support systems, knowledge, skills, material and immaterial resources, culture, traditions and beliefs. To clarify what GRR are available and which can be used and strengthened around the child will liberate other means for strategic interventions when children face divorce.

Also an analysis of society in general could help to identify what kind of societal forces can be mobilized when dealing with children on a macro-level in an attempt to create healthy environments. If the Nordic societies are analysed in this perspective the description in the following paragraph would apply:

The five Nordic countries have stable democratic traditions with a well developed infrastructure including integrated family functions and an extensive support system for families with children. Children are prioritized and respected on the political agenda and special consideration are given in the legislation to strengthen the position of children within the society. All Nordic countries have been actively involved in the development of The *UN Convention on the rights of the child* and also ratified the same. On the other hand these countries have adopted a western, urbanized pattern of living which includes many forces that counteract the value of family and raising children. In spite of generally good economic resources which would enable having children, other interests and values are higher on the agenda. Personal career and development is more important than the value of having more children (Bulatao 1979). Consequently nativity is low; weak and isolated social networks, including less stable family structures, are common. The model for solving family crisis is divorce. Mass media and the general public have accepted fairly high divorce rates. Divorce is socially acceptable, which has both positive and negative consequences; a divorce is no longer a social stigma, which is positive for the parties involved but on the other hand, because of the general acceptance, many couples never try to solve a crisis within the family because divorce is considered the societal model for conflict resolution. Mass media has enforced the image of acceptably high divorce rates. This is partially true but most children still grow up in a nuclear family with the biological parents. A cross-sectional study in 1984, from the Nordic School of Public Health, of 15 000 randomly selected families with children aged 2–18, showed that 85 per cent of children grow up in two-parent families, a figure that has been fairly stable over the last 100 years (Köhler 1990).

Most of the aspects raised in this chapter have dealt with promoting the health of children who are already in some stage of a family breakdown. It would, of course, be desirable to be able to intervene much earlier and improve the basic prerequisites for families and children. A strategic approach using two dimensions: first the stages of breakdown, then the perspectives from the society to the individual level, has been presented by Köhler *et al.* (1986).

Some suggestions for intervention are exemplified in the following text. The long-term programme of educating children in school about human relationships and later about sexual behaviour aim at giving children appropriate knowledge, attitudes, and skills as a protective factor for future needs. Another approach is to give realistic expectations of couple formation, such as organizing a conciliation before cohabitation (which has been a compulsory practice in former

		Pre-breakdown phase	Breakdown phase	Post-breakdown phase
		Cognition Metacognition	Physical breakdown	Reorganization Reorientation
		Underlying factors	Amplifying factors	Resolution factors
Positive development	Process	temporary conflict	problem solving mutual agreement	idem
	Society	stable, accepting good infrastructure integrated family functions family support	means for support (legal, economic, social, health) formal network	supportive system for family functions
	Family	good internal network long cohabitation adapted/flexible existing sensible rules	utilization of support, persons, and network	stable socioeconomic conditions restored or new social network
	Parents	common values healthy, loving, caring, mature, competent power balance child reopeering adequate GRRs	mutual agreement on procedure	existing attachment continues continued contact mutual respect
	Child	first young siblings high self-esteem	informed reacting kept outside the ongoing struggle	in contact with parents
	Carer		competent effective, efficient practical works towards prevention and promotion rather than only therapy	idem
Negative development	Process	ongoing conflict	undecisive loss of parenting child in marital conflict 'strict' legal process	ongoing conflicts
	Society	unstable, rigid lack of infrastructure weak family role	forbidding and unsupportive attitudes	idem
	Family	isolation multichange/multiproblem immature short cohabitation rigid	further isolation lack of support	economic deprivation migration burn out
	Parents	imbalance of power structure destructive patterns psychopathology age difference disrespect of child inadequate GRRs	increased inbalance destructive behaviour indistinguinished hostility	break in continuing parenting (custodial) breaking child contact, especially with opposite sex risk behaviour
	Child	single male handicap age personality disturbances	uninformed apathy blamed victims of violence	break in contact with custodial parents ongoing psycosocial problems/school problems oculated behaviour abusive step-family
	Carer		incompetent too professional/ethnical uses unacceptable approaches	idem

Fig. 24.5 Positive and negative factors influencing the breakdown process as related to the involved parties (societies, individuals, carers).

Yugoslavia, and has now been voluntarily tried in UK and USA (Richards 1990)).

In longitudinal studies of protective factors for children at risk it has been shown that the most unstable link in the family system is the father, especially if he is not mature and of low socio-economic background (Werner and Smith 1982). Therefore efforts to enhance the father's role in a family system, somewhat paradoxically, could be a start in the promotion of child health. As children are at greater risk of losing their fathers in a breakdown situation, there have been attempts to focus on the role of the prospective father in maternity care, using the salutogenic concept; making him understand that his role is meaningful and important, and giving him the skills to participate actively in the delivery and care of the newborn—the result has been that fathers have participated in the care of the child far beyond the first well-baby clinic and are more strongly attached to the child. Instead of having only maternity leave, shared parental leave should be considered, as is occurring in the Nordic countries, but prejudices have made the 'coming of the father' slow. Creating arenas in which fathers can meet and discuss the role of being a father has the objective of increasing awareness and meaning of fathership and improving the skills of parenting among men in peer groups, thus implementing the salutogenic idea. Another approach has been the so called 'couple-or love-enrichment' courses organized by family counselling services for couples who are not in breakdown situations but feel that there is something more to it than the everyday row (Sanden 1991). Creating meeting points and organizations for separated fathers and mothers has been a new development in the post-breakdown process. The next step is to form arenas for children from disrupted families. Discovering that there are shared mutual interests, which ultimately can promote the situation of all involved, instead of fighting former parents, enhances the condition for the children as well. These experiments have strengthened the support networks and increased the possibilities of dialogue between all parties involved. In brief, the role of the professionals is to have the knowledge, skills, and sensitivity to recognize the signals of the children and the parents, raising the awareness of these issues on a community level, mobilizing the different sectors, and creating the necessary arenas for dialogue and intervention. Implementation of the theoretical aspects presented here, e.g. life events, the breakdown process, salutogenesis in the context of the growing child and family, is one way of improving families' and professionals' sense of coherence.

Family breakdown in which children are involved is not an easy issue to deal with in public health. The perspective and voice of children is often forgotten in societal and therapeutic interventions. This chapter has given some guidelines on how to work with health promotion from the child's perspective where the theoretical framework of salutogenesis has been used. In the long term, it seems that most children, in spite of everything, manage family breakdown fairly well and are even inclined to form their own marriages when the time comes. However, much can and must be improved for children in family breakdown where the knowledge and understanding of children's own perspectives must be given more emphasis.

In spite of all the tree of life
grew strong and invincible
and through its branches one can hear
the song of children.
Traditional Swedish Nursery Rhyme

References

Ahrons, C. (1984) *The binuclear family: parenting roles and relationships*, (Seminar Report). Danish National Institute of Social Research, Copenhagen.
Allison, P.D. and Furstenberg E.F. (1989). How marital dissolution affects children: variations by age and sex. *Developmental Psychology* 25, 540–9.
Antonovsky, A. (1979). *Health, stress and coping*. Jossey-Bass, San Francisco.
Antonovsky, A. (1987). *Unraveling the mystery of health*. Jossey-Bass, San Francisco.
Bergstrom, B. and Tengvall, K. (1985). Om det sociala nätverkets betydelse for hälsan. *Socialmedicinsk Tidskrift* 1, 4–9.
Berkman, L.E. (1984). Assessing the physical effects of social networks and social support. *Annual Review of Public Health* 5, 413–32.
Bing, V. (1991). Familjebildning och familjeupplösning. *The Gothenburg Public Health Report* 3, No 2, 92–111.
Bridgewater, C.A. (1984). Divorce, the long-term effect on children. *Psychology Today* 18, 7.
Bulatao, R.A. (1979). On the nature of the transition in the value of children. *Papers of the East–West Population Institute*, No. 60-A. East-West Center, Honolulu.
Coddington, R.D. (1972). The significance of life events as etiologic factors in the diseases of children. II. A study of a normal population. *Journal of Psychosomatic Research* 16, 205–13.
UN Convention on the rights of the child (1990). Ministry of Foreign Affairs, Stockholm.
Douglas, J.W.B. (1970). Broken families and child behaviour. *Journal of the Royal College of Physicians* 4, 203–10.
Elliot B.J. and Richards, M.P.M. (1991). Effects of parental divorce on children. *Archives of Disease in Childhood* 66, 915–6.
Emery, R.E. (1982). Interparental conflicts and the children of discord and divorce. *Psychological Bulletin* 92, 310–30.
Jacobs, J.W. (1982) The effect of divorce on fathers: an overview of the literature. *American Journal of Psychiatry* 139, 10, 1235–41.
Kaplan, H.B. (1983). Psychosocial stress: trend in theory and research. Academic, New York.
Köhler, L. (Ed.) (1990). *Barn och barnfamiljer i Norden. En studie av välfärd, hälsa och livskvalitet*. NHV-Rapport 1990, 1. Studentlitteratur, Lund.
Köhler, L., Lindstrom, B., Barnard, K., and Itani, H. (1986). *Health implications of family breakdown*. NHV-Report 1986, 3. The Nordic School of Public Health, Göteborg.
Lindstrom, B. (1989). Kan en skilsmässa vara hälsosam för barn? In (ed. L. Köhler) *Folkhälsovetenskap—ett nordiskt perspektiv*, NHV-Report 1989, 2. The Nordic School of Public Health, Göteborg.

Nyström, S. (1979). The use of somatic hospital care among divorced. *Scandinavian Journal of Social Medicine*, (Suppl. 17), 1–48.

Pearson Jr, W. and Hendrix, L. (1979). Divorce and the status of women. *Journal of Marriage and the Family*, **41**, 375–85.

Power, M., Ash P., Schoenberg, E., and Sirey, C. (1974). Delinquency and the Family. *British Journal of Social Work* **4**, 13–38.

Rahe, R.H. and Arthur R.J. (1978). Life change and illness studies. Past history and new directions. *Journal of Human Stress* **43**, 3–15.

Richards, M.P.M. (1990). Divorce Cambridge style: new developments in conciliation. *Family Law* **21**, 436–8.

Rutter, M. (1985). Resilience in the face of adversity. *British Journal of Psychology* **147**, 598–611.

Sanden, B. (1991). Samlevnadsfragor i föräldrautbildningen vid MVC och BVC—en framtidsskiss. *The Gothenburg Public Health Report* **3**, 47–58.

Schwarzenberg, L., Shamper, D., and Chalmers, B. (1983) Emotional adjustment and self-control of children from divorced and undivorced unhappy homes. *Journal of Social Psychology*, 121, 305–12.

Statistical yearbook of Sweden 1991. Statistics Sweden, Stockholm.

UN Demographic yearbook 1955–1988. UN New York.

Wallerstein, J.S. (1984). Children in divorce: Preliminary report of a ten-year follow-up children. *American Journal of Orthopsychiatry* **54**, 444–458.

Werner, E. and Smith, R. (1982). *Vulnerable but invincible. A longitudinal study of resilient children and youth*. McGraw Hill, New York.

25 Immigrant and ethnic minority children
John Black

Introduction

In this chapter we are concerned with the needs of children belonging to ethnic minorities, whether of immigrant or refugee origin or descent. Because of ease of availability, much of the data has been taken from the United Kingdom.

People leave their country for a variety of reasons and these reasons influence their willingness and ability to adapt to their new surroundings. Adjustment is a two-way process: the acceptance or rejection of a newly arrived minority family or group affects the behaviour of the minority, and the conduct and behaviour of the newcomers determine, at least to some extent, the reaction of the majority. In most instances an equilibrium is reached, with a variable amount of tolerance on the part of the host population and of adaptation by the minority.

It is generally assumed that minorities are always oppressed and disadvantaged, but this is not so. There are numerous examples of dominant minorities; the British in India, the European colonists in Africa, the Chinese in Tibet, and the whites in South Africa. What started as a minority may become a majority, as in North America, Australia, and New Zealand.

In discussing the patterns of disease and socio-economic circumstances of ethnic minorities, two pitfalls must be avoided. The first is that of stereotyping, which is the assumption that all members of a particular ethnic group have similar characteristics, behave in the same way, and have identical needs. The second is to think that the disease pattern of a minority can be attributed entirely to its genetic constitution or to its dietary and other customs. This pattern is then regarded as an 'ethnic problem', whereas many of these disorders, emotional or organic, arise from socio-economic circumstances, and are the same as those of the host community who live at the same economic level and belong to the same social (occupational) classes.

Definitions

Ethnic minority

An ethnic minority is a group of individuals who consider themselves to be different from the general community, and are seen to be different by the population at large, because of one or more of the following characteristics: common racial or geographical origin, skin colour, physical or facial appearance, language, religious beliefs and practices, mode of dress, and cultural and dietary customs. Some of these, such as mode of dress and dietary customs, are subsidiary to the main attributes, such as skin colour, geographical origin, and language.

Asian

This means anyone who comes from, or whose family originated, directly or indirectly (e.g. from East Africa), from the Indian subcontinent (ISC). The term 'Asian' is synonymous with South Asian, and must be distinguished from the American usage in which Asian indicates someone of South-East Asian origin.

South-East Asian

This indicates someone coming from, or whose family came from, Burma (Myanmar), China, Hong Kong, Malaysia, Singapore, Thailand, Vietnam, and neighbouring countries.

Classification of ethnic minorities

A general classification, including historical examples, is given in Table 25.1. Though we are mainly concerned with recently arrived groups (the last 30–40 years), the persecution of the Jews and Gypsies in Nazi Germany shows that political changes can threaten the stability and even the existence of minorities who were previously tolerated. In present-day western Europe the majority of newly arrived ethnic minorities consist of immigrants and refugees and their descendants, who may continue to be wrongly categorized as immigrants or refugees.

Immigrant

An immigrant is someone who is in a foreign country temporarily or permanently. Strictly speaking, refugees are immigrants but their situation differs in so many ways that they are considered separately. An immigrant may enter a country legally, or illegally, sometimes using an unauthorized route.

Refugee

In 1951 the United Nations Convention relating to the status of refugees defined a refugee as

'any person who owing to a well founded fear of being persecuted for reasons of race, religion, nationality, membership of a particular social group or political opinion, is outside the country of his nationality and is unable, or owing to such fear, is unwilling to avail himself of the protection of that country; or who, not having a nationality and being

Table 25.1 *Classification of ethnic minorities*

Group	Examples
Indigenous minorities	Amerindians in North America, Aboriginals in Australia, Maoris in New Zealand.
Dominant minorities (present day)	Chinese in Tibet, Whites in South Africa.
Long-established immigrant groups	Bretons in France (emigrated from Britain in fifth and sixth Century AD); Gypsies in Europe (first documented in fourteen century, possibly originating from Northern India); Irish in Britain (during the last 150 years).
Forced immigrations	Slave trade from Africa to the West Indies and America (seventeenth to mid-nineteenth century).
Economic immigrants	Afro-Caribbeans and Asians into Britain (1950s to 1980s); North Africans into France (1950s to 1980s).
Immigrants seeking further education	Small numbers, usually temporary, into western Europe and North America.
Persecuted refugees	From Africa, Middle East, South-East Asia, South and Central America, and numerous other countries, into western Europe and North America.
Economic refugees	Some Vietnamese, into Hong Kong (1975 onwards); Albanians into Italy (1991).

outside the country of his former habitual residence, is unable, or owing to such fear, is unwilling to return to it.'

There is also an ill-defined category of economic refugees whose departure may or may not be the result of discrimination by a dominant group. Economic refugees are not recognized as genuine refugees but the distinction is often a difficult one, as with the 'boat-people' from Vietnam.

A refugee may arrive in a country of asylum legally, or may attempt to enter illegally, without the necessary documents, with false documents, or may use an illegal route of entry.

Epidemiology

Immigrants

We are discussing here the immigrations into Western Europe which have occurred in the post-1945 period. It is estimated that there are 15 million immigrant workers in Western Europe. In the post-war economic boom, unemployment was very low and many countries encouraged, or actively recruited, immigration of unskilled labour to fill low-paid jobs.

The main recipient countries have been Germany (West), France, Belgium, Switzerland, Holland, the UK, and to a lesser extent Scandinavia. The majority of workers have come (in descending order) from Turkey, Italy, Portugal, Yugoslavia, and North Africa (Power and Hardman 1984). The UK is a special case (see below) because of immigration from the West Indies, the ISC, and East Africa.

It was initially assumed that economic immigrants would return home when they had earned enough money or were no longer required, but this has not happened. Subsequent economic recessions caused recipient countries to erect barriers to further immigration, and now only dependants are being admitted, usually grudgingly and after long bureaucratic delays.

In the course of the 30–40 years in which immigrant families have established themselves, their social and economic status has improved in some countries and has remained unchanged or has deteriorated in others. In Germany (West) the position of the *gastarbeiter* has remained very unsatisfactory, without proper civil rights, with little possibility of naturalization, and with poor housing. In the UK the Aliens Act of 1919 prevented immigration from non-Commonwealth countries but allowed entry to citizens of the 'New Commonwealth' and Pakistan, but this has been severely restricted by a series of Acts. Now, in the 1990s, in western Europe an increasing proportion of the descendants of the original immigrants have been born in the country of their adoption but do not have full rights of citizenship. These second or third generation descendants have greater social and economic aspirations than did their grandparents or parents, but find, particularly if they are black, the same barriers to advancement still in place.

Demographic changes in the Asian communities in Britain

Because of its large size and the ease with which the various subgroups can be identified from their names and naming systems, the Asian communities can be used as a model for the demographic changes in an immigrant group.

The main groups which entered Britain between 1950 and 1970 were from the West Indies, India, and East Africa (Gujarati Hindus and Punjabi Sikhs), Pakistan, and last of all the Bangladeshis (Bengalis). The first arrivals were economically active young men, but by 1967, 90 per cent of all immigrants from the ISC were dependants. Figure 25.1 shows the pattern of immigration from the West Indies, India, and Pakistan with Bangladesh. The age structures of the three Asian communities in 1985 is shown in Figure 25.2 and the percentage of certain ethnic minorities born 1986–1988 in the UK is shown in Figure 25.3.

Refugees

The number of refugees seeking asylum in western Europe is increasing annually. Figure 25.4 shows the number of asylum applications to the European Community (EC) between 1980 and 1989, and Figure 25.5 shows their regions of origin in 1989. In the world as a whole there are estimated to be 13 million refugees, but only one million are in Europe. In the EC the percentage of rejections of asylum applicants is rising. The UK has imposed a fine on airlines which bring refugees into Britain without valid entry papers (Hooper 1991), though many refugees are in no position to obtain such documents in their own country. Nevertheless, the number of people seeking asylum in Britain continues to rise. In the years after the end of the Second World War refugees have entered Britain from Chile, Cyprus, Czechoslovakia, Eastern Europe, Eritrea, Ethiopia,

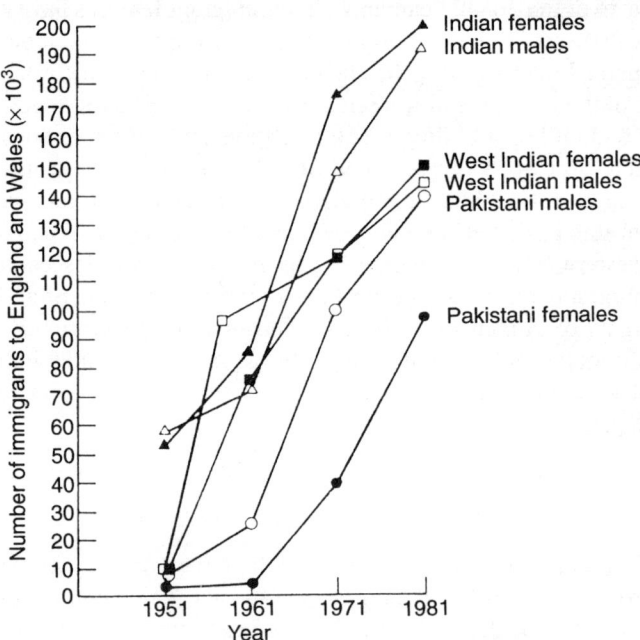

Fig. 25.1 New Commonwealth immigration to England and Wales 1951–81. Figures for Indian females and males include white Indian-born, figures for Pakistan include Bangladesh. (Source: Webster and Fox 1989.)

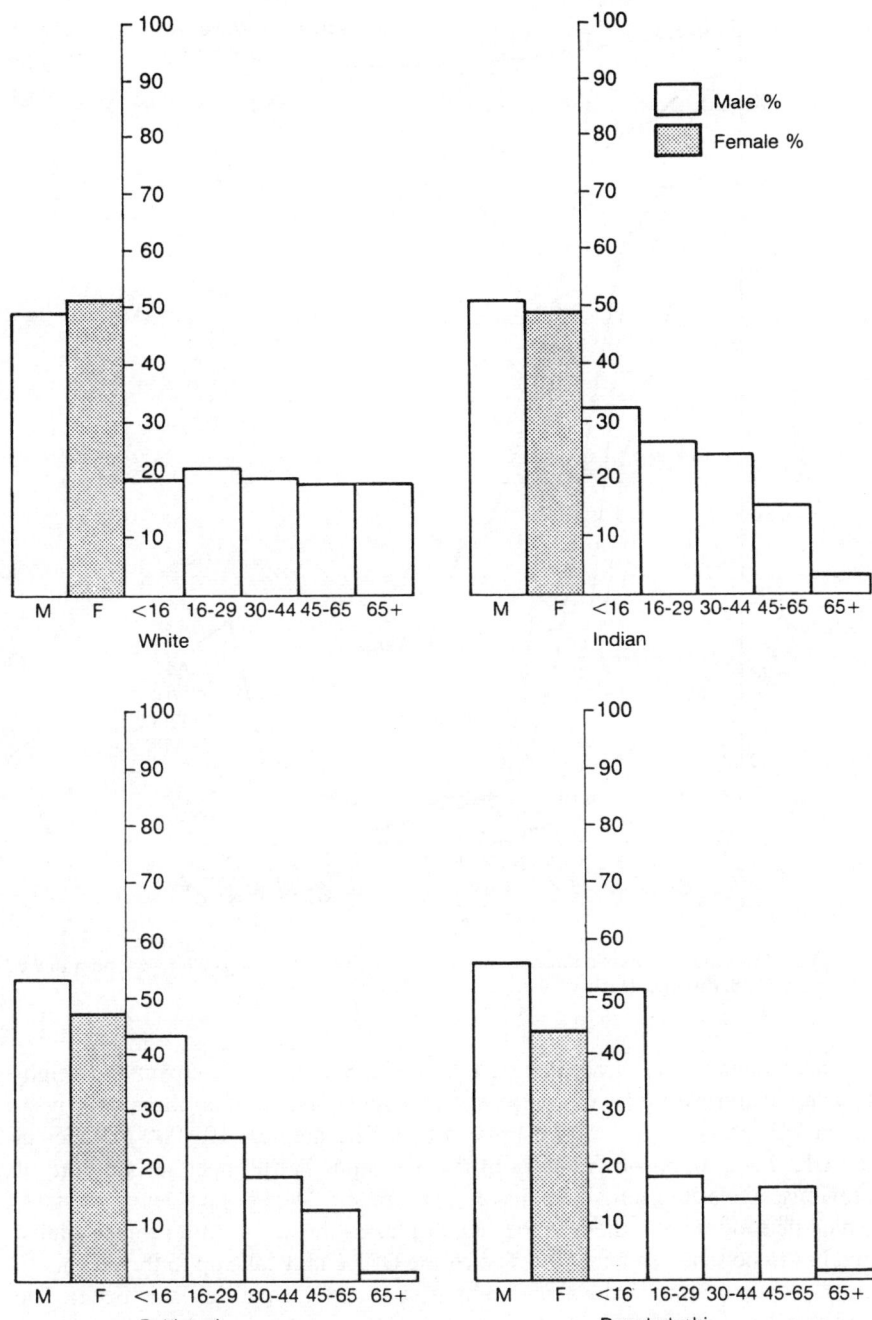

Fig. 25.2 Population of Great Britain by ethnic group, 1985; percentage distribution by age group, and proportion of males and females in each case.

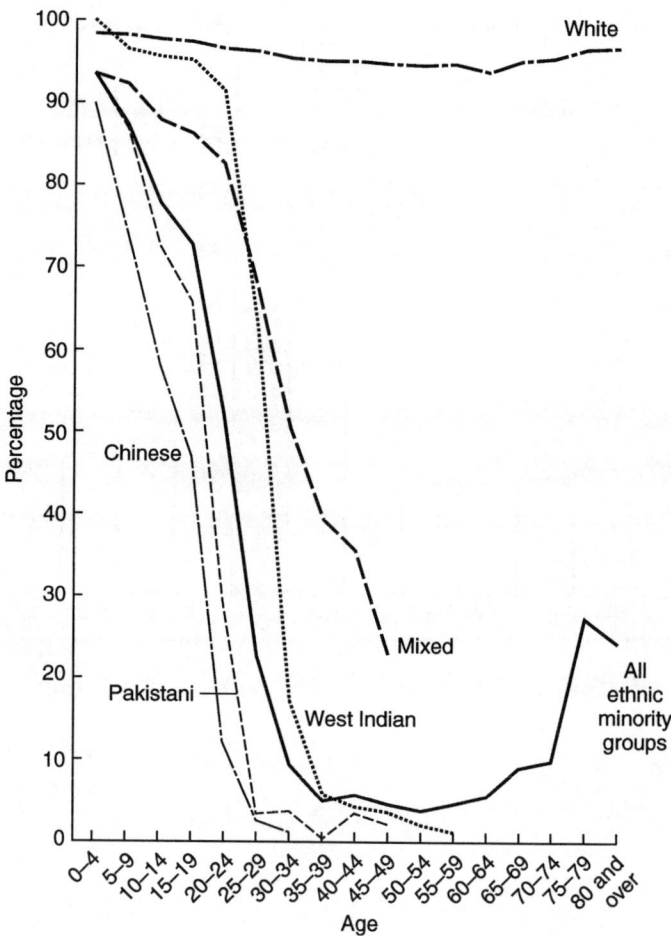

Fig. 25.3 Percentage of ethnic minority population in given age groups who were born in the UK, 1986–1988. (Source: Haskey 1990.)

Ghana, Hungary, Iran, Iraq, Pakistan, Somalia, Sudan, and Vietnam and neighbouring countries (this is of course not a complete list). Not all these have been given full refugee status. It is estimated that there are now 100 000 refugees in the UK. The proportion granted full refugee status has dropped to one third of previous levels; the remainder have been granted 'exceptional leave to stay', which does not entitle them to the same rights as those with full refugee status, and has to be renewed annually. The Home Office may take up to three years to come to a decision, and the situation in most other EC countries is no better. The uncertainties associated with these prolonged, and often unsatisfactory, procedures produces anxiety, depression, psychosis, or suicide, in many refugees, with serious ill-effects on the emotional well-being of their children.

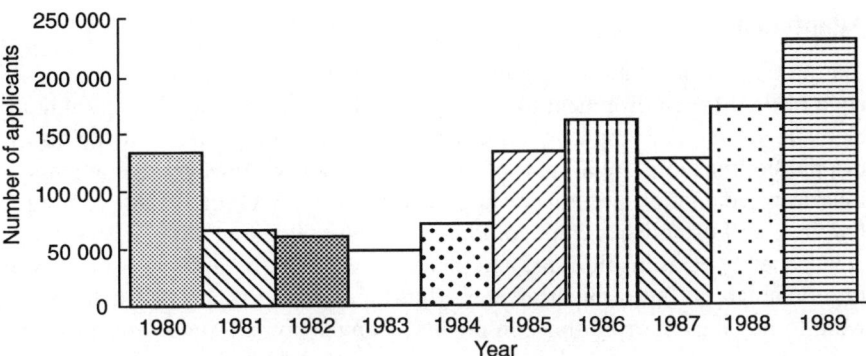

Fig. 25.4 Asylum applications in the European Community. (Source: Crisp 1991.)

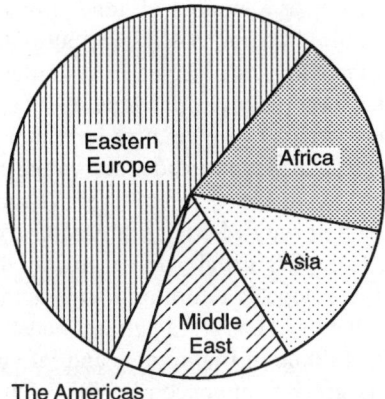

Fig. 25.5 Asylum seekers in the European Community; regions of origin (1989). (Source: Crisp 1991.)

Culture shock, adaptation, acculturation, and assimilation

Culture shock

On arrival the immigrant or refugee may suffer culture shock, the severity being determined by the cultural differences between the entrant's home country and the host country; language difficulties and hostile or degrading procedures by immigration officers make matters worse. The usual manifestations of culture shock are confusion, anxiety, and insecurity, often followed by depression and paranoid feelings. These responses may be transient, long lasting, or permanent.

Adaptation

The process of adaptation involves initially the acquisition of sufficient knowledge of the new environment to survive without undue discomfort; learning the elements of the new language, understanding the currency, and knowing how to use public transport, are all part of this initial process. However, the amount of long-term adaptation necessary varies enormously. A Punjabi Sikh coming to live in a well established Sikh community in West London, with its own shops, newspapers, social institutions, and places of worship, would require relatively little adaptation, but a much greater adjustment would be needed if he or she were to move away from this community. Conversely, a refugee arriving alone from Africa, speaking only his or her native language, and with no family group or community to join, would have to undergo a great deal of adaptation.

Acculturation and assimilation

In the long term, usually over a number of generations, an ethnic minority will acquire some of the cultural characteristics and attitudes of the recipient community, and may become partly or completely assimilated into the host society.

The ability to make these changes depends upon the attitude of the group. Immigrants who choose to stay in a country to which they came of their own free will usually have little difficulty in adapting to the extent necessary for their economic survival and advancement. However, Asians and Afro-Caribbeans have tended to retain their way of life to a greater extent than, for example, Italians or Cypriots. Refugees usually have greater difficulties because they have, initially at least, the hope of returning home, and tend to live in an unreal world centred on past events at home—a cultural bereavement.

The attitudes of the children of immigrants and refugees towards members of the host community is greatly influenced by that of their parents, and stereotyped views acquired in early childhood may be difficult to discard.

The health and welfare of children of ethnic minorities

Though the children of immigrants and refugees have many problems in common, the children of refugees are more likely to suffer emotional or psychological disturbances, not only because of their experiences in their home country, but because of the disturbed or disturbing behaviour of their parents in their struggle to exist in the new environment and their anxieties about their application for asylum.

Oztek (1986) in a survey of the health of Turkish immigrants in West Berlin found that 57 per cent of Turkish children below 15 years were looked after by people other than their mother, and nearly 20 per cent of pre-school children were looked after by slightly older siblings. In West Berlin Oztek found that 24 per cent of Turkish children were malnourished, a higher rate than a comparable group in Turkey.

Patterns of emotional and psychological disorders

Emotional disturbances in a young child are an indication of disordered family relationships or behaviour, or in older children, of difficulties at school or in the wider community. Oztek (1986) found that minor symptoms of emotional disorder, such as stuttering and nail-biting, were commoner in Turkish children in West Berlin than in a similar group in Turkey.

The presenting symptoms of non-organic disease in Asians, Africa, and Turkish patients are different from those in European patients. Depression or anxiety are expressed in purely physical terms (somatization), such as pain in the head, abdomen, or limbs, or as an ill-defined 'body-ache'. 'Fever' may be used as a synonym for feeling unwell. The child presents his or her emotional problems or tensions in this somatic form, but it is important to exclude organic disease such as anaemia, nutritional rickets, tuberculosis, or parasitic disease. Even if an organic disease is not suspected, a blood-count or X-ray may convince the parents that their child's symptoms are being taken seriously. There is often considerable resistance to the diagnosis of emotional disorder, particularly if it appears that this originates in the home.

Until recently it was thought that anorexia and bulimia nervosa were confined to Europeans, but these conditions are now appearing in Asian (Bhadrinath 1990; Mumford *et al.* 1991), and Afro-Caribbean (Thomas and Szmukler 1985) adolescent girls.

The child's reaction to altered or abnormal parental behaviour

The parents' initial reactions to arrival in a new country have already been described. The infant may respond to unusual parental behaviour or to an altered or irregular routine with feeding difficulties, incessant crying, sleep disturbance, or failure to thrive (Fenton *et al.* 1984). The pre-school child may become excessively demanding, or develop food refusal, exaggerated negative behaviour, regression in social development, or difficulties with toilet training. The older child may become enuretic or encopretic, or show negative or disruptive behaviour at home.

School difficulties

Many parents, particularly those of Asian or South-East Asian origin, have very high expectations for their children's school and academic performance. If the child's abilities are not up to parental expectations, he or she may react by truanting, unruly classroom behaviour, elective mutism, or deterioration in school performance. Children of ethnic minorities may be bullied or mocked because of their accent. Teaching staff may be insensitive, unsympathetic, or actually racist in their attitude.

The adolescent's difficulties

Where a group's cultural pattern differs greatly from that of the host country, conflicts may develop between the behaviour expected at home and that of schoolmates and the adolescent's social circle. Asian girls experience special difficulties; they are expected to be the dutiful daughter at home, but may wish to stay out late at night or go to discos. A boyfriend of a different religion or ethnic group may provoke intense parental disapproval. An Asian girl with a western-style social circle may find an arranged marriage difficult or impossible to accept.

The adolescent's reaction to these difficulties may be to develop psychosomatic complaints, or they may abscond from home, or take an overdose as a suicidal gesture. Adolescent boys may join a gang which fulfils their desire to exhibit 'macho' behaviour.

Child abuse

There is no evidence that physical or sexual child abuse is any more or less common in any of the ethnic minorities than in the general population. However, in some communities child abuse may be concealed, because of a refusal to accept the possibility. In Afro-Caribbean families disciplinary physical punishment, with a belt or strap, may be used, but this should not be considered child abuse unless it is administered very frequently, with excessive violence, or from sadistic motives.

Organic disease

With the exception of β-thalassaemia in people from the Mediterranean and Aegean region, it is mainly groups from the West Indies and the ISC who require special provision for conditions such as sickle-cell disease and nutritional rickets.

Antenatal screening

Congenital rubella is more common in the infants of Asian women in Britain than in the general population (Miller *et al*. 1987). This is because many women, born in the ISC, have not been immunized before coming to Britain to get married. Those who are found, at antenatal testing, to have no antibodies should be offered immunization in the immediate postnatal period, while they are still in hospital.

Between three and ten per cent of Asian women and ten and 20 per cent of South-East Asian women are infective carriers of Hepatitis B virus (HBV). Women in these groups should be screened antenatally and the infants of a mother considered to be infective should be protected with immunoglobulin and HBV vaccine according to the standard procedure.

All women belonging to ethnic groups with a high carrier rate (p. 425) for β-thalassaemia and sickle-cell disease should be screened antenatally. In Britain, this means that most antenatal clinics screen for both these conditions all women who are likely (on grounds of the patient's statement, appearance, name, or language spoken) to belong to one of the affected groups. The increasing number of people of mixed race emphasizes the importance of this policy. Genetic counselling and advice on prenatal testing and termination should be given when both partners are found to be carriers of the same condition or one partner is heterozygous for thalassaemia and the other for sickle-cell disease or other abnormal haemoglobin. Neonatal screening should be done in all newborn infants in areas where there is a high proportion of at-risk groups, and in selected cases in other areas. Neonatal testing should be used to confirm the results of prenatal tests, and where antenatal or prenatal testing has not been performed: this is particularly important where there is known to be a risk of sickle-cell disease because the acceptance of antenatal and prenatal testing is much lower than for β-thalassaemia. In Birmingham, Bundey et al. (1991) found an excess of lethal malformations in the perinatal period in the Pakistani community—these had not been recognized on routine ultrasound though the mothers had booked early. They showed that, in contrast to neural tube defects which were not common on this group, these malformations were difficult to detect on routine ultrasound and suggested that Pakistani mothers should be referred to the nearest specialist centre.

The perinatal period

A number of early studies found that the perinatal mortality rate (PMR) was high, compared with that in the white population, in all the Asian communities in Britain. However, MacVicar (1990) showed a progressive decline in the PMR in Leicestershire between 1976 and 1986 (Fig. 25.6) in the Asian community (largely Gujarati Indians); by 1986 the PMR for Asians and non-Asians was the same. MacFadyen (1989) showed a similar fall in PMR in an affluent Asian community in London from 1974 onwards; by 1984 the PMR was the same as that of the indigenous population in the same area.

In contrast to these findings Bundey and her colleagues (1991) showed that the PMR of Pakistanis in Birmingham has remained high and that lethal malformations (see above) accounted for 50 per cent of all perinatal deaths. The risk of a Pakistani woman carrying a fetus with a lethal malformation was one in 100, compared to one in 150 for the Bangladeshis (the numbers for this group were small), one in 250 for Europeans, one in 300 for the Indians, and one in 500 for

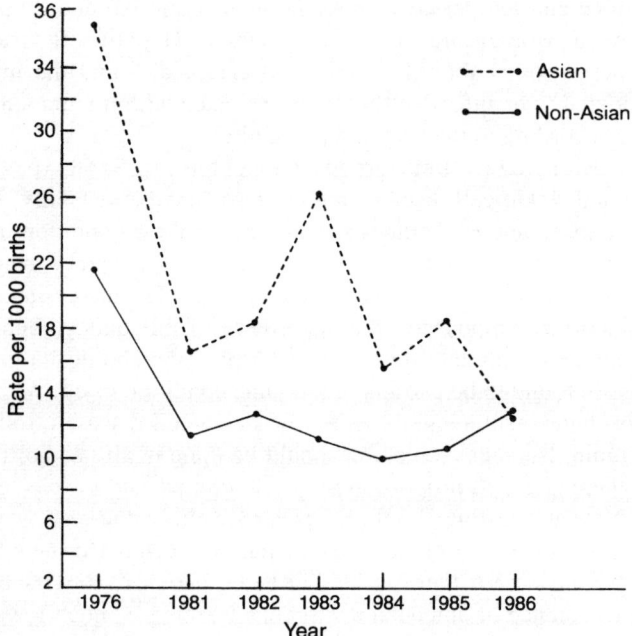

Fig. 25.6 Perinatal mortality rates in Asian and non-Asians in Leicestershire, 1976–86. (Source: MacVicar 1990.)

the Afro-Caribbeans. Consanguineous marriages were common among the Pakistanis and 40 per cent of parents were more closely related than first cousins (mainly uncle–niece marriages). This survey found thirteen deaths from recognized recessively determined conditions (not malformations) in consanguineous marriages and none in the non-consanguineous ones. Consanguinity is therefore an important factor in the high PMR of Pakistanis in Britain and may be related also to some of the lethal malformations.

Birth-weight

Chetcuti *et al.* (1985) found, in all Asian groups, that the newborns were smaller and lighter than in the white population. Punjabi Sikh infants had a mean birth-weight which was only slightly less than that of white infants. Bundey *et al.* (1991) confirmed these findings and showed that Afro-Caribbeans had a mean birth-weight similar to that of Asians.

Alberman (1991) has shown that, while there has been a progressive increase in mean birth-weight of the infants of British born mothers between 1986 and 1989, there has been no change in the mean birth-weight for babies of mothers born in India, Pakistan, and the West Indies. However, there is an increasing proportion of Asian and Afro-Caribbean women of child-bearing age who are born in Britain (Fig. 25.3).

Genetically determined disease

Three conditions are of major importance: β-thalassaemia, sickle-cell disease, and glucose-6-phosphate dehydrogenase (G-6-PD) deficiency; α-thalassaemia of the severe type is largely confined to people from South-East Asia (see below).

The haemoglobinopathies There is a high carrier rate (17 per cent) for β-thalassaemia in the Greek and Turkish Cypriot population in Britain. Carrier rates for people from the ISC are: Gujurati Indians 10 per cent, Pakistanis 5 per cent, Punjabi Sikhs 3 per cent, and Bangladeshis 1.5 per cent. β-thalassaemia also occurs, but less commonly, in the Middle East, North Africa, South-East Asia, Sri Lanka, Nepal, and the Philippines.

As previously described (p. 423) antenatal screening is important, as is education, particularly in schools with a high proportion of affected groups. Advice and testing centres should be available in all large centres of population.

α-thalassaemia (Hb Barts disease) is the commonest cause of hydrops fetalis in infants of South-East Asian origin. For a couple who have had one affected infant there is a one in four chance of a recurrence. Death usually occurs in late pregnancy or shortly after birth; there is no effective treatment. Heterozygote detection is difficult and should be done at a specialist centre, but no screening programmes have been set up and there are no reliable figures for the prevalence of the carrier state. Prenatal diagnosis is now available.

Sickle-cell disease has a negligible incidence in those Asian groups that have migrated to Europe, but the carrier rate for Afro-Caribbeans in Britain is one in ten, so that one in 400 infants are at risk from homozygous sickle-cell anaemia. In Africans, particularly those from west and central Africa, the carrier rate is one in five. Genetic advice and screening should be on the same lines as for β-thalassaemia.

Haemoglobin SC disease (HbC and HbS) and sickle-cell-β-thalassaemia occur but are less severe than homozygous sickle cell anaemia. Haemoglobin D-thalassaemia is found in people from North India and haemoglobin E-thalassaemia occurs in Bangladeshis.

Glucose-6-phosphate dehydrogenase (G-6-PD) deficiency. Though there are numerous genetic variants of G-6-PD deficiency, only three clinical forms need to be considered—the Mediterranean, the Far Easter, and the African forms. The Mediterranean and Far Eastern forms behave in a similar manner clinically and are more severe than the African form. G-6-PD deficiency is transmitted through an X-linked intermediate gene with variable expressions in the heterozygous female. In communities with a high prevalence of the gene, homozygous females are not uncommon and may be as severely deficient in the enzyme as the hemizygous male. The Mediterranean form occurs in 20–30 per cent of males in Greece, and is common in Cyprus, southern Italy, Sardinia, Sicily, and Turkey. The African form is found in African and Afro-Caribbean males; 6–12 per cent of Afro-Caribbean males in Europe are deficient in the enzyme. In South China and neighbouring countries around five per cent of males are affected. The incidence of G-6-PD deficient Indian males is around five per cent and the clinical picture is similar to that in the Mediterranean form. Since the condition is rarely life-threatening and neonatal jaundice in deficient infants can be effectively treated, there is not indication for antenatal screening or prenatal testing.

Acquired diseases

Nutritional disorders. Vitamin D deficiency or (nutritional) rickets is found in the children of all Asian groups living in Europe and occurs occasionally in Afro-Caribbeans.

Contributory factors are a strict vegetarian diet (mainly Hindus), maternal vitamin D deficiency during pregnancy and prolonged lactation, the use of 'door-step' (i.e. cow's) milk for infant feeding, poor uptake of vitamin D supplements by pregnant women and pre-school children, the screening effect from sunlight by pigmented skin, and in Muslim girls, lack of exposure of the limbs to sunlight. In adolescents rickets may be mistaken for a psychosomatic condition. If rickets is discovered in a child, the rest of the family should be investigated.

Anaemia. Iron-deficiency anaemia is common in the children of all Asian groups. Contributory factors are a strict vegetarian diet (Hindus), iron deficiency during pregnancy, short birth interval, prolonged breast- or bottle-feeding, and the late introduction of iron-containing solids. If a child is found to have iron deficiency anaemia, the whole family should be investigated.

Other acquired diseases In Asian communities the following conditions are more common than in the indigenous population: tuberculosis, gastrointestinal infections (rotavirus infection, shigellosis, salmonellosis, typhoid and paratyphoid, giardiasis, and amoebiasis), malaria, hepatitis A and B, hookworm and roundworm infestations. Most of these conditions are acquired during visits to the ISC, but others, such as tuberculosis, rotavirus infection, shigellosis, and salmonellosis may be acquired from other members of the household. A survey in Holland (van Geuns 1986) showed that tuberculosis was 15–20 times more common in Turkish and Moroccan immigrants than in the native Dutch population.

Culturally determined procedures

Female circumcision This operation is performed on nearly all girls in many African countries and the tradition persists in immigrant and refugee groups in

Britain and elsewhere. In the most extensive and mutilating form (infibulation or Pharaonic type) the clitoris, labia minora, and part of the labia majora are removed and the vulval opening is sewn up, leaving a small hole for urine and menstrual blood. There are numerous immediate and long-term complications (McLean and Graham 1985), and fetal death or brain damage may result from a prolonged or obstructed labour.

The operation is illegal in the UK (Prohibition of Female Circumcision Act 1985) but it is almost certainly being performed illegally, and girls are sometimes sent abroad to have the operation. Though female circumcision may be considered as a form of child abuse, social workers have been reluctant to intervene because they do not wish to antagonize communities which believe that they are doing the best for their child. In a few instances the operation has been prevented by invoking child protection procedures, but the best approach to eradicating this operation in ethnic minorities, and in Africa itself, would seem to lie in education.

Health services for ethnic minorities

Uptake of services

It is difficult to say, because of conflicting evidence, whether the uptake of services by ethnic minorities differs significantly from that of the indigenous population. There are still many areas lacking in proper facilities for advice, diagnosis, and treatment of the haemoglobinopathies.

The use of 'indigenous' medicines and 'traditional' practitioners

There are few data on the use of these medicines and practitioners, and it seems probable that those who use them may be unwilling to admit to it when questioned.

Barriers to the use of health services and factors prejudicial to health

Newly arrived immigrants or refugees find an unfamiliar health care system difficult to understand, and need advice on how to get the best out of it. They may be suspicious of a system (e.g. the British National Health Service) which provides most of its services without charge.

Mothers who do not speak the language of the host community find it difficult to obtain appropriate health care for their children. Asian mothers, in particular, have special problems since they spend much of their time in the home and have little opportunity to learn a new language. Hospitals, surgeries, and clinics, should make available multilingual information and instruction leaflets. Language classes can be useful but the house-bound Asian mother may be unable or unwilling to attend classes outside her home. Videotapes for language teaching and health education are particularly useful since most Asian households have a home video.

Interpreters may be necessary at times but are difficult to find and expensive if suitably qualified. Except in an emergency, children should not be used as interpreters for their parents. *Ad hoc* arrangements with hospital staff are unsatisfactory, because they have other things to do, and because of a possible breach of confidentiality in medico-legal or child abuse cases. The most constructive and successful approach has been the employment by health authorities of link, liaison, or advocate workers belonging to the main ethnic groups in the area; they are able to convey the patient's needs and anxieties to medical and nursing staff, and can explain what it is that the staff are doing or wish to do (Cornwell and Gordon 1984).

Ignorance on the part of receptionists, records clerks, nurses, and doctors of the correct pronunciation of a name may result in the patient or parent not recognizing, and therefore not responding to, a mispronounced name. Notes may be lost or misfiled because of a failure to understand the naming system or because of inconsistent spelling. In China and Vietnam the family name is placed before the given name, but many families adopt the European system: it is necessary to ask which system is being used. Muslim names cause much confusion unless their system is properly understood.

Training in the pronunciation of patients' names should be given to all health workers and clerical staff who come into contact with patients. They should be instructed how to record Asian names in a logical and consistent manner; booklets are available for this purpose (National Extension College). Many Asian mothers are unwilling or afraid to take their children for a medical appointment unless accompanied by an adult male. This may involve waiting until the father returns from work, when it is too late for attention except at the nearest Accident and Emergency Department. In addition, the father may be reluctant to take too much time off work for numerous visits in case he should lose his job. Evening outpatient clinics and surgeries would reduce the pressure on the Accident and Emergency Department.

It is not always realized that Asian women and older girls prefer to be examined by a woman doctor; if one is not available the accompanying male relative should be asked to give his permission for the examination to be carried out by a male. In hospital the Muslim child may refuse to eat food which has not been prepared according to Islamic laws. Hospitals should allow parents to bring food into the ward, or should make available meals acceptable to Muslims. Merely to provide an 'Asian meal' is quite inadequate.

Racial harassment

Racial harassment causes severe anxiety and insecurity, or paranoid feelings, in a threatened family. The children may be too frightened to go to school or to leave the house at all. There is evidence, in Britain, that the police response to racist threats or attacks is often slow, unenthusiastic, and ineffective. This reinforces the family's feelings of helplessness and depression.

Housing conditions

In one borough in London there has been evidence of racial discrimination in the allocation of council housing (Commission for Racial Equality 1984). Ethnic minority families are usually allocated the worst housing, particularly if the family is Asian or Afro-Caribbean. Overcrowding is common. In Britain black households are three to four times more likely to become statutorily homeless than are white households, and 80 per cent of families housed in hotel bed and breakfast accommodation in East London are Bangladeshis (Bradshaw 1990).

In a study of a poorly housed, overcrowded Bengali (Bangladeshi) community in the East End of London, Hyndman (1990) found a high correlation between damp housing, poor respiratory health, gastroenteritis, and depression. Khan *et al.* (1986), in a study of gastroenteritis in the same area of London, compared the social and nutritional status of Asian and Caucasian infants with gastroenteritis. Forty three per cent of the Asian infants came from social classes IV and V compared to 28 per cent of the Caucasians, and 10.8 per cent of the Asian infants were admitted to hospital compared to 3.9 per cent of the Caucasians.

Health service policy and ethnic minorities

In Britain, and probably in most western European countries, there is no coherent policy for health services for ethnic minorities. There has been no clear guidance by the Department of Health or the Regional Health Authorities and it has been left to the District Health Authorities to work out their own policies. Part of the difficulty may lie in the number of different communities, each with differing needs, but a more plausible explanation is that governments hoped that the problem would go away if they waited long enough, either the *gastarbeiter* would go home, or in Britain, the Asians and Afro-Caribbeans would somehow blend into the background. Neither of these has happened.

In Britain, various initiatives, such as the 'Asian mother and baby' and 'Stop rickets' campaigns have been sponsored and supported by the Department of Health. Unfortunately, the period when constructive policies should have been worked out coincided with a series of administrative reorganizations and financial cut-backs, which occupied the energies of the administrative and medical staff. McNaught (1988) has described the history and background of the efforts of one District Health Authority in South London to formulate a policy for the health care of ethnic minorities. After a series of ineffective meetings and abortive committees, little was achieved between 1976 and 1985, and the only time when services for the ethnic minorities seemed likely to gain support was when their special needs were invoked in order to prevent a further financial cut-back.

To make adequate provision for the health care of ethnic minorities is not easy. On the one hand authorities may be accused of stereotyping and of discrimination against certain groups, or of telling them how to run their lives, and on the other hand they may be accused of showing a callous disregard for socially and economically disadvantaged groups. What is lacking is an attempt to discover from the ethnic minorities themselves what sort of health provision they would like.

Conclusion

Ethnic minorities, whether immigrants or refugees, are subjected to discrimination in nearly every aspect of their lives. This chapter has examined the effects of this discrimination on the children of various ethnic groups, and has described the patterns of disease which are common to all groups, and those diseases which are peculiar to certain groups. There is a clear need for more humane attitudes to immigration procedures and the processing of applications for asylum.

None of the Western European countries appears to have a clearly thought out policy for the socio-economic future of immigrants and refugees; equally, little has been done to make proper provision for their special medical needs within the national health services.

In all areas there has been a lack of consultation with the ethnic communities on what special provision they would like, and how their aims should be achieved. Representation of ethnic minorities on the relevant health service committees is either absent or inadequate.

References

Alberman, E. (1991). Are our babies becoming bigger? *Journal of the Royal Society of Medicine* **84**, 257–60.

Bhadrinath, B.R. (1990). Anorexia nervosa in adolescents of Asian extraction. *British Journal of Psychiatry* **156**, 565–8.

Bradshaw, J. (1990). *Child poverty and deprivation in the UK*, p. 41. National Children's Bureau, London.

Bundey, S., Alam, H., Kaur, A., Mir, S., and Lancashire, R. (1991). Why do UK-born Pakistani babies have high perinatal and mortality rates? *Paediatric and Perinatal Epidemiology* **5**, 101–14.

Chetcuti, P., Sinha, S.H., and Levene, M.I. (1985). Birth size in Indian ethnic subgroups born in Britain. *Archives of Disease in Childhood* **60**, 868–70.

Commission for Racial Equality (1984). *Race and council housing in Hackney. Report of a formal investigation*. Commission for Racial Equality, London.

Cornwell, J. and Gordon, P. (ed.) (1984). *An experiment in advocacy, the Hackney multi-ethnic women's project*. King's Fund Centre, London.

Crisp, J. (1991). Refugees; debating the E.C.'s role. *Refugees*, No. 83, 14–15.

Fenton, T.R., Bhat, R., Davies, A., and West, R. (1984). Maternal insecurity and failure to thrive in Asian children. *Archives of Disease in Childhood* **64**, 369–72.

Haskey, J. (1990). The ethnic minority population of Great Britain: estimates by ethnic group and country of birth. *Population Trends*, No. 60, pp. 35–8. Office of Population Censuses and Surveys, HMSO, London.

Hooper, E. (1991). Touchdown to trauma. *Refugees* **83**, 31–3.

Hyndman, S.J. (1990). Housing dampness among British Bengalis in East London. *Social Science and Medicine* **30**, 131–41.

Khan, S., Chong, S.K.F., Cullinan, T., and Walker-Smith, J.A. (1986). Gastroenteritis and its impact on nutrition in Asian and Caucasian infants in East London. In *Diarrhoea and malnutrition in childhood* (ed. J.A. Walker-Smith and A.S. McNeish), pp. 129–34. Butterworths, London.

MacFadyen, I.R. (1989). Pregnancy. In *Ethnic factors in health and disease*, (ed. J.K. Cruickshank and D.G. Beevers), pp. 87–94. Butterworth-Heinemann, Oxford.

McNaught, A. (1988). *Race and health policy*, pp. 73–114. Croom Helm, London.

MacVicar, J. (1990). Obstetrics: the Asian mother and child. In *Health care for Asians*, (ed. B.R. McAvoy and L.J. Donaldson), pp. 172–91. Oxford University Press.

Miller, E., Nicoll, A., Rousseau, S.A., Sequerra, P.J.L., Hambling, M.H., Smithells, R.W., *et al.* (1987). Congenital rubella in babies of South Asian women in England and Wales. *British Medical Journal* **294**, 737–9.

Mumford, D.B., Whitehouse, A.M., and Platts, M. (1991). Sociocultural correlates of eating disorders among Asian schoolgirls in Bradford. *British Journal of Psychiatry* **158**, 222–8.

National Extension College (undated). *Asians in Britain: recording and using Asian names*. National Extension College, Cambridge.

Oztek, Z.C. (1986). Social and health problems of migrant workers. In *Migration and health*, (ed. M. Colledge, H.A. van Geuns, and P.-G. Svensson), pp. 128–37. World Health Organization, Copenhagen.

Power, J. and Hardman, A. (1984). *Western Europe's migrant workers*. Report No. 28. Minority Rights Group, London.

Thomas, J.P. and Szmukler, G.I. (1985). Anorexia nervosa in patients of Afro-Caribbean extraction. *British Journals of Psychiatry* **146**, 653–6.

van Geuns, H.A. (1986). Health care in Turkish and Moroccan immigrants. In *Migration and health*, (ed. M. Colledge, H.A. van Geuns, and P.-G. Svensson), pp. 92–102. World Health Organization, Copenhagen.

Webster, J. and Fox, J. (1989). The changing nature of populations. In *Ethnic factors in health and disease*, (ed. J.K. Cruickshank and D.G. Beevers), pp. 7–11. Wright, London.

Further reading

Black, J. (1989). *Child health in a multicultural society*. British Medical Journal Publications, London.

Boyden, J. and Hudson, A. (1985). *Children: rights and responsibilities*. Report No 69. Minority Rights Group, London.

D'Souza, F. and Crisp, J. (1985). *The refugee dilemma. Report* No 43. Minority Rights Group, London

Emecheta, B. (1974). *Second class citizen*. Fontana and Collins, London.
Joly, D. and Nettleton, C. (1990). *Refugees in Europe*. Minority Rights Group, London.
Mo, T. (1983). *Sour sweet*. Sphere Books and Abacus, London.
Tajfel, H. (undated). *The social psychology of minorities*. Report No 38. Minority Rights Group, London.
Tournier, M. (1988). *The golden droplet*. Methuen, London.
UNICEF (1991). *The state of the world's children, 1991*. World declaration on the survival, protection and development of children; the world summit for children, September 30, 1990, pp. 51–74. UNICEF and Oxford University Press, Oxford.
World Health Organization (1988). *The haemoglobinopathies in Europe*. WHO, Copenhagen.

26 Risk and resilience processes in childhood and adolescence

Ian M. Goodyer

Introduction

Over the past two decades substantial advances have been made in delineating those features of family and social relationships that predict maladjustment or psychiatric disorder. These extensive programmes of research have focused on environmental factors that increase the risk of, or protect children from, psychiatric disorder (Rolfe *et al.* 1990; Goodyer 1990; Rutter 1987). Overall it has become apparent that a child's response to adverse environments cannot be fully understood without taking into account their age, stage of development, gender, and the full nature and social circumstances within which they live (Goodyer 1990). In other words, there is a dynamic interplay between a child's constitution and the environment which determines the degree and type of response to environmental demands.

The significance of developmental factors in understanding response to social adversities is well illustrated by a consideration of the impact of chronic parenting difficulties on children of different ages. Thus, chronic parenting difficulties in the first two years of a child's life impairs normal social and cognitive development (Murray 1988). By contrast, the same type of parenting difficulties occurring for the first time in middle childhood results in conduct disorder with modest effects on cognitive development (Rutter 1985).

In addition, risk studies have also demonstrated that, for some children, exposure to adverse social environments does not result in emotional or behavioural disorders (Garmezy 1985; Rutter 1990). Such observations have led to further enquiries aimed at determining why some children are resilient in the face of adversity (Rutter 1987).

These enquiries have indicated that associations between risk 'factors' and adverse outcomes are not always what they seem at first sight. For example, parenting deficits in infancy are explained by parental (usually but not exclusively maternal) neglect of the child often in association with adult psychiatric disorder, generally depression. In middle childhood, parenting deficits associated with conduct disorder are explained by chronic marital disharmony, generally involving aggression between the parents, which is not dependent on adult psychiatric disorder. Parental neglect occurs in both circumstances but is in effect a result of quite different mechanisms, the processes of which have different consequences in relation to the age and stage of the child's development.

From the environmental perspective, it is apparent that measurement of the quality of parenting is a necessary but insufficient first step to delineate the psychopathological mechanisms that operate to determine the adverse outcome for the child. It is clear that a knowledge of the child's age and stage of development is required since the rules that govern an individual's response to environmental demands require an understanding of the person–environment relationship (Hinde 1988). Accordingly, we must ask what personal characteristics the child brings to bear when exposed to environmental demand. Again, however, things are not always what they seem at first sight.

For example, intelligence is a factor continuously distributed amongst the population. Lower intelligence is associated with increased rates of psychopathology and neurological disability. Higher intelligence confers an increased likelihood of lower rates of difficulties and disorders in a similar manner. At IQs of less than 50, however, the main effect on adverse outcomes is directly attributed to mechanisms related to cerebral dysfunction itself, giving rise to manifold neurodevelopmental and behavioural difficulties at any age and stage of development. Above the IQ level of 70, these cerebral dysfunction mechanisms are less apparent or non-existent; why then are some children within this IQ range still subject to similar forms of behaviour disorder as those with IQs below 70? Again, we can see that measuring the personal characteristic of intelligence does not provide an explanation for the underlying mechanisms that predispose an individual to an adverse outcome. Indeed, one may be misled into conferring meaning on the measured factor when the latent (non-measured) mechanisms are different at differing levels of that factor. This example demonstrates that we must take into account the possibility that different mechanisms may exist for a measured personal characteristic dependent on other (non-measured) features of the individual and the environment. We need therefore to determine concurrently a range of environmental demands together with those features of the child that are likely to exert effects, good or bad, on outcome. From this basis we can discuss what is meant by the broad concepts of risk and resilience and subsequently by the more specific notions of vulnerability and protection.

Risk

Put simply, risk occurs when the likelihood of an adverse outcome is increased following exposure to an identifiable variable. This proposes a causal relationship between factor and outcome but, as already noted, does not indicate the nature of such a relationship. The risk process arises as a consequence of adverse person–environment interaction. The nature of risk from the environment will be dependent on the number of adverse variables; the intensity of the stimulus; duration of exposure; and, importantly, the temporal relationship between the event, the person, and the outcome.

The timing of environmental demands

The importance of the timing of adverse environments has received little attention in the literature, yet it is a crucial concept as far as determining the mechanisms of risk is concerned. For example, we must establish that putative causal factors occur prior to the onset of disorder. If this is not done, then adverse environments may be a consequence of the child's disorder. Equally, however, we may wish to determine if illnesses (physical and mental) are themselves increasing the risk for subsequent socio-emotional difficulties. For example, when school-age children and adolescents experience moderate to severe deficiencies in friendships there is, within the next 12 months, a significantly increased risk of occurrence of either anxiety or depressive disorders (Goodyer *et al.* 1989). The presence of depressive disorder may, however, also increase the risk for subsequent deficiencies in friendships (Goodyer *et al.* 1991; Puig-Antich *et al.* 1985).

These findings demonstrate that, when investigating the effects of peer group difficulties, it is necessary to determine the temporal relationship between friendships and disorder, so that the direction of effects between persons and the environment can be elucidated. The findings described above demonstrate that in some cases adverse friendships put children at risk, but, equally, depressed children put their friendships at risk.

Cumulative impact of different risk circumstances

Of course, for most children at risk, more than one set of environmental demands exist at the same time in their lives. In such circumstances we need to determine the associations between risk circumstances as well as the nature of their combined effects. Two somewhat different types of association have so far been described.

Connection between different forms of risk circumstances

Firstly, one type of risk circumstance may significantly increase the risk of a different type of risk circumstance. For example, recent undesirable life events show a tendency to occur in families where there is aggregation of a history of major depression in one or more family members (McGuffin 1988; Goodyer *et al.* 1991). In such circumstances there is (statistically at least) an inextricable link between life events and parental psychiatric disorder, indicating that the two are connected in some as yet unspecified way. Of the few studies to investigate this problem so far, parental depression appears to precede the onset of life events, which tend in the main to be family-related events (Goodyer *et al.* 1991). It appears likely that some children are more likely to be exposed to recent undesirable life events because of previous depression in their parents (Goodyer *et al.* 1988). The precise mechanism of this relationship is unclear; perhaps parental depression results in persistently disturbed family relationships which increases the risk of recent life events. Alternatively, parental depression may decrease parental competence, resulting in more specific undesirable events (such as accidents around the home) without resulting in chronic family disharmony.

Connection of different risk circumstances suggests that some types of risk are causally related. It is important to note, however, that although parental depression may result in increasing the child's exposure to undesirable events, both of these circumstances exert significant additive risk on the likelihood on the occurrence of psychiatric disorder (Goodyer *et al.* 1988). In other words, regardless of the origins of each of the risk variables measured, they exert significant cumulative effects. (The nature of this mechanism is considered again on p. 445).

Additivity of risk circumstances

Not all forms of risk circumstances are causally connected, however. An alternative mechanism may be concurrent exposure to independent and different forms of risk. Under these conditions there may be no connectivity between risk circumstances. For example, some children experience concurrently recent family adversities and recent friendship difficulties. Both of these sets of different undesirable life experiences carry significant risk for the subsequent onset of anxiety or depressive disorders (Goodyer *et al.* 1990). However, the presence of one set of these adversities does not predict the presence of the other. Therefore knowing the relationships between, for example, parental depression and undesirable life events in a family does not provide an understanding of the friendship difficulties a child is currently experiencing. In other words, family and friendship adversities in school-age children are independent domains of risk that arise from different social mechanisms even though they exert effects of the same magnitude. In these circumstances, risk still increases through an additive effect of the two sets of risk circumstances, i.e. via a combination of the known risks carried by each circumstance.

Threshold of risk for psychiatric disorder

When children are exposed to known risks and remain well, two somewhat different mechanisms may be responsible. Firstly, they may possess individual qualities that truly protect them from the risk effects. These personal qualities are discussed in a later section of this chapter. Secondly, the magnitude of risk may be insufficient to provoke clinically meaningful disorder.

For example, a child who is exposed to a single chronic adverse difficulty, such as persistent marital disharmony, is not at significantly greater risk of conduct disorder than other children. Two or more such chronic difficulties, such as parental psychiatric disorder and chronic marital disharmony, does increase the risk for conduct disorder (Rutter 1990). Thus, marital discord exerts important effects on childhood adjustment only if accompanied by other environmental risk variables (Emery and O'Leary 1984). These findings indicate that the likelihood of disorder is predominantly determined by some kind of 'dose response' or threshold effect determined by the increasing intensity of the undesirable stimuli (Rutter 1979, 1990). This threshold is a quantitative concept dependent on the magnitude of risk effects carried by each measured risk circumstance. A knowledge as to how or why such risks arise is not required to investigate whether threshold effects are important. Clearly some risk effects are unlikely to depend on threshold effects. Major community disasters, wars, and terrorism exert major effects on adjustment if the child has been directly involved. Even in such major circumstances, however, individual differences in response and adaptation to the events and their consequences are evident (Goodyer 1990).

Latent risk effects

Threshold effects generally consider (i) risks that have occurred within a similar time frame even if that is over years, and (ii) risks that are a consequence of ongoing difficulties or recent life events. Some children may be at risk, however, because of events or circumstances that occurred at some point distant in time and are no longer occurring. These past events can result in latent or dormant risk (referred to as sensitizing factors in the risk literature) that are below a threshold effect themselves, but carry the capacity to be activated as a risk circumstance at a later point in time. For example, recent findings have suggested that sexual abuse (meaning actual assault not voyeurism) in childhood significantly impairs adult relationships and increases the likelihood of depression even when other forms of social adversity are accounted for (Bifulco *et al.* 1991).

These latent risk effects suggest that some individuals are sensitized to particular types of difficulty as a result of an early environmental experience. This sensitization may have specific associations and may not generalize to all aspects of a person's life. Thus sexually abused women may be directly sensitized to deficiencies in later adult relationships but not to difficulties with employment. There is no evidence that these adults had psychiatric disorders as children. Of course, many children who are sexually abused suffer overt psychiatric disorder, and for those individuals the effects of abuse are direct risks. The mediating mechanisms which determine whether sexual abuse exerts immediate or sensitizing risk effects are not known. The current findings indicate, however, that when the effects are sensitizing, they become apparent (for girls at least) in the post-pubertal period.

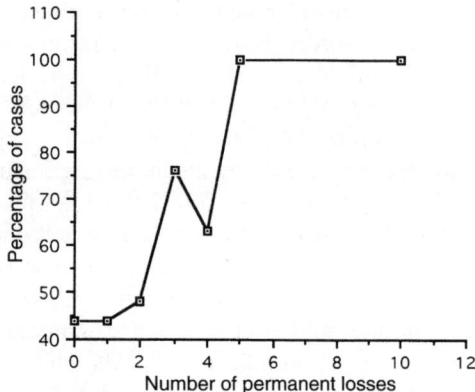

Fig. 26.1

A similar latent effect has been suggested for loss experiences (defined as a permanent exit from the child's social field) in the lives of school-age children and adolescents with emotional disorders (Goodyer and Altham 1991a). Figure 26.1 shows that the greater the number of losses over a child's lifetime, the higher the risk. Firstly, an additive effect is suggested, with emotional disorders becoming increasingly likely with increasing numbers of loss events. Secondly, there is no increase in risk until two or more such events are experienced, indicating a threshold effect for loss experiences.

The effects of such lifetime losses are not explained or subsumed, however, by subsequent other family- or peer-related life events and difficulties which occurred in the 12 months prior to onset of anxiety and depressive disorder (Goodyer and Altham 1991b). This suggests that early multiple loss experiences exert effects for psychopathology in school-age children over and above the risk effects of recent and ongoing social adversities. Could these constitute latent sensitizing effects of early loss for later emotional disorder? We cannot be sure, but the data suggest such a possibility as the majority of these cases were experiencing their first episode of disorder at the time of investigation, i.e. early loss had *not* resulted in immediate psychiatric disorder or chronic family adversities.

The above findings suggest that such sensitizing experiences may operate through cognitive mechanisms resulting in abnormal internal working models or schema that form the basis for subsequent relationship difficulties.

Personal attributes as influences on risk

So far, risk mechanisms have been described as functions and consequences of the social environment. Investigating the environment without considering the intrinsic characteristics of the population under investigation is, however, too narrow a focus for risk research. As already noted, there are (i) marked individual differences in the form and nature of the behavioural response to social stimuli; (ii) no clear specificities between a particular type of psychopathology and a given pattern of environmental risk circumstances; and (iii) substantive age effects on the type and form of response to severe adversities such as chronic marital disharmony. What mechanisms and processes exist in a child which may alter the risk, for better or worse, in the presence of environmental demands has yet to be adequately researched. Some clues are, however, available from the few studies which have measured social adversities and some aspects of individuals concurrently.

Effects of gender

Firstly, there is considerable data to show that boys (particularly prepubertal) are more likely than girls to develop emotional or behavioural disturbances when exposed to family discord (Rutter 1982). The evidence suggests, however, that girls take longer to respond to discord, and that sex differences in the prevalence rates of disorder diminish with time. In addition, sex differences are most prominent in mild and moderate disorders and less evident with increasing severity, especially for emotional disorders.

The risk for boys may be because of biologically determined greater susceptibility to social hazards. Thus the same intensity of family discord may have greater effects on boys than girls. This increase in risk may also lead to greater adverse consequences for boys. Thus boys are more likely than girls to go into care, at the time of family break-up (Packman 1986), and boys are exposed to more parental quarrels than girls (Hetherington *et al.* 1982). Boys are more likely to respond to social adversity with difficult oppositional behaviour, girls are more likely to disengage and withdraw (Rutter 1982; Masten *et al.* 1988).

This male reaction is more likely to elicit a negative response from parents, and may lead to a coercive cycle of disruptive–aggressive response patterns (Patterson 1986*a,b*).

Finally, adults may place a different meaning on aggressive responses in boys and girls. Aggression in boys may be viewed as a desirable response to environmental stimuli, whereas a similar response in girls may be viewed as particularly undesirable. Additionally, adults may respond more positively to girls who disengage and withdraw rather than show aggression (Dunn and Kendrick 1982; Masten *et al.* 1988).

These findings suggest that, for boys and girls, different mechanisms exist for determining the response to the same type of environmental adversity. These gender differences may include the notion that females may be less at risk because of increased biological risk in males. We do not know what these underlying risk mechanisms are but they are likely to involve processes related to central nervous system growth and maturation.

By contrast, girls may be more at risk than boys as a consequence of undesirable events that influence socio-emotional development. For example, girls with a lifetime history of two or more loss events show a somewhat greater tendency to emotional disorders in the school-age years than do boys with a similar number of loss events (Goodyer and Altham 1991a). These latter findings suggest that girls may be more prone than boys to the adverse psychological consequences carried by latent sensitizing effects of multiple losses.

Temperament

The term temperament has become synonymous with the long-held lay notion that people differ in their characteristic styles of behaviour and that, to some extent, these styles have a constitutional origin. In modern times, advances in physiological understanding of the central nervous system have resulted in behaviour being conceptualized in terms of neurobiological and developmental origins. Whilst no firm consensus has yet emerged on the origins, nature, and purpose of temperament, there is good reason to consider this concept, or rubric, as a starting point for understanding the intrinsic mediating mechanisms and processes that influence behavioural responses to environmental stimuli.

What is temperament?

Alexander Thomas and Stella Chess in the 1950s put temperament firmly on the modern scientific map with their New York studies into infants at risk for abnormal behavioural development (Chess and Thomas 1984; Thomas and Chess 1977). In this seminal research programme, temperament was conceptualized as stylistic differences in individual behaviour that appeared early in the first year of life and became the predominant observable behavioural characteristics of that individual across different environmental circumstances. Their longitudinal studies led them to conclude that temperament was best described on a continuum of 'easy' through to 'difficult' behavioural characteristics which were most reliably observed in the presence of environmental demands. Thomas and Chess's notions on the intrinsic behaviour of individuals has resulted in considerable research on both the origins and effects of temperament (Kohnstamm *et al.* 1989).

Currently, temperament is probably best conceptualized as a relatively consistent pattern of behaviour that a child expresses across everyday circumstances. Three groups of behaviour appear to form the core of temperament. Emotionality, meaning the degree of distress; sociability, meaning the degree of interpersonal interest and cooperation; and activity, meaning the amount of physical movement (Buss and Plomin 1984; Plomin and Dunn 1986; Rutter 1987, 1990). There is considerable evidence supporting the validity and stability of these general characteristics across situations and time (Plomin and Dunn 1986; Gibbs *et al.* 1987). These three features remain conceptualized as dimensions of behaviour, i.e. individuals possess all three styles of behaviour to a greater or lesser degree. A child's temperament may therefore be best characterized by the general level and pattern of these three dimensions in differing everyday circumstances rather than as one being more predominant than another. Whilst there is evidence that such behavioural patterns are heritable, the intensity and predominant form of expression of these three dimensions are both shaped by and sensitive to early environmental experiences (Buss and Plomin 1984; Plomin and Dunn 1986; Hinde 1989).

Temperament and psychopathology

In recent years much interest has focused on the possibility that some patterns of temperament may contribute to the risk for subsequent psychopathology. The majority of this work has focused on the role of 'difficult' temperament as increasing risk, rather than 'easy' temperamental styles as protecting children against risk. Thus, in cross-sectional studies, an association has been found between 'difficult' temperament (consisting broadly of high emotionality, poor sociability, and high activity) and emotional and behaviour disorder in three to seven year olds (Graham *et al.* 1973; Earls and Jung 1987; Lee and Bates 1985; Bates *et al.* 1985). In longitudinal studies, difficult temperament at seven has been shown to predict behavioural difficulties at 12 (Maziade 1989). Longitudinal studies have also demonstrated a modest association between deficits in sociability (including the presence of fearfulness and negative mood similar to high emotionality) in infancy with later anxiety disorders (Bates and Bayles 1988; Torgersen 1987; Rosenbaum *et al.* 1988). Recently a number of mechanisms have been suggested to explain the associations noted above, by which adverse temperament may operate to increase risk for psychopathology.

Firstly, temperamental traits may confer direct risk effects on psychopathological disorder. So far, however, findings from twin and case-control studies have demonstrated a lack of specificity between adverse temperamental style and psychiatric symptomatology, suggesting that adverse temperament does not confer direct risk (Graham and Stevenson 1987; Maziade 1989; Maziade *et al.* 1990). Indeed, individuals with the same degree of a particular temperamental characteristic differ considerably on the estimated prevalence of psychiatric disorder (Rutter 1989; Graham and Stevenson 1987). These findings demonstrate that adverse temperament may act as a risk factor for psychopathology but is neither necessary nor sufficient in all cases.

Secondly, temperament may exert its effects through its impact on the relationships of significant others with the child. Thus, it has been shown that children with difficult temperaments (especially boys) are more frequently the target of parental criticism (Quinton and Rutter 1985), and that the nature of parent–child interaction after the birth of a sibling is partly determined by the (older) child's own temperamental style (Dunn and Kendrick 1982). In addition, infant characteristics of activity level and sociability exert marked effects on early parent–child interactions (Bates 1989). On present evidence, this temperament–environment mechanism represents the main link between temperament and psychopathology, particularly for pervasive developmental disorders and behavioural difficulties in boys (Rutter 1987; Maziade *et al.* 1990). The degree to which particular patterns of temperamental style increase the risk for affective disorders of later childhood and adolescence remains unclear.

Overall, the findings on temperament indicate that we cannot consider which child is at risk without a knowledge of the individual's characteristics as well as the social context in which the risk circumstance has occurred. In addition, it is the mechanisms and processes of risk circumstances and situations that require elucidation, and not simply isolated factors. Before turning to a closer inspection of risk mechanisms, it is necessary to discuss a further important concept in relation to risk, namely, that of personal resilience.

Resilience

It is almost two decades since Anthony (1974) presented a paper on 'The invulnerable child' and posed a range of questions about invulnerability, asking whether individuals had within them different, inborn thresholds for coping and stress; whether they required successive masteries of social circumstances in early life to develop this properly; if they had a finite reservoir of resources which, if used up, had deleterious effects later in development; if they had an assortment of specific invulnerabilities, each needing dissection and description and each having particular use for a particular circumstance. These general but central questions have not yet been adequately dealt with. There is, however, increasing evidence to show that resilience and its synonyms such as invulnerability and protection are not easily described in a single unitary theory.

Resilience is concerned with individual variations to risk circumstances and infers differences in personal attributes such as the differential response by boys and girls to family discord. Indeed, resilience implies different responses to the same form and intensity of social stimulus. Resilience is generally inferred as present when a child experiences mild or no undesirable responses when exposed to known adverse environmental stimuli. In a recent review of research into stress-resistant children, Garmezy concluded (Garmezy 1985; Masten and Garmezy 1985) that three broad sets of psychosocial variables operated as resilient factors, as follows:

(a) personality features such as autonomy, self-esteem, and a positive social orientation;
(b) family cohesion, warmth, and an absence of discord;
(c) the availability of external support systems that encourage and reinforce a child's coping efforts.

These psychosocial domains are highly robust predictors of resilience in the face of adversity, but they do not indicate the specific mechanisms that determine individual outcomes. What is needed now is a search for specific developmental and situational mechanisms and processes that indicate how children do and do not negotiate particular types of risk.

The notion of resilience has emerged from a convergence of physiological, psychoanalytic and social cognitive theories of child development. At its core is the premise that a resilient individual is one who exercises the most resourceful response when faced with an environmental demand. This requires the capacity to choose from an availability of personal resources ranging from withdrawal, obsessional, and compulsive behaviour through to problem solving, processing two or more stimuli, or even flight if the circumstance demands! Investigating these qualities presents formidable difficulties and will require many levels of investigation from large-sample research designs to individual case studies where carefully delineated measures of environments and the person have occurred. An example of the latter has been provided recently by Radke-Yarrow and Sherman (1990), who described four children who appeared to 'survive' into middle childhood having been reared in multi-problem families and exposed to well defined risk variables of family discord, adult psychiatric disorder, and economic adversity. They identified three sets of family circumstances that can be found within Garmezy's broad categories of resilience factors, but also noted specific psychological mechanisms which activated the process of resilience.

Firstly, each of the children possessed a quality, psychological or physical, that matched an identified need in one or both of the parents. The child quality in each case appears to be one with which the child was born, and resulted in a positive affiliative relationship with a parent.

Secondly, these children had a clear conception that there was something good and special about him/herself. This 'self-image' may well be derived from the parent–child matching. This quality is then a source of positive self-regard for the child as well as satisfying to the parent. In addition, these four children received the maximum social–emotional resources their families were capable of producing. This parent–child matching appeared early in life and was remarkably different between the four families. One mother identified and therefore valued the health and sturdiness of her daughter; the mother and father of another child valued his gender and male qualities which had given him a special place in his family. A third mother valued the 'placid nature' of her child. In each case we see specific identifications serving to facilitate the general pathway to resilience through the development of positive self-esteem and the maintenance of positive family relations, at least with one parent. A confiding relationship with one parent has been shown to decrease the risk of conduct disorder even in the presence of chronic family discord (Rutter 1985). Surviving long-term family adversities may depend on the possession of personal qualities that can promote a good enough degree of intimacy with another person, particularly at times of acute distress.

Clearly the vignettes of these four children do not suggest a single unitary pathway or process for the evolution of resilience. In other words, resilience is not a fixed attribute of a person or a circumstance, rather if circumstances and/or perception change, risk alters.

Vulnerability and protection

Vulnerability and protective mechanisms are particular examples of risk and resilience respectively. They need to be considered together because they represent different examples of a single underlying mechanism. The essential defining feature that such mechanisms are operating is that there is an alteration in an individual's expected response to a known risk situation. A vulnerability mechanism increases risk, and therefore increases the likelihood of an adverse response. A protective mechanism decreases risk, and therefore decreases the likelihood of an adverse response. In both circumstances, however, this potentiating or ameliorating influence is not discernible in the absence of another risk circumstance.

Vulnerability mechanisms

Potentiating an existing risk process

In recent years substantial research attention has focused on the concept of some risk circumstances rendering individuals vulnerable to psychiatric disorder. In its simplest form, a social circumstance may result in a vulnerability mechanism by acting as a catalyst on a known risk process. For example, in research on depressed women, chronic absence of a confiding relationship acting alone exerts only a marginal risk for the onset of depression until an undesirable life event (provoking agent) occurs (Brown and Harris 1978). Under these circumstances the combined risk is significantly increased beyond the known risks carried by either of these two social adversities. The social mechanism does not indicate that a chronic lack of confiding has 'no risk', rather that its risk is not sufficient alone to cause depression under any circumstances.

This 'lack of confiding' social vulnerability model does not appear to be present in young persons. Indeed, the same broad measure of 'lack of confiding' in a woman's life has been shown to have a direct (provoking) risk effect on the likelihood of anxiety or depressive disorders occurring in a school-age child (Goodyer *et al.* 1988). In other words, the same risk circumstances exert their effects via different risk mechanisms at different ages and stages of development.

Overall, the current findings suggest that for the age range 8 to 16 the risk mechanism arising from recent (i.e. in the 12 months prior to disorder) severe family adversities or friendship difficulties are direct 'provoking' and not 'potentiating' vulnerability mechanisms. In school-age children, at least when risk circumstances arise in the environment, they exert direct effects sufficient to cause psychiatric disorder. In the majority of cases two or more such adversities frequently occur. Since each carries a significant degree of risk, the likelihood of disorder is substantially increased (Goodyer *et al.* 1988; Goodyer 1990). Whether or not the same variables exert a potentiating vulnerability or direct provoking effect in younger children is not known.

Facilitating the occurrence of risk circumstances

In some circumstances a vulnerability mechanism arises through a connective process (see p. 436 for examples of connectivity) in which the presence of one social adversity facilitates the occurrence of another, and both exert direct effects on the likelihood of disorder. In this example the original risk circumstance may exert direct effects on the risk of disorder when occurring alone. More important, however, is the increase in the likelihood of exposure to a subsequent and different form of social adversity.

For example, children may be exposed to greater rates of adverse life events when they live with distressed mothers who lack a confiding relationship in their own lives (Goodyer *et al.* 1988). Similarly, mothers with a previous history of psychiatric disorder may be prone to adverse life events (Goodyer *et al.* 1991). In both these examples, already existing maternal risk circumstances for the child (maternal distress and lack of confiding) increase the likelihood of a further direct risk circumstance occurring. This is a 'facilitative vulnerability model' in which one or more risk circumstances causes the likelihood of further risk circumstances to occur.

Public health programmes (often with limited budgets) concerned with prevention of psychiatric disorder in school-age children may be more efficacious if resources were targeted directly at young people who are exposed to known provoking/vulnerability risk circumstances. Such an approach may achieve better value for money than a blanket educative programme aimed at all young persons.

Enhancement of existing risk effects

A somewhat different indirect mechanism to those of vulnerability is illustrated by the risk mechanisms that arise from two non-familial social experiences, friendships and desirable social achievements. The principle of effects is the same in that there is a high and low or neutral risk variable whose combined effects are not explained by a knowledge of either occurring alone. Unlike either vulnerability mechanism, however, the neutral or low risk variable occurs following the high risk or (provoking) variable, thereby enhancing the already existing risk. The crucial notion here is the temporal relationship between the risk circumstances, i.e. vulnerability circumstances occur prior to provoking circumstances; enhancing circumstances occur following provoking circumstances. Both mechanisms occur before onset of disorder.

For example, in the 12 months prior to the onset of their disorder, anxious and depressed school-age children are as likely as well children to report one or more episodes of social achievement. This indicates that recent social achievements do not exert any moderating (i.e. protective) effects on the risk for these disorders (Goodyer *et al.* 1990). Alternatively, it can be said that the absence of achieving carries no risk for the onset of such disorder.

In the presence of poor friendships, however, the absence of social achievements exerts a significant catalytic effect as shown in Fig. 26.2. In other words, absence of social achievement enhances the existing risk of poor friendships. It is not possible to say that the absence of social achievements exerts a vulnerability effect, as poor friendships preceded the lack of achievements. The magnitude of risk is increased markedly and is not simply a combination of the known risks of these two social circumstances (particularly as absence of achievements carries little or no such risk). In other words, the psychological mechanism involved may be different from those where the overall risk (as found with maternal adversities and life events) is a combination of the known risks carried by each social adversity.

This enhancing mechanism is specific to friendship experiences since no such enhancing effect occurs between adverse life events and the absence of social achievements. In other words, when a child experiences an absence of social achievement and one or more adverse life events concurrently, the former exerts no enhancement effect and the magnitude of risk of the latter remain the same. This absence of enhancing is shown in Fig. 26.3. These findings demonstrate the importance of determining specific risk pathways and processes for different patterns of social risk circumstances.

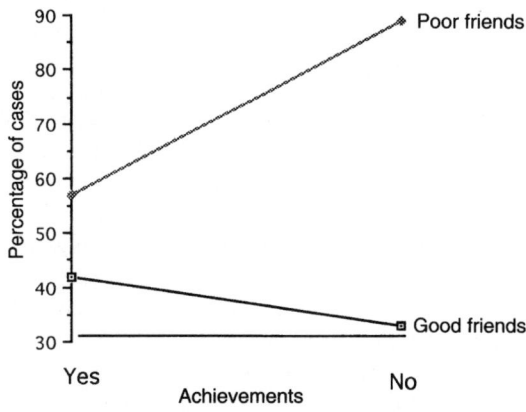

Fig. 26.2 Enhancement of poor friends.

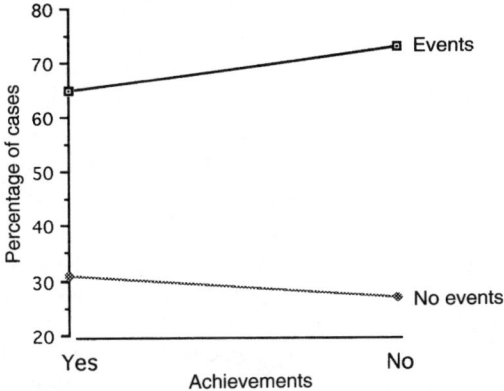

Fig. 26.3 No enhancement of life events.

The personal impact of adverse social experiences

Surprisingly few studies have investigated which aspects of the individual are adversely influenced by social risk processes and mechanisms.

Studies on depressed adults have proposed a psychological mechanism in which social adversities decrease self-esteem and increase thoughts of hopelessness and helplessness about their own lives and thereby increase the risk for depression (Brown and Harris 1978; Brown 1988).

Although we know that low self-esteem occurs in children with psychiatric disorder, we do not know if this is a consequence or cause of disorder, nor do we know whether social adversities directly result in low self-esteem. The current evidence suggests, however, that ongoing chronic family and social difficulties do adversely influence factors related to an adequate sense of self (Rutter 1985, 1987). The mechanism may arise as a result of perceived personal failure through consistently poor social function and educational under-achievement. Whilst the data are sparse, it appears that these risks may be at least as great in social and school settings as they are for family adversities (Rutter 1990; Fergusson et al. 1990).

This model seems very plausible for frequent and long-term family and social adversities which result in low self-esteem and are associated with behavioural disorder. It is less clear how such mechanisms may apply to young persons with low self-esteem who do not become behaviourally deviant but suffer from developmental or emotional disorders. In these types of affective disorders, exposure to chronic long-term family adversities has often not occurred. Whilst there are no firm findings, some clues are available. For example, it is possible that in anxious and depressed children, family risk processes influence self-reflection, resulting in the child carrying an impaired view of his or her capacity to produce or maintain close personal relations in adolescent and adult life. By contrast, friendship risk processes may influence self-competence and self-efficacy, resulting in a child carrying an impaired view of his or her capacity to participate and/or complete tasks. These psychological mechanisms involving alterations to different components of the self-system, whilst speculative, are now testable on the basis of our understanding of the different risk processes and mechanisms that arise from the manifold social adversities to which children and adolescents are exposed. The impact on self-esteem may, nevertheless, be important, perhaps as much through the intensity of the stimulus as via duration. Finally, previous episodes of psychopathology, particularly depression, are themselves potent adverse influences on self-esteem and peer relations (Kazdin 1989; Goodyer *et al.* 1991). Thus in some individuals social adversities may affect a child already at risk with low self-esteem through previous episodes of psychopathology, particularly past episodes of depression.

Protective mechanisms and processes

The notion that children may be protected from the impact of undesirable events and difficulties by other social circumstances is problematic because invariably the desirable protective effect is the polar opposite of the risk circumstance. Thus the presence of a good friendship can be considered as protective, whereas its absence can be considered as a risk. Similarly, a confiding relationship with a parent decreases the risk of behaviour disorder, and may be considered as protective, whereas the absence of such a confiding relationship may be considered a risk.

In the latter example it is the lack of a normal aspect of parenting that represents the risk. Is it appropriate to consider normal components of child development (such as a good relationship with a parent) as protective rather than normative? Indeed, children need to experience certain types of undesirable events in early life, such as illness and separations, for their own good, and perhaps to assist in evolving resilience to later adversities. Similarly, there may be necessary undesirable social events, such as hearing marital disagreements inside a secure family, that children should be exposed to so that they may learn at all such experiences do not result in negative impacts or alter the *status quo* in their lives. There are many compelling scientific reasons to investigate the normative social processes of development but not, 'as if', they represent protective circumstances. When then is it preferable to speak of protection as a separate process to risk or normal development?

First, when previous experiences confer the opportunity for an improved outcome in the face of a current novel event. For example, children who are securely attached to their mother in infancy are less likely to withdraw from new peer-group exposures and may be more socially competent in the presence of such peers (Belsky and Isabella 1988). These findings suggest that secure attachment is protective for some children facing new social demands. Not all children classified as insecure (using a systematic laboratory model known as the Ainsworth strange-situation test) are incompetent, however. Indeed, some children classified as insecure go on to become social and competent individuals (Grossmann *et al.* 1988; Grossmann and Grossmann 1991). In other words, the absence of secure attachment does not allow the inference that a child is at risk. Second, when previously successfully negotiated undesirable events are repeated; for example, previously successful separations from parents (likely to be viewed by the young child as a potentially negative experience) decreases the likelihood of the child reacting adversely to the undesirable event of hospital admission (Stacey *et al.* 1970).

The protective mechanism may result from the implication that a previous successful negotiation alters the child's cognitive appraisal of the event. Altering cognitive appraisal as a protective process does not have to depend on previous experiences. For example, the various ways of preparing children for admission to hospital probably do the same (e.g. Ferguson 1979). Developing cognitive processes that anticipate the likelihood of risk circumstances or ameliorate the impact of risk are probably a fundamental feature of protective mechanisms (Lazarus and Folkman 1984; Goodyer *et al.* 1991).

Finally, protection may be inferred when the main effect seems to be derived from the positive end of a variable. For example, the presence of a supportive harmonious relationship to women in adult life who had been in care in childhood had a marked protective effect on the quality of their parenting (Quinton *et al.* 1984). Whilst lack of support (the other end of the pole) for these women operates as a vulnerability process for their well-being, there is some advantage in focusing on the positive pole because it forces one to ask what a confiding relationship does as a protective effect for good parenting.

Rutter (1990) has succinctly noted that the crucial difference between vulnerability and protection is that the psychological processes involved are different even where the presence of absence of a single variable suggests (incorrectly) the presence or absence of a single process.

Temperament, personality, and protection

Protective processes are perhaps more readily seen in the way individuals mediate the impact of adverse environments. Individuals who demonstrate personal competence when exposed to intensely difficult environments are often cited as possessing protective characteristics (Goodyer *et al.* 1991; Garmezy 1985).

These characteristics may reside in an individual's behavioural or temperamental style. For example, the possession of a temperamental style which increases the chance of successful engagement with risk may also foster the development of a cognitive set of self-esteem, itself a positive factor in socio-emotional development (Bates 1989). Werner and Smith (1982) in their important publication of longitudinal research on resilience in childhood, *Vulnerable but invincible*, found the expression of an active, sociable temperament to be associated with improve outcome in a situation of long-term deprivation, possibly mediated via the increased social support which these children experienced.

Radke-Yarrow and Sherman (1990), in their account of children who survived, noted that the children shared a cluster of positive features that are universally valued and potentially protective. These included being alert, curious, and having a 'zest for life'. In addition, they all had winning smiles, were physically attractive and socially engaging, and possessed an attribute that their parents could closely identify with which resulted in love and non-judgemental positive regard.

Restitution

Rutter and Quinton (Rutter and Quinton 1988; Quinton *et al.* 1984) carried out a longitudinal study of women raised in care and demonstrated that some were restored to normal adult functioning through a number of important interpersonal mechanisms. Firstly, although the institution-reared girls had a worse outcome than the comparison group, it was found that their adult functioning was closely related to their marital situations at the time. The level of good parenting by the ex-care women who had supportive spouses was as high as that in the comparison group. The presence of a supportive spouse appeared less critical for good parenting in the comparison group. The implication here is that marital support acts as a crucial protective mechanism for good parenting only in high-risk groups.

Secondly, women who planned their choice of spouse were much less likely to marry deviant men and therefore more likely to receive marital support. Such women were also good at planning for work and appeared to possess greater all round levels of competence although raised in care (Quinton and Rutter 1988). (Planning meant they did not marry for a negative reason to escape intolerable family or care circumstances or because of illegitimate pregnancy and they had known their spouse for more than six months.) Planning was associated with a significantly lower rate of teenage pregnancies in the institution-reared women. Overall planning was less relevant for the comparison group because they received greater family support and were exposed to less deviant men in their peer group. Planning seems less necessary in low-risk groups. Perhaps some women made good use of care to learn how to plan for the future. Why some high-risk girls, and not others, exhibited the ability to plan is not clear. The capacity to plan, however, does appear crucial to the avoidance of further risk circumstances in adult life. A clue to the origins of planning, however, was found in past school experiences. In the ex-care group successful planning was significantly associated with positive school experiences but not examination success *per se*. This association was not found in the comparison group presumably because of good family experiences. The findings again suggest that important components of self-esteem are derived from the non-familial environment. Again, these may be more relevant for high-risk groups. Overall this important study demonstrates that restorative processes in adult life can become available to some women whose childhood was impaired by persistent social difficulties.

Conclusions

It is clear that all studies note marked individual variations in response to risk situations. Some children succumb easily and rapidly, while others escape. Some maintain adaptive functioning in the presence of severe hazard and are termed resilient. The processes that promote resilience are poorly understood. The overall level of risk is one important feature, but even in conditions of severe privation some children appear to survive. There are mediating processes that determine the nature and form of response to risk. Vulnerability and protective processes are such examples, and are clearly implicated in the degree of resilience an individual may have when exposed to risk circumstances. Developmental factors are important in determining the type and form of response that arise from the same risk circumstances occurring at different ages. Cross-sectional and longitudinal studies are much needed to investigate the impact of life transitions, such as leaving home or school, on personal adjustment. Such studies will need to discriminate high- and low-risk groups of children because the mechanisms and processes that predict adjustment may be different both within and between these populations. So far, protection appears to involve reducing the impact of risk circumstances and providing social opportunities for improving self-esteem. The evidence also indicates, however, that personal qualities in the child substantially influence who is likely to take up and make best use of such opportunities. Protective processes are not synonymous with normal development but are to be found in the way children negotiate the risks in their lives and steer their way through the manifold social adversities to which they are exposed. Particular attention needs to be paid to delineating the mechanisms that result in an adverse developmental trajectory and those that redirect children to a more adaptive path.

References

Anthony, E.J. (1974). The syndrome of the psychological invulnerable child. In *The child in his family, Vol III: children at psychiatric risk*, (ed. E.J. Anthony and C. Koupernik), pp. 529–44. John Wiley, New York.

Bates, J. (1989). Concepts and measures of temperament. In *Temperament in childhood*, (ed. G. Kohnstamm, J. Bates, and M. Rothbart). Wiley, Chichester.

Bates, J. and Bayles, K. (1988). Attachment and the development of behaviour problems. In *Clinical implications of attachment*, (ed. J. Belsky and T. Nezworski). Erlbaum, Hillsdale, NJ.

Bates, J.E., Maslin, C.A., and Frankel, K.A. (1985). Attachment security, mother–child interaction, and temperament as predictors of behavior problem ratings at age 3 years. In *Growing points of attachment theory and research*, (ed. I. Bretherton and E. Waters). Society for Research in Child Development, Monograph No 209, Vol. 50, pp. 167–93. University of Chicago Press, Chicago.

Belsky, J. and Isabella, R. (1988) Mother, infant and social–contextual determinants of attachment severity. In *Clinical implications of attachment*, (ed. J. Belsky and T. Nezworski), pp. 41–95. Erlbaum, Hillsdale, NJ.

Bifulco, A., Brown, G.W., and Adler, Z. (1991). Early sexual abuse and clinical depression in adult life. *British Journal of Psychiatry* **159**, 115–22.

Brown, G.W. (1988). Early loss of parent and depression in adult life. In *Handbook of life stress, cognition and health*, (ed. S. Fisher and J. Reason). John Wiley, Chichester.

Brown, G.W. and Harris, T. (1978). *The social origins of depression*. Tavistock, London.

Buss, A. and Plomin, R. (1984). *Temperament: early developing personality traits*. Erlbaum, Hillsdale, NJ.

Chess, S. and Thomas, A. (1984). *Origins and evolutions of behaviour disorders*. Bruner/Mayel, New York.

Dunn, J. and Kendrick, C. (1982). *Sibling: love, envy and understanding*. Harvard University Press, Cambridge, MA.

Earls, F. and Jung K.G. (1987). Temperament and the home environment. Characteristics as causal factors in the early development of childhood psychopathology. *Journal of the American Academy of Child and Adolescent Psychiatry* **26**, 491–8.

Emery, R.E. and O'Leary, K.D. (1984). Marital discord and child behaviour problems in a non-clinic sample. *Journal of Abnormal Child Psychology* **12**, 411–20.

Ferguson, B.F. (1979). Preparing young children for hospitalisation: a comparison of two methods. *Paediatrics* **64**, 656–64.

Fergusson, D.M., Horwood, L.J., and Lawton, J.M. (1990). Vulnerability to childhood problems and family social background. *Journal of Child Psychology and Psychiatry* **31**, 1145–60.

Garmezy, N. (1985). Stress-resistant children—the search for protective factors. In *Recent advances in developmental psychopathology*, (ed. J. Stevenson). Pergamon, Oxford.

Gibbs, M.V., Reeves, D., and Cunningham, C.C. (1987). The application of temperament questionnaires to a British sample: issues of reliability and validity. *Journal of Child Psychology and Psychiatry* **28**, 61–77.

Goodyer, I.M. (1990). Family relationships, life events and childhood psychopathology. *Journal of Child Psychology and Psychiatry* **31**, 161–92.

Goodyer, I.M. and Altham, P.M.E. (1991a). Lifetime exit events and recent social and family adversities in anxious and depressed school-age children and adolescents—I. *Journal of Affective Disorders* **21**, 219–28.

Goodyer, I.M. and Altham, P.M.E. (1991b). Lifetime exit events and recent social and family adversities in anxious and depressed school-age children and adolescents—II. *Journal of Affective Disorders* **21**, 229–38.

Goodyer, I.M., Kolvin, I., and Gatzanis, S. (1985). Recent undesirable life events and psychiatric disorder in childhood and adolescence. *British Journal of Psychiatry* **147**, 517–23.

Goodyer, I.M., Wright, C., and Altham, P.M.E. (1988). Maternal adversity and recent life events in childhood and adolescence. *Journal of Child Psychology and Psychiatry* **29**, 651–69.

Goodyer, I.M., Wright, C., and Altham, P.M.E. (1989). Recent friendships in anxious and depressed school age children. *Psychological Medicine* **19**, 165–74.

Goodyer, I.M., Wright, C., and Altham, P.M.E. (1990). The friendships and recent life events of anxious and depressed school-age children. *British Journal of Psychiatry* **156**, 689–98.

Goodyer, I.M. Germany, E., Gowrusankur, J., and Altham, P.M.E. (1991). Social influences on the course of anxious and depressive disorders in school-age children. *British Journal of Psychiatry* **158**, 676–84.

Graham, P. and Stevenson, J. (1987). Temperament and psychiatric disorder: the genetic contribution to behaviour and childhood. *Australian and New Zealand Journal of Psychiatry* **21**, 267–74.

Graham, P., Rutter, M., and George, S. (1973). Temperamental characteristics as predictors of behaviour disorders in children. *American Journal of Orthopsychiatry* **3**, 328–39.

Grossmann, K.E. and Grossmann, K. (1991). Attachment quality as an organizer of emotional and behavioral responses. In *Attachment across the life cycle*, (ed. C.M. Parkes, P. Marris, and J. Stevenson-Hinde). Routledge, New York.

Grossmann, K., Fremmer-Bombik, E., Rudolph, J., and Grossmann, K.E. (1988). Maternal attachment representations as related to patterns of infant/mother attachment and maternal care during the first year. In *Relationships within families: mutual influences*, (ed. R.A. Hinde and J. Stevenson-Hinde). Oxford University Press.

Hetherington, E.M., Cox, M., and Cox, R. (1982). Effects of divorce on parents and children. In *Non-traditional families: parenting and child development*, (ed. M.E. Lamb). Erlbaum, Hillsdale, NJ.

Hinde, R.A. (1988). Continuities and discontinuities: conceptual issues and methodological considerations. In *Studies of psychosocial risk: the power of longitudinal data*, (ed. M. Rutter). Cambridge University Press.

Hinde, R.A. (1989). Temperament as an intervening variable. In *Temperament in childhood*, (ed. G. Kohnstamm, J. Bates, and M. Rothbart). Wiley, Chichester.

Kazdin, A.E. (1989). Childhood depression. *Journal of Child Psychology and Psychiatry* **31**, 126–60.

Kohnstamm, G., Bates, J., and Rothbart, M. (1989). *Temperament in childhood*. Wiley, Chichester.

Lazarus, R.S. and Folkman, S. (1984). *Stress, appraisal and coping*. Springer, New York.

Lee, C. and Bates, J. (1985). Mother–child interaction at age 2 years and perceived difficult temperament. *Child Development* **56**, 1314–26.

Masten, A.S. and Garmezy, N. (1985). Risk, vulnerability, and protective factors in developmental psychopathology. In *Advances in clinical child psychology*, Vol. 8, (ed. B. Lahey and K. Kaden). Plenum, New York.

Masten, A.S., Garmezy, N., Tellegen, A., Pellegrini, D., Larkin, K., and Larsen, A. (1988). Competence and stress in school children: the moderating effects of individual and family qualities. *Journal of Child Psychology and Psychiatry* **29**, 745–64.

Maziade, M. (1989). Should adverse temperament matter to the clinician. In *Temperament in childhood*, (ed. G. Kohnstamm, J. Bates, and M. Rothbart), pp. 421–37. Wiley, Chichester.

Maziade, M., Caron, C., Coté, R., Boutin, P., and Thivierge, J. (1990). Extreme temperament and diagnosis: a study in a psychiatric sample of consecutive children. *Archives of General Psychiatry* **47**, 477–84.

McGuffin, P. (1988). Major genes for major affective disorder. *British Journal of Psychiatry* **153**, 591–6.

Murray, L. (1988). Effects of post-natal depression on infant development: direct studies of early mother–infant interactions. In *Motherhood and mental illness*, (ed. R. Kumar and I.F. Brockington). Wright, London.

Packman, J. (1986). *Who needs care?* Blackwell Scientific, Oxford.

Patterson, G.R. (1986a). The contribution of siblings to train for fighting. A microsocial analysis. In *Development of antisocial and prosocial behaviour. Research theories and issues*, (ed. D. Olweus, J. Block, and M. Radke-Yarrow), pp. 235–61. Academic, New York.

Patterson, G.R. (1986b). performance models for antisocial boys. *American Psychologist* **41**, 432–44.

Plomin, R. and Dunn, J. (eds) (1986). *The study of temperament: changes, continuities and challenges*. Erlbaum, Hillsdale, NJ.

Puig-Antich, J., Lukens, E., Davies, M., Goetz, D. Brennan-Quattrock, J., and Todak, G. (1985). Psychosocial functioning in prepubertal major depressive disorders. I: Interpersonal relationships during the depressive episodes. *Archives of General Psychiatry* **42**, 500–7.

Quinton, D. and Rutter, M. (1985). Family pathology and child psychiatric disorder: a four year prospective study. In *Longitudinal studies in child psychology and psychiatry*, (ed. A.R. Nicol). Wiley, Chichester.

Quinton, D. and Rutter, M. (1988). *Parenting breakdown: the making and breaking of intergenerational links*. Avebury, Aldershot.

Quinton, D., Rutter, M., and Liddle, C. (1984). Institutional rearing, parenting difficulties and marital support. *Psychological Medicine* **14**, 107–24.

Radke-Yarrow, M. and Sherman, T. (1990). Hard growing: children who survive. In *Risk and protective factors in the development of psychopathology*, (ed. J. Rolfe, A.S. Masten, D. Cicchetti, K.H. Nuechterlein, and S. Weintraub). Cambridge University Press.

Rolfe, J., Masten, A.S., Cicchetti, D., Nuechterlein, K.H., and Weintraub, S. (eds) (1990). *Risk and protective factors in the development of psychopathology*. Cambridge University Press.

Rosenbaum, J.F., Biederman, J., Gersten, M., Hirschfield, D.R., Menninger, S.R., Herman, J.B., *et al.* (1988). Behavioural inhibition in children of parents with panic disorder and agrophobia. *Archives of General Psychiatry* **45**, 463–70.

Rutter, M. (1979). Protective factors in children's response to stress and disadvantage. In *Primary prevention of psychopathology. Vol. 3: Social competence in children*, (ed. M.W. Kent and J.E. Rolfe). University Press of New England, Hanover, NH.

Rutter, M. (1982). Epidemiological–longitudinal approaches to the study of development. In *The concept of development*, Minnesota Symposia on Child Psychology, Vol. 15, (ed. W.A. Collins). Erlbaum, Hillsdale, NJ.

Rutter, M. (1985) Family and school influences. Meanings, mechanisms and implications. In *Longitudinal studies in child psychology and psychiatry*, (ed. A.R. Nicol). Wiley, Chichester.

Rutter, M. (1987). Psychosocial resilience and protective mechanisms. *American Journal of Orthopsychiatry* **47**, 317–31.

Rutter, M. (1989). Temperament: conceptual issues and clinical implications. In *Temperament in childhood*, (ed. G. Kohnstamm, J. Bates, and M. Rothbart), pp. 463–82. Wiley, Chichester.

Rutter, M. (1990). Psychosocial resilience and protective mechanisms. In *Risk and protective factors in the development of psychopathology*, (ed. J. Rolfe, A.S. Masten, D. Cicchetti, K.H. Nuechterlein, and S. Weintraub). Cambridge University Press.

Rutter, M. and Quinton, D. (1988). Long term follow-up of women institutionalized in childhood: factors promoting good function in adult life. *British Journal of Developmental Psychology* **2**, 225–34.

Stacey, M., Dearden, R., Pill, R., and Robinson, D. (1970). *Hospitals, children and their families: the report of a pilot study*. Routledge and Kegan Paul, London.

Thomas, A. and Chess, S. (1977). *Temperament and development*. Brunner/Mazel, New York.

Torgersen, A.M. (1987). Longitudinal research on temperament in twins. *Acta Geneticae Medicae et Gemellogiae* **36**, 145–54.

Werner, E.E. and Smith, R.S. (1982). *Vulnerable but invincible: a longitudinal study of resilient children and youth*. McGraw-Hill, New York.

PART VIII

Service and intersectoral issues

Traditional approaches to child health work based in the one-to-one consultation with child and parents remain useful in some aspects of social paediatric practice but are inadequate in dealing with many of the problems highlighted in the foregoing parts. Child health services have tended to respond to parental request; child health promotion, prevention, and services based on the identification of need require initiative form the services, preferably in collaboration with parents and communities and an orientation to child populations as well as individual children and their families. This part outlines some important elements of these approaches.

27 Planning and managing child health services

Luis Martín Alvárez and Joaquín Uris Sellés

Historical background to child health services

As with many other special and legal child regulations, child health services have been implemented later or with less relevant development than those for other age or social groups in the majority of the European countries. This development has followed a course characterized by several stages (Nordio 1978; Arbelo Curbelo and Arbelo López 1980; De Miguel 1984), the first of which coincided with the existence of high infant and maternal mortality rates, and took place during the end of the nineteenth century and the first two decades of the twentieth century. The principal characteristics of this period were as follows:

- legislation aimed at the protection of childhood and pregnancy was developed;
- paediatric hospitals with a curative approach and funded by charity were set up;
- paediatrics as a medical specialty, along with 'well-baby' care, was initiated and consolidated during this period.

During the second period between the First and Second World War, it became necessary to cope with increasing social needs and demands. This fact meant the implementation of a significant number of paediatric preventive services all over Europe (WHO 1985). These services focused on minimizing the infection–nutritional hazards and also on reaching certain risk groups, generally targeting groups of low socio-economic level. The activities provided were directed at increasing family knowledge and abilities in healthy feeding and care-giving. The vaccines available at that time represented the starting point for future immunization programmes.

The protection approach of the former periods were followed by a third period characterized by a marked development of curative care, both in hospital and in ambulatory settings. Then, the mostly hospital-based care services invested heavily in the development of diagnostic–curative procedures. Subsequently, rehabilitation and disabilities became important issues of the medical care and social services. Another characteristic of this period and the attitude to child health care was of 'universal' medical coverage, which occurred in parallel with the establishment of the welfare state and social security allowances in the majority of European countries. This predominantly curative model of child health care, in association with preventive services, has been a feature common to almost all the European countries from the post-war period to the seventies (Pritchard 1981), despite differences in the various socio-political regimes operating throughout Europe. Present and future strategies for the planning and management of child health services in Europe should undoubtedly build on this commonality and consider Europe as a whole, in terms of socio-demographic data and shifts in the child health profile.

Socio-demographic influences on child health services

As far as the socio-demographic pattern is concerned, the most useful information is of changes in birth rates, family structures, lifestyles, and educational facilities (Köhler and Jakobsson 1987).

The birth rate has been decreasing in all European countries, more so in the more industrialized ones. Whereas the one-child family has become prevalent, extended families have become scarce and the previously notable differences in family models among nations and regions have ceased to exist. Nevertheless, the 0–18-year age group still represents one quarter of the total European population. The family as the cornerstone of society has obviously faced and undergone important changes which have resulted in a different family model. The 'one-parent' family is now a rather frequent situation, constituting as much as one third of the families in northern Europe. The increasing or stabilized divorce rate has played an important role here. The consequences of family breakdown on child health have been delineated in the Nordic countries (Köhler et al. 1986; Barnard 1989; see also Chapter 24).

The improvement of economic life standards in the majority of European countries and the consumer-oriented attitudes of society have modified the lifestyles of many citizens, and this wealthy lifestyle has become an aim of the underprivileged groups as well. The diet in a wealthy lifestyle involves a higher protein and calorie intake together with a decreased cereal intake, which may have implications for health.

The former socio-economic standards are not equally distributed among the different social groups (Black Report 1980). An example of these inequities is unemployment, which has increased with marked national and regional differences, and has affected young people most intensely. Unemployment rates range from 25 per cent to 60 per cent in the 14–24 year age group and unhealthy consequences have been registered in terms of drug addiction, suicide, and unwanted pregnancies. Another change in lifestyles concerns increased smoking and alcohol consumption among youngsters all over Europe

(Ministerio de Sanidad y Consumo España 1988; WHO 1990a; Spykerelle and Herberth 1991). Another fact which reflects changes in lifestyles is the increasing demand for family planning and sexual orientation services. Although these services are spread throughout Europe they are still insufficient and/or under-utilized by those adolescents and socio-economically disadvantaged groups who most need them.

Education and child health services

Education is compulsory all over Europe and reaches all children from 6 to 15 years of age. Pre-school education is a common experience for many European children, and years of attendance at school have increased. The school atmosphere has been modified in quantitative terms, with fewer children per classroom, and also in qualitative terms, with teachers being more aware of family and developmental difficulties. However, cognitive learning is still more predominant than social training and career orientation, and personal choices play an important role in the last school years, which can cause increased competition and stress. This stress is sometimes aggravated by an excessively intolerant attitude by parents and teachers, which can create a demand on the individual's responsibilities before the child is ready (WHO 1989).

Information and information systems

Concerning information on child health in Europe, mortality data are available and reliable, permitting an outline of gender and cause distribution together with geographical differences to be determined. Information on morbidity is less available and reliable but there are still some sources which can provide information, namely the primary health care registers (patients and family demands), infectious diseases monitoring, and specific registers (congenital abnormalities). The paucity of information about 'positive' indicators (child development, social factors, etc.) is even more marked. Nevertheless, the data available are sufficient to create a profile of the European child which will serve as a general framework for the planning and management of child health services. This European child health profile can be described by four main points (Manciaux *et al.* 1987):

- declining mortality rates;
- a shift in the morbidity pattern;
- the increasing relevance of chronic diseases;
- the emerging challenge of mental health and psychosocial problems.

Mortality

Mortality rates decreased tremendously in the 50s and 60s in the 0–14 year age group, mostly in the post-neonatal period (Fig. 27.1). In terms of the planning of services, this fact has obviously modified family demands and the child health services offered. In the last two decades this tendency reached the perinatal and neonatal period in which mortality stabilized and morbidity (sequelae and risk children) became the challenge for child health services. It also made professionals realize the necessity of teamwork and intersectoral coordination. Because of its importance in prevention strategies in childhood, special attention should be paid to the dramatic increase in the mortality rate of 15–18-year-olds due to accidents and violence (WHO 1986).

This shift in mortality rates is even more marked if mortality rates by sex are analysed, showing that the male mortality rate (15–18 years) is twice the female rate. Another fact to be considered in terms of the planning of child health service is the comparison of mortality rates among countries and regions. The different times taken to reach optimal rates illustrate the impact of socio-economic development versus the results of health interventions.

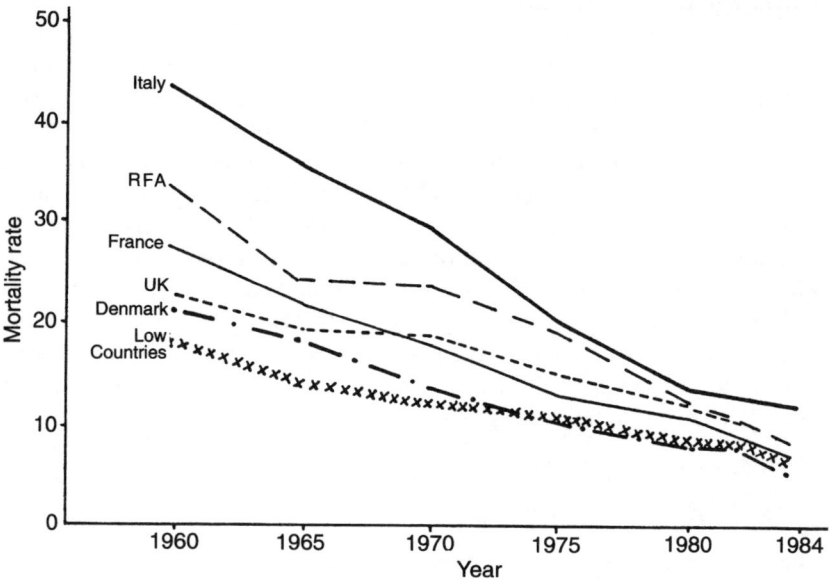

Fig. 27.1 Child mortality in several European countries (WHO 1986).

Shift in morbidity patterns

According to the existing data on infectious diseases and nutritional problems, these are now rare, except among deprived groups. However, this trend has reversed, with increasing prevalence and incidence of infectious diseases for which the social component is crucial in terms of contagion and prognosis (e.g. viral hepatitis, AIDS) (WHO 1990*b*).

Increasing influence of chronic diseases

Chronic diseases, congenital abnormalities, and handicaps have became important issues for both clinical and social paediatrics. Their importance is related to the awareness of those children's 'special needs'. These special needs cover a wide spectrum from early detection to rehabilitation as well as the consideration of the social component, both in terms of the social impact of these problems in the family as well as the influence of social factors in the prognosis and outcomes of these health problems (Köhler 1987; INE España 1987).

A child health profile is not merely a list of health problems; children are to be considered along with their community in which there are differences and inequities between nations, regions, and social groups. Fortunately, we now have sufficient data to find out what these inequities are. However, any child health care model should include a continuos monitoring system able to detect these inequities. It is well known by professionals and citizens who advocate for children how seldom the impact on child health financial restraints or the reorganization of health services or other social services (e.g. education, social security allowances, etc.) is measured (Miller *et al.* 1985).

Mental health and psychological problems

Because of the generalized development of child health surveillance programmes along with an increased social and professional sensitivity to mental health problems, these and psychosocial disturbances are becoming increasing components of primary health care, specialized care, and socio-educational services. However, they should not be forgotten in the planning and management of child health services; however difficult, they ought to be included not only in curative and rehabilitative care but also in promotive activities (Ten and Pedreira 1988).

Planning and managing child health services

Some negative aspects

Together with the panorama of child/family needs and demands mentioned above which should in the future, influence decision-making priorities, it is important to point out some managerial aspects which, in general, have characterized child health services in Europe and which, conversely, have widened the gap between a child's needs/demands and the response to them (programmes and services). These two negative managerial aspects, which should be overcome in any child health services plan are described below.

- Evaluation of child health services/programmes has been absent or incomplete and, if performed, based mainly on negative indicators. However, there are some evaluative studies which have delineated reliable child screening procedures together with procedures for routine and opportunistic screenings in primary health care and health promotive activities (Macfarlane *et al.* 1989; Butler 1989).

- Child care has undergone a process of fragmentation into different institutions, professions, and community agencies (medical, educational, and social, services etc.) which has resulted in overlapping and/or duplication of programmes and services, and accordingly an increase in the cost of child care.

Besides these managerial difficulties there is another circumstance outlined in the needs–demands profile which adds more complexity to the content of child health services and consequently to its planning and management. This complexity is related to the necessity of facing the biopsychosocial basis of child health problems, which becomes even more evident if child development surveillance is taken as the core of child health care. This necessary integration of the different factors influencing child health should also be viewed with the relative influences of family, school, and community throughout the life of the child (Fig. 27.2) (Nordio 1978).

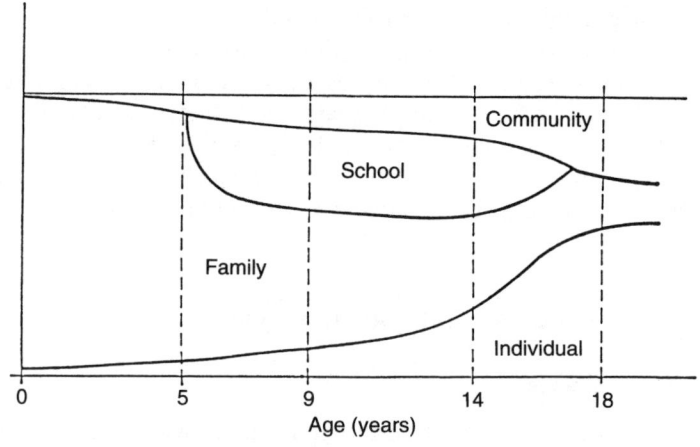

Fig. 27.2 Individual development and social factors (Nordio 1978).

Steps in planning and managing child health services

The planning and management of child health services follows the same steps as the planning of general health services. However, there are some aspects which are characteristic of child health services alone and, if not fully developed, would mean that actual needs and demands would not be met. These requirements are for

- 'holistic' child health care;
- integration and coordination of services;
- community participation.

'Holistic' child health care

Child health care must be 'holistic' by addressing the biopsychosocial background of child health problems and also taking into account the varying role in child development of the family, school, and community. In terms of management, this issue raises the need for multidisciplinary functioning, which does not mean that every professional should be part of the health team but that effective coordination with other disciplines and professionals is necessary, whether or not they belong to the health sector.

Integrated child health care

Child health care must be integrated and coordinated so that there is coordination between

- health promotion and preventive programme; curative care and rehabilitation;
- primary health care, specialized care, and hospital care;
- health, social, and educational services and their specific programmes.

In order to develop this issue it is necessary to reach political agreement between different administration levels (national, regional, local) and the agencies involved in different health care services and programmes.

Community participation

Together with political and administrative agreements, it is important that at the community level (country, town), the professionals and institutions involved in child care have a 'platform' in the form of a 'child health committee' which will oblige professionals to meet and discuss child and family needs and demands. This coordination strategy will be different in each country depending on its 'child care model', but a practical approach would be to concentrate on a child problem for which the biopsychosocial components are evident throughout the different sectors and professionals, such as child abuse and children handicapped by chronic disease.

The development of community participation as a tool for the identification of child and family needs and demands rather than an ideological issue, is strongly related to the promotion of coordination between professionals and sectors. Problems related to the accessibility, acceptability, and flexibility of services are best determined by the community, which is often more able to identify the difficulties in these general principles of adequate management. (See also Chapter 34.)

Conclusion

Figure 27.3 shows the relationship between the child health care model, needs and demands, and planning and management of child health services. These

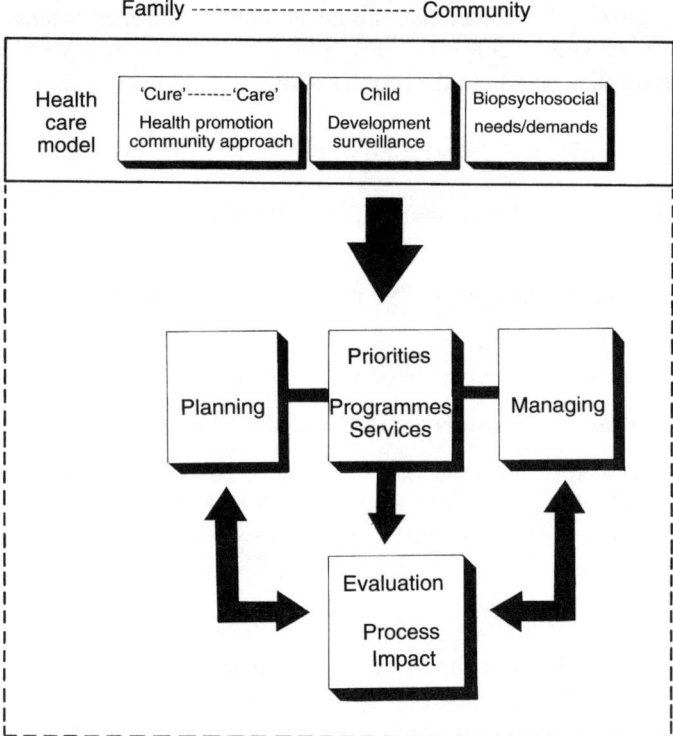

Fig. 27.3 Relationship between child health care model needs/demands and planning and managing child health services.

three issues will turn out to be different according to the prevailing economic, political, and health care model in each European country. Thus, the development of child health services and programmes will require, in the majority of European countries, a reorganization in terms of structure and content of the existing services and programmes at the national, regional, and local levels. However, in all countries it is necessary to implement short-term and medium-term evaluation systems to measure both the process outcomes (accessibility, acceptability, flexibility) and health impact (negative and welfare indicators and cost effectiveness). This reorganization process should develop alongside the educational programme which will permit a long-term evaluation of child needs and demands and the response to them from the perspective of the planning and management of child health services.

References

Arbelo Curbelo, A. and Arbelo López de Letona (1980). La salud del niño a través de la mortalidad del lactante y mortalidad perinatal. *Anales Españoles de Pediatría* **13**, 5–10.
Barnard, K. (1989). Health of youth. A view on youth and health from the Nordic Countries. *Technical Discussions*. Nordic School of Public Health, Gothenburg.
Black Report (1980). *Inequities in health*, Report of the Research Working Group. Department of Health and Social Security, London.
Butler, J. (1989). *Child health surveillance in primary care*. Department of Health, London.
De Miguel, J. (1984). *La amorosa dictadura*. Anagrama, Barcelona.
INE (Instituto Nacional de Estadística) España (1987). *Encuesta sobre discapacidades, deficiencias y munusvalias: un primer comentario de los resultados*.
Köhler, L. and Jakobsson, G. (1987). Children's health and well-being in the Nordic countries. *Clinics in developmental medicine*, Vol. 98, pp. 1–58. Blackwell Scientific, Oxford.
Köhler, L., Lindström, B.G., Barnard, K., and Itani, H. (1986). *Health implication of family breakdown*, NHV Report, No 3. The Nordic School of Public Health, Gothenburg.
Manciaux, M., Lebovici, S., Jeanneret, O., Sand, A.E., and Tomkiewicz, S. (1987). *L'enfant et sa santé*. Doin, Paris.
Macfarlane, A., Sefi, S., and Cordeiro, M. (1989). *Child health. The screening tests*. Oxford University Press.
MSC (Ministerio de Sanidad y Consumo) España (1988). *Los escolares y la salud*, M-2816. MSC, Madrid.
Miller, C.A., Coulter, E.J., Schorr, L.B., Fine, A., and Adams-Tailor, S. (1985). The world economic crisis and children: United States case study. *International Journal of Health Services* **15**, 95–134
Nordio, S. (1978). Needs in child and maternal care. Rational utilization and social-medical resources. *Rivista Italiana di Pediatria* **4**, 3–20.

Pritchard, P. (1981). *Manual of primary health care. Its nature and organizations.* Oxford University Press, London.

Spykerelle, Y. and Herberth, B. (1991). In *Comportements alimentaires d'adolescents francais*, Fifth Congress of the International Association for adolescent health. Montreux, France.

Ten, G.H. and Pedreira, J.L. (1988). Cases register and epidemiology in mental health of children. *Revista de al Asociación Española de Neurolgía* **26**, 373–90.

WHO (World Health Organization) (1985). *New perspectives in prevention in childhood*, Working group on today's health—tomorrows. WHO, Geneva.

WHO (World Health Organization) (1986). *Annuaries de statistiques sanitaries mondiales*, 1, No 1. WHO, Geneva.

WHO (World Health Organization) (1989). *The health of youth. Technical discussions*, A-42. WHO, Geneva.

WHO (World Health Organization(1990*a*). *Adolescent health. The WHO Approach.* WHO, Geneva.

WHO (World Health Organization) (1990*b*). *Aids surveillance in Europe*, WHO–EC collaborating Centre on AIDS. Quarterly report, No 28. WHO, Geneva.

28 Intersectoral approaches to promoting healthy families and children
Bob Chamberlin and Barbara Wallace

Promoting the health and development of children on a community-wide basis requires an ecologic framework. Healthy children require healthy families. Families in turn need support systems of relatives and friends and sometimes human service agencies. To function effectively these support systems must be encouraged by the policies of local government, businesses, and other community groups. These local efforts need to be positively reinforced at the regional and national level through legislation which provides the resources and structures necessary to make them work. This interdependent system is shown in Fig. 28.1.

Since family and child functioning is affected by a variety of factors, no one provider or agency can meet these multiple needs and therefore some kind of intersectoral approach becomes essential. This chapter will present a review of experience in developing intersectoral support for promoting healthy families and children in several US and UK sites with which the authors are familiar and compare this with the experiences reported by a number of cities participating in the WHO *Healthy cities* project. Finally the experience of establishing and working with an intersectoral approach by an insider in a specific community will be described.

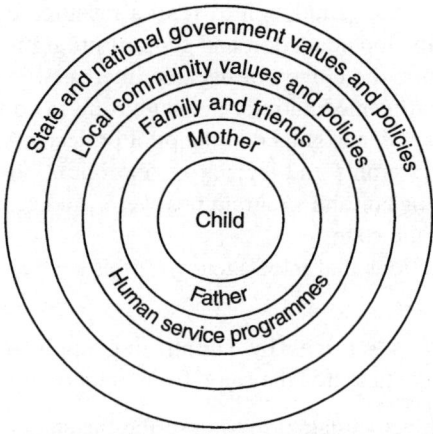

Fig. 28.1 Interdependent system for promoting the health and development of children.

Experience in US and UK communities

At a recent conference looking at how to implement community-wide approaches to promote the health and development of families and children, it was clear that one of the essential ingredients for success would be to build up a broad-based coalition with representatives of key community providers, organizations, local government, and influential citizens. This was accomplished in a number of different ways.

In the US there is the Federal Government for the whole country, State governments for each of the 50 states, County governments that are generally limited in scope, and local city or community governments of several different kinds. The main interaction between governing bodies is usually between the state and local levels. Federal money goes to the states and is generally funneled to the local communities through state agencies overseeing health, education, social welfare, and environmental protection. Communities can also apply directly to various Federal agencies for grants to fund a specific project.

Top down approaches

In some instances the energy for establishing an intersectoral approach comes from the governor of a state who becomes interested in some problem such as adolescent pregnancy. He or she then gives an executive order requiring all the state agencies dealing with adolescents to form an inter-agency task force to study the problem and come up with specific recommendations about how to better coordinate existing services and what service gaps need to be filled. An example of this kind of approach is the 'ounce of prevention' and 'parents too soon' programmes in the state of Illinois. In this instance a state agency matched a donation from a private foundation to fund a resource centre to help several pilot communities develop education and support programmes for new parents. At about the same time the Governor became interested in the problem of adolescent pregnancy and formed an inter-agency group to coordinate programmes and expand on the experience gained in the pilot projects. Additional funds were found through federal grants and legislative appropriations. A request for proposals (RFP) was sent out and programmes were funded in about 35 different communities around the state.

Some specific functions that inter-agency groups such as this have performed are listed below.

1. Increase access to services by simplifying application procedures and making eligibility standards the same from one programme to another.
2. Build a comprehensive database to describe the status of children and adolescents and their families in communities. For example, with adolescents,

we would like to know, for a given community, how many are getting pregnant out of wedlock, are contacting sexually transmitted disease, are involved with juvenile crime or substance abuse, are dropping out of school, are committing suicides and homicides. We would also like to know what types of basic preventive programmes of proven value are operating in a given community to prevent these kinds of problems.

3. In addition to building a comprehensive database, inter-agency groups can combine resources to develop a pool of money that can be applied for by local communities through a 'request for proposal mechanism' (RFP) and used to start up basic primary preventive programmes or improve existing services. This group can also provide the technical assistance necessary to do this such as how to write proposals, conduct baseline surveys, implement specific programmes, use social marketing techniques to sell prevention to the community, and monitor progress.

'Bottom up' approaches

An example of a 'bottom up' approach to intersectoral coordination is the Buddle Lane Family Centre in Exeter, UK. This programme, initially, was a child care centre located in a working class neighbourhood in Exeter. Children were accepted from all over the city and there was little orientation toward or interaction with the surrounding community except that the centre was experiencing a good deal of vandalism. The centre was then taken over by a person who, in a period of three or four years, turned it into a family centre that was integrated into the neighbourhood. She did this by making a proposal to the local education authority to develop a community-based programme through collaboration and support by social services, the local health authority, and the department of education. Social services agreed to pay for maintenance of the facilities, transportation costs, and family counselling. Education agreed to furnish educational materials and books and pay the salaries of two teachers. The health authority provided no money, but had a physician visit on two afternoons a month to examine children, answer parents' questions, and facilitate interaction with the community health nurses visiting in the area. To reach into the community a neighbourhood catchment area was established for two of the child care groups and teachers made home visits to become better acquainted with the families and neighbourhood. Toddler play-groups were started in several locations around the town. A parent's room was established at the centre which was used as a neighbourhood meeting place and sponsored activities such as an exercise programme and video club. Relationships were established with five schools in the area in terms of sharing resources and having visits by children approaching school age, so that they could become better acquainted with the teachers and the facility. Various community fund-raising activities gave further visibility and opportunities for community participation. The centre is now advised by a panel of advisors with representatives from education, social service, health service, the play-groups, and two centre parents.

The success of a 'bottom up' approach often depends on the readiness of a community to change. Sometimes local government officials and agency heads who have not been very receptive to intersectoral approaches are jolted into action by some dramatic occurrence (sentinel event). This can be a flagrant case of a 'tip of the iceberg' type problem such as child abuse, drug abuse by a child of a prominent family, a report exposing high rates of preventable problems in a community, or gross inequalities in access to services. An example of the latter is a 'bottom up' approach from Weston, UK that was described by Dr Sarah Stewart Brown at a recent ESSOP Congress on urban health. This community contains about 8000 people and consists of a post-war council estate on the urban fringe of the city of Bristol. The initiating factor for the project was a report showing high rates for infant mortality and child abuse and neglect in this area when compared with the rest of the city. The report received quite a lot of publicity and the Health Authority covering the area was put under a fair amount of pressure to do something about it. A local branch of a national advocacy group (The pre-school play-group association) came forward with a proposal that the Health Authority agreed to support. This group had been aware for some time that there were few resources in the area to relieve the isolation and loneliness expressed by many of the young parents living there. They proposed that a community centre be developed in the area to educate and train parents, provide social support, and improve access to and coordinate community services. The Health Authority agreed to fund it and a half-time community development worker was hired. She persuaded the city council to delegate one of the flats on the estate for use as a 'drop-in' centre with facilities for both parents and children. A fenced-in outdoor play area was later added.

The centre served as a focal point for meetings of local groups, recreation and skill-building activities, and adult education. In addition, the health and social service authorities used it as a meeting place to coordinate services and help families solve problems. Additional play-groups were started in other parts of the estate. Funding was provided by the Health Authority, the City Council, and through foundation grants. The centre was highly successful in terms of its use by community residents. No figures on infant mortality and child abuse are provided, but the centre had only been in operation several years at the time of this report so one would not expect dramatic results in this short period of time. Also, at the time of this report, funding for the centre had been cut back and the paid position of the community developer could no longer be sustained. Volunteers had taken over some of these functions, but the centre was surviving on a hand-to-mouth basis.

This brings up the great weakness of a 'bottom up' approach. While they are very successful in mobilizing energy and participation at the local level, some mechanism for sustained long-term funding must be built into the system, or 'burn out' of community volunteers all too often ends the project. Getting and keeping adequate funding generally requires the development of an advocacy group which must be ever alert to attempts by politicians or agency heads to cut back the funding of primary prevention programmes such as these in times of shrinking budgets.

Combining 'top down' and 'bottom up' approaches

What appears to be needed for maximum community participation and sustainability is some combination of 'top down' and 'bottom up'. For instance in Maine, a state in the north-eastern section of the US, a group of parents and service providers formed a state-wide advocacy group and sponsored two bills in the legislature to mandate services for children aged 0 to 5 years with developmental disabilities. The bill was heard by the education committee of the state legislature which then required the three main state agencies involved with the care of children with disabilities to report back on what they were doing. This led eventually to legislation setting up an 'Inter-Departmental Coordinating Committee for Pre-school Handicapped Children' at the state level, involving the departments of education, health, and social services. On this committee are also three parent representatives and a representative of the originating advocacy group. It also provided funds for an RFP mechanism requiring local communities or regions to set up a similar interdisciplinary coordinating committee in order to receive funds that could be used to enhance or expand services.

Another example of a successful combination of 'bottom up' and 'top down' approaches is from Vermont, another small state in the north-eastern US. Here a local group started a parent/child centre in one town. They gradually spread out programmes into the surrounding towns throughout a semi-rural county of 32 000 people. After about seven years of operation, evaluation studies showed significant drops in child abuse, infant mortality, adolescent pregnancy, and school drop-out. A state-wide advocacy group convinced the state legislature to appropriate funds to help start up other centres in other counties throughout the state. When the appropriations are voted on each year there is a mass turn out of parents and children to the state capital to lobby for continuation of the funding of these highly successful programmes.

In Britain, the 'healthy communities' project in Newcastle has forged an unusual partnership between the Health Authority, the City Council, Save the Children Fund, and several of the city's most deprived communities. The aim of the project was to address the links between child health, poverty, and the environment. A video which takes a child's eye view of growing up in the 'West-End' of Newcastle is being produced in the first stage of the project. The video, based around the hopes and fears expressed by the community's children, will also provide hard information about the extra burden of morbidity which these children face. The video will be the focus for local people to identify priorities in child health, and will enable them to draw up a 'community plan for child-health' to spell out the strategies needed. Health and local government services have committed themselves to reshaping the delivery of their services in the West-end of Newcastle to put this plan into action. The project reverses the order of traditional strategic planning: the plan is developed at grass-roots level, with policy makers committed to ensuring that the strategies determined by local needs and perceptions receive adequate and sustained support. The project also builds upon earlier experiences in Newcastle of working directly with children to identify community problems in devising innovative strategies for change.

Experience in 'healthy cities' projects

It is interesting to compare the more spontaneous experiences just described with the more systematic 'healthy cities' approach as reported in two recent publications (Tsouros 1991; Ashton 1992). All the healthy cities projects started with cities whose leadership had already expressed support for healthy public policies and the creation of supportive environments which develop and sustain the health of all citizens. In the Milan Declaration of 1990, Mayors of project cities expressed political support for 'the strengthening of intersectoral action on the broad determinants of health' and 'establishing effective intersectoral mechanisms for developing healthy public policies'. This was further defined as establishing 'an intersectoral political committee to act as a focus for and to steer the project'. In this sense, then, they all started with a 'top-down' approach to intersectoral cooperation. How this evolved in actual practice varied considerably from one city to the next.

In some cities different sectors such as health and social services have similar geographic catchment areas which facilitates cooperation. It becomes considerably more complicated when different sectors have responsibility for different catchment areas and decisions are made at different political levels.

Not all these cities achieved this state of readiness spontaneously. The general approach has been to start off with a report indicating which areas of the city have an excess of health problems and a deficit in resources, or to hold a workshop looking at the concept of healthy cities and providing examples of good practice to create a vision of what can be done, or both. If the mayor and city council sign on to the concepts, the next step is usually the formation of an intersectoral planning committee who develop an overall framework and find funding to establish the position of a coordinator. Because intersectoral work is so time-consuming, almost all cities that have achieved some measure of success have established an office and hired a coordinator to facilitate the process. Individual projects are then developed through task forces. The process is, however, often considerably more complicated. For example, the experience of the city of Sheffield, UK illustrates some of the complexities of intersectoral work even in a city with a good track record of interest in prevention and planning and collaboration between the Health Authority and other local authorities.

This project started with a report commissioned by the city council which showed inequalities in health in different segments of the city. This was followed up by a report from the Sheffield Health Authority that linked health status with indicators of deprivation such as unemployment and poor housing. This lead to the formation of an intersectoral planning team who initially tried to orient their activities around the 38 WHO *Health for all* (*HFA*) targets. However, it was found that these predetermined targets did not fit their circumstances. Rather than define specific targets from the start, the planning team decided to develop an overall framework based on basic WHO principles and allow interested participants to develop their own targets. A coordinator position was funded in part through pooled funds from the different authorities with some additional money added by the Health Authority. Administrative support in the form of two part-time positions was funded by the city council. For specific projects a 'lead officer' within one organization was designated to act as the coordinator. Each participating agency would then 'lend' workers for specific projects as needed. Projects were financed by contributions of participating organizations. Communities could also apply for pooled resources for short-term projects, but had to seek external funding for bigger, long-term ones. In reading the progress reports of this city and others one is struck by the complexity of the undertaking, which often takes several years to develop the basic infrastructure necessary for successful action and long-term sustainability.

Some large cities such as Barcelona and Zagreb have not only managed intersectoral cooperation at the city level but have taken this one step further by dividing the city into districts. Each district has an intersectoral board or council made up of representatives of health, social services, education, other city departments, and voluntary organizations. These district boards then convene task forces to study and work on improving some aspect of city life in their district.

In some areas academic institutions have initiated the process and played a key role in spreading the concepts over a wide area. For example, in one region of Spain (Valencian community) containing about four million people and 59 cities, the 'healthy city' idea was introduced by a group of academics from the Department of Community Health of the University of Alicante and the Valencian School of Public Health. They spread the *HFA* concepts among public health workers, politicians, and the country at large. Support was obtained from local city governments and the regional government who jointly funded a coordinating office. This, in turn, led to the formation of a network of 34 member cities with two coordinating offices staffed by two full-time professionals trained in public health and two part-time honorary senior consultants. Intersectoral groups were created in each city to develop a community diagnosis (a profile of problems and resources and good practices) (see Chapter 34). These concepts and reports then become part of the curriculum for training social workers, nurses, and for those seeking a masters degree in public health. A Healthy Cities Association composed of all these different elements meets once a month and includes representatives of the media who further spread the information.

Keeping political commitment has been one of the most important activities of 'healthy cities' advocates because this gives the project visibility and legitimacy and provides help in obtaining resources and intersectoral cooperation. Strategies that have helped gain political support include independence of any one political party, and avoidance of identification with any one administrative department such as the Department of Health. Rather it was found helpful to be located, administratively and physically, in a central location with ready access to senior politicians. Other important elements were to define roles and activities, so that the project can be easily understood, and to show links between different departments and the overall plan. It was also important to make projects relevant to current political concerns and to pick some short-term projects having a high likelihood of success. Being able to show that the project has a broad-based constituency and maintaining high visibility are other ways of attracting and keeping political support.

In summary, intersectoral collaboration is essential for an ecologic approach to promoting healthy families and children. This process is complicated and it takes time to work out an appropriate infrastructure to facilitate the working together of diverse groups. The funding of a full-time coordinator increases considerably the chances of success. Keeping this position funded, in turn, requires maintaining political support for the project as a whole so that in developing projects one needs to consider political needs as well as community needs.

Decentralization and 'bottom up' approaches are very effective in mobilizing community participation and support for specific projects but must be combined with 'top down' efforts to ensure stable long-term funding and sustainability. Successfully involving academic institutions has been helpful in getting technical assistance from the faculty and participation of students in carrying out surveys, building a database, social marketing, and other types of help that would often be too expensive for the city to carry out on its own.

Further reading

1. Chamberlin, R. (ed.) (1988). *Beyond individual risk assessment: community wide approaches to promoting the health and development of families and children*. The National Center for Education in Maternal and Child Health, Washington, DC.
2. Chamberlin, R. (1992). Preventing low birth weight, child abuse, and school failure: the need for comprehensive, community-wide approaches. *Pediatrics in Review* **13**; 64–71.
3. Brown, Sarah Stewart (1989). Community action and health promotion. In: *The child in an urban environment*, (ed. M. Lordeiro). ESSOP, Portugal.
4. Tsouros, A. (ed.) (1991). *World Health Organization healthy cities project: a project becomes a movement. Review of progress 1987 to 1990*. Fadl, Copenhagen.
5. Ashton, J. (ed.) (1992). *Healthy cities*. Open University Press, Philadelphia.

29 Outcome and performance measures in child health

Aidan Macfarlane

'The ideal should never stand in the way of the merely good'
                                                        Anon.

Introduction

This chapter will deal with 'outcome measurements in child health' as it relates to the work of medical professionals. It will also be useful to managers, politician, administrators, and the public in general.

So why measure? First because health professionals, working in the field of child health, will, or should, know whether the work they are doing is worthwhile and effective. To answer this they will want to know first what it is that child health services are seeking to achieve and then whether they are actually achieving it. Secondly, because those people given the responsibility both nationally and locally for distributing resources towards various health interventions when setting priorities, will need to know as much as possible about the costs and effectiveness of all the interventions available in the health field.

What are the child health services seeking to achieve?

> *'The goals may be broadly specified as lowering child mortality and certain types of acute morbidity, correcting or minimising disability, promoting optimum growth and development and perhaps achieving a longer and fuller life'* (Yankauer 1973)

More specific aims are outlined in *Measurement of child health*, a report of the UK working party of the Executive Committee of the Community Paediatric Group in association with the British Paediatric Association (1989) and are a summary of the present overall aims of the World Health Organization's *Health for all by the year 2000* programme, as it related to children, which are summarized below.

1. Reducing rates of death;

    reducing rates of acute illnesses;

    reducing prevalence of chronic illness and disability;

reducing the adverse psychological consequences of disability or chronic illness;

reducing the prevalence of psychological and behaviourial disturbance.

2. Promoting healthy lifestyles in children;

promoting the optimal development of children;

reducing social and geographical inequality in health.

The target of the first five aims involves a decrease in the incidence and prevalence of 'diseases' causing mortality and morbidity. At least part of this is achieved by decreasing individual case fatality and case morbidity via treatment (e.g. eight per cent of deaths in children in 1940 were due to pneumonia, but with the advent of antibiotics this is now virtually zero). The last three aims seek to achieve, in the absence of disease, an increase in the overall health status of children in terms of being bigger, cleverer, more adaptable people with emotionally richer, more fulfilled, and longer lives.

Obviously, to 'decrease' or 'increase' something, we have to have some measurement of its present status. Change can only be assessed from the basis of knowing what the current situation is in some kind of objective way.

Are the child health services achieving these aim?

Overall, most countries know very little about whether they are achieving their aims. What we do know is that the main factors influencing both the prevalence of diseases and the overall health status of children concern the social, cultural, economic, educational, and environmental circumstances of the individual child and the child's family. As a result, in most European countries, as social conditions improve, so overall mortality rates are improving. Compared with this, the influence of the work of the professionals involved in the child health services is relatively small, though we do also know that in some specific areas, direct health service interventions do affect outcome. Screening for phenylketonurea and hypothyroidism with subsequent dietary or drug management are two examples where social and economic factors are secondary to direct medical interventions.

However, what is most difficult to measure in many cases, is *how much* a decrease in mortality and morbidity or improvement in health status is brought about by direct medical intervention and *how much* by other factors, such as improving socio-economic circumstances.

Some would claim that it does not really matter, as long as mortality and morbidity are on the decrease and health status is improving (British Paediatric Association 1939). However, if large quantities of resources are being channelled into one area of the health service on the grounds that they are effective—this must, if possible, be validated by research, or the money (which is a limited resource) should be reallocated elsewhere where effectiveness has been demonstrated (Department of Health 1991; Welsh Office 1991). However, there is a dilemma here that needs taking into account—sometimes, a study indicating lack of effectiveness of an intervention is the fault of the validation study design (often including faults in techniques of the representativeness and sampling) rather than that of the intervention itself.

The most searching attempt at dealing with this paradox is outlined in *Children's health in Sweden* (Kohler and Jakobsson 1991). This book attempts, using data collected in a country with more experience than any other of trying to formalize the measurement of the health of the children, to unravel some of the problems that are faced in both defining need and measuring the effects of medical intervention and social change. Even here the authors conclude, when looking at 'methods and data quality' that 'one looks in vain for a systematic, continuous and comprehensive reporting of children's health, viewed in a child perspective and related to a social context'.

Nevertheless, with the measurements available to them, the Swedish researchers draw many real and fundamental conclusions with considerable implications for resource distribution. These include that for Sweden

- mortality at all ages during childhood is low, often the lowest in the world, and is still declining;
- children make extensive use of public-caring resources, hospital and out-patient care, dental care, and drugs;
- care utilization mainly concerns minor health problems and is of brief duration;
- caring costs are low compared with other sectors of the population;
- chronic illness and disability have grown in importance, partly because certain conditions have become more frequent while survival prospects have improved for others;
- accidents still occupy a dominant position as a cause of mortality and morbidity amongst children, despite a conspicuous decrease during the past few decades;
- use of alcohol and narcotic drugs is low amongst Swedish youngsters by international standards;
- police reports of maltreatment and sexual abuse of children increased during the 1980s.

These are not just 'nice generalized statements' plucked from the air, but well researched findings on which social, political, and resource distribution decisions should, and must, be made.

A model for child health measurements

There are a number of specific steps to setting up a practical system to measure child health within a population. These are listed below.

1. To define, by epidemiological studies, what health problems affect the population of children. A less sophisticated and more practical approach is to question those working in the field of child health as to what they see are the major health priorities and to take the common problems that are identified.

2. To review available research and carry out new research (if possible using specific controlled trials) to find the optimal forms of intervention available in order to improve outcomes (these forms of intervention can be social, environmental, political, medical, etc.).

3. To define the most appropriate personnel (parents, politicians, teachers, social workers, community nurses, doctors, etc.) to carry out the interventions.

4. To set priorities for the interventions in the light of (i) the severity of the health problem because of the mortality and morbidity it causes, (ii) the prevalence of the problem, (iii) the effectiveness of the intervention, and (iv) the resources available.

5. To set strategic objectives in the light of 1–4 above. These objectives should also include measurable targets—e.g. reducing the rate of death of children from accidents by five per cent per year.

6. To monitor whether the interventions are being implemented and the cost and quality of the interventions.

7. To develop outcome measures by which to judge whether the prioritized interventions are effective if applied to whole populations.

The main measures involved in the above scenario are therefore concerned with the health needs of a population, the effectiveness of the interventions, monitoring the implementation of outputs (interventions), the inputs needed to achieve the outputs, and the outcomes. Even the step of setting strategic objectives, which also involves setting priorities, can only rationally be done using available measurements. The step are summarized in Fig. 29.1.

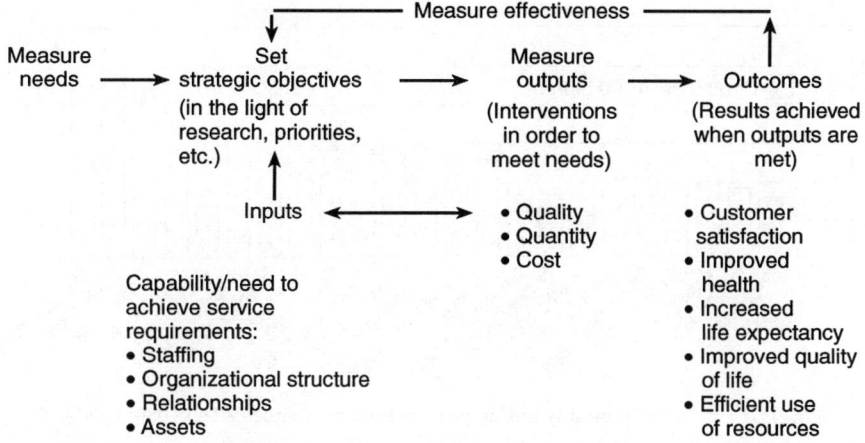

Fig. 29.1 Measurements in child health.

Current measures including mortality, morbidity, and background factors

Mortality rates

Mortality has the advantage that it is absolute. There is no grading of mortality as there is with morbidity. The normal artificial time divisions and definitions of mortality rates in the first year of life are shown below. (OPCS 1991a)

- still births and late fetal deaths (i.e. deaths after 28 completed weeks of gestation per thousand live and still births).
- Perinatal deaths (i.e. still births and deaths in the first week of life per thousand live and still births).
- Neonatal deaths (i.e. deaths under 28 completed days of life per thousand live births).
- Infant deaths (i.e. deaths at ages under one year per thousand live births).

Comparative examples of some of these rates are shown in Figs. 29.2 and 29.3. After one year, mortality rates by age are not standardized but may be given as (OPCS 1991b)

(1) deaths between 28 days and 4 years;

(2) deaths 5–14 years;

(3) deaths 15–24 years.

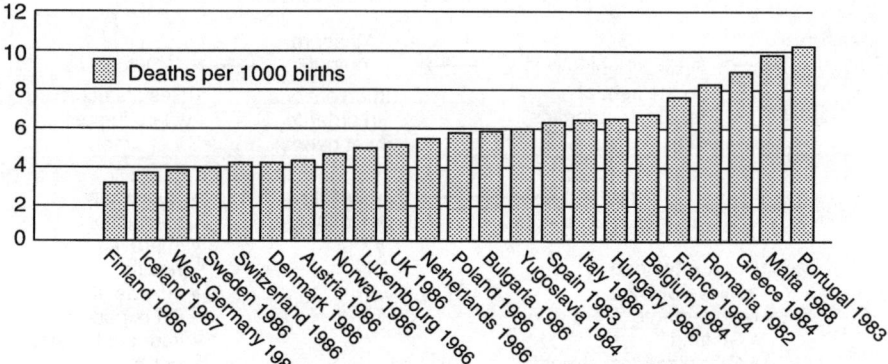

Fig. 29.2 Perinatal mortality in European countries. (Source: WHO 1989; OPCS.)

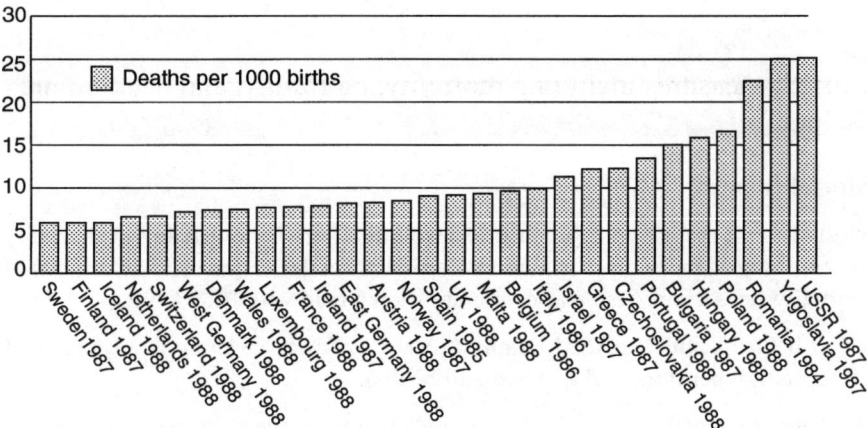

Fig. 29.3 Infant mortality in European countries. (Source: WHO 1989; OPCS.)

Causes of mortality

For accuracy of diagnosis there is no short cut to having well qualified paediatric pathologists carrying out as many as possible routine post-mortem examinations on babies that die. This is because of the poor correlation between what is written on death certificates and what is found at post-mortem examination. However, there is a great shortage of paediatric pathologists in many countries in Europe. Examples of the kind of data concerning death by cause which can then be provided, are shown in Figs. 29.4–29.6.

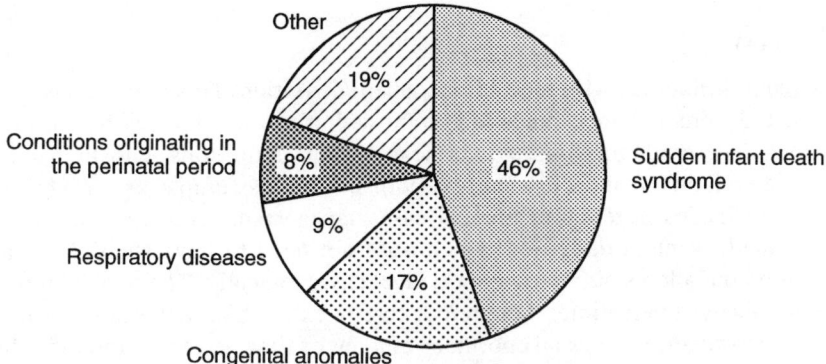

Fig. 29.4 Other infant deaths (28 days to under one year old) in the UK, 1989. (Total = 2536.)

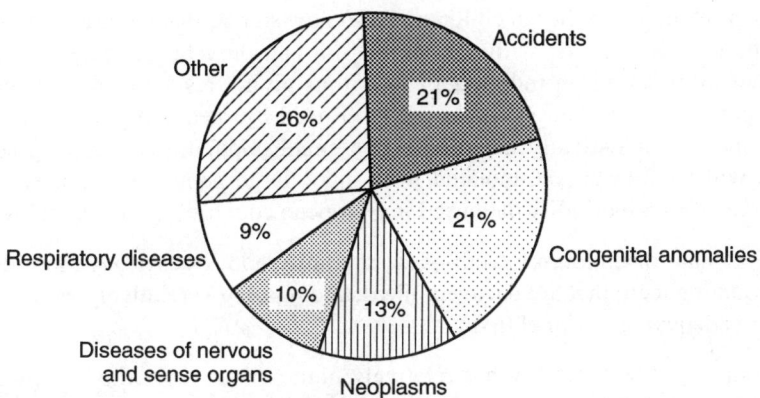

Fig. 29.5 Deaths at age 1–4 years in the UK, 1989. (Total = 1078.)

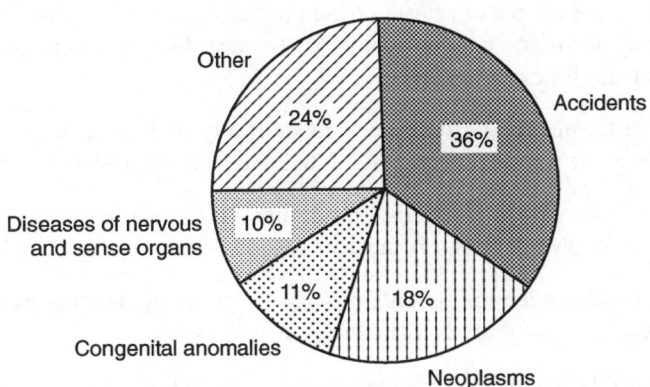

Fig. 29.6 Causes of death at age 5–14 years in the UK, 1989. (Total = 1175.)

Morbidity

The main difficulties with morbidity concern definition. This will always be so because different professionals will want definitions of illnesses for different reasons. The epidemiologist wants neat, simple definitions with high inter-observer reliability and clear cut-off points, with less emphasis on what the definition means in terms of clinical case management. The clinician, on the other hand, wants a definition which does not need to have such clear case definition but allows him to treat individual cases logically. The two definitions are not always compatible, though to a certain extent both definitions relate to 'need'. However, it saves an enormous amount of time and frustration if, when settling on 'a definition', it is first decided what exactly the definition is required for—epidemiological data collection concerning prevalence, a clinical definition to develop a treatment protocol, a definition to look at resource needs, and so on.

Much severe morbidity in children is also now so rare that significant baseline data of resource 'need' within a population can only be collected by using detailed information on individual cases, thus giving resource implications as 'cost per case'. To then estimate the total need by measuring the number of cases may be statistically meaningless in small populations, and in practical terms will have to be extrapolated from much large population studies. Some high-prevalence morbidity data used in European countries are listed below.

1. The state of children's teeth—low mortality and low serious morbidity—counting teeth that are decayed, filled, and missing is relatively easy if there are adequate personnel to do it.

2. Asthma—low mortality but relatively high serious morbidity—difficult to define although some definitions are available.

3. Injury rates—relatively high mortality (see Table 29.1) and morbidity—it is difficult to collect data because of the multiple treatment points from 'self-treatment' through 'parent treatment' to 'accident and emergency' and 'hospital admission'.

4. Serous otitis media—virtually absent mortality and level of morbidity is conflicting—it is moderately difficult to have clear definitions.

5. Enuresis—absent mortality, low morbidity—relatively easy to define, but difficult to collect data as it is mostly 'coped with' within the family.

6. Mild to moderate learning problems—absent mortality, level of morbidity is difficult to assess—there is difficulty over definitions.

7. Psychiatric/behaviourial problems—low mortality, high morbidity—difficult definitions.

Table 29.1 *Risk of children under six being killed as car passengers. Averages, 1985–1987*

	Deaths	Population 1000	Risk
France	117	4554	25.7
USA	539	21 729	24.8
Denmark	6	320	18.8
Finland	7	385	18.2
Spain	52	2906	17.9
Austria	9	539	16.7
Hungary	12	771	15.6
Belgium	10	729	13.7
Former GDR	15	1365	11.0
Former FRG	39	3601	10.8
Norway	3	310	9.7
UK	41	4404	9.3
Greece	7	772	9.1
Netherlands	8	1059	7.6
Sweden	4	584	6.8

Source: *Statistics of Road Traffic Accidents in Europe*, 1989.

Some low-prevalence morbidity include the following.

- Cerebral palsy—high mortality, high morbidity—difficulty over definitions.

- Cystic fibrosis—high mortality, high morbidity—no difficulty over definitions.

- Severe learning problems–low mortality, high morbidity—clear definition, but not always accurate.

- Congenital heart disease—with appropriate treatment, relatively low mortality and morbidity—relatively good definitions.

- Diabetes—with treatment, relatively low mortality but still high morbidity—good definitions.

Background factors

Background factors can be seen as measures of resources or components of existence that may influence a child's health, and of course also influence outcomes for long term morbidity where it already exists. Many of these will relate to a single factor—poverty (see Chapter 22). Thus housing, dietary habits, family relations, recreation, access to care, and education will all be influenced by the economic circumstances surrounding the child, the family, and the country. Therefore some measurements of threats to children's health and well-being will include the following:

(1) poverty—number of children living in families with below-average earning power, number of children living in families below a specified poverty line;

(2) Family breakup—number of divorces and number of unsupported single-parent families;

(3) use of narcotic drugs—age-specific drug-taking rates;

(4) use of alcohol—age-specific alcohol usage rates;

(5) child abuse—rates of child abuse (from questionnaires to adults and report to the police, social services, or medical system);

(6) poor diet—total calorie intake and relative proportion of diet from fat, protein, and carbohydrate;

(7) use of tobacco—age-specific smoking rates;

(8) subjective general satisfaction with life rating (see Figs. 29.7, 29.8);

(9) environmental factors such as availability of safe play areas.

Related, but more difficult to measure and understand, are 'protective' factors—those characteristic of children who, although they grow up under extreme circumstances, nevertheless show good adjustment and competency in

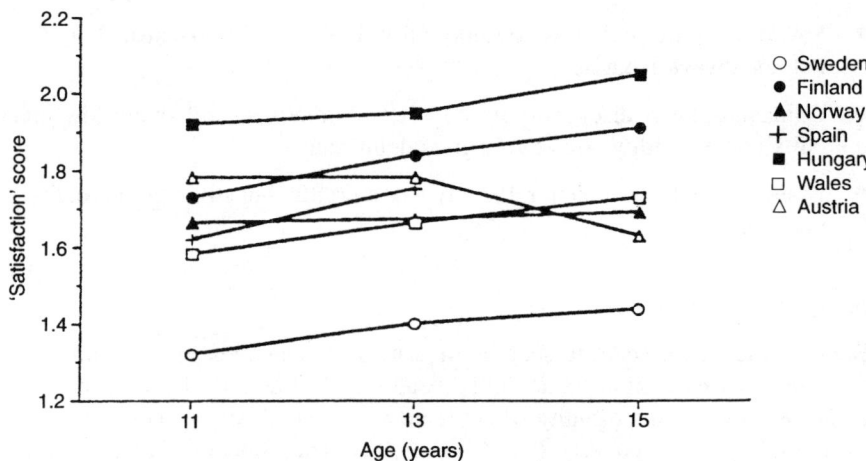

Fig. 29.7 General satisfaction with life, boys. Average score on a scale from 1 = 'very good' to 4 = 'not at all good'. (Source: Marklund and Strandell 1989.)

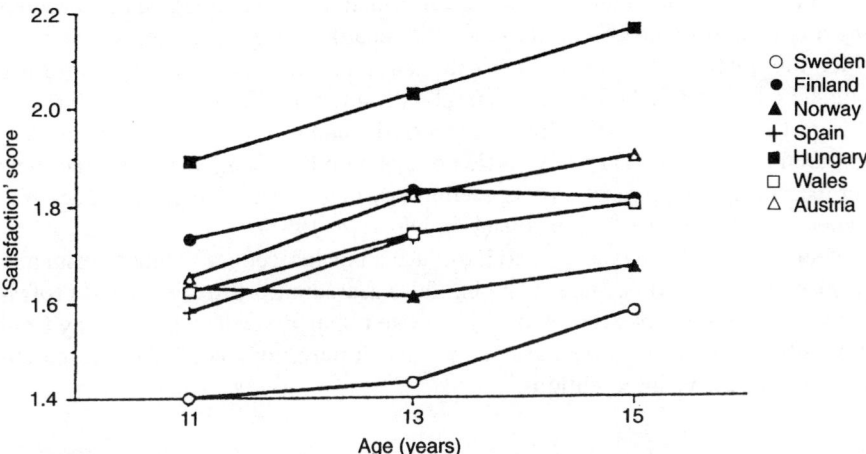

Fig. 29.8 General satisfaction with life, girls. Average score on a scale from 1 = 'very good' to 4 = 'not at all good'. (Source: Marklund and Strandell 1989.)

later life (Wernes 1989). These include the fact that this group of successful children never lack friends, have a feeling of independent power, think and act independently, and invariably score well in creativity tests. How much of this 'protection' is nature, how much is nurture, is probably less important than the interaction between the two.

It is worth reflecting, however, that if one protective factor can be singled out—it is probably the child having a close human confidante of any age with whom they can discuss their most intimate problems.

The effectiveness of interventions

The interventions offered by the child health services are no different from most other medical interventions provided elsewhere within the health services, or for that matter social and economic interventions, in that many of them were implemented before the concept of proper research into effectiveness and efficacy had been introduced. Thus most of child health surveillance using regular routine checks to assess a child's health and development, although carried out in many countries, has not been evaluated for effectiveness. There remains, therefore, a dilemma for the health professionals carrying out these programmes. Should they continue to carry out child health surveillance procedures which are of unknown benefit, using up considerable resources, where the outcome is unknown, or should they cease the procedures and risk losing something that might be of benefit even if this has not been established?

On the other hand, there is now a clear principle to be applied when introducing a new, untried procedure into the child health service: (1) that, where possible, the intervention must be evaluated on a limited scale by carefully conducted research before its general introduction; (2) where possible this should be by using double-blind control trials; and (3) where it is not possible, research must still be carefully carried out using other recognized research tools for measuring effectiveness, i.e. epidemiology in the case of relating cot death to the position babies are laid in cots (Wigfield *et al.* 1992).

It should now be inexcusable to introduce a new procedure without evaluating its effectiveness, (a) because of giving false reassurance to patients and professionals where it is not warranted; (b) because it may divert resources away from more effective interventions; and (c) because it may stop people from researching more effective interventions.

Setting priority strategic objectives

Having measured the effectiveness of an intervention, there is then the different, but equally difficult, decision as to whether to introduce the intervention or not. With ever-increasing emphasis on cost and effectiveness and 'health gain' (Welsh Office 1991), this is an area of great importance, but limited information is available. Resources can be seen in terms of people's time, actual material (equipment, etc) required, and so on, or in terms of their actual cost. What are the resources needed to prevent, say, injury, against treating the injury once it has occurred? It is an area of measurement that holds many paradoxes—not only of 'prevention versus crisis intervention' but the fact that death itself can frequently be much less demanding on resources than continuing life. An obvious example is in the field of neonatology with its ever-increasing demand on resources as it seeks to achieve better survival figures for lower and lower birth-weight babies. The increased demand for resources extends beyond that required for the unit itself to that needed for the management and treatment of the 1 in 10 babies who will end up with handicaps, and for the possibly increased long-term 'needs' of the other nine whose 'needs' will also have to be evaluated into adulthood.

Making decisions on priorities in the child health services therefore involves taking a number of different factors into account—the list below being by no means exhaustive:

(1) political priorities, which tend to be an unknown element, but frequently over-ride other considerations;

(2) importance, as seen by the general public—this can be measured;

(3) resources needed for introduction, which can be estimated;

(4) Severity of the disease in terms of mortality and morbidity, which can be measured;

(5) prevalence of disease, which can be measured;

(6) effectiveness of intervention, which can be measured (see below);

(7) ease of controlling the quality of intervention, which can be measured;

(8) monitoring the extent of intervention after introduction, which can be measured;

(9) resources (medical, nursing, or other staff) already available in the area of work, which can be measured;

(10) resources required for long-term 'side-effects' of an intervention (e.g. neonatal care), which can be measured.

It is worth noting that 'can be measured' does not mean that it 'will be measured'; that the only way of *not* allowing political considerations to over-ride everything else when setting priorities is by providing suitable data to argue for a more rational approach (assuming that in the majority of cases political decisions are made on a 'vote getting' rather than on a 'health gain' basis) and that the effectiveness of the service's 'curing elements' will always be easier to measure than the 'caring elements' (de Mare 1990).

Quantity and quality measures

For services already in place, or for new interventions being put into place—whether these are political, social, or medical, etc., but have been accepted as both effective and a priority—there then needs to be a programme to examine how the services are actually being delivered. Part of the programme will have to monitor uptake and part will monitor quality (Kaplan and Anderson 1990). For instance, in implementing a new medical screening programme, say for the early identification of children with sensori-neural hearing loss, there needs first to be some way of monitoring whether it is actually reaching as near 100 per cent as possible of the children it is designed for, and secondly, an assessment as to whether the field workers carrying out the test are performing at the same standards of quality as were obtained during the original research trials.

Measurements of outcomes

'Outcome' can be defined as 'that which comes out of something: visible or practical result, effect, or product' (*SOED* 1973). However, a 'health outcome' has been defined as 'a direct measurement of an aspect of health in which improvement is sought'. Unfortunately this particular definition (British Paediatric Association 1989) goes on to suggest 'It will be influenced by services and/or social, economic and environmental circumstances but *understanding of the separate contribution of these influences is not relevant to the measurement*'. But going back to the original dictionary definition of 'outcome' being 'that which comes out of *something*'—the 'something' must be relevant. 'Outcomes' occur because of something—and, as far as is possible, we need to know 'how much' of which of the 'somethings' is responsible for the changes in outcome. If resources are being used in a specific intervention on the grounds that they are effective in contributing to an improvement in a health outcome, then we need to know that it is actually so.

Where a specific 'outcome' is causally closely linked with some form of definite intervention, the intervention is known as an 'output' (British Paediatric Association 1989). The link between decreased prevalence of some infectious disease (outcome) appearing to be closely linked with immunization cover of a population (output) is usually given as an example. 'Inputs' are the staff, equipment, etc. that are needed to produce an 'output'.

A good example of a specific outcome measure used for a fairly specific output is demonstrated by a decision made on the island of Cyprus where, by 1976, treatment for thalassaemia with blood transfusions and desferrioxamine had begun to use up one-fifth of the island's total medical budget. It was therefore decided to introduce a fetal screening programme for the disease, coupled with a liberal abortion policy (the two coupled medical outputs). The resulting decrease in the number of babies born with thalassaemia is shown in Fig. 29.9. It is worth noting that prior 1977, the rate had already begun to drop due to the counselling of heterozygote carriers about marriage, and this probably still contributes to a small apart of the fall although this form of intervention proved to be less than optimal because of resistance to the limitations on 'freedom of choice' of a marriage partner (Fig. 29.10).

Of primary interest to the health professional, therefore, is knowing whether their own personal output is having any discernible effect on 'outcome'. On an individual basis, this will almost always have to be subjective. At best, the individual professional may be aware that an intervention they are carrying out has

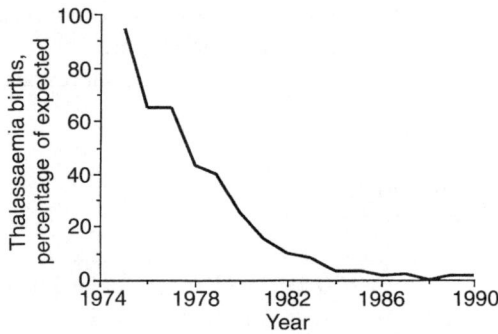

Fig. 29.9 Prevention of thalassaemia in Cyprus, 1977, illustrating the effectiveness of fetal diagnosis.

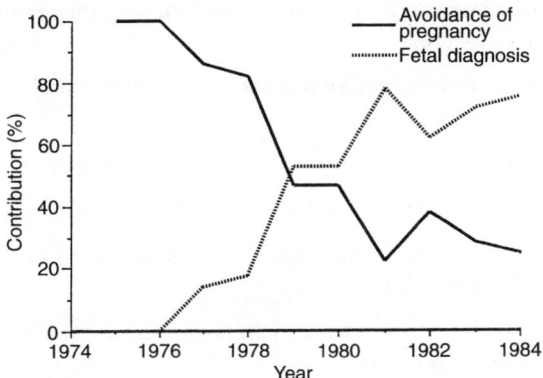

Fig. 29.10 Percentage contribution to the reduction of thalassaemia births of avoidance of pregnancy and fetal diagnosis.

been shown, by case-control studies, to be effective. However, they will also need to be aware that different people will want different measurements in order to judge outcomes. Doctors and patients will want to have outcomes judged mainly in terms of the effectiveness of the intervention and their own personal satisfaction (doctors' and patients') resulting from the intervention. Politicians and managers may want to know the cost-effectiveness of interventions and patient satisfaction.

It would be of obvious value to develop health outcome measurements for a range of specific interventions in paediatrics and child health. However, these measurements are fraught with problems for two main reasons—(i) because many of the health problems being measured are so rare that variations in prevalence may well occur because of chance rather than a specified intervention, and (ii) even if there does appear to be a significant improvement in the prevalence of the health problem it may be extremely difficult to link this improvement with a specific intervention. These problems will be dealt with further when individual outcome measures are discussed below.

Measurements of health outcome are, however, important for the following reasons:

(a) they are necessary to inform judgements on priorities;

(b) they are necessary to try and determine how the effect of interventions in the health, social, or other services relate to changes of health;

(c) they help informed decisions about whether a service should be retained, expanded, altered, or abandoned;

(d) they aid in judging the effectiveness of 'outputs' in achieving strategic objectives;

(e) there is a need to measure patient satisfaction with the services provided as one specific outcome;

(f) they can allow some objective measurement of the overall 'health status' of a population of children.

Some criteria of outcome measures include the following:

(a) the measurement must be able to be defined unambiguously;

(b) the direction in which the measurement should move to indicate improved health must be unequivocal;

(c) the data from which the measurement is derived should be generally available or feasible to generate;

(d) each measurement should be able to be made regularly for trends to be identified and for regular feedback to staff;

(e) there should be some concept as to what interventions are likely to be influencing a significant trend.

Some general rules for data collection[†] are to

(1) keep it simple—collect as few items as possible;

(2) define the measure clearly and unambiguously (preferably the definition should be the same as everyone else's);

(3) make sure that the staff responsible understand the point of data collection;

(4) provide feedback on the results in an intelligible form.

Some suggested child health outcome measures[†] for populations of between 100 000 and 600 000 were drawn up by a working party of the British Paediatric Association (1990), and were proposed for district level (100 000 to 600 000 population), these are listed below.

1. Health outcome measures:

- day one and neonatal mortality in four birth-weight bands;
- notification of cause of measles and mumps;
- asthma admissions to hospital lasting over 72 hours.

2. 'Implied' outcome measures:

- late fitting of hearing aids for congenital deafness;
- late recognition of congenital dislocation of the hip;

[†] Many of the suggestions given in these sections are either adapted or taken directly from a paper entitled 'measuring child health' by Stuart Logan (1991). I am indebted to him for permission to use his excellent material in this way.

- late recognition of congenital hypothyroidism;
- late recognition of developmental problems;
- immunization uptake;
- proportion of children with insulin-dependent diabetes mellitus whose control is poor, as measured by glaciated haemoglobin concentrations.

3. Descriptions of patterns of service:
- proportion of admissions of children aged less than thirteen years who are admitted to adult wards;
- proportion of operations of hernia and squint done as day cases.

These suggestions have been criticised (Logan 1991) both because in many of these measurements the link between the intervention and a specific outcome is likely to be limited, and because the very small numbers involved within a population of between 200 000 and 600 000 mean that the 95 per cent confidence limits will be very broad, so that even quite large changes of, say neonatal mortality, may be due to chance. Some of these problems for the individual measures suggested are shown in Table 29.2.

Table 29.2 *Problems associated with proposed outcome measures for use by District Health Authorities*

Measurement	Problem	
	Link between service and outcome uncertain or likely to be limited	Small numbers
Useful:		
Immunization coverage	No	No
Admissions for asthma	No	No
Useful but interpret with caution:		
Notifications of measles and pertussis	No	No
Late recognition of developmental problems	No	No
Not useful in this form:		
Neonatal mortality	Yes	Yes
Mortality on day one	Yes	Yes
Late fitting of hearing aids	No	Yes
Late recognition of congenital dislocation of hips	No	Yes
Congenital hypothyroidism	No	Yes
'Poor control' of insulin-dependent diabetes mellitus	Yes	Yes

(From Logan 1991.)

However, there is a further use of the 'implied' outcome measures shown above which has considerable significance for the actual management rather than measurement of the services. By identifying individual children who have had late fitting of hearing aids for sensorineural deafness and late diagnosis of congenital dislocation of the hip, congenital hypothyroidism, and developmental problems, it is possible to examine in detail if, and where, there has been a failure in the surveillance services and then take appropriate action, i.e. retraining staff implementing a screening technique.

Some child health measurements in populations of between 2000 and 100 000

The aim of this section is to suggest some kinds of information, relative to child health, which may be useful to collect on a relatively smaller population that a group of family doctors or health centre might deal with.

Needs

(1) Number of children in the population, as part of an age/sex register;

(2) frequency of consultation;

(3) reasons for consultation.

Monitoring interventions

(1) Immunization uptake rates;

(2) child health surveillance rates of under fives;

(3) referral rates from surveillance programmes.

Outcomes

(1) Audit of child and parent satisfaction with services;

(2) Age-related smoking rates;

(3) Age-related alcohol use;

(4) Teenage pregnancy rates;

(5) Number of hospital referrals;

(6) Number of hospital admissions.

The same problems that exist with the larger population measurements will also apply.

Health status outcome measures

These are measurements taken on every member (or a properly randomized representative sample) of a whole population to look at the overall distribution of a certain measurement. They will depend mainly on socio-economic levels and distribution of wealth within a country. They are only useful if done on large populations.

Some measurements of overall population health status are as follows:

(1) birth-weight distribution;

(2) age-specific height and weight distribution;

(3) age-specific development/intelligence quotient distribution;

(4) age at death;

(5) age of onset of puberty;

(6) age-specific general satisfaction with life measures.

A social and/or scientific judgement is made within the population as to what the optimal normal distribution should be. Obviously the factors influencing these measures are far more to do with the overall 'care', whether provided by the parents, environment, political situation, etc. than by the health professionals.

Targets

As well as measuring 'outcomes' it is possible to set specific target to be achieved by health service interventions. Such targets have to be based on available information; be realistic; have a specified time period within which they should be achieved; and have a specific measurable ambition. Targets, by necessity, need to be set for individual populations but below are a few examples from one health district (total population 550 000) in England. Over one year aims were

(1) to achieve and maintain breast-feeding rates at two weeks, eight weeks,and eight months at 75, 60, and 30 per cent respectively;

(2) to achieve a five per cent fall in attendances of children at local accident and emergency departments;

(3) to decrease smoking amongst 15-year-old children from the present level of 21 per cent to 19 per cent.

Conclusion

Trying to develop reliable measurements in the field of child health is essential (Dunnel 1990). Although our ability to actually produce such measurements and to understand their significance is still developing, the fact that they are not yet perfect should not deter us. It should rather encourage us to use what is available to develop more sophisticated indices. The ideal should not stand in the way of the merely good.

References

British Paediatric Association (1989). *Measurement of child health*. Report of a Working Party of the Executive Committee of the Community Paediatric Group. Available from the British Paediatric Association, 5 St Andrews Place, London NW1 4LB.

British Paediatric Association (1990). Report of the outcome measure Working Party of the British Paediatric Association Health Services Committee, British Paediatric Association, London.

de Mare, J. et al. (1990). *Objective, principles and outcome measures in preventive child health care for children from 0–4 years*. Report to the Dutch Working Party on preventive child health care, WP010UK. Utrecht.

Department of Health (1991). *The health and the nation: a consultative document for the health of England*. HMSO, London.

Dunnel, K. (1990). Monitoring children's health. *Population Trends* **60**, 16–22. HMSO, London.

Kaplan, R.M. and Anderson, J.P. (1990). The general health policy model: an integrated approach. In *Quality of life assessments in clinical trials*, (ed. B. Spiker). Raven, New York.

Kohler, L. and Jakobsson, G. (1991). *Children's health in Sweden*, an overview of the 1991 Public Health Report; Socialstyrelsen. The National Board of Health and Welfare, Stockholm. (Available from Allmanna Forlaget, Kundtjanst, S-106 47 Stockholm, Sweden.)

Logan, S. (1991). Outcome measures in child health. *Archives of Disease of Childhood* **66**, 745–8.

OPCS (Office of Population Censuses and Surveys) (1991*a*). Document DH3 91/2. OPCS. HMSO, London.

OPCS (Office of Population Censuses and Surveys) (1991*b*). Document DH4 91\5. OPCS. HMSO, London.

SOED (1973). *The Shorter Oxford English Dictionary*. Oxford University Press.

Werner, E. (1989). Protective factors and individual resilience. In *Handbook of early intervention*. Cambridge University Press.

Welsh Office (1991). Protocol for investment in health gain; maternal and early child health. Welsh Office Planning Forum, Welsh Office, Cardiff.

Wigfield, R., Flaming, P., Beny, P., Rudd, P., Golding, J. *et al* (1992). Can the fall in Avon's sudden infant death rate be explained by changes in sleeping position? *British Medical Journal* **304**, 282–3

Yankauer, A. (1973). Child health supervision—is it worth it? *Paediatrics* **52**, 272–9.

30 Implementing immunization programmes
Stuart Logan and Helen Bedford

Introduction

There has been a dramatic decline in the morbidity and mortality associated with infectious diseases in the richer countries of the world. In the UK, infectious disease was the third most common cause of death in childhood in 1920, the fourth most common in 1955, and is now the sixth. Much of this decline preceded the availability of either therapeutic or preventive measures and was the result of improvements in standards of living and of public health measures such as provision of safe water and efficient sanitation. The introduction of safe and effective vaccines has, however, played an important role.

Polio, diphtheria, and tetanus have virtually disappeared from Europe and the other preventable diseases have declined in importance. None the less, our inability to achieve sufficiently high rates of immunization means that pertussis and measles remain important causes of morbidity in childhood in England and Wales and are still responsible for a few deaths every year; between one and five children die each year from pertussis and in the decade 1980–89, 126 children died from measles. In the Third World, widespread poverty and low immunization coverage result in a huge and continuing burden of mortality and morbidity from preventable diseases: measles alone is said to kill one and a half million children per year in the world.

Although much remains to be done, immunization has been one of the great public health successes of the last 20 years. Since the inception of Expanded Programme on Immunization (EPI) by the World Health Organization (WHO) in 1974, it is estimated that the proportion of children in the developing world who are being reached by a protective course of immunization in the first year of life has risen from five to 80 per cent. The global eradication of poliomyelitis and elimination of neonatal tetanus have become realistic goals. In 1984 the WHO Regional Committee for Europe adopted, as one of its 'health for all' targets, that there should be no indigenous measles, poliomyelitis, neonatal tetanus, congenital rubella, diphtheria, congenital syphilis, or indigenous malaria by the year 2000. With wholehearted and sustained effort all of these targets are within our grasp.

Theoretical considerations

Immunization protects the individual against infection but also has effects on the dynamics of the spread of disease within the community. As the proportion of susceptible individuals falls the circulation of the wild organism in the community slows. When the proportion drops below a level determined by the characteristics of the specific infection and of the population, circulation may cease and the organism disappear from the community even though many individual remain susceptible. Indigenous polio virus, for instance, has disappeared from most of Europe, in spite of vaccine coverage rates that are often below 90 per cent. It is important to recognize, however, that the unimmunized remain at risk of disease from imported infection. In 1978 an outbreak of polio in Netherlands was reported in a religious group who had low immunization uptake and in 1978/88 a small outbreak occurred in Spain in children of low socio-economic class, mainly gypsies, who had very low uptake rates. This emphasizes the danger of complacency in the face of high coverage rates in the general population and the importance of reaching all social groups.

In some circumstances the effects on the spread of the infection may lead to the paradoxical situation in which immunization, while of benefit to the individual, may actually increase the burden of disease in the community. For example, complications associated with measles infection are most common in the very young and in older children and adults: low rates of measles immunization may lead to an increase in the peak age of incidence thus increasing the total number of individuals with severe disease. Similarly, low rates of rubella immunization in childhood may slow the circulation of wild virus, leading to a delay in acquiring the infection until the child-bearing years, and thus to an increase in the number of congenitally infected children. This is not an argument against immunization but rather a further reason to ensure high levels of coverage at the earliest possible age. The minimum level of immunization uptake for each disease which will prevent these effects can be estimated by the use of mathematical modelling. It has been calculated that for the UK it will be necessary to achieve coverage rates of rubella vaccine in infancy of at least 60–70 per cent to ensure that the community as a whole benefits from the vaccine (Nokes and Anderson 1988).

It is important to acknowledge that, in the face of very high vaccine coverage rates, the risk associated with acquisition of infection may, theoretically, be outweighed by the risks associated with the vaccine; in this case immunization will be of benefit to the community but not to the individual. With the increase in movement across borders, however, even in countries with very high uptake rates, the risk to unimmunized individuals probably continues to outweigh the very small risks associated with immunizations.

Immunization and infection in Europe

The WHO European Region comprises 31 members, including the Scandinavian countries, members of the European Community, the former USSR, and the countries of Eastern Europe. There is, unfortunately, no common policy throughout all of them on which vaccines should be used nor when to give them. All member states use vaccines against diphtheria, poliomyelitis (either oral polio vaccine (OPV) or inactivated polio vaccine (IPV)), tetanus, and measles; virtually all immunize against pertussis, and 17 continue to use BCG. Eighteen countries have now introduced combined measles, mumps, and rubella (MMR) vaccine and most of the rest offer measles vaccine. By 1990, three countries, Finland, Germany, and Iceland, had introduced *Haemophilus influenzae* b (Hib) vaccine.

Immunization coverage is generally high in the European region. By 1988, coverage of diphtheria and tetanus toxoids was over 80 per cent in all countries except Ireland and some parts of the former USSR, and of polio, was over 80 per cent in all but four—Ireland, Spain, Turkey, and the former USSR. Rates of coverage of pertussis and measles vaccines were much lower, with a number of countries reporting less than 80 per cent uptake. The result of these efforts has been that the incidence of all of the immunizable disease has declined in the region and eradication of some is a reality.

Poliomyelitis

The progress a country has made towards polio eradication is classified into three stages by WHO. Stage A is classified as high immunization uptake and no indigenous cases of polio associated with wild virus infection in the last three years; stage B, immunization coverage over 80 per cent and less than 10 indigenous cases per year in the last three years; and stage C, more than 10 indigenous cases per year. In 1989 23 European region countries were in stage A, six in stage B, and only two, the USSR and Turkey, were in stage C. The morbidity from polio has been declining since 1974 (Fig. 30.1), reaching a nadir of 134 cases in 1989 but rising to 350 cases in 1990 (figures from 1990 are preliminary). Well over 90 per cent of the indigenous cases in this period were reported from either the former USSR or Turkey (Oblapenko 1991).

During 1990, 15 vaccine-associated cases of polio were reported in the region (Oblapenko 1991). Most countries in the region use oral polio vaccine (OPV) but some use inactivated polio vaccine (IPV) to avoid the possibility of vaccine-associated cases. However, although both vaccines are effective, OPV is thought to have advantages in the struggle to eradicate wild virus from the community. There is now considerable discussion in many countries which have reached stage A about combining OPV and IPV in the routine immunization schedules, a policy already adopted by Denmark. This policy retains the advantages of OPV while successfully preventing vaccine-associated disease: the major problems are cost and the need for an extra injection although this could be avoided by the use of combined IPV and diphtheria, tetanus, and pertussis vaccine (DTP) in a single injection.

Tetanus

The incidence of tetanus in Europe has declined sharply (Fig. 30.2) and the majority of cases now occur in adults, with the highest rates being found in

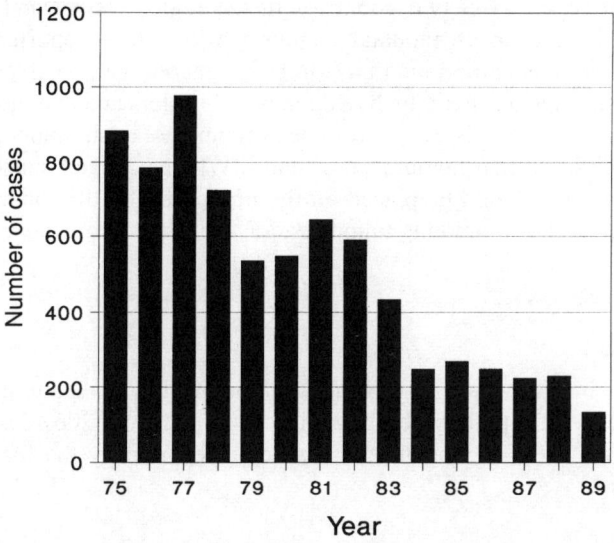

Fig. 30.1 Number of reported polio cases in Europe. (Source: WHO 1990*a*.)

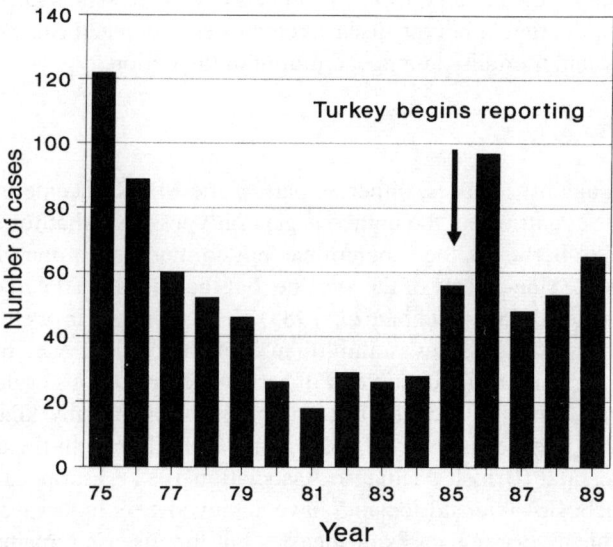

Fig. 30.2 Number of neonatal tetanus cases in Europe. (Source: WHO 1990*b*.)

southern Europe. In 1989 two countries in the region, Israel and Romania, reported one case each of neonatal tetanus while Turkey reported 69 cases (WHO 1990*a*). It is important that adults be encouraged to maintain their immunity against tetanus toxin by having regular boosters and that those in older age groups, who are less likely to have been immunized in childhood, should be encouraged to check their immunization status. Where neonatal tetanus remains common, emphasis should be placed on the immunization of women of child-bearing age as well as promoting immunization of infants to prevent problems in the future.

Diphtheria

The generally high coverage of diphtheria immunization has led to the reported annual incidence of diphtheria in the region declining from 2067 cases in 1974 to 889 cases in 1988, 873 of these cases being reported by the former USSR (WHO 1990*a*).

Pertussis

A few countries, including Czechoslovakia, Hungary, and Switzerland have virtually eradicated pertussis by achieving high rates of coverage of pertussis vaccine. Most countries have had difficulty in achieving high uptake as a result of concerns among both parents and professionals about vaccine safety. The evidence suggests that these concerns are misplaced; serious side-effects are extremely uncommon and the benefit of immunization enormously outweighs the risk of side-effects (Cherry 1990). Eradication of pertussis is not one of the WHO goals for the region but the disease remains common and causes considerable morbidity and mortality amongst children in the region.

Measles

Immunization against measles, either as part of the MMR vaccine or alone, is offered in most countries but the uptake is generally less than that for most other vaccines. Unlike pertussis, the problem has not so much been one of concerns about the possible side-effects of the vaccine, but the widespread perception that measles is a mild disease (Blair *et al*. 1985). It is true that in well nourished populations measles is less devastating than in malnourished ones but even in rich countries it carries a significant risk of serious complications or death. It has been estimated in the UK that the rate of complications of any kind amongst notified cases of measles is 1 to 10, while 1 in 70 children with the disease are admitted to hospital (British Paediatric Association 1991). European countries, including Czechoslovakia and Iceland, have achieved very high vaccine coverage and now have very few cases of measles but the disease remains common across most of the region.

Measles is a highly infectious disease and eradication will require extremely high coverage with a very effective vaccine. The experience from the USA, which has very good coverage of measles vaccine at school entry, suggests that outbreaks of the disease can still be expected from time to time as susceptibles who either avoided immunization or failed to seroconvert accumulate, especially if they are concentrated in geographical areas or social groups. The most hopeful sign is that in most European countries which have introduced MMR this has led to an increase over the previous coverage rates for measles immunization.

Rubella

Rubella is of considerable theoretical interest as it is a mild disease whose peak age of incidence in the unvaccinated population is in early childhood and is of importance only when contracted during the first 18 weeks of pregnancy, facts which must be considered when designing immunization strategies. There are three possible strategies, each used in some countries in the region: to immunize schoolgirls, hoping that most will acquire will virus infection before this time and that the immunization will mop up those who remain susceptible; to immunize all children at around 12 to 18 months hoping to interrupt spread of the wild virus, protecting the unimmunized as well; or to combine infant and schoolgirl immunization, the most effective method. The second option may result in the slowing of wild virus circulation, raising the peak age of incidence and thus leading to more cases of congenital rubella syndrome (CRS). The likely increase in cross-border movements of people in Europe means that the lack of a common approach to the prevention of CRS may lead to complex changes in the patterns of rubella infection. These changes might potentially lead to either an overall increase in CRS or to swings in incidence over time. These effects are difficult to predict using mathematical models as they are crucially dependent on the degree of mixing that occurs as well as the coverage of rubella immunization at different ages in different countries.

The coverage of rubella vaccine at the different ages varies greatly from country to country. We have only limited data as to the effects of these programmes, as rubella is notifiable in only 24 countries and CRS in only 13. In the UK, which does have a good system for the notification of CRS, it is encouraging to note that with reasonably good coverage of schoolgirl vaccination, the rates of CRS and rubella-associated terminations is now low (Miller *et al*. 1991). The addition of universal immunisation in childhood in 1988 is already having impact on reducing reports of rubella infection; although rubella was not a notifiable disease before the introduction of MMR, other schemes already show a significant decline in rubella reports (Miller *et al*. 1991).

The measurement of immunization coverage and the incidence of infection

In the preceding section we have discussed immunization rates as report to WHO: it must be recognized that these reported rates may not be strictly comparable nor completely accurate. The methods of estimating immunization coverage vary from country to country. Ideally, coverage figures should be based on cohorts of children in whom the record of immunization can accurately be linked to the denominator. Few countries approach this ideal: even where this approach is attempted, as in the UK, there are frequently serious doubts about the quality of both the numerator and denominator data. For instance, a recent national study of immunization in two-year-olds found that up to 20 per cent of the children were not recorded on the district immunization record system (Peckham *et al.* 1989). In some countries the numerator for estimating immunization coverage is based on counting the number of doses of vaccine distributed, a method which is inherently imprecise and cannot provide good estimates of coverage in different areas.

Estimates of the incidence of infection are even less accurate and even more difficult to compare. For a disease to be notified, it must be correctly diagnosed, the practitioner convinced that notification is worthwhile, and an effective system must exist for registering the notifications. Not surprisingly, even within countries, there are large differences between diseases and between areas in the proportion of incident cases notified. For more serious diseases this proportion is generally high: it is believed that virtually all cases of poliomyelitis in most European countries are notified although if eradication is to be achieved the system of notification and investigation needs to be strengthened even further. For the less serious disease such as measles and pertussis, the proportion of cases notified is generally low. In the UK it has been estimated that only about 25 per cent of pertussis cases are notified (Clarkson and Fine 1985).

These differences make it difficult to compare countries across Europe. In a recent paper Galazka (1991) summarized the present situation with regard to pertussis control. He clearly showed that countries with very similar reported immunization coverage have widely varying rates of pertussis notifications. Although it is possible that this reflects real differences in the patterns of infection, it seems more likely that this is an artefact due to variations in reporting. There are also problems in comparing different areas in the same country: a district which has high immunization coverage may, paradoxically, have high disease notification rates because the enthusiasm of the local health care workers leads to a high proportion of cases being diagnosed and notified.

If we are to move from disease control to disease eradication then these data systems will have to improve. This is particularly important when cases reach very low levels and it becomes essential to record and investigate each case. For poliomyelitis it is now recommended by WHO that every case of acute flaccid paralysis in childhood should be investigated for the possibility of polio. Fortunately, governments across Europe are now recognizing the need for better information and the quality of the data is generally improving, although much remains to be done.

Factors influencing immunization uptake

Compulsory immunization and immunization linked to school entry

In some countries immunization is either compulsory in the absence of valid contraindications or required before admission to school or nursery. All provide an option for parents with specific objections to refuse immunization for their children. Not surprisingly, the level of uptake in these countries is high. Interestingly, however, in France the uptake of diphtheria, pertussis, and polio, which are compulsory, is high while the uptake of measles, which is recommended but not compulsory, is less than 60 per cent (Williams 1990).

In the United States proof of immunity is required before school entry, and vaccine coverage at school age is very high (95 per cent). In the early 1980s, largely as a result of this policy, measles notifications fell dramatically with only 1500 in 1983. However, in 1989 and 1990 there has been a marked increase in measles cases, with almost a half occuring in unvaccinated pre-school children. The principal cause for the epidemic is failure to immunize pre-school children, particularly in deprived inner city areas such as New York where coverage at two years of age is as low as 50 per cent (Hinman 1991). This demonstrates the importance of immunizing children as early as possible; school entry legislation ensures a highly immunized school population but it may result in delay in obtaining protection.

In other countries without such policies, the level of vaccine uptake in a community is determined by a complex interaction between parental attitudes, social factors, and service provision.

Parents' perceptions

Factors which may influence a parent in the decision to immunize their child have been described in Becker's 'health belief model' (1974). These include perceptions of the infectivity and severity of the disease and the safety and efficacy of the vaccines. Studies in the UK have found these factors to be significantly associated with vaccine uptake (Peckham *et al.* 1989). It is, however, clear that this model is at best only a partial explanation of parental actions: families act within a social context and their beliefs and actions are influenced by objective conditions as well as by professionals, the media, and family and friends.

Social factors

In the UK, socially deprived districts, particularly inner city areas, generally have the lowest vaccine coverage (Begg and White 1988). Many studies have shown that people from lower socio-economic groups and marginalized sections of society are less likely to use preventive services of all kinds (Rosenstock 1986). It has been suggested that this is because lower status groups accord greater priority to immediate rewards than to long-term goals (Simmons 1958): a more plausible explanation is that the demands made on them by everyday life are such that activities which do not contribute to some immediate need must necessarily be accorded a lower priority. This explanation would be consistent with the finding by Peckham *et al.* (1989) that factors such as social class, family size, and the presence of a chronically ill child in the family continued to have significant effects on the probability of immunization even after taking account of parental attitudes.

The importance of social influences is demonstrated by the fluctuations in uptake of pertussis vaccine. In spite of a paucity of evidence, some consider this vaccine to be associated with an increased risk of brain damage. During the 1970s in the UK a great deal of media attention was devoted to supposed dangers of the vaccine, and pertussis uptake rates in 1978 fell to 30 per cent. A combination of diminished attention from the media, an increase in the incidence of the disease leading to greater awareness of the potential hazards, and sustained attempts by professionals eventually overcame much of the opposition and the rates have risen substantially, although they still remain below target levels.

Health professionals

One of the strongest factors found to influence vaccine uptake is health professionals' knowledge of contraindications to immunization; a number of studies have shown that many health care workers advise against immunization on the grounds of spurious contraindications (Hull 1981; Wilkinson 1986; Peckham *et al.* 1989) and this has been shown to have a detrimental effect on vaccine uptake (Peckham *et al.* 1989). This not only leads to children being unnecessarily deprived of protection but can also result in parents receiving conflicting advice, the consequences of which may be a loss of faith in health professionals and the service generally.

Organization of services

Whether or not families have their children immunized is a result of an interaction between the strength of their beliefs as to the importance of immunization and the 'costs' of immunization. These costs may include both financial costs, although free immunization is available for virtually all children in Europe, and the difficulties involved in obtaining immunization. Impressive improvements in immunization coverage have been achieved in general practices in the UK that are committed to providing a flexible service and immunizing all the babies in their practice (James *et al.* 1986; Ross 1986).

Strategies for improving immunization programmes

Immunization is one of the few medical interventions whose benefits unequivocally outweigh its costs. It can be argued that if we do not make every effort to ensure that all children are immunized, we are denying them one of their basic rights.

Promotion of immunization

Immunization programmes are in danger of becoming a victim of their own success: as the diseases they prevent become less prevalent, both professionals and parents are less likely to be aware of the potential dangers of infection and more inclined to focus on the rare side-effects of immunization. Those responsible for immunization programmes must be aware of the need for social mobilization to achieve and maintain the high levels of coverage required for disease elimination. Parental refusal is a relatively uncommon reason for missed immunization but there is a difference between passive acceptance and the positive demand for the service which we should encourage.

Campaigns should be carefully planned so that they reach all the target groups, including health professionals as well as parents. Imaginative use of different vehicles for health education is important if we are to convince members of disadvantaged groups who are otherwise least likely to be protected. In addition to nationally run campaigns, much can be achieved through local initiatives involving community or religious leaders and making use of the media and local organizations.

Organization of services

Convincing parents of the importance of immunization is only one component in the creation of an effective programme. Even the most enthusiastic parent will find it difficult to obtain protection for their child if immunization services are inflexible and the providers are unenthusiastic or poorly informed. Auditors of the service must consider whether immunization is available in accessible places at convenient times, and decisions about such practicalities should be made following consultation with service users. Where possible, immunization services should be part of the primary health care system.

Opportunistic immunization is an important approach in the provision of a flexible service. Health care workers in a variety of setting such as clinics, surgeries, hospitals, and schools should use every contact with children as an opportunity to review their immunization status and if necessary offer protection (Peckham *et al.* 1989). Similarly, the provision of domiciliary immunization may be important for some vulnerable groups who, for a variety of reasons, have difficulty in attending clinic or surgeries (Jones 1984).

A greater involvement by community nurses in administering immunization increases the feasibility of providing both opportunistic and domiciliary services. In the UK an increasing number of health authorities are providing the appropriate training and encouraging nurses to adopt this role (Jefferson *et al.* 1987).

Health professionals

Programme managers must ensure that all health workers involved in immunization have access to clear guidelines on immunization policies, procedures, and contraindications and that staff training is provided on a regular basis. Ultimately the success or failure of an immunization programme depends on the skill and enthusiasm of the people who work in the service. Time spent on staff training and motivation is never wasted. It is also useful for health professionals to have a readily available source of expect advice if they have uncertainties about immunization for a particular child (Hall and Williams 1988).

Computer systems and records

A reason often advanced by health professionals for not making use of contacts with children to check immunization status is that the appropriate records are not available when they see the child. One method of overcoming this problem is to give parents their children's main health record or at least to provide each child with an immunization card. These practices are becoming more common in Europe. It has been reported that parent-held records enable parents to feel more in control of their children's health and that parents are less likely to lose notes than either hospitals or clinics (Saffin and Macfarlane 1991). They have also been shown to lead to increased uptake of immunization and child health surveillance (Polnay and Roberts 1989).

The accuracy of record keeping in a district is crucial for evaluation of vaccine coverage. Most districts in the UK now use computerized information systems (Nicoll *et al.* 1989), but these are only valuable if the database is accurate. Increasing social mobility between districts results in rapidly changing child registers and it is important that there are effective channels for communicating information about such movements and the immunization administered. Much of this information will be notified manually, although many clinics and surgeries now have direct on-line links with the district computer.

Monitoring vaccine coverage and disease incidence

Vaccine coverage and disease incidence should ideally be determined at both a national and a local level. Feeding the local immunization coverage figures back to those responsible is a useful way of encouraging better performance, provided that this is done in a cooperative rather than in a threatening context (Nicoll *et al.* 1989). Even where the overall coverage is high it is necessary to ensure that pockets of low coverage do not occur. Any unusual increase in incidence or clusters of cases should trigger an investigation. For those diseases such as neonatal tetanus and poliomyelitis where we are close to achieving elimination, any suspected case must be thoroughly investigated. To facilitate this, each country must develop and disseminate protocols which explain the system of notification and what samples should be collected, they should ensure that appropriate laboratory facilities exist.

Audit of immunization services

Continual evaluation is an important component of any immunization programme. An effective programme requires that parents want to have their children immunized, that an effective vaccine is available, and that potential barriers to immunization are minimized. Immunization programme managers should conduct regular audits of their system which examine all three aspects as well as collecting data on vaccine coverage and disease incidence.

The audit must also address practical considerations such as the supply of vaccine and adequacy of the vaccine 'cold chain'. Computer software developed by WHO to assist with the assessment of the cold chain has been shown to be effective in identifying subtle deficiencies in the system and should be more widely used.

Managers must regularly review their programmes to identify possible barriers to immunization. In part, this should consist of going through a checklist which would include many of the items discussed above, including the level of staff commitment and training, the existence of up-to-date guidelines, the accessibility of clinics and the availability of effective vaccines, and consideration of any structural barriers such as financial costs associated with immunization. It is also important to undertake periodic investigations of the reasons why parents have not had their children immunized so that any deficiencies in the system can be addressed.

The future

Over the next few years the challenge is to eradicate poliomyelitis, measles, and hopefully, pertussis and to eliminate neonatal tetanus and diphtheria from Europe. Thereafter it will be to maintain the necessary high levels of vaccine coverage while public perception of the threat of these diseases diminishes. Part of our task will be to develop common approaches to immunization to cope with the trend towards increasing migration and European integration and to establish reliable methods of disease surveillance across the region.

Some countries have already introduced Hib and hepatitis B vaccines or plan to do so and the rest will need to consider whether to follow suit. It is likely that in the near future we will also be called upon to consider the introduction of varicella vaccine and probably others not yet in production. The introduction of any new vaccine must be preceded by careful cost–benefit analyses which take account of the effects on the individual and on populations. The temptation to introduce a vaccine simply because it is available must be resisted.

Finally we will need to take account of changing patterns of disease in the region when developing strategies. In particular, the spread of HIV infection may change the pattern of other infectious disease, especially tuberculosis.

References

Becker, M.H. (1974). The health belief model and sick role behaviour. *Health Education Monographs* **2**, 409–19.
Begg, N.T. and White, J.M. (1988). A survey of pre-school vaccination programmes in England and Wales. *Community Medicine* **10**, 344–50.
Blair, S., Share, N., and McKay, J. (1985). Measles matters, but do parents know? *British Medical Journal* **290**, 623–4.
British Paediatric Association (1991). *Manual on infections and immunizations in children*, (ed. P. Rudd and A. Nicoll). Oxford University Press, Oxford.
Cherry, J.D. (1990). 'Pertussis vaccine encephalopathy': it is time to recognise it as the myth that it is. *The Journal of the American Medical Association* **263**, 1679–80.
Clarkson, J.A. and Fine, P.E.M. (1985). The efficiency of measles and pertussis notification in England and Wales. *International Journal of Epidemiology* **14**, 153–69.
Galazka, A. (1991). Pertussis control in the Europe region. *World Immunization News* **7**, 27–9.
Hall, R. and Williams, A. (1988). Special advisory service for immunisation. *Archives of Disease in Childhood* **63**, 1498–500.
Hinman, A.R. (1991). What will it take to fully protect all American children with vaccines? *American Journal of Diseases of Children* **145**, 559–62.
Hull, D. (1981). Interpretation of the contraindications to whooping cough vaccine. *British Medical Journal* **283**, 1231–3
James, J., Clark, C. and Rossdale, M. (1986) Improving health care delivery in an inner-city well baby clinic. *Archives of Disease in Childhood* **61**, 630.
Jefferson, N., Sleight, G., and Macfarlane, A. (1987). Immunisation of children without a doctor present. *British Medical Journal* **294**, 423–4.
Jones, A.E. (1984). Domiciliary immunisation for pre-school child defaulters. *British Medical Journal* **289**, 1429–31.
Miller, E., Waight, P.A., Vurdien, J.E., White, J.M., Jones, G., Miller, B.H.R., *et al.* (1991). Rubella surveillance to December 1990: a joint report from the PHLS and

National Congenital Rubella Surveillance Programme. *Communicable Disease Report* **1**, R33–7

Nicoll, A., Elliman, D., and Begg, N.T. (1989). Immunisation: causes of failure and strategies and tactics for success. *British Medical Journal* **299**, 808–12.

Nokes, D.J. and Anderson, R.M. (1988). The use of mathematical models in the epidemiological study of infectious diseases and in the design of mass immunization programmes. *Epidemiology and Infection* **101**, 1–20.

Oblapenko, G. (1991). Elimination of poliomyelitis in Europe: activities in 1989–90 towards polio zero, ICP/EPI 027/6 WHO, Copenhagen.

Peckham, C., Bedford, H., Senturia, Y., and Ades, A. (1989). *National Immunisation study: factors influencing immunisation uptake in childhood*. Action Research, Horsham.

Polnay, L. and Roberts, H. (1989). Evaluation of an easy to read parent-held information and record booklet of child health. *Children and Society* **3**, 255–60.

Rosenstock, R.M. (1986). Why people use health services. *Millbank Memorial Fund Quarterly* **44**, 94–127.

Ross, S.K. (1986). Childhood immunoprophylaxis: achievements in a Glasgow practice. *Health Bulletin* **44**, 370–3.

Saffin, K. and MacFarlane, A. (1991). How well are parent held records kept and completed? *British Journal of General Practice* **41**, 249–51.

Simmons, O.G. (1958). *Social status and public health*, Pamphlet Number 13, Social Science Research Council. SSRC, New York.

WHO (World Health Organization) (1990*a*). *Expanded programme on immunization—Progress report*, EUR/RC40/12. WHO, Genera.

WHO (World Health Organization) (1990*b*). *Expanded programme on immunization: information system summary for the WHO European Region*, WHO/EPI/CEIS/90.2 EU. WHO, Copenhagen.

Wilkinson, J.R. (1986). Measles immunisation—contraindications perceived by general practitioners in one health district. *Public Health* **100**, 144–8.

Williams, B.C. (1990). Immunization coverage among preschool children: the United States and selected European countries. *Pediatrics* **86**, 1052–6.

31 Child health promotion in Europe
Concha Colomer

'Man cannot hope to find another paradise on earth, because paradise is a static concept whereas life is a dynamic process.
.... growing in the midst of danger is the fate of mankind.'

Rene Dubos

The emergence of health promotion

In recent years we have been in the process of witnessing, on a worldwide scale, new approaches towards the issues of health, illness, the determinants of both these processes, and strategies to promote the former and prevent the latter. In the 60s there were great developments in health services with an increase in resources destined for them, something which will probably go down in history as unique. However, both scientific and technological advances in that era, as well as development in services and investment in resources, were almost exclusively confined to the diagnosis and treatment of illnesses.

When the world economic crisis began in the 1970s, with hindsight it seems inevitable to reflect upon the cost and effectiveness of paying so much attention to illness. Thus appear the works of McKeown,[1] Illish,[2] and Cochrane,[3] developing hypotheses which question the possible positive role of medicine in the state of population's health. McKeown suggests that the improvements in the health of the inhabitants of England and Wales from the eighteenth century onwards is owed more to the effects of improved environmental factors (nutrition and hygiene) and to the changes in certain types of behaviour (fall in birth rate) than to the contributions of scientific medicine.

At the same time, it is also apparent that the pattern of illness and death in industrialized countries' populations in the last few decades of the twentieth century is unlike that which has been observed previously. Accidents, cancer, chronic illness, and psychosomatic illness are presently the issues which concern professionals and the population as a whole.

In this atmosphere of crisis of the paradigms of prevailing services, and based on the emergence of new ideas, the Canadian health minister, Lalonde, in 1974, proposed a framework strategy for health promotion and illness prevention among Canadian people.[4] The Lalonde report has been—and still is—one of the most influential governmental documents on health policy in the modern world ever published. Its importance emerges basically from the recognition that the determinants of health are numerous and diverse ('health field concept'). Apart from the importance of the organization and the quality of medical care, hereditary factors (human biology), lifestyles, and environmental factors play important roles in the making and promotion of health. This report created the basis for what is now known as the 'new public health', placing emphasis on action for the environment and understanding it not only as physical, but psychological and social at the same time. In it, the importance that lifestyles have on health and illness is recognized, while at the same time the role of public policy is highlighted, thus avoiding falling into the trap of blaming the victim for his or her poor state of health and/or unhealthy lifestyle.

At the same time, the World Health Organization has played a very important part in the development of healthy public policy since the early 1970s. As a result, in 1977, the World Health Assembly decided that the main social target of governments and the WHO in the coming decades should be the attainment, by all the citizens of the world by the year 2000, of a level of health which would permit them to live a socially and economically productive life. It was agreed to strive for the attainment of each of the goals of *Health for all by the year 2000 (HFA 2000)*.[5] Primary health care was to be a leading principle in this development, and in 1978 a conference was held in Alma-Ata to discuss it.[6] The most important idea present in the Alma-Ata Declaration is that primary health care is not only concerned with health care but also with its surrounding social and economic environment.

The specific problems of the industrialized European countries called for an operational programme which would take into account the problem of inequalities in health (between groups within countries and also between countries themselves). With the first and foremost aim of reducing this inequality, the majority of countries have been developing their own programmes along similar lines over the course of the past few years.

In light of this European regional strategy for *HFA 2000*, WHO developed a 'health promotion' programme which is based on the social concept of health. Now health is defined in more operational terms instead of the classic WHO definition of 'complete physical, mental and social wellbeing'. Health is now treated as 'the capacity by which the individual or group is able to realize his aspirations or satisfy his needs, and at the same time is also capable of changing or coping with the environment in which he lives'.[7] The focal point is on health and not illness and also on health as a resource for everyday life, not as an ultimate goal to attain. Health is a social idea with psychological, cultural, economic, political, and biological elements. This concept of health is not new, neither does it emerge from the health service sector. The popular view of health is fundamentally and naturally holistic and seeks improvements in the very community sources that are characterized by their lack of paternalism, their respect for popular knowledge, and for strengthening individual or group capability on a pragmatic level.[8] There are many examples of attempts on the part of the population to win control over their health e.g. feminists, ecologists).

Health promotion has been defined as 'the process of enabling individuals and communities to increase control over health determinants and, thereby, improve their health'.[7] This process uses various complementary approaches such as health education, facilitation, and regulation. Its focus is on advocacy, enabling, and mediation of health; building healthy public policy; creation of supportive environments; strengthening community action; developing personal skills; and reorienting health services.[9]

Children and young people as a focal point

If we refer to children and young people, who are the focus of this chapter, it is apparent that they are populations of special interest for health promotion for a variety of reasons. The classic and most referred to reason is that 'they are tomorrow's adults' and that their behaviour and attitudes during this period of their lives will determine their state of health in the future. This argument, without being mistaken, is too restrictive and 'selfish' (those who claim this are of course adults) because it forgets, or at least minimizes, the most important issue in the spirit of health promotion—i.e. the present, the here and now. That is to say, good health implies good quality of life for children and young people during their childhood and youth, or a time when they should live in the most healthy way possible so that they are able to enjoy life.

In the past 100–150 years a series of changes have taken place in the physical and social aspects of children and adolescents. The socialization of children occurs very early nowadays, and this implies elements which are fundamental for establishing behaviour, such as access to information and subjection to group pressure, which begin to exercise their influence much earlier than before. Schooling from an earlier age and for longer periods, along with intensive television viewing (the adult window of the world) play their role in creating values and attitudes and in the establishment of behaviours.

At the same time, the family, another fundamental element of lifestyles, has changed not only its composition (there are more and more nuclear families and in some European countries a high number of one-parent families) but also in the role of each separate component, mainly the role of the mother, and that of family life in general.

Lifestyles versus individual risk behaviour

The case of AIDS as an example

In recent years, and to a great extent thanks to epidemiology, a whole series of risk factors have been discovered to be linked to the different illnesses which affect today's men and women. Many of these factors are related to certain individual behaviour which has been qualified as risky. In some cases behaviour is discussed which is linked to the so-called 'new' lifestyles and basically refer to sedentariness, the consumption of toxic substances, and in general to the type of activities and relations which are developed or which can be developed in a society like ours which is technological, well communicated, and fundamentally urban. These are also patterns of behaviour known as the 'rich' way of life, although this is not true in many cases.

Some of the risks detected are associated with behaviour which is a deep-rooted, classic element which is often fundamental and peculiar to different cultures. This is the case, for instance, with nutrition, which, because of the risks attached to its different components, has given rise in recent years to recommendations for certain kinds of food or diets which may be healthier than others. In an already difficult situation (i.e. of attempting to promote a change in behaviour of this type), it must be noted that the messages transmitted tend to be paternalistic and often accusatory and on some occasions, even contradictory.

But perhaps the most important fact in this sense has been that related to sexuality and the events which have produced the emergence of AIDS and the spread of this epidemic. More than 10 years ago the Gottlieb *et al.* article[10] was published, through which AIDS was to acquire medical naturalization. Since then, discoveries have been made and numerous measures and debates have taken place which have shocked society as a whole and have obliged all sectors to take part, take sides and act (judges, teachers, doctors, clerics, politicians and so on).[11] After this first decade, one of the great AIDS debates has emerged: that of the spread of the infection by heterosexuals.

For some years it has been accepted that it was possible to contract AIDS from heterosexuals, but up to now attempts to quantify the risk linked to different types of sexual practice have failed (except apparently in case of anal penetration, where the receiver is exposed to a high risk of becoming infected). This, together with the diversity of possibilities of sexual practice, and the frequent combination of these in a sole sexual encounter, makes attempts to classify them somewhat illusory.

For all this, the preferred slogan of the moment is 'safer sex' instead of the too-optimistic 'safe sex' which is beyond our capabilities.

It is this aspect of safety which is the most important when we approach the issue of AIDS from the point of view of health promotion. AIDS is a disease, and the actions developed have been aimed logically at its prevention. But these actions, by their very characteristics, have repercussions on everyone's lifestyle. If we understand and accept that sexual relations, in any of their manifestations, are a fundamental element in the quality of life of young people and adults, information that is given out on this issue and the behaviour and attitudes induced then imply that changes are necessary in the basic elements of interpersonal relations and self-esteem.

Some of the 'safe sex' messages undermine human relations, which are built on a basis of maximum personal security, so that couples dare not share intimacy at all. The underlying theme is distrust of a partner or partners. And this is where the dilemma occurs[12]—'If totally avoiding the small risk of contracting a very serious infection means rejecting a friend, an embrace or the trust in a look, what should the choice be?'.

This is the fundamental question in the process of preventing an illness which has been developing over the past years. An approach which, due to its being based on a biomedical model, is centred on the illness and does not have as its ultimate aim the absence of the illness. Not having health as its aim has brought about a paradoxical situation in which, as a preventive measure, we interfere negatively in the quality of life and health of those on whom a positive action should be proposed. We have seen this in some screening programmes which have been incorrectly set up from the point of view of their suitability, sensitivity and/or specificity, confidentiality in the results, or possibilities of intervention. Too often irreparable damage has been done to the mental health or social acceptability or self-esteem of some people, at worst without even having been of benefit to anyone.

Another example is the anti-smoking campaigns based on preventing lung cancer and founded on the changing of individual behaviour and negative or 'blameful' messages. Amongst the effects achieved by these campaigns are investigation of smoking patterns linked to social characteristic (the poor, the poorly educated, and in some cases women and young people continue to smoke to the same or possibly even greater extent despite the campaigns)[13] and social pressure has attached stigmas to individuals who have not altered their behaviour. In some cases, especially vulnerable and socially sensitive situations have been used, such as pregnancy, in a dramatic way and with a restricted and rigid view of the issue, thus increasing the stress which pregnancy holds for some women, especially those in the lower echelons of society.[14]

There is more and more evidence to show that peoples' feelings, values, and attitudes are the determinants of their behaviour and that a change in the latter will not come about unless accompanied by a change in the former. Besides, certain types of messages, principally ones which are negative, 'blameful', and based on arousing fear, have a limited effect only on that sector of the population with most motivation to change. For the other sectors, the opposite effect occurs, making subsequent messages difficult to get across.[15]

In the case of AIDS prevention, although what has been mentioned above is true, reactions take on a different hue, owing almost definitely to the fact that feelings, values, and attitudes are very specific. In order to illustrate this we can comment on the reaction in the USA to the Surgeon General's annual report on two separate occasions dealing with two separate issues. In 1986 the report recommended the use of a latex condom for each sexual relation among those people whose partners had been exposed to the AIDS virus. Over the following year the sales of this type of condom rose by 20 per cent. On the other hand, the sale of cigarettes, after the publication the following year (1989) of a report on tobacco and health, fell by only 2.4 per cent.[16]

AIDS arouses a series of contradictory feelings and fears which give way to reactions that are difficult to anticipate or control. In the majority of countries and for reasons linked in some way to morals and sex taboos, programmes and activities have been developed with unclear objectives and confused messages which have given rise to certain sections of the population feeling unaffected by the issue. The 'AIDS = male and homosexual' stereotype has been encouraged, although on many occasions unintentionally. But it has meant the loss of prevention opportunities in the rest of the at-risk population i.e. women and heterosexual male.[17]

At the same time the equation 'AIDS prevention = condom use' has also created problems, above all for young people who must accept the message and convert it into behaviour in their everyday lives; lives which are already full of complications as far as their sexuality and interpersonal relationships are concerned. For those young people the issue cannot be simplified in such a way.[18-20]

A good example of this took place in Australia in 1987 with the education campaign on AIDS in the mass media ('The grim reaper').[21] In the evaluation of the results obtained, the campaign considered that it had been successful since the proportion of population who were aware of the risks of AIDS increased significantly—although among the high-risk population the effect was much less significant. However, at the same time it was also seen that a series of unplanned or unwanted effects were produced, due to the use of fear of death by AIDS as the main message of the campaign. Among many people considered to be at low risk the anxiety provoked did not produce the response of a request for more information, as we thought would happen; instead greater numbers of diagnostic tests were carried out and an increase in the discrimination and isolation of HIV-infected people took place. The educators denied that an atmosphere of inhibition and anxiety in people's sex lives has been crated because of the link between sex, AIDS and death, which is easily shortened to 'sex = death'. The campaign was not repeated and at present, work on community involvement and participation in AIDS prevention is going on.

Multiple actions versus health education

People's behaviour, including of course, children and young people, is the result, not only of personal choice, but also of the framework of society, of group pressure, and the conditioning factors of prevailing patterns of thoughts, feelings, and actions. The possibilities of choice are very limited and difficult to determine in individual cases. People establish a behaviourial pattern because it gives them intention. In the majority, influence on health is secondary or collateral. Even for people who state health as among their prized possessions, other values such as prestige and personal and collective recognition, economic success, and emotional satisfaction are often a greater priority in everyday life.[15,22]

The challenge which, at the moment, is set for us by the *Health for all* strategy is how to turn didactic approaches into participative ones and how to transfer them from unisectoral to multisectoral.[23]

In recent years there have, without doubt, been great developments in health education, which have been implemented in schools in all European countries to a greater or lesser extent. All governments, national and regional, have been sensitive to the need for reporting health and how to maintain it (although more often than not, on illness and how to prevent it). But up to now, practically all efforts to promote child health have been dedicated exclusively to health education.

The results of all these programmes and activities for health education in schools have been highly contradictory and have given rise to a method crisis, which has deceived even those who, at first, defended these innovative initiatives. The analysis of these results should take into account the aims of health education, which are to transmit information and create favourable attitudes towards certain healthy behaviour. These aims are within reach of this technique. The problem and the deception have arisen when aims to modify behaviour or even create certain lifestyles have been suggested, based exclusively on didactic methods. This has occurred due to lack of knowledge of factors which intervene in the establishment of lifestyles; maximizing individual values and forgetting the effect that environmental and political aspects have. Obviously these factors do not alter with health education approaches towards children, but they require specific multisectoral action.[24]

At the same time, the same didactic approaches have lacked a fundamental element for their effectiveness, which is the participation of those involved in its definition and execution. It has been shown that the impact of school health education programmes improves when the children themselves are the ones to define the priorities, aims, and methods of the programmes.[25-27]

Another fundamental element necessary for the success of promoting healthy lifestyles is that of not tackling the different aspects which compose it separately (e.g. sexuality, nutrition, exercise, etc.) as if they were divisible parts of everyday life. Given the falsity of this separation, the danger for the results is logical. The most appropriate strategy is one of empowerment of individual values, strengthening the capacity of people so that they are able to face up to situations and to decide freely their best option.

However, decisions in real life are almost never independent, they are interrelated and take into account the assessment of an apparently partial element, the individual and social factors of the environment.[28] In fact, there are examples of health promotion programmes aimed at young people, which have been planned, either specifically for this population group or as part of a more general programme for the population as a whole, which combine the principles of treating health globally with an intersectoral approach, considering the environment, with clear effects on the change of behaviour towards more healthy behaviours.[24,19-31] On the other hand there are also examples that both school education programmes[32-34] as well as publicity campaigns,[35] correct from the technical and methodological point of view, have failed in their aim of modifying behaviours due to their not being designed properly and being carried out without help from the population.

In any case, efforts to promote health should adopt alternative strategies, with aims that assume that experiments and exploration into risky behaviour arise inevitably as part of the normal development of the adolescent. According to Jessor,[28] some of these alternative strategies could include 'minimization' (the aim being to limit involvement in risky behaviour to simple exploration or monitored moderate or responsible levels); 'insulation' (avoiding long-term serious, irreversible, or negative consequences); 'delay the start' (the aim being to postpone the initiation of risky behaviour so that greater maturity and skill has been reached as far as handling risks is concerned).

Evidence exists which seems to indicate that those political measures aimed at creating atmospheres which make certain behaviours considered harmful to health difficult bring about a drop in their practice.[33,36-38] Thus, restrictions and punishments for smoking on school premises at least reduces this practice among young people. The same effect occurs with the ban on selling tobacco to young people, as long as the legislation is enforced.[39]

The 'healthy cities' initiative

In the sense of creating favourable atmospheres for health, reference has to be made to the *healthy cities project*.[40] This movement, which began in Europe in 1986 and to which many cities from all over the world belong, has created the framework for the development of health promotion programmes in children and young people. One of its fundamental principles is the improvement of health among its citizens by means of their own participation in taking decisions. In Seattle (USA), children have had the opportunity to take part in defining their city's problems and finding solutions. After years of experience in participation in municipal affairs, 'The greater Seattle kidsboard'[41] has been created—a children's organization which evaluates the needs of children in the community, develops proposals and programmes to deal with them, and maintains contacts with organizations, institutions, and individuals. The city of Seattle recognizes the contributions children make towards the provision of services and gives them the chance to learn important social and political skills. Experiences of this type demonstrate that children are capable of developing these skills if they are given the opportunity to do so.

Conclusion

In summary, if the aim of promoting health among children and young people is to be achieved, we must apply the principle of health promotion developed in the Ottawa Charter.[42] That is to say, we have to train them, from a very young age, how to look after themselves, how to look after others, and how to participate in their community; help them to develop the skills and values necessary for repairing what does not work for them or in society—let them acquire skills in order to lead a healthy everyday life. For this, school and the family have an important part to play and should work together to design and implement a curriculum which develops in children the skills for taking decisions, facing up to problems (coping), and interaction with the community. The approach of these programmes should be global and integrating in both senses, those of involving all participants (community, parents, teachers, and children) and of treating health and lifestyle as a whole and not only as certain behaviours isolated from one another. The most effective orientation is that aimed at promoting positive and healthy alternative behaviours, not that centred on avoiding those harmful to health.

At the same time the influence of the environment on decision-making and in determining behaviours and lifestyles should not be forgotten. Thus it is advisable that, in order to achieve greater effectiveness, any educational activity should coincide with public policies (school, local, national, and/or international), oriented in such a way that the mass media and other agencies, legislation and the rest of possible environmental measures are able to support the informed choice of the healthiest options.

A clear consequence of these new approaches is that care of the child, in health and in illness, at present includes wider reaching objectives and requires different methods. In order to handle this new situation, professionals need to know the basic aspects and techniques related to lifestyles, the environment, and health. Along with this, they will require personal skills in order to work with professionals from different disciplines, away from the health sector and with the community, acting as catalysts for a change towards health.

References

1. McKeown, T. (1971) *The role of medicine: dream, mirage or nemesis*. Nuffield Provincial Hospitals Trust, London.
2. Illich, I. (1976). *Limits to medicine: medical nemesis, the expropriation of health*. Marion Boars, London.
3. Cochrane, A.L. (1972). *Effectiveness and efficiency*. Nuffield Provincial Hospitals Trust, London.
4. Lalonde, M. (1974). *A new perspective on the health of Canadians*. Department of National Health and Welfare, Ottawa.
5. WHO (1977). World Health Assembly Resolution 30.43: *Health for all by the year 2000*. WHO, Geneva.
6. WHO (1978). *Alma-Ata 1978: primary health care*, Health for all series No 1. WHO, Geneva.
7. WHO (1986). *Health promotion—concept and principles In Action. A policy framework*. WHO, Copenhagen.
8. Levin, L.S. (1987). Health empowerment: an approach to community-controlled self-care development. In *Issues and trends in health*, ed. Rick Carlson and Brooke Newman. CV Mosby, St Louis.

9. Ottawa charter for health promotion (1986). *Health promotion* **1**, iii–v.
10. Gottlieb, M.S., Schroff, R., Schanker, H.M., Weisman, J.D., Fan, P.T., Wolf, R.A. *et al.* (1981). Pneumocystis carinii pneumonia and mucosal candidiasis in previously healthy homosexual men. *New England Journal of Medicine* **305**, 1425–31.
11. Novello, A.C. and Wise, P.H. (1991). Public health issues. In *Paediatrics AIDS*, (ed. Philip A. Pizzo and Catherine M. Wilfart), pp. 745–55 Williams and Wilkins, Baltimore.
12. Segura, A. (1991). SIDA: Tres anecdotas para un aniversario (in Catalan) *Quadern Caps* **15**, 42–44.
13. Silvestre, A., Colomer, C., Nolasco, A., Gonzalez, L., and Alvarez-Dardet, C. (1990). Nivel de renta y estilos de vida: ¿Hacia una ley de prevención inversa?. *Gaceta Sanitaria* **20**, 189–92.
14. Graham, H. (1989). Women and smoking in the UK: The implications for health promotion. *Health Promotion* **4**, 371–82.
15. Research Unit in Health and Behavioural Change (1989). Health related behavioural change. In *Changing the public health*. Wiley, London.
16. Moran, J.S., James, H.R., Peterman, T.A., and Stone, K.M. (1990). Increase in condom sales following AIDS education and publicity, United States. *American Journal of Public Health* **80**, 607–8.
17. AIDS prevention (1990). Facts from the countries. *Hygiene* **9**, 39–43.
18. Wenzel, E. (1990). Health promotion for young people about the prevention and control of HIV transmission and AIDS. *Hygiene* **9**, 13–17.
19. Soskolne, C.L. and Robson, E. (1989). A preventive response to AIDS in a low prevalence region: a multisectoral, multistrategy approach. *Canadian Journal of Public Health* **80**, 319–24.
20. Martin, J. (1990). Les jeunes *et al* 'constellation' des questions suscitées par le SIDA quels thémes aborder? *Hygiene* **9**, 22–4.
21. Winn, M. (1991). The grim reaper: Australia's first mass media AIDS education campaign. In *AIDS prevention through health promotion: Facing sensitive issues*. WHO, Geneva.
22. Hunt, S.M. (1988). Health related behavioural change—a test of a new model. *Psychology and Health* **2**, 209–30.
23. Kickbusch, I. (1981). Involvement in health: a social concept of health education. *International Journal of Health Education* **24**, 4–10.
24. Nutbeam, D. and Catford, J. Welsh heart programme evaluation strategy: progress, plans and possibilities. *Health Promotion* **2**, 5–18.
25. Green, L.W. (1984). Health education models. In *Behavioural health*, (ed. J.D. Matarazzo, S.M. Weiss, J.A. Herd, N.E. Miller, and S.M. Weiss). Wiley, New York.
26. Conell, D.B., Turner, R.R., Mason, E.F. (1985). Summary of findings of the school health education evaluation: health promotion effectiveness, implementation, and costs. *Journal of School Health* **55**, 316–21.
27. Arborelius, E. and Bremberg, S. (1988). 'It is your decision!' Behavioural effects of a student-centred health education model at school for adolescents. *Journal of Adolescence* **11**, 287–97.
28. Jessor, R. (1984). Adolescent development and behavioural health. In *Behavioural health*, (ed. J.D. Matarazzo, S.M. Weiss, J.A. Herd, N.E. Miller and S.M. Weiss). Wiley, New York.

29. Practical program experience from Europe, United States and Australia (1991). In *Youth health promotion: from theory to practice in school and community*, (ed. Don Nutbeam, Bo Haglund, Peter Farley, and Per Tillgren). Forbes, London.
30. Walter, H.J. and Wynder, E.L. (1989). The development, implementation, evaluation and future directions of a chronic disease prevention program for children: the 'know your body' studies. *Preventive Medicine* **18**, 59–71.
31. Bush, P.J., Zuckerman, A.E., Theiss, P.K., Taggart, V.S., Horowitz, C., Sheridan, M.J., and Walter, H.J. (1989). Cardiovascular risk factor prevention in black schoolchildren: two-year results of the 'know your body' program. *American Journal of Epidemiology* **129**, 466–82.
32. Lachapelle, D., Desaulniers, G., and Bujold, N. (1989). Dental health education for adolescents: assessing attitude and knowledge following two educational approaches. *Canadian Journal of Public Health* **80**, 339–44
33. Cleary, P.D., Hitchcock, J.L., Semmer, N., Flinchbaugh, C.J., and Pinneg, J.M. (1988). Adolescent smoking: research and health policy. *Milebank Quarterly* **66**, 137–71.
34. Effectiveness of a health education curriculum for secondary school students—United States, 1986–1989 (1991). *Morbidity and Mortality Weekly Report* (MMWR) **40**, 113–16.
35. Bauman, K.E., LaPrelle, J., Brown, J.D., and Padgett, C.A. (1991). The influence of three mass media campaigns on variables related to adolescent cigarette smoking: results of a field experiment. *American Journal of Public Health* **81**, 597–604.
36. Pierce, J.P., Macaskill, P., and Hill, D. (1990). Long-term effectiveness of mass media led anti-smoking campaigns in Australia. *American Journal of Public Health* **80**, 565–9.
37. Reid, D. (1985). Prevention of smoking among school children: recommendations for a policy development. *Health Education* **44**, 3–12.
38. Porter, A. (1982). Disciplinary attitudes and cigarette smoking: a comparison of two schools. *British Medical Journal* **285**, 1725–6.
39. Altman, D.G., Rasenick-Douss, L., Foster, V., and Tye, J.B. (1991). Sustained effects of an educational program to reduce sales of cigarettes to minors. *American Journal of Public Health* **81**, 891–3.
40. Ashton, J., Gray, P., and Barnard, K. (1986). Healthy cities—WHO's new public health initiative. *Health Promotion* **3**, 319–24.
41. European Case Studies (1992). In *Healthy cities*, (ed. John Ashton. Open University Press, Buckingham.
42. Hart-Zeldin, C., Kalnins, I.V., Pollack, P., and Love, R. (1990). Children in the context of 'Achieving health for all: a framework for health promotion. *Canadian Journal of Public Health* **81**, 196–8.

Further reading

Green, L.W., Kreuter, M.W., Deeds, S.G., and Patridge, K.B. (1980). *Health education planning. A diagnostic approach*. Mayfield, Palo Alto.

Green, L.W. and Kreuter, M.W. (1985). *Measurement and evaluation in health education and health promotion*. Mayfield, Palo Alto.

Ashton, J. and Seymour, H. (1988). *The new public health*. Open University Press, Milton Keynes.
WHO Europe (1990). *The European Network of Health Promoting Schools*. WHO Regional Office for Europe, Copenhagen.
Handbook for a modular course in health promotion and health education (1991). (ed. Lee Bariá). Barus, Altrincham.

PART IX

Exploring solutions and practical positive change

This part explores new approaches and innovations such as community participation and diagnosis and active partnership with parents. The final chapter explores the implications of measuring and enhancing quality of life for children; this is likely to be an essential task for all child health workers in the future with a shift of emphasis from illness and disease to well-being and life quality.

32 Can we create a more optimal hospital environment?

Berlith Persson

The care of children in hospitals has changed remarkably in recent years.[1] When a child is hospitalized, the hospital has to take on tasks beyond those of healing so that the rhythm of life, growing, playing, and learning can go on.[2] As early as the fifties, Bowlby[3] reported on the nature of the child's tie to the mother, and the psychological disturbances a child could suffer due to a separation caused by a stay in hospital.

Parents' unlimited presence throughout all stages of care is, therefore, important, as is the necessity of structured, age-related information prior to investigation and treatment of the child.[4] Many hospitals also have specially trained teachers for 'play therapy'.[5]

What about our youngest patients? There have been dramatic developments, both medical and technical with regard to the caring of the neonate, the result being that more prematurely born and/or very low birth-weight infants now survive. However, there is growing concern for their long-term developmental and behavioural outcome. In addition to medical complications, another increasing area of concern is that regarding iatrogenic effects occurring during the separation of mother and infant,[6,7] in the high technology environment of a hospital with its bright lighting, noise, and hectic activity.

The birth of a premature infant is also known to be a time of stress and crisis for parents, involving feelings of guilt or failure due to the inability to carry the pregnancy to term,[8] problems with breast-feeding,[9] uncertainty about the infant's early health status, and anxieties and fears of parenting the infant at home. Recent studies shows that dramatic improvements are made in the outcome of these infants, when individualized supportive care is provided in the hospital, such as developmental care[10,11] and 'skin-to-skin' care.[12,13,14] This can result in reduction of ventilator use, decreasing the need for incubators, oxygen therapy, and gavage feeding; and increased breast-feeding success.[15] The psychological, clinical, and societal significance of these methods of care cannot be overemphasized.

However, the implementation of these care-giving philosophies demands a restructured environment and improvement in the quality of the methods used for diagnosis, treatment, clinical organization and education, and repeated evaluations.

Local development work

I shall describe an attempt at improvement of the clinical work in this direction. It is a development project from the Paediatric Clinic, Helsingborg, Sweden. The project began on the neonatal ward and has been developed into a model which, with some adjustment, may even suite other types of childrens' wards. The model (Fig. 32.1) is the result of a critical evaluation of care routines and methods.

With the aim of working with the family as an inseparable entity, a series of studies began whose purpose was to understand better childrens' and parents' needs, and to integrate these in the methods and organization of the neonatal ward. Frequent interviews and questionnaires with the families were carried out. The fact that a large number of the staff members were engaged in compiling the questionnaires and/or analysing the results, led to an increased awareness of the questions being asked. This made development and change a necessary outcome of these market researches.

The theme has been: 'The caring chain—the family's journey through the caring process after a premature birth'. What happens? How is it experienced?

Using semi-structured interviews under this heading, families were asked to describe the baby's stay in hospital. The following are some typical accounts from parents of babies with birth-weights below 1500 g, and the use of these descriptions as a base for caring development.

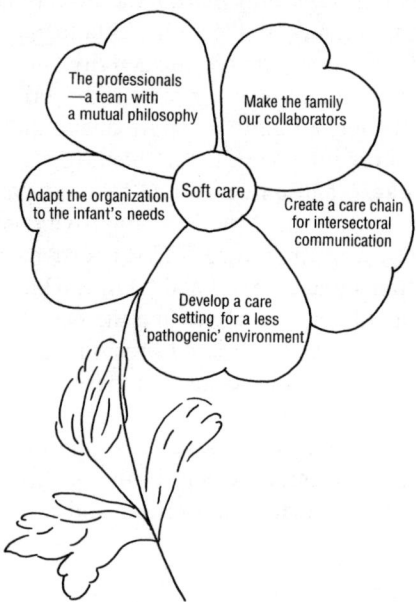

Fig. 32.1 A care model for the neonatal ward.

Prepared during pregnancy?

Our findings:

- Few parents were prepared for the premature birth.
- Doctor/Midwife information was mainly focused on the pregnancy and the delivery.
- To be admitted to hospital for a longer time during the pregnancy created family problems for a lot of the women.

Kristin

When I was admitted for premature labour, it was with mixed feelings. I felt guilty for the family at home, and for my husband's increased responsibility for the other children. At the same time, I was also worried about the baby and what was taking place. I was not much informed about: How small a baby can survive? What are the risks? How will the baby be born? I tried to remember all I had read about premature babies in weekly magazines, but its seems so unreal and I didn't dare to ask.

How was the delivery?

Our findings:

- The delivery was often acute and/or dramatic, with a lot of staff and a lot of technical equipment.
- Parents were disappointed because of 'the delivery one did not get'. For example, the father did not always arrive in time; the baby was quickly taken away.
- The staff's behaviour often created negative feelings regarding the infant's chances of survival.

Maria

I had been a patient on the maternity ward for two weeks when my twin daughters were born in their 27th week. I had been led to understand the risks by my doctor and the nursing staff. I gave birth to them early one morning, and luckily my husband arrived in time. We were by now completely exhausted. When they were born, I neither wanted nor managed to lift myself up to watch while the midwife cut the cord. I just held on to Sten, my husband, and we both cried, convinced that we had lost our babies.

   After a while the door opened, and in walked a doctor. He came towards us with a big smile on his face and said: 'Congratulations on your two mini-girls, 800 g a piece. They look strong and we will now do what we can for them, taking it hour by hour'. These words became a real lifeline. He was the first person who dared to give us a little hope. He was the paediatric doctor. I sat up. I wanted to see them immediately, and make the most of every minute I could as their mother.

Contact with the staff?

Our findings:

- Most parents gave an honest, friendly opinion about the staff, but the majority felt that they were 'so many people'.
- The criticism which arose can be called 'negative professionalism' or lack of empathy.
- On our high-tech wards, there is an image of 'urgency' and 'effectiveness' which can often become an obstacle for good relationship with parents.

Anna

I felt a continual guilt for what I had caused my son; at being born too soon and having to remain in a plastic box, with tubes in his throat, and exposed to painful procedures. When I was able to care for him, it was as if I could not, as I did not know how. It all looked so simple, when the effective nurses cared for him, but when I tried, it all went wrong. My hands were too big, the diaper was not straight, and he just cried. I had the same feeling when I started to breast-feed. I didn't do it. The nurse took my breast and his head, and they did it.

Taking part in the daily care and planning for the infant?

Our findings:

- Early contact between the mother and the baby increased the breast-feeding rate.
- Parents who were active in the caring of the baby at an early stage had less problems after discharge from hospital.
- The staff gave good information regarding changes in the nursing routines, but it was seldom given in advance, so that parents felt that they were participating in the planning stage.

Per

You were all so clever when informing us about why and what you did on the ward. What the cords and tubes were for, how the incubator was adjusted, and all the different routines. Yes I think I could almost work as a childrens' nurse after my 'ten-week introduction-course'.

But when you ask about planning, that was completely taken care of by the doctor and the nurses and we were informed afterwards. I remember, for example, one morning he was taken from his incubator and placed in a bed. We did not arrive that day until the afternoon, and we were so disappointed. My wife had picked out special clothes just for this special occasion and we would like to have taken a photo. At a time like this, we would have liked to have been part of the planning stage.

How did you experience the clinical environment?

Our findings:

- The physical environment was primarily suited to the ward equipment and the staff, and not much to the needs of a family.
- An environment full of technology can create hostile feelings, with a risk of less participation from the parents.

Katrin

The ward frightened me. When I arrived in the corridor I was met by a long row of technical equipment. I found this somewhat contradictory, because they were both life-saving and threatening to my little, little son. I was very tired during the first period after delivery, so I did not manage to visit my child as often as I wanted. It was so hot in the room, the chair by the side of the incubator was uncomfortable, and there was no place to take a rest when I felt dizzy or sad.

Your contact with the baby?

Our findings:

- Early close contact with the child led to an increased presence of the parents.
- The mother's presence and participation in the care of the baby increased her milk production.

Karin

I came to the ward everyday. I opened the incubator and carefully touched her with my finger tops. I was so afraid of disturbing her, she needed all the rest she could get. I was afraid of doing something wrong to the monitors or the tubes, but I was continuously longing to be able to hold her close to me. A longing that was almost painful.

Eva

I never really felt that she was my daughter during the period spent in the incubator. The walls kept us apart. There was one thing during this period which became my life-saving duty, and that was breast-feeding her. No one else could do that for her. I felt a kind of pride, a motherly instinct, when I arrived on the ward with my few drops of milk.

However, the amount of breast milk did not increase, and after some weeks a young nurse said to me: 'You have done very well in producing milk all this time, but it does not appear that it is going to be sufficient. I think you should give it up, it is so difficult for you.' To think that she did not understand, that this was the only thing I could give my daughter for the moment.

The family's reactions?

Our findings:

- Family relationships suffered when a prematurely born child was in the hospital for weeks or months.

Lars

It was a difficult time for all of us. We were torn between home, the hospital, and between our two children. When we came home from a visit, my mother-in-law or some other relation would usually phone, and we had to try to explain what was happening to our son. His older sister was not permitted to visit the ward at that time, and she soon began to protest. There was nothing to keep her occupied in the corridor outside the ward while waiting for her mother. At about this time she began being fussy with the food, and I think it was really the whole family situation which had influenced her.

Lisa

My husband and I were divorced a few months after Jonas was discharged. He was our first child, and we had not known each other for too long. It was such a burden on our relationship, with all those weeks of emotional strain. I lived only for Jonas and for him to survive, and for a long time I did not speak to anyone around me, not even to his father.

After discharge?

Our findings:

- The necessary 'overprotection' on the ward sometimes even continued at home, with worry and apprehension about, for examples, the amount of food to give the child, weight increase and general development.

- Many babies had problems with nourishment, infections, sleep, and general restlessness.

Ann

I had so looked forward to putting on his own clothes, laying him in his own bed, and being a completely normal mother. It was like planning a honeymoon for us. I planned to drive him around the town and show him where he was going to grow up, and delight in the long nightmare being over at last. But it was not so. He screamed, or it appeared so to me, all day long. I was worried about his weight and his poor appetite. I felt suddenly very much alone without all the nurses and doctors around.

Elisabeth:

I studied him carefully everyday. The first period at home I sometimes even counted his respiratory rate, as in the hospital. The anxiety was always there. Was everything as it should be? He was a very restless baby compared to his older sister. He seldom slept deeply. He awoke whimpering after just a few hours sleep. I think it was due to the fact that incubator babies are not left in peace for very long.

There is always so much to do. Suctioning every other hour, naso-gastric feeding according to the schedule, tests, examinations, and so on. He was never allowed to finish his sleep.

A comprehensive care model unfolds

After conducting interviews, dealing with the families process of caring, we began to create a model. (Fig. 32.1)

Using the parents' accounts, the main theme was drawn up.

This took place at both ward and group meetings, and was the beginning of process which was to bring about radical changes in the ward routines.

Soft care—uterus life

The premature baby is born into a world which differs totally from the secure uterus life. The daily pattern, the darkness, and the well-known voices are suddenly replace by the continuous noisy activity of the intensive care ward. Bright lights, sounds from incubators, ventilators and monitors, and all the unfamiliar voices. Investigations and blood tests interrupt the infants' sleep, and food is given at regular times, without any sign of hunger needing to be shown.

Much of the work in an intensive care ward is necessary and lifesaving, but perhaps the medical and technical progress has made us too eager, so we forget the therapeutic value of rest and deep sleep. We must, and we can, create a balance between the medical procedures, and good primary care, by consciously planning our ward routines and training ourselves to be aware of the infants signals of worry, stress, and pain. With the help of a few simple nursing methods, we can create a nursery life which more closely resembles the secure intrauterine life, maybe we can even help to reduce the risk of stress and relationship problems which may occur after the patient's discharge due to the hospital environment that we create.

The infants' right to rest, darkness, closeness, pain relief, and individual care

- The incubators are made cosy by using sheepskins or soft towels, folded, and placed to form a little 'nest'.
- The infant is helped to remain in a flexed, uterus position while being nursed, in order to maintain a neurological balance (Als 1982).
- Incubator tops are covered to protect the baby from bright light, alarms, and telephones ringing. Conversations are kept to a minimum.

- Any manipulation of the deeply sleeping baby is avoided and if he must be woken, this is done by gently holding him, and maintaining the flexed position.

- The staff are trained to continuously observe the baby for signs of stress and restlessness.

- Painful procedures and blood tests are coordinated so as to allow the infant longer periods of uninterrupted sleep. Pain relief and/or sedation should be administered with more complicated procedures, for example, intubation.

- All blood tests, investigations, and treatment which are not acute, are carried out in the mornings, as well as cleaning and other activities of daily living. In the evenings and at night, the light is dimmed, and individual light is used only for those infants requiring intensive care.

- As soon as the baby is healthy enough to be moved around a little, he is removed from the incubator and placed 'skin-to-skin' with the mother's breast for warmth and mutual stimulation. The upright position facilitates the process of breathing and bowel activity, and the skin contact gives both warmth and closeness.

The early contact gives rise to:

- More parental participation in the care of their baby.
- The mothers respond emotionally toward their infants.
- A greater number of infants are entirely breastfed.

Table 32.1 *Age when first taken out of incubator, Weight gain, Days in incubator and hospital and proportion breast-fed at discharge by group status*

Variables	K-group ($n = 33$)		SPC-group ($n = 33$)			
	$\bar{X}$	(SD)	$\bar{X}$	(SD)		
First time out of incubator, age in days	4.36	(4.7)	8.0	(5.9)	$t =$ 2.80	$p = <0.01$
Weight gain per week, (grams)	237.48	(96.4)	195.5	(82.9)	$t =$ 1.90	$p = <0.05$
Days in incubator	20.9	(13.9)	30.5	(15.7)	$t =$ 2.61	$p = <0.05$
Total days in hospital	41.6	(16.9)	49.4	(18.9)	$t =$ 1.76	$p = <0.05$
	n	(%)	n	(%)		
Breast-fed upon discharge frequency	27	(82)	15	(45)		
	$x^2 = 7.92$		$p = 0.005$			

Source: Wahlberg *et al.* (1992).

- The time in the incubator is reduced.
- Earlier discharge.

'Open doors'—to enable us to create a care chain

Every effort should be made to establish an early contact with the future parents so as to inform them about the ward. For example, all pre-natal classes should make a short visit to the neonatal ward and receive the necessary information. Women who are admitted to the maternity ward due to a complication of the pregnancy should be given the opportunity to visit the neonatal ward, or to meet a paediatrician. When the risk of a premature birth is high, the family should be encouraged to meet the staff. Together with the information they receive, and from visiting the ward, the future parents are better able to visualize what may take place.

Eva

When I was lying in the maternity ward with premature labour, there were so many tests and examinations that the baby inside me seemed unreal. It wasn't until I visited the childrens' ward and saw the small ones in the incubators, that the baby became real, and I dared to hope.

The family—our 'collaborators'

Competent, experienced paediatric staff should be present at any high-risk birth in order to determine the infant's condition, and to take the necessary measurements. Every effort should be made not to remove the baby from the room and the parents.

If possible the baby should lie 'skin-to-skin' on the mother for this important first contact (Whitelaw 1990). Warm towels, an infra-red lamp if necessary, and in some cases an incubator placed beside the mother's bed, help to reduce the possibility of heat loss. Heart and respiratory rates, transcutaneous monitoring, etc., may also be checked without separating mother and infant. The father should come with the baby, if it is to be transferred to the intensive care ward, in case the mother is too tired. He is the best contact link until they can meet again.

Per

I still find that I feel something special for Daniel. I was the first to hold him and to carry him to the incubator. When the nurses had taken a polaroid photo of him, I went up to Carina, who had just woken up after the caesarean section in the post-op ward, and told her about our baby. Carina was very tired the first few days, so I had to nurse him in the incubator. I think that I got a sort of 'advantage', similar to that which mothers get in the first week.

The maternity ward and the neonatal ward should ideally be situated side by side. You can create a 'family-area' on the ward, where children can play while waiting and where it is possible to take a rest, have a bite to eat, or chat with other parents.

The family should be actively involved in the care work as soon as possible.

Lena

I really felt that she was mine when I started to change diapers, turn her around, and feed her by the tube with my milk. I especially remember one evening when she was to be weighed. Bengt, my husband, was present. The nurse let him disconnect the flexes and carry her to the scale. It was her first weight over 1000 g. He still talks about how he felt when holding his little daughter in his big clumsy fists.

A care plan should be done once a week together with the parents. Weekly parent meetings are arranged for informing, educating, and, if necessary, to meet the social worker or psychologist. Slides and videos may also be shown at this meetings, dealing with, for example, premature babies, breast-feeding.

Discharge is done by a soft approach, through home leaves and by close contact and collaboration with the district nurse. The end to our 'care chain' is planned individually, and always leaves the door open for telephone contacts, home visits, and out-patient visits on the ward.

Lena

After discharge, I was terrified. I continued to give her the kind of 'protection' you had given her. I was preoccupied with her food and increase in weight. I did not dare to give her a bath and hardly went outside. The telephone number to the wards was my life-line during the first few weeks.

Creating a more human environment—a care setting

In an effort to attain this comprehensiveness in our work, we have to remember the impression which the physical environment has on children and their parents. Neonatal wards are usually planned as common intensive care units, which in other words means a sterile and rather boring environment, which from the first impression usually brings to mind the very sick. It is therefore an important part of the work to try and create better surroundings for the family. We need to create a kind of a day nursery for the sick children, where the families are capable of spending as much time as possible near the baby.

It is not impossible to create a ward environment with both a high standard of hygiene, good practical working conditions and a worm, friendly, and cosy environment for the families. This type of ward can even have a positive effect on the staff. For example, a touch of colour and lighting can help to give a peaceful impression in an otherwise stressed atmosphere. Textiles, pictures, babyclothes and toys can give a more homely feeling and comfortable chairs and sofas allow the parents moments of relaxation and rest. A kitchen allows them to prepare meals. Play corners for siblings, and television, radio, and tape-recorders help pass the time and give a little cultural stimulation.

Eva

When I first came to the room, I saw the cords, tubes, and flashing lights. Suddenly I caught sight of a little red cloth toy lying beside my little boy. That little cuddly toy somehow made him more real. He was, despite his tiny size and weakness, still a child.

Developing the professional role by inter-disciplinary collaboration between the medical and nursing professions

Every child/family is assigned their own doctor and contact-nurse (primary-nurse). They are responsible for the medical care, support, information, and the individual care plan of each child. With repeated discussions about the care plan, which take place regularly throughout the hospital stay, the parents are given the chance to be part of the planning. They also have the opportunity to ask questions and make requests.

The contact team is enlarged as and when necessary, with, for example, a psychologist, a physiotherapist, or district-nurse. Decisions on any measurements taken are continuously documented in both the medical and nursing record, to enable the remaining staff to keep themselves informed.

Through 'soft' discharges, by way of day leave and early contact with the district-nurse, there is still a supportive link for both the parents and their nurse during this first period. In some cases, it is more suitable to have the first out-patient visits back on the ward.

Adapting the organization and leadership to the care philosophy

To enable the entire staff to strive after a mutual care philosophy and a mutual goal, it is necessary that any development in organization and leadership is a joint-effort. Ward staff are divided into teams, which makes it more possible for the contact persons to develop a sense of responsibility for the patient and allows for better continuity. Every nursing team is lead by an experienced nurse, an instructor, who serves as a role figure and a support to less experienced nurses. The team follow their patients during the entire hospital stay, from intensive care to discharge and out-patient visits. In this way it is more satisfying to the staff who thus have a complete picture, on a ward which is mentally tough and where there is a risk of so called 'burn out syndrome'.

The nursing team also have their own doctor, and they hold regular team meetings where the contact persons receive supervision. On a ward where the doctors are highly specialized, it is also important that the nurses are given the opportunity to develop their skills in different fields. It may be, for example, in the area of medicine, technology, child development, breast-feeding, baby-massage.

These specialized nurses are responsible for educating, supervising, and keeping the methods up to date in the chosen area.

The head nurse, in the long-term, has to maintain and develop the competence of the nursing staff to enable the care philosophy to be achieved. This requires competent leadership which 'takes care of the carers' and is amenable to the continuous evaluation of routines and methods for quality assessment and improvement.

Future challenges for creating a more optimal hospital environment

- *To provide individualized supportive care*, where each manipulation that may be stressful or painful to the infant will be evaluated for need, and if needed, for frequency.

- *To avoid mother–infant separation*, by facilitating and supporting the opportunities for closeness, mutual stimulation, and breast-feeding.

- *To develop intersectoral cooperation*, for strengthening a mutual, comprehensive, infant care philosophy among all professions.

Neonatology

A strange word
maybe it means
the art of leaving alone
minimal handling
as softly as possible
support the vital force
take care of the will to live
to gently nurse
take fear in hand
and discharge a family

References

1. Petrillo, M. and Sanger, S. (1980). *Emotional care of hospitalized children*, (2nd edn), pp. 245–8. J.B. Lippincott, Philadelphia.
2. The Nordic standard for children's need of care in hospital. Statement from: Nordic Society for the Needs of Sick Children (NOBAB), Chairman Bengt Lindström, the Nordic School of Public Health, Box 121 33, 402 42 Sweden.
3. Bowlby, J. (1958). Nature of a child's tie to his mother. *International Journal of Psychoanalysis* **39**, 350–73.

4. Edwinsson-Månsson, M. (1992). The value of informing children prior to investigations and procedures. Doctoral dissertation. Dept. of Paediatrics, University of Lund, Sweden.
5. Betz, C.L. (1983). Teaching children through play therapy. *AORN Journal*, **38**, 709–24.
6. Klaus, M. and Kennell; (1982). *Parent–infant bonding*. C.V. Mosby, Ontario, Canada.
7. Minde, K., Whitelaw, A., Brown, J., and Fitzharding, P. (1983). Effects of neonatal complications in premature infants in early parent–infant interactions. *Developmental Medicine and Child Neurology*, **25**, 763–77.
8. Kaplan, D., Mason, E. (1960). Maternal reactions to premature birth viewed as an emotional disorder. *American Journal of Orthopsychiatry* **30**, 539–52.
9. Meier, P., Cranston-Andersson, G. (1987). Responses of small preterm infants to bottle and breastfeeding. *Maternal and Child Nursing* **12**, 97–105.
10. Als, H. Lawhon, G., Brown, E., Gibes, R., Duffy, F.H., McAnulty, G., *et al.* (1986). Individualized behavioral and environmental care for the VLBW preterm infants at high risk for bronchopulmonary dysplasia: NICU and the developmental outcome. *Pediatrics* **78**, 1123–32.
11. Lawhn, G. and Melzar, A. (1988). Developmental care of the very low birth weigh infant. *The Journal of Perinatal and Neonatal Nursing* July, 56–65.
12. Whitelaw, A. and Sleath, K. (1985). Myth of the marsupial mother. *Lancet* **i**, 1206–8.
13. Affonso, D., Wahlberg, V., and Persson, B. (1989). Exploration of mothers' reactions to the kangaroo method of prematurity care. *Neonatal Network* **7**, 43–51.
14. Whitelaw, A. (1990). Kangaroo baby care: just a nice experience or an important advance for premature infants? *Pediatrics* **85**, 604–5.
15. Wahlberg, V., Affonso, D., and Persson, B. (1992). A retrospective comparative study using the kangaroo method as a complement to the standard incubator care. *European Journal of Public Health* **2**, 34–7.

33 Partnership with parents
Nick Spencer

Introduction

This chapter considers the possibilities and problems of making parents partners in the health care of their children.

Partnership with parents will be defined with reference to the variance of this approach from most current European child health practice. The theoretical and historical background to partnership will be outlined and specific examples examined. In conclusion, future developments towards partnership will be considered.

Definition

Partnership with parents and related concepts such as parent involvement and participation have become fashionable in recent years constituting a central theme of some UK Government commissioned reports ('Court report', DHSS, 1976; Warnock report, DES 1978).

In practice, these concepts remain ill-defined and rarely applied. Definition and application have varied according to the theoretical and practical perspective of the professionals; in essence, whether the partnership is conceived as a means of teaching parents to be better child carers or as a means of enabling parents to take greater control of their lives by enhancing parental confidence and skills.

Pugh and De'Ath (1989) define partnership as 'a working relationship that is characterised by a shared sense of purpose, mutual respect and the willingness to negotiate. This implies a sharing of information, responsibility, skills, decision making and accountability'. This challenges the underlying assumption of most current European child health care practice that professional knowledge and guidance are the key elements in ensuring optimal child health care. Partnership does not seek to devalue the professional role but to recognize and nurture the unique role of parents in the care of their children

Theoretical and historical background

Though the partnership or participation 'movement' has never been as powerful as at present, the phenomenon of the 'active patient' is not new. Steele *et al.* (1987) suggest that it has fluctuated over two centuries in line with broader societal change and, in the form of traditional folk medicine and mutual self help, had a greater role in the lives of most people in nineteenth century England than medical and health professionals (Woodward and Richards 1977). The end of the nineteenth and most of the twentieth centuries have been dominated by the explosion of scientific medicine and the accompanying revolutions in diagnosis and treatment. However, the major improvements in health of populations are attributable to public health measures based on scientific knowledge rather than individual diagnosis and treatment (Rose 1990).

The medicalization of child care has arisen out of the dominance of scientific medicine and the accompanying protective organization of the health professionals. Child health professionals expect, and are expected, to comment and advise on all aspects of child care and an extensive literature of books, journals, and pamphlets has been generated. Parents are encouraged to rely on professional skills and to reject 'lay' advice; the majority of health education leaflets related to infant feeding given free to parents in the UK encourage parents to seek professional help and some stress that non-professional advice is often conflicting and confusing (Perkins and Spencer 1980).

Conflicting messages have been given by health professionals as well; at the same time as being encouraged to seek advice in the event of uncertainty, parents are persuaded to use their own judgement in order to reduce consultations for conditions viewed as trivial by the professionals (Roberts 1983). According to Mayall (1986), mothers negotiate this contradiction by acknowledging the importance of professional advice whilst retaining a certain scepticism, acquiring knowledge from a range of sources and regarding their own judgements as the principal guides to action.

The growing interest in partnership and participation has acted as a counterbalance to professional domination of child care, challenging some of the underlying assumptions. It has developed under the influence of a number of processes (Hickey 1986). In Western Europe, tailing the USA, the growth of consumerism has brought with it pressure for greater participation and protection for patients, shifting the focus from the professional's right to direct and the patient's obligation to comply with consumer's rights and professionals' obligations. Professional skills and knowledge no longer go unchallenged and the concept of 'iatrogenesis' (Illich 1974) is now widely accepted. The post-war challenges to established orthodoxies, particularly through the women's movement, have created a climate in which deference to professional standing is undermined. Of equal importance is the recognition, within and outside the health professions, of the crucial role of self-help groups, established by families, in the management of chronic diseases affecting children.

The perception of limitless demand for health care at a time of financial stringency has encouraged the view that greater participation will lead to reduced costs (Pistorius 1983). Though controversial and unproven in rich countries, parent participation in the primary health care of children in countries without adequate resources is of established and proven benefit (Sanders 1985). The success of parent participation in developing countries has stimulated interest in developed countries; this is particularly true of 'parent-held records' which will be considered in detail below. The declaration of Alma-Ata (WHO 1978) reflects and advances this international experience:

'The people have the right and duty to participate individually and collectively in the planning and implementation of their health care. This is clearly a basic human right and is supported by current ideas on the nature of health and illness.

Health can never be adequately protected by health services without the active understanding and involvement of the individuals and communities whose health is at stake. Action to promote health therefore depends on a partnership, based on mutual understanding and trust, between those working in the health sector and the community.'

WHO has subsequently adopted this approach as the basis for its *Health for all 2000* initiative. Whilst *HFA 2000* targets charge governments with responsibility for ensuring their achievement, community participation and involvement is seen as the means to this end. The *UN Convention on the rights of the child* addresses the rights of the child within the context of the rights and responsibilities of the parents and the State. Article 18 recognizes the primary role of parents in child care and charges signatory states with the responsibility of assisting parents in the task of child rearing. Article 12 safeguards the right of the child to an independent opinion in a manner consistent with the child's age and maturity. The Convention, then, accepts parents as full and active participants in the care of their children.

Alongside these pressures for change, a considerable literature in sociology, health, and education has accumulated which confirms the essential and skilled role of parents in child care. Davis (1963), in a sensitive and beautifully observed study, described the process by which parents had arrived at the conclusion that their child's illness (in this case, polio) was serious and not just a transient 'flu-like' illness. Subsequent studies (Alpert et al. 1967; Spencer 1984; Locker 1981) have confirmed the skilled process by which parents identify significant illness in their children and manage the majority of symptoms without recourse to professional assistance.

The key role of parents in the identification of children with hearing impairment and other developmental problems is now widely accepted (Hall 1990). Parents have been shown to be as effective as the services in the maintenance of their children's health records (Saffin and Macfarlane 1990).

In pre-school education parents can fulfil a variety of roles successfully from supporters and fund raisers to policy makers and managers (Pugh and De'Ath 1989). Whilst parental skills and the potential for partnership are increasingly recognized, the capacity and desire of some parents for partnership, especially those whose children are particularly vulnerable, has been questioned (Bax and Whitmore 1990). Further, it is evident that parents do not always respond appropriately to the needs of their children, either as a result of lack of knowledge or of conflicting pressures and needs which distort their response.

Abusive and neglectful parents are the extreme example but even here, as discussed below, a partnership approach which empowers parents is more likely to be successful than a professionally led approach which excludes them.

Current experience

Though practical experience of partnership is limited and the application of the theoretical concepts variable, experience and an associated literature is accumulating. The examples discussed here are chosen to show the application of the concepts of partnership at different levels; individual parent/professional contacts, and work with identifiable groups and general service approaches. They are based primarily on the UK experience but have wider applicability.

Individual parent/professional contacts

Nicholl (1986) identifies three elements as essential in a parent–professional relationship based on partnership: the relationship must be equal, with parents and professionals as colleagues and confidants; the relationship must be active with an active role for both parties; the relationship must be responsible, with mutual trust and shared responsibility. Another approach stresses the rights of parent and child (Davis 1985) to information, consultation, representation, and negotiation, placing more emphasis on the duty of professionals to respect these rights rather than the development of an equal active sharing of skills. The sharing of skills is the implicit message of the Warnock report:

'Parents can be effective partners only if the professionals take notice of what they say and of how they express their needs, and treat their contribution as intrinsically important.'

Wolfendale (1983) goes a step further, explicitly stating that partnership requires parents to be 'active and central to decision-making and its implementation; perceived as having equal strengths and equivalent expertise; able to contribute as well as receive services (reciprocity); able to share responsibility, so that they and the professionals are mutually accountable'.

Skilled decision making by parents has been explored (Spencer 1984; Locker 1981) as has the process of mutual skill sharing within the medical consultation (Spencer 1985). This analysis of consultations illustrates the ease with which the professional, even one striving to put the concepts of partnership into practice, can revert to the time-honoured techniques of obfuscation and opinionated monologue in order to negotiate a 'tight corner'. Apart from removal of the obvious various barriers between professional and parent such as the imposing and interposing desk and the protective receptionist, in order to nurture partnership through the consultation the professional must learn to 'tune in' to parental skills, acknowledge them and enhance parental confidence in themselves as skilled carers by mutual skill sharing.

Work with identifiable groups

Pre-school education

The principles outlined above for partnership in parent–professional contact apply equally to initiatives for partnership involving identifiable groups. In pre-school education, parent participation, sometimes falling short of partnership as envisaged by Wolfendale (1983), is widely accepted as beneficial to the educational progress of children. Participation functions at a number of levels from parent as supporter (in the UK the fund-raising activities of parents have taken on more importance as a result of financial stringency) through parent as teaching aide/volunteer, to parent as policy maker and partner (Gordon 1969; Smith 1980). Thus, many participation initiatives in pre-school education appear to be driven more by service and professional needs than by those of the parents. In the UK, day nurseries, which are run by local social service departments, have developed work with parents characterized by van der Eyken (1984) as 'contractual involvement' where the family is involved only in a compulsory relationship which is initiated by the services and arises because of concerns about the parents' child-caring abilities. However sensitively carried out, this 'contractual involvement' cannot achieve equality in the relationship necessary for partnership.

From their extensive study of pre-school centres in the UK, Pugh and De'Ath (1989) cite examples of good practice and identify what they call 'partnership proneness'. Ten factors are listed which can help or hinder the partnership process: type, function, and overall philosophy of the centre; presence or absence of a policy on working with parents; type of management and type of parental involvement; source and adequacy of funding; location and premises; time allowed for partnership to develop; methods and strategies employed by the centre and their degree of flexibility; ability of professionals to change their roles and develop new skills; level of training and support for the staff; and the attitudes, expectations, and roles of the parents. Partnership needs time to develop, challenges established attitudes (parental as well as professional), and implies the development of new skills.

Children with handicapping conditions

Parents of children with chronic handicapping conditions have been in the forefront of the pressure for partnership. The magnitude of their needs for support and services, the experience and skill they develop in coping with the constant demands of caring, and, initially at least, the lack of professional interest or sensitivity to the physical and psychological strains of caring have led to the development, over the past 50 years, of highly effective self-help groups, such as the Spastics Society, which have a major role in care for children with special needs. The self-help groups, with the assistance of enlightened professionals, have obliged the professions and the services to take account of the views and needs of parents. As a result, many parents now have a detailed knowledge of their child's condition and a role reversal takes place with the parent as expert (Brimblecombe and Russell 1988).

In many parts of Europe, services for children and families with special needs have recognized the need for more involvement of parents in the management of their children's problems. Respite care is widely practiced and, in the UK, most services have improved the information given to parents. However, examples of true partnership, as defined above, remain rare. The Honeylands Family Support Unit in Exeter in the south-west of England is one such example (Brimblecombe and Russell 1988). It has developed from a district therapeutic and assessment centre for handicapped children into a family resource centre with maximum parental involvement in the planning and use of the services. The unit coordinates all the services for children with handicapping conditions in the district. Key elements in the approach of the unit are a commitment to partnership, with a recognition of the delicate balance which has to be achieved to protect the interests of all parties; an 'open-door' policy for parental access; and the identification of a 'named person' for each family to act as a family resource and a link between the family home and the unit.

Children living in social deprivation

A similar approach has been developed as part of interventions to reduce adverse health outcomes in socially deprived communities. The family worker, based on the French model of the 'travailleuse familiale', has been used to reduce stress and increase social support in expectant mothers (Spencer *et al.* 1989) and parent advisers have been introduced for Bangladeshi families in the poorest part of London coping with handicapped children (Davis and Choudhury 1988). Both initiatives depend on a close partnership between the worker, who is not usually a professional, and the parents. Initiatives based on community participation and community diagnosis, described in detail in Chapter 34, take this approach a step further; the community and the professionals start as equal partners and the community decides the priorities for intervention. This approach, developed in Third World countries, appears to have particular relevance for deprived areas of developed countries.

Child abuse and neglect

Families in which abuse has taken place or children are at serious risk of abuse constitute the most serious challenge to the concept of partnership. Legal constraints frequently limit the freedom of the parents and the professionals and impose a framework in which voluntary and informed cooperation is not possible. In addition, the normally accepted unity of interest between parent and child may not apply and most professionals are committed to the concept of the interests of the child as paramount. Despite these difficulties, participation and cooperation initiatives are developing under the twin pressures of the 'family rights' lobby and perceived failure of the traditional management strategies such as exclusion of parents from decision making and separation of the child from the parents to offer a more satisfactory outcome for the child or the family. In the UK, parent participation in case conferences has been legally enshrined in the 1989 Children Act and the Act insists on parental participation at all levels of decision making related to their children as well as imposing a duty of parental responsibility on parents even when the child is not in their direct care.

A number of initiatives in primary and secondary prevention of child abuse (Chamberlin 1988; Mitchell et al.1988; Pound and Mills 1985) utilize the partnership/participation model and emphasize the value of mobilizing untapped community and personal resources for support with child rearing and child care and avoiding the stigmatizing and labelling effects of statutory interventions by social and child health workers to 'protect' the child. Hard data are difficult to collect in such projects but accumulating evidence suggests that they may succeed in offering positive protection to children by strengthening social support (Wolfe 1991).

General service approaches

Parent-held records

One of the most important general service approaches to partnership has been the development of parent-held records.

Developed initially in France as the Carnet de Sante and in some Third World countries, they are now being adopted in a number of European countries. The essential premise upon which they are based is that parents have a positive interest in the health and progress of their children and given responsibility for the primary record they will become more involved and interested in the well-being of their child. Experience so far with parent-held records indicates that parents are more efficient at maintaining the records and producing them at the appropriate times than the services and the responsibility of record maintenance does enhance parental interest and involvement in the progress of their children (Saffin and Macfarlane 1990). Professional concerns about recording negative findings related to parenting and the availability of records for legal purposes have not been borne out by experience and professionals have been obliged to share their concerns more actively with parents. Parent-held records would seem to have become an essential part of any child health service committed to the concept of partnership with parents.

Developing, evaluating, and researching partnership

Partnership strategies will usually be initiated by professionals but their success will depend, to some extent, on the degree to which parents are consulted and involved in the planning and establishment of the strategy. For example, the introduction of parent-held records without prior preparation or explanation to parents of the importance of their role in the maintenance of the record is likely to lead to confusion and misunderstanding, which may threaten the future of the whole project. Experience in the UK suggests that, given adequate preparation, parents are enthusiastic about greater involvement (or greater recognition of their role) in the health care of their children and resistance tends to come from professionals. Thorough preparation and groundwork with parents and professionals is likely to enable both to adapt more readily to the changes implicit in partnership. For some partnership strategies, prior consultation and planning with parents is difficult; partnership in established child abuse is one such example. In these circumstances professional preparation and commitment to the strategy is the best way of ensuring its success alongside a flexible, sensitive approach to parents faced with the daunting task of cooperating with professionals who are questioning their parenting skills and their capacity to protect their child. Despite the problems inherent in this situation, parents appreciate involvement in decision-making and the tensions generated by parental exclusion are avoided. Community participation strategies, though initiated by professional agencies, can only develop if consultation and planning involves the community from the outset as is emphasized in Chapter 34.

Evaluation and research into partnership presents particular problems. Measurable health outcomes are difficult to identify and even more difficult to attribute to the partnership initiative. Evaluation and research are essential, however, if partnership is to flourish. The challenge is to develop methods and measures which reflect the changes anticipated as a result of partnership. These may have more to do with parent satisfaction than dramatic changes in child health outcomes.

Measures of satisfaction, improved service use, and increase in parental confidence have been used in the evaluation of parental participation in developmental assessment, parental perceptions of professional communication related to their child's disability, and the effect of support programmes for mothers experiencing severe child care problems (Pound and Mills 1985).

To dismiss such measures as 'soft' is to miss the point; these are precisely the kind of changes partnership is aiming to promote. The danger is that, in their enthusiasm for the concept of partnership, advocates will avoid the difficulties of evaluation or inappropriately design or interpret evaluative data.

Conclusions

Considerable experience has been gained in parent participation and partnership though the principles are not universally accepted or applied. It seems likely that pressure for an increased parental role will continue. Social paediatricians could contribute to the development of imaginative, well evaluated partnership initiatives, especially in the fields of parent-held records and the prevention and management of child abuse.

Knowledge of the experience accumulated so far and a flexible, sensitive approach based on sound principles of evaluation are essential if this potential contribution is to realized. Social paediatricians should promote understanding of partnership among their medical colleagues and introduce consideration of the theoretical and practical concepts into undergraduate and postgraduate training.

References

Alpert, J.J., Kosa J., and Heggarty, R.J. (1967). Medical help and maternal nursing care in the life of low income families. *Paediatrics* **39**, 749–55.
Bax, M.C.O. and Whitmore, K. (1990). Health for all children controversy. *Archives of Disease in Childhood* **65**, 141–2.
Brimblecombe, F. and Russell, P. (1988). *Honeylands: developing a service for families with handicapped children*. National Children's Bureau, London.
Chamberlin, R. (ed.) (1988). *Beyond individual risk assessment: community wide approaches to promoting the health and development of families and children*. The National Center for Education in Maternal and Child Health, Washington, DC.
Davis, F. (1963). *Passage through crisis*. Bobbs-Merrill, Indianapolis.
Davis, J. (1985). Sharing care in hospital. In *Partnership, Paper 4*, (ed. E. De'Ath and G. Pugh). National Children's Bureau, London.
Davis, H. and Choudhury, P.A. (1988). Helping Bangladeshi families: Tower Hamlets parent adviser scheme. *Mental Handicap* **16**, 48–51.
DES (Department of Education and Science) (1978). *Special educational needs. A report of the Committee of Enquiry into the education of handicapped children and young people* (The worn out report). HMSO, London.
DHSS (Department of Health and Social Security) (1976). *Fit for the future*, report of the Committee on Child Health Services (The Court report). HMSO, London.
Gordon, I.J. (1969). Developing parent power. In *Critical Issues in Research related to disadvantaged children*, (ed. E. Grotberg). Educational Testing Service, Princeton, NJ.
Hall, D. (1990). *Health for all children*. Oxford University Press.
Hickey, T. (1986). Health behaviour and self care in later life. In *Self care and health in old age*, (ed. K. Dean, T. Hickey, and B. Holstein). Croom Helm, London.
Illich, I. (1974). *Medical nemesis: the expropriation of health*. Calder & Boyars, London.
Locker, D. (1981). *Symptoms and illness*. Tavistock, London.
Mayall, B. (1986). *Keeping children healthy*. Allen and Unwin, London.
Mitchell, S.K., Magyang, D., Barnard, K., Summer, G., Booth, C. *et al*. (1988). A comparison of home-based prevention programmes for families of newborns. In *Families in transition: primary prevention programmes that work*, (ed. L. Bond and B. Wagner). Sage, Beverly Hills, CA.
Nicholl, A. (1986). New approaches to child health and care: is there a role for parents? In *Partnership, Paper 8*, (ed. E. De'Ath and G. Pugh). National Children's Bureau, London.

Perkins, E.R. and Spencer, N.J. (1980). Clinic booklets: help or hindrance in parent education? In *Education for childbirth and parenthood*, (ed. E.R. Perkins). Croom Helm, London.

Pistorius, G.J. (1983). The case for more patient participation. In *Common dilemmas in family medicine*, (ed. J. Fry). MTP, Lancaster.

Pound, A. and Mills, M. (1985). A pilot evaluation of 'Newpin' home-visiting and befriending scheme in south London. *Association for Child Psychology and Psychiatry Newsletter*, Vol. No 4.

Pugh, G. and De'Ath, E. (1989). *Working towards partnership in the early years.* National Children's Bureau, London.

Roberts, C.R.I., P.B., Turner, J.D., Hosokawa, M.C. and Alster, J.M. (1983). Reducing physician visits for colds through consumer education. *Journal of the American Medical Association* **250**, 1986–9.

Rose, G. (1990). Reflections on the changing times. *British Medical Journal* **301**, 683–8.

Saffin, K. and Macfarlane, A. (1990). Do general practitioners and health visitors like 'parent-held' child health records? *British Journal of General Practice* **40**, 106–8.

Sanders, D. (1985). *The struggle for health*. Macmillan Education, London.

Smith, T. (1980). *Parents and pre-school*. Grant McIntyre, London.

Spencer, N.J. (1984). Parents' recognition of the ill child. In *Progress in child health*, (ed. A. Macfarlane), Vol. 1. Churchill Livingstone, London.

Spencer, N.J. (1985). *Developing partnership with parents: strategies for the consultation. Practical Paper 11*. Notingham University Department of Adult Education, UK.

Spencer, B., Morris, J., and Thomas, H. (1989). The south Manchester family worker scheme. In Seedhouse D. and Cribb A. (eds) *Changing ideas in health care* (ed. D. Seedhouse and A. Cribb). Wiley, London.

Steele, D.J., Blackwell, B., Gutmann, M.C., and Jackson, T.C. (1987). The activated patient: dogma, dream or desideratum? *Patient Education and Counselling* **10**, 3–23.

Van der Eyken, W. (1984). *Day nurseries in action: a national study of local authority day nurseries in England 1975–1983*. Department of Child Health, University of Bristol, Bristol.

Wolfe, D. (1991). Preventing violence towards children: recent developments. In *Abstracts of First National Congress on the Prevention of Child Abuse and Neglect, University of Leicester*, (ed. K. Browne and M. Lynch). BAPSCAN in association with the Continuing Education Unit, University of Leicester, UK.

Wolfendale, S. (1983). *Parental participation in children's development and education*. Gordon and Breach, Reading.

Woodward, J. and Richards, D. (1977). *Health care and popular medicine in nineteenth century England*. Croom Helm, London.

WHO (World Health Organization) (1978). *Primary health care; report of the International Conference on primary health care, Alma-Ata*. WHO, Geneva.

34 Community diagnosis and participation
Jon Cook, Michel Pechevis, and Tony Waterston

Introduction

In a recent review of progress in 'health for all' in the European region, Curtis *et al.*[1] note that 'La région est bien pourvue en institutions, en personnel et en ressources de santé: il n'en reste pas moins beaucoup à faire sur les plans de la qualité des services, et de la satisfaction et de la participation des consommateurs, de la gestion et de l'usage des moyens, et de la réduction des disparités' (p.20). 'The region is well provided with facilities, personnel, and health resources: however, there is still much to do in the areas of quality of service, satisfaction and participation of consumers, management and use of resources, and in the reduction of disparities.'

In this chapter we would like to present the notion of community participation, in particular community participation in the assessment of children's health needs, and suggest this approach as one way of improving health programmes in the region. An important caveat should be mentioned, however. Community participation programmes, like other actions involving people on a local level, do not lend themselves well to global recipes on 'how to do it'. This is especially true when the concept is to be applied to diverse social and cultural settings such as those found in the European region. Rather, community participation programmes must be conceived and built locally, using and adapting local definitions and practices of participation. As work in other parts of the world has shown, the very concept of community participation held by community members may differ considerably from that held by programme planners (see Stone[2] for a discussion of this point). We wish therefore to present a model of community participation in the assessment of children's health needs which is flexible enough to be adapted to different settings, but with sufficient structure to be useful for programme planning.

Background discussion of community participation

Programmes of economic and social change have for many years recognized the importance of involving community members in various aspects of the development process. Foster[3] has reviewed this trend and identifies its early beginnings in the cooperative movements in the United Kingdom and the Scandinavian countries in the latter half of the nineteenth century. Rural development efforts in the United States, post-war colonial governments, and, more recently, national and international aid programmes, especially in the developing world, have all espoused variations on the theme of community participation in development to spur economic and social progress.

The Alma-Ata conference in 1978 specifically outlined those features of a primary health care programme which were considered important: '...essential health care made universally accessible to individuals and families in the community by means acceptable to them, *through their full participation* and at a cost that the community and country can afford'[4] (italics added). The nature of participation in development programmes in general, and health programmes in particular, has rarely been adequately defined. Green[5] has shown the evolution of the concept of participation as it relates to health education in national and international agencies. The image of the ideal participatory role of the population has shifted from one of implementing specific health programmes conceived by health professionals towards a decentralized planning role covering several objectives, particularly those relating to '...building self-awareness, community involvement, and a variety of organizational, economic, and environmental supports for behaviour conducive to health' (p. 219).

The nature of participation

Recently, the problem of the definition of participation has been addressed by Rifkin[6,7] through a review of literature describing community participation. Answers to three questions appear central to an understanding of the role of participation in health programmes according to Rifkin (ref. 7, pp. 10–15).

Why should there be participation in a health programme?

Rifkin notes several reasons given in the literature for desiring participation in health programmes: (i) prevention programmes have the potential for improving health beyond what medical technology alone can do for a population—attempts to change behaviour and life style to improve health can only succeed through peoples' conscious participation; (ii) participation of users in the planning and running of services should improve their appropriateness for the population; (iii) communities have untapped resources which may be directed to health concerns through the involvement of community members in the financing, building, and running of health facilities; (iv) it is the right and duty of people to participate in activities affecting their daily lives.

Who should participate?

The answer to this question depends on the objectives of the health programme. For example, Maternal and child health (MCH) programmes may require the participation of a different set of people from those needed for a programme in the prevention of vascular disease. The more people involved who may contribute to the programme, the more resources will be available for reaching programme objectives.

How should they participate?

Rifkin recognizes five levels of participation of community members in health programmes, each higher level including participation at the preceding level(s): (1) as simple **beneficiaries** of programme activities (passive patient role); (2) as contributors of **work** or **resources** to programme activities; (3) in the **implementation** of programmes with limited managerial responsibilities, but not involved in determining objectives; (4) in **monitoring** and **evaluating** programmes to ascertain the extent to which they meet their objectives; (5) as programme **planners** who determine objectives, find resources, and manage the programme.

Factors influencing MCH programmes

In addition to these important questions on the nature of community participation in health programmes, Rifkin (ref. 7, pp. 16) lists two sets of factors that influence the success of Maternal and child health/family planning (MCH/FP) programmes, which she identifies as '**descriptive factors**' and '**action factors**'. The former refers to the local and national context within which programmes are carried out, including cultural, economic, social, political, and historical factors, as well as questions relating to the degree of centralization or decentralization and the flow of communication between the centre and the periphery. These descriptive factors define the limits or potentialities inherent in the society under consideration.

While attempting to change these descriptive factors is often considered outside the responsibility of MCH services, they should be identified and their relative importance for child health and health programmes in a community should be clearly established. In health programmes where community participation is an important element, community members themselves have the potential for bringing about changes in the local context which in turn may affect the success of health programmes (see Eng and Blanchard[8] for an example of community involvement in changing the local context).

In addition to these descriptive factors, action factors are variables upon which programmes planners may act more directly in order to achieve programme objectives. Rifkin (ref. 7, p. 17) lists six main action factors which '... reflect:

- how community needs are assessed;
- how community organizations are developed;

- how programmes are managed;
- how financial and human resources are mobilized;
- how leadership is developed;
- how the problems of the poor, especially the very poor, are dealt with.'

Participation in the context of these action factors may be evaluated to determine the degree of community as opposed to professional participation in health programmes. To the extent that participation is considered a key element in the success of primary health care programmes, measuring and monitoring participation is essential for programme planning (see Rifkin et al.[9] for a discussion of the measurement of participation in health programmes).

Participatory community diagnosis

Indeed, some writers consider community participation as indispensable for successful primary health care programmes. For example, Green (ref. 5, p. 229) states: 'the effective adaptation by people to their own needs for health protection and health enhancement (E) is a function of their degree of active participation (A) in identifying their own goals and needs (I), setting their own priorities among goals or needs (P), controlling the implementation of programs or solutions (C), and evaluating or otherwise obtaining feedback on their own progress (F).' Green believes that each element (A to F) contributes in a multiplicative and not an additive fashion to health enhancement, and therefore the presence of each one is essential.

How can active community participation in child health programmes be achieved? We would like to suggest a first step in community participation, the assessment of child health needs, by presenting a model for assessing health needs known as 'community diagnosis'.

What is community diagnosis?

The meaning of the term

'Diagnosis' is a well known term among health professionals and the public. For any patient, before treatment is prescribed, and before any decision is reached on what action should be taken, an effort is made to diagnose the patient's disease. In the same way, before health activities are developed in a particular community, an evaluation needs to be made of the situation in that community—its problems, its needs, its resources, as well as its traditions, its history, etc. Only when all this is known is it possible to take appropriate measures.

The term 'diagnosis', however, may be considered too heavily weighted with medical connotations, and too static. In the case of a community, what is needed is not only to obtain a 'snapshot' of the current situation, but also to add progressively to the information obtained and to follow the situation as it develops. Furthermore, clinical diagnosis all too often implies a somewhat passive role by the individual being 'diagnosed'. Here, on the contrary, as we shall see below, the community participates fully in its own diagnosis.

It is also necessary to clarify precisely what is meant by 'community'. The definition proposed at the Alma-Ata Conference on primary health care would seem to come closest to what is required:

'A community consists of people living together in some form of social organization and cohesion. Its members share in varying degrees political, economic, social and cultural characteristics, as well as interests and aspirations, including health. Communities vary widely in size and socio-economic profile, ranging from clusters of isolated homesteads to more organized villages, towns and city districts' (ref. 4).

The term 'community' thus refers to a comparatively homogeneous group of individuals. By its very nature, it masks internal social differentiation, the position of groups, and even conflictual relationships existing between them. In village communities, neighbours are often rivals. It will thus be necessary to identify, and draw distinctions between, the groups and possibly subgroups that make up the 'community' and to determine the different problems and needs accordingly.

Furthermore, the term 'community' is more apt than 'population' or 'group of people', because what is involved is not simply a collection of individuals, but the nature of the relationships that these individuals establish, and the development dynamics that such relationships make it possible to achieve.

As we will see below, community diagnosis does not refer to a simple assessment of needs performed by health professionals. The term 'community' implies that the diagnosis is undertaken in close collaboration with the community. It is a joint venture!

The meaning of the process

To make a community diagnosis is to identify the problems, needs, and the resources of a community in order to develop appropriate solutions to these problems. This process can be seen as the first step in community health programme planning as shown on Fig. 34.1.

This diagram is well known and is attractive because of its apparent logic. In fact, however, it may lead health professionals to set up services and activities that have no connection with the real needs of the population if the first step is not in the right direction. Needs that are wrongly identified may result in health programmes condemned to failure from the start because they do not coincide with the problems that the members of the community consider to be of priority. As an example: in a small town in a developing country, the health authorities had decided to set up a family planning centre, whereas the population was

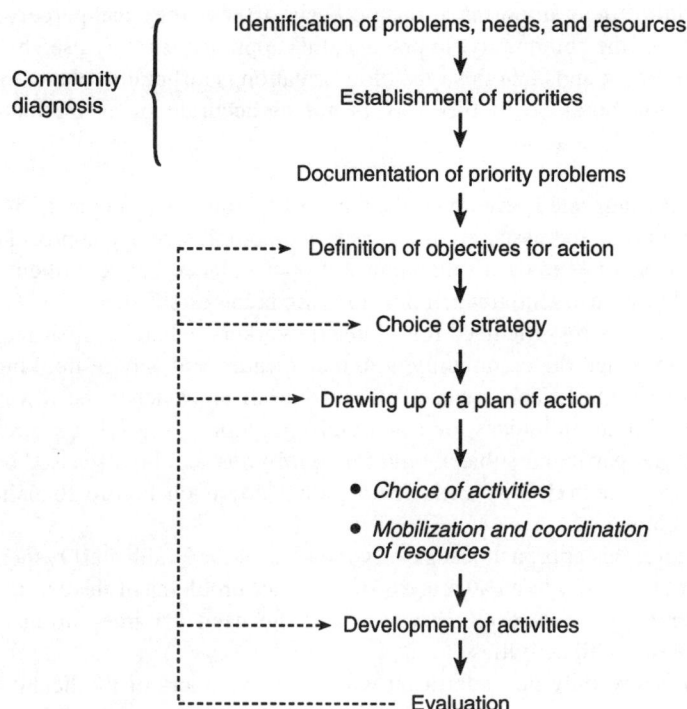

Fig. 34.1 Steps in the planning of a community health programme. (Source: Pineault,[10] with modifications.)

faced with a serious water supply problem for which they had been requesting assistance from the very same authorities for many months. They very much resented the establishment of the family planning centre, which had been imposed on them from above and which had no impact. Community diagnosis must therefore be seen not as diagnosis *of* a given community, but as diagnosis *with* the community.

The needs of a population may indeed differ considerably according to whether they are defined and identified by health professionals alone or in close collaboration with the members of the community and with their participation.

As we are reminded by Raynald Pineault,[10] two main approaches may be used to identify health problems :

- the first approach is based on the *epidemiological* concept of need, and uses various ways of measuring the health status of a population, such as indicators of mortality and morbidity;
- the second approach corresponds with the *psycho-sociological* concept of need. This approach consists of identifying a population's problems and

determining their importance on the basis of how they are perceived by members of the community. In practice, this approach is rarely used by planners, on the grounds that this type of information is difficult to obtain, or that information obtained in this way is not as accurate or as meticulously scientific as it should be.

The process suggested here under the name of 'community diagnosis' is actually a combination and association of these two complementary approaches, in which every effort is made to maintain a proper balance between them. This balance will also be essential when priorities are being established.

We would also stress the need for all health workers, whatever their responsibilities, to approach the community with the attitudes and way of thinking of a 'general practitioner'. This means that an overall approach must always be maintained without prejudices, narrow mindedness, or a 'specialist's' preoccupation with one particular subject. And this is why (as will be discussed below) the (proposed) methodology calls for a global approach before focusing on specific problems.

Furthermore, this approach leads every member of the health staff responsible for a particular activity to an awareness of the other problems of the community, the complementary nature of activities, and the need for integration of the various family health activities.

It can therefore only be undertaken with other members of the health team, the other professionals concerned, and the population, and provides an excellent opportunity for developing intersectorial cooperation and teamwork.

Another essential characteristic of community diagnosis is that it is a *local* process. Whatever the health policy defined at the central level and the broad outline of activities planned, the activities themselves are going to be carried out in the field, at the local level. They will thus have to be adapted to local circumstances and to the real needs of the population (or communities) concerned.

If appropriate objectives for action are to be set, if activities based on the resources of a community are to be developed, and if the activities thus undertaken are to be evaluated accurately, it is necessary for local data to be available.

Information collected by the primary health care services and sent in the form of periodic reports to the regional or central level are all too rarely used at the local level of the planning and evaluation of activities. Community diagnosis, however, helps to restore the full value and significance of data collection, which is an essential activity of basic health services.

Community diagnosis is therefore clearly a preliminary step which is essential in order to apply a true policy of primary health care. *In community diagnosis, the role of health professionals is first and foremost to 'give the floor' to the community, listen attentively to what it has to say, and in this way help it to express its needs.*

The attitude which makes this approach possible will help to transform relationships between health personnel and the members of the community.

Strategy and methods of community diagnosis

If the diagnosis is to truly have a community orientation, health professionals must involve both the community and professionals of other disciplines concerned, from the preparatory phase onwards.

It is indeed essential to avoid confronting the community and its representatives with a '*fait accompli*', and asking them to 'participate' in a project which has already been planned without them.

One means of ensuring this collaboration from the start is to set up a working group[11] or a committee bringing together professionals and members of the community. It will be for the working group to decide on the successive steps, define the objectives of the community diagnosis, determine how it is to be carried out and the methods to be used, mobilize the necessary resources, evaluate the results, and make the preliminary contacts required.

Once the preparatory phase is completed and the working group or committee set up, the following steps will need to be taken in succession:

- definition of the objectives of the proposed community diagnosis;
- compilation of the list of information or data to be collected;
- identification of sources of data, choice of the most appropriate methods of data collection, and, if necessary, the preparation of tools for data collection, taking available resources into account;
- collection of data;
- analysis and interpretation of the data collected, and identification of the problems, needs, resources, and groups at risk;
- establishment of priorities;
- documenting of priority problems.

The collection of information

Once it has been decided what kind of information should be collected, all the possible sources of information will need to be identified, and the most suitable methods of collection chosen, in order to proceed with data collection itself.

It is necessary to determine

- what information is already available;
- what information needs to be gathered;
- where the information may be found and/or who to contact to obtain it.

The committee will have to make an index of all existing information on the community or on the area in which the community is located. This may require a great deal of work and tedious searching, but it is often surprising to find out how many little known or insufficiently used studies, reports, and documents exist. This search also provides an opportunity to make contact with administrations and services with which it may be useful to collaborate later on.

Several techniques, which are complementary with one another, may be used to collect specific information on the community. In the first place, all relevant information on life in the community should be collected. This covers both quantitative and qualitative data, the latter corresponding to what we have termed the psychosocial approach to needs and problems.

For this purpose, it will be necessary

- on the one hand, *to observe* the community: observation is indeed one of the best ways of learning about a community's activities, problems, and needs, but it requires much more careful and meticulous work than would appear at first sight, including the preparation of observation guides;

- on the other hand, to *collect the views expressed* by key persons and groups in the community. This may be done through conversation on particular themes, focus group meetings, semi-structured interviews, or by using formal survey methods.

It may also be useful to hold *meetings* with large or small groups, such as the community forum which is open to all members of the community. This technique can be used to complete data obtained from key persons, or to ascertain how valid and representative these data are.

Visits can also be paid to various services and public places (health services, social centres, schools, professional training centres, cultural centres, places of worship, markets, shops), and the workshops and factories in the area, etc.

Furthermore, precise and *quantifiable data* need to be collected on the community itself, in order to confirm and complete the items of information uncovered or surmised as a result of the informal methods mentioned above, or identified through a study of existing documentation. For this purpose, systematic surveys of an epidemiological or sociological nature will be required.

With regard to the choice of methodology and techniques, it will be necessary to make do with the means—and particularly the skills—that are available.

The methods chosen must therefore be those that can be planned and carried out with local personnel, even if this means some loss of precision in the information.

The differences between a community diagnosis and a classical epidemiological or sociological survey lie not only in the objectives, the people involved, or the kind of information to be collected, but also in the methods of collection to be used. During the past decade, simplified methods of data collection have been developed, with the help of epidemiologists, which can be utilized by local non-specialized staff (see Lemeshow and Robinson[12])

Community diagnosis also involves *identifying resources*. These are of course existing health, social, or educational facilities, and the personnel available and their qualifications. But the resources of the community itself are also involved:

- the skills of one or another of the members or groups in the community which might be used to solve problems;
- existing community networks, both formal and informal (e.g. different associations, and also welfare networks);
- formal and informal channels of communication and meeting places used by the community.

However, all this information, although necessary, is not sufficient for developing sustainable community solutions to health problems. If limited to these data, the diagnosis will fail to reveal the collective dynamic and the functions of relationships within a community, and interactions between a community and the society at large will not become evident. That can impede or promote the conditions and skills required to make decisions and take action.

As pointed out by Eng and Blanchard,[8] without the participation of the community, a health programme can undermine the problem-solving capacity of a community by ignoring existing social structures and introducing competing ones, and by replacing functions of local organizations with dependency on external ones.

They also feel that action-oriented community diagnosis is as much solution focused as it is problem focused. While information is gathered on the conditions contributing to disease and illness, data is also collected to assess the problem-solving history and skills of community-based groups and organizations, networks of communication and influence, and individual leaders. (For further information regarding the methodology of community diagnosis see Pechevis)[13].

What child health problems can be address using a participative community diagnosis approach?

The answer to this question depends on who defines the problem. To a parent, the main child health problems may be poor housing, lack of play areas, inadequate pre-school child care, a crying baby, or a child who 'plays up'. To a GP, the main problems may appear to be upper respiratory infections, asthma, and babies who cry at night or won't sleep. To an epidemiologist, the list might include accidental injury, child abuse, congenital anomalies, and cerebral palsy. The process of community diagnosis allows both lay and professional perspectives to be addressed on a locality basis.

Certain criteria may be used to judge which problems will benefit from a participative approach. Essentially, they are problems which are multifactorial in origin, often with social causes predominant ; problems which require intervention from a number of directions, including from outside the health service; and they are problems which are of perceived importance to both parents and professionals. It would also be important that intervention on a local level would have some likelihood of success. These criteria may be summarized as follows:

- multifactional origin (partly social/environmental);
- interventions require interdisciplinary collaboration;
- seen as important by parents and professionals;
- local interventions have a reasonable chance of success.

It should be accepted that any problem identified by members of a local community would be considered for a participative approach. All the problems mentioned above would fall into this category. What about the child health problems as identified by an epidemiologist? Professionals may consider that only the problems with a high mortality and morbidity are of significance. The preceding discussion has shown why a 'community' as well as a 'scientific' perspective must be adopted if common problems are to have any chance of alleviation.

Even defining epidemiologically important conditions is not that easy. Listing the conditions which cause death is straightforward (Table 34.1). Those which fulfil the criteria for a participative approach are starred. On a national scale, one may also list the conditions which present most commonly to general practitioners (Table 34.2).

Again an asterisk identifies those fulfilling the criteria. Handicapping conditions comprise a further list to consider—the top 10 most common are shown in Table 34.3. Problems as defined by a health visitor might be rather different and would include parenting difficulties, under/over-nutrition, conduct disorder, growth delay, and child abuse. A public health physician might add lifestyle factors such as smoking, lack of exercise, poor nutrition, drug ingestion, and inadequate health knowledge as health problems contributing to disease in later life.

An accumulated list of the conditions identified by professionals in these different ways is shown in Table 34.4.

Table 34.1 *Commonest causes of death in children in the UK (0–14 years)* [14]

Condition
Birth injury
Congenital malformation
Pneumonia*
Accidents*
Malignant neoplasm
Infection of newborn
Gastroenteritis*

Table 34.2 *Childhood morbidity in general practice* [14]

Condition		Percentage of consultations
Respiratory diseases*	Infections, asthma	28
Symptoms*	Cough, vomiting, abdominal pain, rash, otitis media	13
CNS diseases	Epilepsy, migraine, conjunctivitis	11
Infective/parasitic*	Diarrhoea, measles, rubella, pertussis	11
Skin diseases*	Eczema, impetigo, boils	10
Accidents, poisoning*		7
Digestive diseases	Constipation, hernia	3
Emotional disorders*	Behaviour, enuresis	3
Genito-urinary diseases		2

Table 34.3 *Top 10 disabilities in school entrants* [14]

Dental caries*
Diseases of tonsils
Refractive error
Enuresis*
Asthma*
Speech disorder*
Strabismus
Hearing impairment
Pes planus

Table 34.4 *Summary of problems amenable to participative approach*

Accidents
Infections (gastroenteritis, immunizable disease)
Emotional/behavioural disorders
Dental caries
Asthma
Speech disorder
Under/over-nutrition
Child abuse/parenting difficulties
Smoking
Drug ingestion
Lack of exercise

The necessary components of a health services approach to these same problems are

(1) a high level of accessibility of the service;

(2) availability of health knowledge in accessible form;

(3) professionals who work in partnership with parents;

(4) professionals who work together effectively across disciplines.

Examples of community diagnosis

Full participation by community members in all aspects of a primary health care programme appears to be infrequent. Most programmes achieve participation in fewer areas, than the five or six discussed above (p. 552) and considered to be essential by both Rifkin[7] and Green[5]. Two examples of participation by community members illustrate how these programmes work in the context of local situations.

Belgium

An article written jointly by a health professional and a community member[15] describes an initiative by a local patient participation group to study what kind of participation community members consider appropriate for themselves. The setting is a poor suburb of Ghent, Belgium, where the population is relatively elderly (20 per cent over 65 years) and modestly educated (70 per cent have only a primary education). Unemployment is high and housing substandard.

In 1981 a local group practice with three GPs was transformed into a multidisciplinary community health centre with a team of four physicians, two nurses, a social worker, a dietitian, and an administrative worker. It was hoped this change would help achieve integrated primary health care which included participation by the local population.

Participation by the population at the time of the study was of three kinds

1. Participation as consumers:
   - subscribing to a centre newsletter;
   - attending health exhibitions and reading health education material;
   - participating in information meetings for patients with specific illness;
   - participating in health related courses (cooking, smoking cessation, etc.).

2. Participation in centre activities:
   - producing the newsletter;
   - preparing health education materials 4 times yearly on selected topics, in collaboration with health staff;
   - encouraging voluntary work (unsuccessful);
   - redecoration of the centre.
3. Participation in policy-making:
   - participation in determining centre hours, road safety, and financing measures for health care;
   - annual meetings to discuss topics of interest to patients and formation of a 15 member advisory committee to translate discussions into suggestions;
   - running the centre through an executive committee of six patients and two health workers.

In 1985, the advisory committee decided to try to find out what patients' views on participation were by preparing a questionnaire which was filled out, mostly in the centre waiting room, by 200 patients during a one-month period. The sample thus obtained was not completely representative of the total centre-served population (which the authors do not enumerate), being somewhat younger, better educated, and with a higher percentage of women.

The questionnaire was designed to obtain the following information:

- identifying characteristics of the respondent;
- knowledge of health care and participation activities;
- views about and priorities for patient participation;
- prospective participation envisaged by the respondents.

The results showed that better-educated and more frequent centre users had better knowledge of the centre's services and activities. Of the group, only 13.5 per cent said they took part in centre activities. While most respondents favoured participation in decision making and cooperation between patients and health workers, only 21.5 per cent said they would participate in centre activities in the following months and 72 per cent said they would not. Older people and those using the centre more frequently were more likely to say they would participate. Most people (58 per cent) who would not participate cited lack of time, 17 per cent cited lack of interest, and an equal proportion said they were unavailable evenings while eight per cent lived too far away. The results of prioritization of 12 suggested participatory activities is shown in Table 34.5 (ref. 15, p. 452).

Table 34.5 *Patients' views on the importance of various kinds of patient participation*

Order of priority	Activity	Percentage[*]
1	Organizing clinics for the early detection of illness	56.5
2	Organizing groups where patients with similar illnesses can exchange ideas and give support	52
3	Visiting and helping the sick, elderly, and disabled	51
4	Organizing health education while in the waiting room	51
5	Providing transport for those who cannot reach health facilities	48
6	Arranging first-aid classes	45
7	Organizing information and discussion evenings	43
8	Campaigning for better health services	43
9	Organizing a counselling service for family and educational problems	37.5
10	Actions concerning the payment system	32.5
11	Organizing social events where patients and staff can get to know one another	24.5
12	Providing a child-minding service during surgery hours	18

[*]Percentage of respondents who indicated the activity should be a priority.

In discussing the results of the survey and the past years of functioning of the centre, the authors note that people are often unwilling to participate in health care activities because they are not often sick. Chronic patients participate more and are more motivated. Motivation appears to be the major problem in obtaining participation from people in health activities. They conclude that 'The development of an appropriate structure for patient participation is a permanent process of trial and error and consumes large amounts of energy' (p. 453). However, in spite of difficulties in aligning patient and professional objectives, the authors feel patient participation contributes to health education programmes, to giving support to sick people, and may effect health policy positively.

The following example focuses more directly on children's health problems and shows how a similar attempt at community prioritization on a different theme reveals differences between health professionals and the population which need to be understood if primary health care programmes are to succeed.

England

An inner city area estate of Newcastle upon Tyne was well known to have many health problems and a high rate of social deprivation. Demographic indices related to figures for the city as a whole, are given in Table 34.6.

Table 34.6 *Demographic indices (from Newcastle household survey 1986, mimeo)*

	Estate (%)	City (%)
Children in one-parent families	33	14
Children < five years old	9	6
Families with children	44	29
Families with three or more children	14	5
Full-time education > 17 years	4	31
Unemployment, male	48	27
Council-rented housing	83	40
Use of car	12	38
Access to telephone	43	81

In 1988, the possibility that funding might be withdrawn from a community-based midwifery project[16] lead to discussions among health workers and members of the community about the type of health service that was required in the area. A population of around 3000 is served by

One single-handed GP practice based in the estate;

One Health Authority child health clinic;

One mobile shop;

One public telephone;

One primary school with a nursery class;

One children's centre funded by Save the Children, Social Services, and Health.

The nearest shopping centre is across a busy dual carriageway. There is no pharmacist on the estate. There is a high crime rate. Although there is only one GP practising on the estate it is served by over 20 additional GPs, the majority with small numbers of patients.

A group of health workers met regularly at the children's centre, which, together with a drop-in centre for local families, became a focus for discussion on heath needs in the area.[17] Health workers (GPs and health visitors) considered the main health problems to be inappropriate use of emergency services (e.g. excessive call outs at night for minor ailments), infectious diseases, especially cough and ear infections, inadequate parenting, accidents, conduct disorders, poor nutrition, and child abuse. However, it is apparent from discussion with mothers attending the children's centre that local people's views about health problems were not at all the same. The opportunity of visiting health students was taken to carry out a health survey in 1990, the content of which was agreed upon with parents. Forty households with young children were selected

Table 34.7 *Major problems affecting health of families (1990)*

Problem	Number	Percentage
Law and order	36	27
Personal health	22	16
Housing	18	13
Environment	16	12
Dogs	12	9
Roads	11	8
Recreation	7	5

by cluster sampling and parents were asked what they considered to be the main problems affecting the health of families on the estate. The results are shown in Table 34.7.

One of the recommendations following the survey was the formation of a health committee with local residents. A health forum was established and has discussed the problems identified by local people. These have included dogs, water purity, hepatitis, and asthma. Leaflets have been prepared by the group on hepatitis and asthma, and a meeting with the water board has been held on water purity. As a result the water pipes on the estate are now being replaced.

It has now been agreed that a health worker will be appointed jointly by the Health Authority and the Family Health Services Authority, to work with a project manager funded by Save the Children. The worker will liaise between the primary care teams and the local population and assist them in developing a service more relevant to local needs.

Evaluation

Not all stages described by Rifkin have been encompassed. The population is participating as beneficiaries, as contributors (parents assisted the students with their survey), and to some extent, in implementation. However, the lead has mainly come from health professionals and community workers, and formal evaluation has not yet been performed. The 'action factors' of programme management, mobilization of resources, and leadership development have not been tackled systematically. Also the real issues of poverty and unemployment have yet to be tackled head on. However, there is considerable enthusiasm for the approach, and it is apparent that some local parents are becoming empowered and more able to take decisions in their own lives. This attempt at community diagnosis in one area has stimulated more systematic work with the same aim in other parts of the city, with the full cooperation of the local authority.[18] In our view, the model is still relevant even if not all components are tackled on the first occasion. It is better to start simply than not at all! On subsequent occasions, the team's approach may approximate more closely to the ideal.

Community diagnosis and training of professionals

If community diagnosis is to be adopted more widely then it needs to enter the training of health professionals. Medical undergraduates and postgraduates need to understand the process of working with a community to resolve problems.

Undergraduates

It is easy for community medicine, as presently taught, to seem boring to medical students, as it is very theoretical and usually accompanied by technical lectures. Human relationships are lacking and there is none of the excitement of seeing an ill person recover, nor the intellectual satisfaction of making a good diagnosis, when the subject is confined to the lecture room. If community diagnosis is to be taught effectively then students should be in the field using a problem-solving approach. It is far more satisfying actually talking to people about the problems they face, and hearing their ideas on how to tackle them, than to read about the problems in a textbook. The logistics of such an exercise may be daunting. However, students who have heard from families first hand, then put their views on paper or to a group, will never forget the experience. The following steps could be undertaken by medical students (perhaps working with students from another discipline):

(1) identify a neighbourhood (1000 families);

(2) allocate groups of four students;

(3) Distribute tasks:

   (a) collect demographic information and health statistics;

   (b) interview non-health professionals;

   (c) interview health professionals;

   (d) interview selected members of the local population.

(The interviews would collect views on a specific topic—for example, mental health; elderly health; family planning; child health; youth problems; women's problems. This would ensure that the area could be used again for a different topic on a future occasion.)

(4) allocate a time period (two weeks?) and a tutor who would provide back-up and point to references;

(5) write up and present the project: (i) to the local community; (ii) to tutor and colleagues. Marks would be allocated accordingly.

The projects when collected together would provide a fine database for health planning in the district.

Postgraduates

All paediatric trainees should understand the community diagnosis approach and hence it should enter the curriculum for qualifying examinations. The subject would most suitably be included within an epidemiology or public health module (or ideally a community health module), of which few are available at present. Practical experience will be less easy to obtain than theoretical—even community paediatric training does not always include direct contact with members of a local community. All community paediatric trainees should, if possible, be attached to a community development project for a period to learn about how to work closely with community groups.

As with bedside clinical training, training for community diagnosis should follow certain precautions and rules of ethics. No community should be considered as a simple field-training site where students come to practise their analytic skills and to collect data for academic ends, however noble these ends may be. A community is a living entity, in a way similar to an individual patient. Therefore, it is important, for example, not to raise false hopes for solutions while inquiring about existing problems.

The best way of avoiding such pitfalls is to integrate and initiate the training process within health service activities. One way this can be done is by drawing up contracts between training institutions and health services. One may then speak of 'action learning', that is learning which is designed not just to teach problem identification or assessment of needs, but becomes simultaneously part of the mechanism for developing and implementing the solutions with the local health personnel and authorities and the local community.[19]

This is what 'community oriented medical education' (COME) attempts to achieve, COME is a means of assuring educational relevance to community needs and of implementing a community-oriented educational programme. It consists of learning activities that take place within the community and in which not only students but also teachers, local health professionals, members of the community, and representatives of other sectors are actively engaged throughout the educational experience.[20]

References

1. Curtis, S.E., Taket, A.R., and Thuriaux, M.C. (1990). Vers la Santé pour tous dans la Région européenne de l'OMS—Surveillance des progrès accomplis, IV. Résponses des systémes de santé. *Rev. Epidém. et Santé Publ.* **38**, 19–26.
2. Stone, L. (1989). Cultural Crossroads of community participation in development: a case from Nepal. *Human Organisation* **48**, 206–13.
3. Foster, G. (1982). Community development and primary health care: their conceptual similarities. *Medical Anthropology* **6**, 183–95.

4. WHO/UNICEF (1978). *Primary health care. Report of the International Conference on primary health care, Alma-Ata, USSR, 6–12 September 1978*, WHO Geneva.
5. Green, L.W. (1986). The theory of participation: a qualitative analysis of its expression in national and international health policies. *Adv Health Educ. Promotion* **1**, 211–36.
6. Rifkins, S. (1986). Lessons from community participation in health programmes. *Health Policy and Planning* **1**, 240–9.
7. Rifkin, S. (1990). *Community participation in maternal and child health/family planning programmes*. WHO, Geneva.
8. Eng, E. and Blanchard, L. (1991). Action-oriented community diagnosis: a health education tool. *International Quarterly of Community Health Education* **11**, 93–110.
9. Rifkin, S.B., Muller, F. and Bichmann, W. (1988). Primary health care: on measuring participation. *Soc. Sci. Med.* **26**, 931–40.
10. Pineault, R. (1976). Eléments et étapes d'elaboration d'un programme de santé communautaire. *Union Médicale du Canada* **105**, 1208–14 (In French only.)
11. Lecorps, P. (1986). *Le diagnostic communautaire*. Communication personnelle, National School of Public Health, Rennes, France.
12. Lemeshow, S., and Robinson D. (1985). Surveys to measure programme coverage and impact: a review of the methodology used by the expanded programme on immunization. *World Health Quarterly* **38**, 65–75.
13. Pechevis, M. (1991). Community diagnosis. In *Diseases of children in the subtropics and tropics* (4th edn), (ed. P. Stanfield, M. Briorton, M. Chan, J. Parkin, A. Waterston *et al.*), Edward Arnold, London.
14. Forfar, J.O. (1978). Demography and vital statistic. In *Textbook of Paediatrics*, (ed. J.O. Forfar and G.C. Arneil). Livingstone, Edinburgh.
15. De Maeseneer, J. and Debunne, M. (1988). Patients: a health care resource. *World Health Forum* **9**, 449–53.
16. Evans, F. (1987). *The Newcastle community midwifery care project: an evaluation report*. Newcastle Health Authority.
17. Stacy, R. (1990). *Cowgate children's centre: evaluation report 1987–89*. Save the Children Fund, Newcastle upon Tyne.
18. Save the Children (1991). *Child health strategy*. Newcastle Health Authority/Local Authority (mimeo).
19. Gabbay, J. (1991). Courses of action. The case of experiential learning programmes in public health. *Public Health* **105**, 39–50.
20. Hamad, B. (1991). Community-oriented medical education: what is it? *Medical Education* **25**, 16–22.

35 Measuring and improving quality of life for children

Bengt Lindström

Children's quality of life in a public health perspective

Most studies that claim to deal with children's health focus on the opposite, i.e. death, disease, disadvantages, and disabilities. These approaches are understandable in the light of the research traditions involved in clinical medicine, public health, and sociology where the focus generally is on risk factors and risk populations. Unfortunately these studies often fail to consider the positive aspects of health. What is needed, in contrast to the above descriptions, is a complementary approach where health is seen as a resource that enables people to reach their full capacity and lead an active and productive life. Concepts like 'well-being' and, more explicitly, 'quality of life' bring forward these aspects.

People in general express their preferences as their definition of quality of life (QoL). Some prefer listening to music, some the harmony of life, some the intimacy of their partner, some to have candy every day, and so on. In everyday language the preferences are usually connected to positive values. The preferences are individual and cannot serve as a definition but they have to be considered when applying quality of life in practice if the objective is to satisfy needs or making resources available.

Most sciences argue for a positive value when approaching quality of life, therefore a QoL theory should be constructed around a positive value system. In principle one may argue that a wide definition of health has much in common with quality of life. In the last decades more interest has been directed towards issues that enhance peoples' possibilities of improving their health potential and thereby promoting their health. Recently such research into so-called salutogenic factors has begun also in the context of children. The scope of studying these factors will bring a new quality and focus to health.

The global health policy and QoL

Since WHO started to develop a global health policy, starting in 1977, leading to the *Health for all* strategy, an increasing consideration has been given to quality of life issues. Basically, WHO is striving for a positive view on health, making an inventory of the health resources available both on an individual and on a societal level. The shift from the medical focus towards the social and psychological context of health started much earlier. In its constitution in 1946 WHO defined a health concept based on the three dimensions of physical, mental, and social well-being. The spiritual dimension was later added as a fourth dimension. There has also been a shift from a health service approach towards a population and societal approach where health is considered to be a general political issue concerning all. The focus has moved from a curative approach through protective and preventive issues to health promotion which offers the possibility of developing and investigating the health resources available rather than dealing with health problems only. The WHO policy documents also indirectly give indications of quality of life issues when stating that: 'it is not only a question of adding years to life but adding life to years.' A specific target on QoL was added in 1991: 'By the year 2000 all people should have the opportunity to develop and use their health potential in order to lead socially, economically and mentally fulfilling lives.' In WHO's interpretation, QoL is to lead such a fulfilling life but no other definition is given.

In health science, QoL has mainly been used in the assessment of the well-being of patients with chronic disease or analysing the cost/benefit of medical interventions. It seems, from the orientation of quality of life research in the health sector, that there is a risk of weakening the potentially positive value of QoL through this disease-orientated research. This can ultimately lead to the same fate as that of the health concept which, to the general public, is strongly linked with disease. Therefore it would be important to address QoL from the positive side, investigate the resources of the population instead of analysing problems only. It would be important to try to find a definition that would create a common framework and thus enable interdisciplinary approaches. The definition of QoL within medicine has often been neglected, probably because of its complexity, but this greatly reduces the possibilities of comparative research.

This chapter will make an overview and analysis of some of the different views on quality of life and relate it to children.

What is quality of life?

Semantics

In dictionaries quality is defined as the degree of a capacity, often in the sense of a good or first class capacity. In philosophy, the word 'quality' means capacities in general. Psychology uses the term as a capacity that can be perceived by our senses (e.g. form, taste, size). Life has been described as a series of physiological processes between birth and death and said to be the opposite of death. Biological life can be seen, in its most reduced form, as mere physiological survival while all additions can be considered as adding qualities to life. The combination of the two words, quality and life, can be understood as the essential characteristics of life which, to the general public, often has been interpreted as the positive values of life or the good parts of life.

Historical aspects—in search of the 'good life'

Creation, meaning of life, survival, and death form some of the central questions that have engaged mankind throughout history. Ideas about these issues have been expressed in early myths, religion, and philosophy which have later influenced the societal attitudes of life and formulated general norms for ways of living.

In western tradition, Plato stated that protected life, where man lives beyond reach of destiny and chance, was the only worthwhile condition for the good life. Logical reasoning and contemplation of truth were the highest values in life where man was supposed to escalate above human feelings and perspectives. On the contrary, Aristotle, a pupil of Plato, stated that a life without challenge and engagement in human relationships, even when this involved risk taking, was worthless.

A parallel to the different views of Plato and Aristotle can easily be seen in different definitions of health. The WHO health definition that describes as state of complete well-being in a physical, mental, and social sense resembles Plato's thinking, while modern dynamic health theories that include risk or stress as natural parts of life resemble Aristotle's definition of the 'good life'.

Sociology—'being happy'

A seminal work in the development of a scientific approach to quality of life was a sociological study on welfare called 'Having, loving and being'. Allardt's innovation was to combine both objective and subjective perspectives to material and immaterial resources and needs when describing welfare.

In Allardt's study, quality of life was defined as the immaterial resources and needs of people, or people's relationships to others people, society, and nature (loving and being) and the subjective perceptions of the same. The corresponding material needs and their perceptions (having) were called 'level of living'. Allardt's ultimate objective was to describe welfare where the level of living forms the contextual framework of quality of life. Later, a tradition of describing subjective perceptions has developed where satisfaction or happiness have been the essential components. The argument for using such an approach has been that subjective well-being can be interpreted as a total outcome measure of an individual's situation. Problems arrive in comparative studies, since subjective perceptions are to a large extent individually or culturally determined. Children create a special problem because it seems that subjective perceptions are less stable in childhood and therefore considered less reliable. They also require more sophisticated methods of measurement.

Economics—'being rich'

Gross National Product (GNP) per capita has been the traditional measurement of economic growth and as such often regarded as a QoL measurement on a country level. There are, however, several reasons to question the use of GNP other than as a measurement for economic growth. First, GNP does not consider the distribution of the economic resources within a population. Second, conditions such as an extended health and social insurance including, for example, parental leaves, employment for weak groups such as the disabled or mentally retarded, reduced working hours for parents of small children, are all factors that lower the GNP per capita. On the other hand they may make it easier to live in a society and improve the citizens' quality of life. A fact often neglected is the lack of evidence that quality of life always corresponds positively to economic growth. There is initially a somewhat linear correlation between an increase in economic standard and QoL which then levels out and there is a possibility of a decrease in QoL in spite of economic growth.

Reacting to the use of a country's GNP as a measure of QoL of its citizens the World Bank developed an index called 'physical quality of life index' (PQLI) which include social and health-related variables: infant mortality, life expectancy at the age of one, and general literacy rate. Later an index focusing on the needs of children was developed by adding two more variables: children in the labour force (as a health risk factor) and female literacy rate (as a factor enhancing child health).

The greatest use of these indices has been in the comparison of conditions between poor and developed nations. Several UN agencies have used similar variables to describe health resources or quality of life in their annual reports (such as UNICEF's report, *State of the world's children* and the UNDP 'human development index'. However, the value of children seems to change with socio-economic development; in less developed countries children are considered as an economic asset while they are more of an economic burden in developed countries.

Industrialized nations tend to hold the top positions in these indices but in contrast to the use of GNP only there are several nations having low GNPs that score well on these indices. One example is Costa Rica, which competes with some of the richest nations of the world. Outcome measures such as under-five-year survival of children, accident rates among children, tend to correlate positively to high ratings on these indices.

The medical view—staying normal on the disease–health axis

The development of nursing science, new intervention methods and technology have increased the possibilities of survival for people suffering from diseases that previously caused premature death. Attempts to improve the quality of the survival time has also increased research interest in quality of life issues. The medical specialties that have taken the greatest interest in quality of life have usually been related to chronic disease, such as cancer care, medical rehabilitation, and psychiatry, but lately many other medical specialities and policy makers have joined. A wide variety of different assessment schemes have been developed both for self-administration or in the form of interviews.

In a different voice

When structuring a model for quality of life that responds to the above requirements there is a need to look into studies where the primary purpose has been to investigate or establish resources for the population. Such examples can be found within behaviourial science, where attempts to set objectives for good mental health have been made. The foundation for good mental health is intimately connected to conditions of early development in childhood. An individual who is given optimal conditions for physical, social, mental, and spiritual development will also find it easier to obtain good quality of life. This would indicate that the coming generations, or children, would be a strategic entry point when considering quality of life issues. This fact is also stated in the European *Health for all* document. Jahoda, one of the early researchers in this field, goes one step further stating: 'When individuals are assured good conditions for mental health, they will also be able to improve their quality of living' which, according to Jahoda, means that mental health has a higher priority than other dimensions.

The criteria for good mental health were: having a positive self-perception, being active and able to develop one's capabilities, being an integrated person, being able to take independent decisions and actions without isolation from other people, having a good sense of reality and emphatic skills, being able to create deep and lasting relations to other persons out of which at least one should be with the opposite sex.

In the Nordic countries the Norwegian psychologist Siri Naess developed Jahoda's model further when creating the concept 'inner quality of life'. The starting point for Naess is assigning values to aspects of quality of life. The quality of life increases to a higher level when an individual is

(1) active;

(2) has good inter-personal relations;

(3) has high self-esteem;

(4) has a basic mood of joy.

These values are not ranked in a hierarchy but are considered as being equally important.

The criticism against Naess is that the value system may create strong individuals that have little solidarity towards society as a whole. A further development of Naess's ideas towards a system taking into consideration both the psychological inner quality of life concept and the societal factors has been made by Kajandi in 1981 who included three spheres of life: the external conditions, the inter-personal conditions, and the inner psychological conditions.

A framework for a quality of life definition

People in general find it difficult to define QoL because they use unique personal preferences and perceptions as their own references for QoL. These cannot serve as a general definition. A QoL definition should be applicable on an interdisciplinary level, therefore the general definition of QoL has to be broad. Since it is difficult to give the QoL concept an exact definition it has been suggested that framework definitions be used which can serve as sensitizing concepts that encompass people's experience of QoL. Such a framework can give guidance to empirical applications and is supportive of interdisciplinary research.

It is suggested here that the following framework be used for a definition:
Quality of life is the total existence of an individual, a group or a society.

This framework requires a specification of the essential life spheres and a breakdown into research variables. It is suggested here that spheres shown in Table 35.1 be used.

The general QoL model is universal and includes the essential components human existence. The life spheres as such are interdependent but function as a clarifying structure to QoL. Societies have different levels of requirements within the spheres, depending on the culture and stage of development. Preferences and subjective perceptions of people are also to a large extent determined by cultural and individual traits. These facts make comparative research difficult because there will always be components that cannot be exactly defined but only put into a general framework (Table 35.2).

Table 35.1 *A general quality of life model, life spheres, and dimensions*

Spheres	Dimensions (objective/subjective)	Examples
Global	1. Macro environment 2. Human rights 3. Politics	Clean environment Democratic rights Culture
External	1. Work 2. Economy 3. Housing	Employment Income Type of housing
Interpersonal	1. Family 2. Intimate 3. Extended	Structure and function of social relationships
Personal	1. Physical 2. Mental 3. Spiritual	Growth, development activity, self-esteem, meaning of existence

Table 35.2 *Three components of quality of life: the objective conditions, the subjective perceptions, and the cultural or individual preferences*

Objective conditions	Preferences	Subjective perceptions
Global, external, interpersonal, personal* (material, immaterial)	Freedom of choice, solidarity+, to read, to exercise, make politics, play music, contemplate, relax	Perceived satisfaction of objective conditions (happiness, general satisfaction)

Children in the context of quality of life

Children are seldom given a value of their own which is reflected in laws, policies, and attitudes towards the child population. Therefore a QoL model for children particularly should respect the intrinsic value of this target group. In principle, QoL for children should be based on the same criteria as for any other age group and be given the same independence and dignity. As such, children may need special considerations and support but this has to be based on their own needs and perspectives, as stated in the child Convention: 'for the best interest of the child'. The role of the supportive social network and society at large is to create an environment which stimulates the child's growth and development in combination with the long-term objective of creating a good QoL for the child. It is not a question of describing the dependency of the child but to define what factors are important for the child and set what ever base values are used in a QoL instrument in a child's perspective.

The main difference of childhood as compared to others periods of life is the rapid development that occurs in a physical, mental, and social perspective. Different development scales makes it possible to evaluate how well the child has developed in relation to its genetic potential as of length and weight, and to estimate neurosensory, cognitive, emotional, moral, an social development by measuring the deviations from the 'normal'. A joint interdisciplinary evaluation will give an approximation of the age appropriateness of the child's development. The child's socio-economic background is not included in these assessment scales although such background factors are known to influence development. Another important aspect is the difference in development between the sexes. Any study of children requires an understanding of children's development including emotional and cognitive development. However, these developmental scales mainly give a quantification of the development of the child. QoL studies of children on the individual or small group level require qualitative methods which enable descriptions of individual preferences and subjective perceptions. In population studies, quantitative methods such as questionnaires are more practical but can be combined with qualitative approaches.

Global conditions

Starting from a very broad perspective, one can discuss in terms of the 'macro' environment. Even then the growing individual is at greatest risk of exposure because of an increased vulnerability. Environment pollutants, such as dioxin, can be found in growing bone and human milk. Questions of legal justice and equity are also made explicit through the vulnerability of children. The protection of the child has been considered to be important enough to require special international agreements apart from the *UN Declaration of human rights*. The declaration of child rights of 1924, recently completed with the *Convention on the rights of the child,* are the present international guidelines. Countries that have ratified the child convention have committed themselves to report on children's development every fifth year and an international committee has been appointed by UNICEF to control and enforce the convention in practice. This convention was for the first time included in the revised WHO *Health for all* targets in 1991 emphasizing a joint effort to improve the conditions of children from two UN organizations. Recently, human rights, also for the first time, have been included as in indicator in the UN human development index.

External conditions

The optimal external conditions for a child are difficult to define since they are dependent on the interaction between the child's own resources and capabilities and the surrounding resources within the family and society. A base requirement for the human being is food, shelter, and a social structure that enables development of the skills needed for survival and growth. Transformed to children in a modern society it is a question of the family with its education, occupation, and housing as well as the parent's genetics, their personalities, and knowledge through life experiences that will form the first social and economic structure around the child. Ultimately any societal support aimed at the family will be to the benefit of the child. The resources available create the external environment and give the child a possibility to obtain certain kinds of material conditions such as food and housing but also stimuli and models for the child's own future pattern of living.

It has been shown that the number of families with dependent children are increasing among the poor in Europe. The EC Observatory on National Family Policy has commented that any family with dependent children is underprivileged by comparison with households not have dependent children. Another new feature is that no longer do larger families predominate in this group but a new dimension in poverty is emerging where smaller families are increasingly vulnerable. In the period 1980–85 children became relatively worse off and the rates of poverty among children are significantly higher than for the population as a whole.

A Norwegian comparison of governmental expenditures on children (aged 0–16) as compared to the elderly (aged 67–99) showed that although the children comprised 23 per cent of the population, they received just 17 per cent of the total budget while the elderly received 42 per cent, comprising only 14 per cent of the total population. In Norway, expenditure per capita on children in local communities has been estimated to be only a third of what is spent on the elderly.

Urban areas create environments that can cause problems for the child such as environmental pollution, physical health hazards such as traffic, social restrictions, and isolation. Traffic accidents, for instance, are a main cause of child mortality and morbidity all over the world. Constructing means of transportation that are safe for the child and run on non polluting energy would be a major advantage not only for children but for the whole population. Children can have worse housing conditions in terms of space and convenience than their parents in spite of living in the same flat or building. Outcome measures such as the mental health of children can be correlated to the type of housing, where children living in high storey buildings seem to have more mental problems. Conflicting ideals between adults and children can occur; an adult might consider living in the centre of a big city ideal, giving easy access to work, social contacts, services, and recreation while the same setting for the child can lead to a total dependence on the parents and an increase in the health hazards. As an example, a high-storey building makes it difficult for a four year old child to contact a friend in the adjacent block because of traffic and elevators.

In a socially segregated society, external conditions have a further impact on the child's life, since the patterns of living are set by the above factors and they influence the child's future education, social contacts, and ways of living as an adult. There are several studies on child health that point in this direction, also in developed countries.

Education as such can be seen as a power structure in society and the education level and occupation of the parents affect the child's choice of education. In spite of free education in the Nordic countries, children tend to follow an educational path similar to that of their parents, thus preserving their social stratification which makes social migration an uncommon event. Most outcome measures related to health correlate positively to social class, which is usually based on the father's social class. As an indicator of children's social class it has been suggested that the combined professions of the parents be used but it seems that the father's occupation still correlates better with the child's health status.

Interpersonal conditions

The interpersonal conditions include the structure and function of the social networks. The family of origin, its individuals, values, and resources form the social basis for the development of the child. The key persons involved are the parents and siblings living in the household. The parents and the child form the primary social group where the mother, initially, is the key person in a biological and psychological sense, acting as the child's social interface. Later, other members of the family, the extended family, peers, and society at large influence the child and play different roles in the various developmental stages.

Siblings are potentially the longest lasting relationships. In many developed countries the sizes of families are decreasing and family life patterns are changing, leaving children with fewer close relatives. There is an extensive literature on the negative effects of single parenthood on children's material and social conditions. Today both fathers and mothers are often employed outside the family. The positive effects of high employment can have negative consequences for children simply because the parents' available time for family life is reduced, especially when inconvenient working hours or long trips to work are involved.

Personal conditions

The personal conditions include physical, mental, and spiritual dimensions. Physical growth is multifactorial, depending on genetics, environment, nutrition, and social conditions. Even affluent societies have differences in growth between the social classes. The prerequisites for mental and spiritual well being are perhaps even more complex, functioning as an outcome of genetics, personality, temper, experience, preferences, physical, and social environment. There is strong evidence that the prerequisites for mental health are important components of the conditions that promote health as a whole. Models for the development of personal conditions can be found in research focusing on health as a resource, i.e. salutogenic research identifying general resistance resources (i.e. economy, social structure, knowledge, experience, intelligence, culture, belief systems). A new concept has lately been introduced, the sense of coherence, which is a capacity that enables people to maintain their health in spite of negative life events and hardships. The central components are being able to understand a situation (the cognitive component), having a sense of control (the behavioural component), and finding a meaning (motivational component). This framework has also been developed for studies of children and young people. Rutter has studied resilience in childhood focusing on protective factors which support the individual in crisis situations (i.e. social functioning, self-esteem, basic mood). Werner and Smith have studied socially deprived children in longitudinal studies trying to find out why some children are able to develop normally, do well in school, and later as adults, to hold jobs, create stable relationships, and raise children who also do well in spite of so-called high-risk life conditions. These factors of resilience are, for instance, the capability to find social support, to elicit positive feelings and empathy. It has been shown that the salutogenic factors correlate positively to QoL.

The QoL spheres mainly have a practical importance to structure and organize the components into an entity, but many of the various components are interdependent. Self-esteem is, for instance, not only a personal factor, it can be enhanced by the acceptance and support of the social network.

Child development as related to quality of life

A description of the quality of life instrument used in this chapter is related here to different stages of childhood development.

The newborn

External conditions

The external conditions are initially completely dependent on the immediate environment, i.e. the conditions of the parents and the society they belong to. The family conditions (housing, social status, and economy) rule the child.

Interpersonal relations (family, friends, intimate relations)

Initially the relation to the primary carer (usually the mother) is the most important factor but the indirect relations to the social environment are also mediated through her (child–mother–father–siblings–extended network).

Inter-psychological conditions

It is essential for the newborn child to develop and stimulate his senses (vision, hearing, touch, smell, taste) in order to be able to be active and activate others. Self-image and the basic mood is, as far as is known, little developed. External and internal stimuli are modified by temper and personality and serve as a basis of developing the psychological conditions.

Toddlers

The external conditions are much the same as for the newborn, i.e. parental conditions are important. The child's 'work' is the function the child has in the family or in the institution. Housing conditions are basically the same as the parents' but in a child perspective they may serve quite a different function. Within the house the child may have different living conditions compared with the adults, as described earlier. Also the possibilities for a child may be limited by traffic, elevators, stairs. There is no independent economy.

Interpersonal relations are still greatly influenced by the nuclear family. Parents and siblings serve as the platform for basic trust, while the child also seeks the contact of the other children and adults.

The inner psychological conditions are already broad-based enough to allow interpretation of new experience. The way the child handles dramatic experiences and the immediate environment will play a major role in the development and integration of the child's personality. For instance, it may be impossible to explain the idea of a painful medical intervention (such as a vaccination) to the child, but if it is performed in a way that enables the child to prepare, react, and feel comfort and support in spite of the pain, we may form a basis for acceptance. The values and attitudes of the immediate environment are of utmost importance.

School age

This period will, for most children, introduce some form of external socialization as the child enters school. It is also represents the first societal demand on the child. The workplace of the child is the school where he gains knowledge and learns to socialize in a broader context. The child receives no economical support but in many countries primary school is free of charge, which is recommended in the UN Convention. Housing and economy is still dependent on the family.

There is also an expansion of the social network. Peers gain an increasing influence and relationships to friends are made. The intimate relation is still linked to the parents.

Activities are intense in the form of playing and a need to master skills. Competence in the activities strengthen the self-esteem. Basic mood seems, on the surface, to be harmonious since the child gives very few expressions, which has been interpreted as a 'calm period' (named 'the latency' by Freud). Present knowledge is more inclined to discuss a more conflicting internal life where psychosomatic symptoms become common.

Adolescence

School is still the dominating arena in working life. Employment in leisure time also occurs which enables a greater independence as of economy, but basically the economy and housing is still dependent on the family.

The family influence on social life decreases and reaches its minimum in the middle of this period. Peers are the major group of influence. Sexual maturation also increases interest in forming intimate relations.

Activities are dominated by sports, music, and other cultural expressions. The self-image is influenced by success in these activities as well as by the physical and psychological changes in conjunction with sexual maturation. There are great variations between individuals and the genders and the spread in onset may vary up to five years. Basic mood is often relatively unstable and rapidly shifting.

An example: children's QoL in the Nordic countries

Depending on the society the child is living in there will be different basic conditions depending on, for instance, the cultural values and the socio-economic circumstances. The extreme is a country where there is a great risk of not surviving the early years of life compared to a country where this risk is negligible. The differences can of course be more subtle. Therefore the base values will vary depending on what society is studies but the QoL framework as such can be applied universally to any society.

An analysis of society in general could help to identify what kind of societal forces can be mobilized to create conditions that enhance the children's QoL. Here the five Nordic societies are analysed in a child QoL perspective.

In international comparative statistics on economics, welfare, and health the five Nordic countries (Denmark, Finland, Iceland, Norway, and Sweden) generally have fairly positive outcomes. The human development index presented by the United Nations development fund place three Nordic countries among the top ten. The physical quality of life index developed by the World Bank in the late 1970s ranked four Nordic countries first. The only existing quality of life index for children, the national index of children's quality of life, is based on infant mortality, life expectancy, general literacy rate, women enrolled in primary school, and child work, and ranks Iceland first. Further singular health indicators such as life expectancy, infant mortality, and perinatal mortality usually rank the Nordic countries among the top ten in the world. Risk factors such as child abuse and neglect are as common as in other developed countries. Accident rates, especially traffic accidents, are low. Self-destructive patterns, i.e. suicide rates, are comparably high, especially among young males in Finland.

These countries have stable democratic traditions with a well developed infrastructure including integrated family functions and an extensive support system for families with children. Children are given priority and respected on the political agenda and special considerations are given in the legislation to strengthen the position of children within the societies. All Nordic countries have been actively involved in the development of the *UN Convention on the rights of the child* and also ratified the same. On the other hand, these countries have adopted a Western urbanized pattern of living which includes many forces that counteract the value of family and raising children. Employment rates are high also among women. In spite of generally good economic resources which would enable families to have children, other interests and values are higher on the agenda; personal careers and development are more important than the value of having more children. Consequently nativity is low, and weak and isolated social networks, including less stable family structures, are common.

The model for resolving family crises is divorce. Mass media and the general public have accepted fairly high divorce rates. Divorce is socially acceptable, which has both positive and negative consequences; a divorce is no longer a social stigma, which is positive for the parties involved, but on the other hand because of its general acceptance, many couples never try to solve a crisis within the family because divorce is considered the societal model for conflict resolution. The mass media has enforced the image of high divorce rates. This is partially true but still most children grow up in a nuclear family with their biological parents.

In these countries a study of children's quality of life has been carried out. It was directed at 15 000 randomly selected children and also to about 3000 children with specific disabilities. The information was collected through questionnaires.

Sweden

Among the Nordic countries, children in Sweden had the highest overall quality of life. Both the objective life conditions and the perceived subjective satisfaction were high. Although Norwegian children had equally high objective conditions and Finnish children had equally high subjective conditions, Sweden rated high in both aspects. Swedish children had the highest self-esteem, the highest activity level, and the best basic mood of all, thus having the best quality of life among Nordic children. This is so in spite of not having the highest incomes or the highest educational level of Nordic families nor living in the best houses and not even having the best social networks (in fact, they were the most likely to face a major negative life event).

Denmark

Danish parents had the lowest educational level and only intermediate jobs and income levels but the parents had most time to spend with their children and Danish children were most likely to live in a spacious house and have a room of their own.

Major negative life events were almost as common as in Sweden and only Finnish children had fewer siblings. The self-esteem and basic mood was second only to that of Swedish children.

Norway

Norwegian parents had the best employment and their children were most likely to live in detached houses with a housing standard equalling that of the Danes. The children were the ones most likely to have two parents and also lived in the biggest households having most siblings. This was also indicated in the perceived well-being, as Norwegian families had the highest level of satisfaction with family life and the best conditions regarding family networks. However, Norwegian families were least satisfied with societal support. The self-esteem and basic mood of Norwegian children were equal to the Danes but the activity levels were lower.

Finland

The Finnish families expressed the second highest level of satisfaction and they were the ones who were most pleased with extended networks and the societal support. Contrary to the Norwegians, Finnish children were living in the smallest households having the fewest siblings and they were the least likely to have a room of their own. Major negative life events were least frequent in Finland but peer acceptance was lowest.

Iceland

Most strikingly, the level of satisfaction was much lower in Iceland, influencing all quality of life spheres. Icelandic parents had the best education and the highest incomes but they also expressed the lowest degree of satisfaction with these conditions as with most other quality of life aspects considered here. The basic mood of the children equalled the Finnish but activity levels and self-esteem, especially, were low.

When the conditions of the children with cystic fibrosis and myelomeningocoele were compared with the average children, the inequities for children with disabilities in the Nordic countries as compared to their normal peers were rather small in terms of material well-being. This result differs from most previous research which claims that families with disabled children have lower socio-economic resources than average families. Literature generally claims that social support networks are less developed and family breakdowns more common in families with disabled children. This result was partly repeated but the differences were smaller than expected. The greatest differences occurred among the personal conditions. It seemed that a visible motor handicap such as myelomeningocoele reduced peer acceptance while children with cystic fibrosis had more psychosomatic symptoms. The self-esteem of the disabled children was rated much lower by the parents than among the control group. It also decreased for the disabled the older they were.

A high level of satisfaction towards the various aspects of life was found in the reference population. Over 60 per cent indicated they were satisfied. The proportion that indicated they were 'very satisfied' was higher in the disability groups.

Conclusion

Although concepts such as health, welfare, and quality of life basically carry positive values, they have most usually been used in descriptions of disease, problems, and misery. The world of science has to a large extent oriented itself towards problem descriptions to the extent that the positive aspects of life are forgotten. On the other hand, when people are asked about their general satisfaction of life, much to the researchers surprise, many seem to be pleased and even enjoy their lives. There has been increased demand to find ways of creating arenas for interdisciplinary research. The UN and WHO have stated this need specifically in their global health strategy called *health for all*. QoL is here developed into an interdisciplinary research model emphasizing the positive values of life. In many respects children are an extremely vulnerable group in society. Therefore, a QoL model for children could serve as a sensitive indicator of society's human investment and a powerful tool in health policy making because it is designed 'for the best interests of the child'.

References

An extensive list of references can be obtained through the following articles:

Lindström, B. (1992). Quality of life: a model for evaluating 'health for all'. *J. Sozial und Präventiv Medizin* **37**, 301–6.

Lindström, B. and Eriksson, B. (1993). Children's quality of life in the Nordic countries. *Journal of Quality of Life Research* **2**, Vol 1.

Geographical index

Africa
  accidents   177, 183
  aid programmes   63
  debt   48
  desertification   46
  ethnic minorities   412–13, 415, 425–7
  HIV   128, 130, 133, 135–6, 139–40
  literacy   60
  morbidity   52–5
  mortality   48, 50–1, 177
  nutrition   55–6
  population   46
  refugees   61, 420
  special needs   341
  see also names of individual countries
Albania   22, 177
Americas
  accidents   176
  special needs   341
  see also Central America; Latin America; North America; South America; United States of America
Antilles   342
Asia
  accidents   176
  ethnic minorities   413, 415–16, 420–9
  HIV   128
  literacy   60
  morbidity   52, 53, 55
  mortality   48, 50, 51
  nutrition   56
  population   46
  special needs   342
  see also names of individual countries
Australia
  ethnic minorities   412
  health promotion   517
  poverty   365
  special needs   341
Austria
  accidents   178
  child abuse   313
  iodine deficiency   284
  social paediatrics   22
  special needs   341

Bangladesh   415–16, 423, 425, 429, 545
Belgium
  accidents   178, 179
  community diagnosis   562–4
  ethnic minorities   415
  nutrition   274
  poverty   364
  social paediatrics   22
Bosnia   112
Brazil
  adolescent risk-taking   233, 246
  child abuse   319
  HIV   142
  morbidity   52
  poverty   368
Britain, *see* United Kingdom
Bulgaria
  accidents   178, 179, 181
  infant mortality   97
  social paediatrics   22
Burma   342, 413

Canada
  adolescent risk-taking   230–1, 241, 247
  health promotion   512
  HIV   132, 142
  poverty   365
  special needs   341, 343
Cape Verde Islands   341
Central America
  aid programmes   64
  debt   48
Central Europe
  accidents   177, 178
  family demographics   81, 91
  social paediatrics   22
  special needs   338
Chile   416
China
  accidents   177
  adolescent smoking   233
  ethnic minorities   413, 426, 428
  infant mortality   51
Costa Rica   51, 573
Croatia   22
Cuba   368
Cyprus   416, 420, 425–6, 490
Czechoslovakia (former)
  abortion   87
  immunization   502
  infant mortality   71–5, 78
  poverty   364
  refugees   416
  social paediatrics   22, 24

Denmark
  accidents   178, 183, 185
  family demographics   78, 83
  immunization   500
  infant mortality   97

Denmark (*cont.*)
  nutrition 273
  poverty 364
  quality of life 582, 583
  sexual abuse 105
  social paediatrics 22
  special needs 344

Eastern Europe
  accidents 177–9, 181, 183
  family demographics 81, 86, 89, 91
  immunization 499
  infant mortality 77–8, 97
  pollution 104, 157
  poverty 364
  refugees 416
  social paediatrics 22
  special needs 338
El Salvador 122–3
England and Wales, *see* United Kingdom
Eritrea 416
Ethiopia 233, 341, 416
Europe
  abortion 259
  accident mortality 174–91
  adolescent risk-taking 226, 231, 233, 235
  child abuse 312
  community participation 550
  demographic trends 69–108
  doctors per inhabitants 45
  family breakdown 397–9, 401
  growth and development 215
  health promotion/services 459–60, 462, 464, 467, 512–23
  historical aspects of childhood 199
  HIV 50, 128–9, 134–5, 137, 140
  immunization/infection 498–509
  infant mortality 50, 51, 97
  low birth-weight 381, 383, 389
  nutrition 270–91
  outcome/performance measures 478, 482, 484–5
  parent participation 540, 545–6
  pollution 154, 156–8, 169–70
  poverty 362–8, 373, 377
  quality of life 577
  refugees 418
  SIDS 297–9, 306
  social paediatrics 22–35
  special needs 42, 333–4, 337–8, 341
  see also Central Europe; Eastern Europe; Northern Europe; Southern Europe; Western Europe; *names of individual countries*

Fiji 341
Finland
  accidents 178, 183
  immunization 500

infant mortality 97
low birth-weight 381
nutrition 276
quality of life 582–4
social paediatrics 22
special needs 343
war 116
France
  accidents/injuries 178, 185, 229–31
  child abuse 312
  ethnic minorities 415
  family demographics 81
  historical aspects of childhood 196
  immunization 505
  low birth-weight 381, 383
  mortality 97, 99, 101
  nutrition 274, 275, 277
  parent partnership 545, 546
  poverty 364
  social paediatrics 22, 24

Gaza Strip, *see* Israel
Germany
  accidents/injuries 101, 183
  adolescent risk-taking 229, 237
  ethnic minorities 415, 420
  family demographics 89
  immunization 500
  infant mortality 78
  nutrition 276, 278, 284
  poverty 364, 366
  social paediatrics 22, 24, 26
  special needs 333, 334, 337–8
Ghana 418
Greece
  accidents 178, 179
  adolescent risk-taking 233, 234, 237
  family demographics 81, 89, 92
  G–6–PD deficiency 426
  infant mortality 97
  nutrition 274, 279, 284
  pollution 166, 167, 168
  poverty 364, 373
  social paediatrics 22, 24
Guyana 341

Haiti 134
Holland, *see* Netherlands
Hong Kong 413
Hungary
  accidents 178
  family demographics 87, 89
  immunization 502
  low birth-weight 383
  nutrition 282, 284
  poverty 364
  refugees 418
  satisfaction with life 105
  social paediatrics 22, 24

special needs 334–5

Iceland
  accidents 178
  immunization 500, 502
  quality of life 582, 584
India
  ethnic minorities 412–16, 422–6
  infant mortality 51
  pollution 156
Iran 418
Iraq 156, 418
Ireland
  accidents 178
  immunization 500
  poverty 364, 366, 372
  special needs 341
  see also Northern Ireland
Israel
  accidents 178
  immunization 58–9, 502
  nutrition 57
  war 111, 113, 116–18
Italy
  accidents 178
  adolescent risk-taking 233
  ethnic minorities 415, 420, 426
  family demographics 89, 92
  nutrition 274, 276, 284
  pollution 156
  poverty 364, 367, 369
  SIDS 297
  special needs 343

Jamaica 368
Japan
  accidents 177
  adolescent smoking 229, 233
  infant mortality 98
  pollution 156
  poverty 377

Kiribati 341
Korea 233

Latin America
  debt 48
  HIV 128
  morbidity 53, 55
  nutrition 56
  see also names of individual countries
Latvia (Lettonia) 97
Lebanon 111, 113, 116–17, 122
Lettonia (Latvia) 97
Lithuania 97, 370
Luxembourg
  accidents 178, 179
  poverty 364, 365
  social paediatrics 22

Madagascar 63
Malawi 134
Malaysia 413
Mali 341, 342
Malta 178
Mauritania 63
Mediterranean Region
  accidents 176
  organic disease 422, 425–6
  see also names of individual countries
Monaco 177
Morocco 426
Mozambique 111, 120

Nepal 425
Netherlands
  accidents/injuries 100–1, 178, 230–1
  ethnic minorities 415, 426
  immunization 499
  low birth-weight 383, 385–6, 388
  nutrition 272, 273, 287–8
  poverty 364
  SIDS 297, 301
  special needs 333
Netherlands Antilles 342
New Zealand 343, 412
Nicaragua 50
Nigeria
  adolescent smoking 233
  immunization 58
  poverty 368
  special needs 344
Nordic countries
  accidents 175
  families 81, 397, 399, 407, 409
  health service planning 460
  morbidity 100
  quality of life 574, 578, 581–4
  see also Denmark; Finland; Iceland;
          Norway; Sweden
North America
  ethnic minorities 412
  family demographics 86
  HIV 134
  nutrition 274
  special needs 332, 338
  see also Canada; United States of America
Northern Europe
  adolescent smoking 235
  families 81, 401
  health service planning 460
  nutrition 284
  pollution 155, 157
  social paediatrics 22
Northern Ireland 113–14, 116, 118–19, 367
Norway
  accidents/injuries 178, 230, 231
  childhood mortality 99, 100
  morbidity 105

Norway (*cont.*)
   nutrition   276
   poverty   364
   quality of life   578, 582, 583
   SIDS   300
   social paediatrics   22

Pakistan
   ethnic minorities   415–16, 418, 423–5
   special needs   342, 343
Palestine, *see* Israel
Panama   64
Philippines   342, 425
Poland
   accidents   178, 183
   family demographics   83–94
   infant mortality   97
   nutrition   272
   poverty   364
   social paediatrics   22
Portugal
   accidents   177, 178, 179
   child abuse   312
   ethnic minorities   415
   family demographics   81, 89
   iodine deficiency   284
   poverty   364
   social paediatrics   22, 24

Romania
   abortion   89, 319
   accidents   177, 178
   HIV   130
   immunization   502
   iodine deficiency   284
   orphans   198, 319
   social paediatrics   22

Sardinia   426
Saudi Arabia   368
Scandinavia
   community participation   550
   ethnic minorities   415
   immunization   499
   infant mortality   98
   nutrition   272, 275
   SIDS   297
   see also names of individual countries
Scotland
   adolescent risk-taking   240
   HIV   143
   low birth-weight   385
   nutrition   279, 281
   poverty   370
Senegal   233, 368
Sicily   284, 426
Singapore   413
Somalia   63, 418
South Africa   113–14, 117, 412

South America
   HIV   128
   morbidity   52, 55
   mortality   48, 50
   nutrition   56
   population   46
   special needs   341
   see also names of individual countries
Southern Europe
   family demographics   89, 92
   illegitimacy   78
   immunization   502
   pollution   155
   social paediatrics   22
   see also names of individual countries
Soviet Union (former), *see* USSR (former)
Spain
   accidents   178, 179
   family demographics   81, 89, 92
   immunization   499, 500
   intersectoral approaches   475
   nutrition   274, 277, 284
   poverty   364, 367, 373, 375
   social paediatrics   22, 24
Sri Lanka   51, 368, 425
Sudan   418
Sweden
   accidents   174, 177–8, 181, 184–7
   adolescent risk-taking   234, 239
   child abuse   312, 313
   families   81, 216, 398–400
   HIV   141
   hospital neonatal care   528
   infant mortality   71–4, 78, 97, 98
   morbidity   100, 103, 105
   nutrition   272, 273, 276, 277
   outcome/performance measures   479
   poverty   364, 366, 370, 377
   quality of life   582, 583
   social paediatrics   22, 24
   war   116
Switzerland
   accidents   178, 179, 183
   child abuse   313
   ethnic minorities   415
   family demographics   82
   immunization   502
   social paediatrics   22, 24

Tagikistan   97
Tahiti   233
Taiwan   156
Tanzania   46
Thailand   177, 185, 413
Tibet   412
Trinidad and Tobago   341
Tunisia   341, 342
Turkey
   accidents   177

ethnic minorities 415, 420–1, 426
immunization 500, 502
nutrition 279
Turkmenistan 97, 370

Uganda 114, 119, 139–40
United Kingdom
  accidents 99, 101, 178, 179
  adolescent risk-taking 229, 230–1, 235
  child abuse 311, 312, 313
  community participation 550, 564–6
  dental caries 103
  ethnic minorities 412, 415–18, 420, 423, 425–9
  families 81, 409
  health promotion 512
  height trends 102
  historical aspects of childhood 202
  HIV 130, 132
  immunizations 498–9, 502–8
  intersectoral issues 469–75
  in vitro fertilization 261
  low birth-weight 383, 385
  mortality 97, 99, 101
  nutrition 270–81, 285–7, 289
  parent partnership 541, 543–7
  poverty 362–8, 371–6
  SIDS 299, 304, 306
  social paediatrics 22, 24
  special needs 343, 349
  speech disorders 217
  wartime 116
  see also Northern Ireland; Scotland
United States of America
  accidents/injuries 177, 187
  adolescent risk-taking 225–6, 229–35, 239–49
  child abuse 311, 312, 314
  child soldiers 43
  community participation 551
  family breakdown 398, 399, 401–2, 409
  growth and development 203, 221

health promotion 516, 519
HIV 50, 128, 131, 134, 137–9, 142–3
immunization 503, 505
infant mortality 97
intersectoral approaches 469–70, 473
low birth-weight 381, 383–4
nutrition 272–5, 280, 281, 283, 291
parent partnership 541
poverty 365, 372
SIDS 301
special needs 341, 343, 344
temperamant studies 440
Uruguay 177, 233
USSR (former)
  accidents 177–8, 181, 183
  family demographics 88, 91
  immunization 499, 500, 502
  infant mortality 97
  nutrition 278
  pollution 156, 158, 168
  poverty 370
  social paediatrics 22

Venezuela 341
Vietnam 413, 414, 418, 428

Wales, *see* United Kingdom
Western Europe
  accidents 100, 177–9, 181, 183
  ethnic minorities 415, 416, 429
  family demographics 81, 86, 89
  parent partnership 541
  special needs 338
West Indies 415, 416, 422, 424

Yugoslavia (former)
  ethnic minorities 415
  family breakdown 407, 409
  war 112

Zaire 130

Subject index

abortion
  adolescents 235, 241
  demographic trends 78–9, 83, 87–9
  ethnic minorities 423
  fetal rights 259
  HIV infection 133, 134
  in vitro fertilization 260
  legislation 202–3
  outcome/performance measures 490
  prevention of disability 389
  rubella-associated 503
abuse, *see* child abuse
accidents 99–101, 174–91
  child abuse 312, 314, 315
  burns 164, 176, 181, 315, 318
  community issue 184–90, 559, 565
  developing countries 57, 176–7, 183, 185, 187
  drowning 100, 177, 181–3, 187, **230–1**, 234
  falls 99, 176–7, 180–1, 187, 234
  firearms 100, 231
  fires 100, 181, 187, 234
  health promotion 512
  homicide 100, 177, 231, 240
  outcome/performance measures 479, 484, 488, 495
  poisoning 99, 177–83, 370
  pollution 155–6, 165, 168, 170
  poverty 370, 372, 377
  prevention of 27, 174–6, 179–80, 183, **184**, 185–90
  quality of life 183, 573, 578, 582
  risks 185–9, 436
  road, *see* traffic accidents
  social paediatrics research 27
  teenage, *see* adolescents
  see also safety
acid rain 155, 157, 158
addiction, *see* drug abuse
adolescents 9, 196
  abuse of 246, 315, 316
  accidents **174–91**, 225–6, **229–31**, 234, 239–40, 245–9
    health service planning 462
    suicide 100, 231, 240
    Third World 57
  alcohol 227, 230, **233–4**, 235–44, **245**, 246–8
  developing countries 54, 57
  divorce sequelae 236, 403
  ethnic minorities **235**, 421, **422**, 426
  growth and development 214–15, 219, **227–9**, 249, 279

  health promotion/services 461, 514, 519
  HIV infection 140, **141–2**, 225, 240–8
  nutrition 242, **279**, 280, 283–6, 344
  pollution 165
  pregnancy 225, 235, 240, **241–2**, 245–9
    child abuse 316
    health promotion 470–3
    outcome/performance measures **494**
  preventive care 246–9, 471
  psychiatric problems 227, 238, 246, 343–7
  puberty 215, **344–5**, 346–7, 353, 495
  quality of life 581
  risk/resilience 225–56, 433–55, 519
  sexual behaviour 141–2, 225–7, **231–3**, 235–48, 345, **347–8**, 581
  special needs 334, 341–57
  war 113
adoption and fostering 25, 143, 261, 319
advocacy 377, 473, 514
Afro-Caribbeans 289, 420–2, 424–6, 429
age factors
  accidents 177–81, 183, 184, 188, 249
  adolescent risk-taking 226, 231–4, **235**, 240–3, 249
  child abuse 312, 313
  control of children 207
  dietary reference values 271
  divorce sequelae 403
  gestational 380–2
  growth and development 210, 213–14, 576
  HIV infection 141
  immunization/infections 499, 503
  outcome/performance measures 494, 495
  poverty 366
  risk/resilience 433, 434, 439, **444**
  sexual behaviour 81
  SIDS 298, 299, 301
  special needs 332, 346, 350
  toxic effects 162
  see also adolescents; fetus; infants; maternal age; pre-school children; school-age children; young adults
aggression 119, 320, 439
  see also violence
aid programmes 63–4, 551
AIDS, *see* HIV infection
air pollution 153–6, 157, 161–2, 165, 169–70
  respiratory illness 372
  rickets 279–80
alcohol
  adolescents 227, 230, **233–4**, 235–44, **245**, 246–8
  cardiovascular disease 88

Subject index

child abuse 313–14, 321
child health services 460
fetal alcohol syndrome 245
low birth-weight/prematurity 389
outcome/performance measures 479, 486, 494
poverty 373
SIDS 299
alienation 103, 143, 288
allergies 95, 100, 159, 162–6, 275
anaemia 112, 289, 421–5, **426**, 490–1
see also iron deficiency
anorexia nervosa 315–16, 351, 421
antenatal care **132–3**, 138, 242, 389, **422–6**, 490–1, 535
anxiety
  adolescents 227, 238, 345
  child abuse 321
  ethnic minorities 418–21, 428
  growth and development 211
  health promotion 517
  pollution 165
  premature babies 267, 527, 532
  risk/resilience 435–8, 441, 444–7
  SIDS 306
  war and children 112–15, 117, 120–1
apnoea 299, 300, 306, 317
Aries, P. 196, 197, 198, 201
Asians 413, 415–16, 420–9
  nutrition 276, 279–82, 286, **289**
  substance abuse 235
asbestos 157–9, 161–2, 166
asthma
  adolescents 343, 346, 351
  community participation 559, 566
  morbidity trends 104, 484
  outcome/performance measures 492
  pollution 162
  poverty 372
attitudes
  breast-feeding 272
  changing 373
  child abuse 322–3
  to childhood 198, 204
  community participation 556
  demographic trends 83, 86
  divorce 403
  ethnic minorities 420
  family/parental 211, 215, 216, 461, 506, 544
  health promotion/services 459–60, 514–18
  HIV infection 143
  immunization 506
  personal relationships 401
  quality of life 572, 576, 581
  reproductive technologies 263, 264
  risk-taking 226
  satisfaction 105–6, 486–7, 491–5, 547, 572, 583–4
  to special needs 331, 338, 349, 353

war 118–19
see also cultural issues; priority setting; religious belief
auxology, *see* growth and development

babies, *see* infants
BCG vaccination 54, 58, 138, 500
behavioural factors
  accident prevention 186
  adolescents 226–7, 239, 244, 247–8, 349, 353
  child abuse 314–16, 320–2
  community participation 551, 560, 565
  divorce 402
  ethnic minorities 412, 420, **421**, 422
  growth and development 218, 222
  health inequalities 373
  health professionals 529
  health promotion 512–20
  HIV infection 141
  low birth-weight 380, 386, 388, 527
  outcome/performance measures 484
  parental 211, 322, 372, **421**
  pollution 163, 164
  quality of life 579
  risk/resilience 433–43, 447–8
  sexual, *see* sexual behaviour
  SIDS 305
  special needs 334, 349, 353
  war 112–15, 118–20
see also lifestyle factors; risk factors/risk-taking; violence
bereavement 114, 305
biopsychosocial factors 464–6
see also genetic factors; psychological issues; social/socioeconomic issues
birth, *see* childbirth
birth control
  adolescent risk-taking 232–3, 235–8, 240–1
  community participation 552, 554–5
  condoms 241–2, 246, 248, 516–17
  developing countries 64
  demographic trends 77–8, 82, 86–9
  health service planning 461
  HIV infection 133, 141–2
  see also abortion
birth rates
  adolescents 241–2, 249
  developing countries 45, 59
  Europe 82, 84, 85, 89
  health promotion/services 460, 512
  see also fertility and infertility
birth-weight, *see* low birth-weight
blacks, *see* racial factors
blood transfusions 130, 141
'boat people,' Vietnamese 414
body mass index 286
bonding 135, 213–14, 325, 384

Subject index

bottle feeding 138, **273–5**, 298, 426
  see also formula feeding
boys, *see* gender issues
brain damage 163, 284, 320, 427, 506
breast-feeding **272–3**, 275, 280–3, 286–90
  developing countries 51, 56, **57–8**, 64
  ethnic minorities 426
  HIV infection 129–30, 138
  outcome/performance measures 495
  pollution 159, 162
  premature babies 266–7, 384–5, 527, 530–1, 534–8
  SIDS 298
bulimia nervosa 421
burns 164, 176, 181, 315, 318

cadmium 156–7, 161–2, 164
caesarian sections 260
calcium 160, 274, 277–8, 287–8, 290
calorie intake 50, 56, 62, 460, 486
cancer
  adolescents 346
  developing countries 55
  health promotion 512
  lung 162, 164, 516
  pollution 154, 162, 164, **165**, 166, 167
  substance abuse 245
candida 136, 137, 141
carbon gases 154, 157, 160–3, 169
caring elements
  in hospital 527–8, 530, 533–8
  outcome/performance measures 489, 495
  see also child care/rearing; health care/services
cataracts 154
cereals 275–6, 282, 290, 460
cerebral palsy
  adolescents 347
  child abuse 317
  community diagnosis 559
  demographic trends 95
  growth and development 222
  outcome/performance measures 485
  poverty 372
  premature babies 262, 386, 388, 389
chemical pollution **153–4**, 155–8, 161–5, 168, 171
chickenpox immunization 510
child abuse 25, 29, **105**, **310–30**
  accidents 183
  adolescents 246, 315, 316
  community issue 326–7, 466, 559, 560, 566
  ethnic minorities 422, 427
  growth and development 211, 214, 316, 320–2, 325–7, 433
  historical perspectives 198–9, 208, 310, 319, 322

intersectoral approaches 472, 473
  outcome/performance measures 479, 486
  parent partnership 545–7
  quality of life 582
  risk of 304, 312, 324–6
  ritual 318
  sexual, *see* sexual abuse
  torture 43, **114**, 310, 318
  wartime 122
childbearing, *see* birth rates; childbirth; pregnancy
childbirth
  developing countries 51, 53
  HIV transmission 129
  maternal mortality 51, 89, 139, 183
  neonatal intensive care 73, 262, 265, 381, **384–5**, 388–9, **527–39**
  pre-term, *see* prematurity
  see also maternal age
child care/rearing
  and abuse 310, 314, 319, 322, 325
  accidents 179
  education in 290
  fathers 409
  historical perspectives 198, 200–7, 459, 464
  medicalization v. parental role 540–2, 544–6
  premature babies 388, 530, 537
  see also health care/services
child development, *see* growth and development
child health, *see* health
childhood v, 193–209
child labour 4–5, 42, 573, 582
childlessness
  intentional 77, 82
  unintentional, *see* fertility and infertility
child protection
  child abuse 311, 319, 326–7
  ethnic minorities 427
  historical perspectives 207, 260
  legislation 459
  multidisciplinary teams 327
  parent partnership 546
  quality of life 571, 577
  social paediatrics research 29
  wartime 116, 121–3
  see also prevention; resilience; safety
children
  abandoned 25, 55, 139–40, 198, 319, 323
  abuse of, *see* child abuse
  adopted 25, 143, 261, 319
  and adults 196–208, 265, 287, 578
   see also families
  'backward' 42, 163, 222–3, 262, 332
  battered, *see* child abuse
  'best interest' principle 39–40, 576
  birth-weight, *see* low birth-weight

Subject index

care of, *see* child care/rearing; health care/services
childhood   v, 193–209
  control of   **199**, 203–7, 320, 351, 405–6, 579
    see also punishment
  death of, *see* mortality
  definition of   39
  dependency of   200
  deprived, *see* deprivation, social
  development of, *see* growth and development
  'difficult'   218, 325, 334, 440–1, 559
  disabled, *see* special needs
  emotional problems, *see* psychological issues
  employed   4–5, 42, 573, 582
  exploited   38, **43**, 319, 323
  extermination of (!)   319
  feeding, *see* nutrition
  fostered   25, 143, 261, 319
  friends, *see* interpersonal relationships
  growth of, *see* growth and development
  handicapped, *see* special needs
  health of, *see* health
  ill, *see* morbidity
  illegitimate   77–8, 81–2, 86, 369–70
  illiterate   50, 59, **60–1**, 96, 183, 573, 582
  image of   202
  immigrant, *see* ethnic minorities
  injured, *see* accidents
  as interpreters   428
  in literature   202
  maltreatment of, *see* child abuse
  mental health, *see* psychiatric factors
  needs of, *see* needs
  neglect of, *see* child abuse
  obese   100, 104, **218–21**, 275, 278, **286–7**
  orphaned   25, 55, 139–40, 198, 319, 323
  'ownership' of   261
  poor, *see* poverty
  premature, *see* prematurity
  protection of, *see* child protection; resilience
  refugee, *see* refugees
  retarded   42, 163, **222–3**, 262, 332
  rights of, *see* rights
  safety of, *see* safety
  schooling, *see* education
  sex, *see* gender issues; sexual behaviour
  single   286
  socialization of   200–3, 206, 332–4, 401, 514, 581
  as soldiers   43, 112, **120**, 123
  survival of, *see* life-expectancy
  teenage, *see* adolescent
  Third World, *see* developing countries
  tortured   43, **114**, 310, 318
  unborn, *see* fetus
  vaccination of, *see* immunization
  value of   576
  vulnerable, *see* risk factors
  at war   43, 109–27, 285
  welfare of, *see* quality of life
  working   4–5, 42, 573, 582
  see also adolescents; families; fetus; infants; pre-school children; school-age children; young adults
Children Act (1989)   363
Chinese   289–90
chlamydial infections   243, 316
chronic illness, *see* special needs
cigarettes, *see* smoking
circumcision, female   130, 426–7
cirrhosis of the liver   55
cities
  child abuse   314, 324
  community participation   564
  developing countries   45
  family breakdown   402
  health promotion   515
  healthy cities projects 16, 363, 469, **474–6, 519**
  immunization   505–6
  nutritional deficiency   285–6, 291
  pollution   155, 157, 169
  poverty   370, 372
  quality of life   578, 582
cocaine   142, 233–4, 238, 240–2, 245
cognitive factors
  adolescents   227, 238, 242, 244, 461
  child abuse   320, 321
  growth and development   211, 218
  nutritional deficiency   283, 284
  prematurity   262
  quality of life   576, 579
  risk/resilience   433–4, 449, 579
  special needs   332, 334, 336
  see also intelligence
cohabitation   75, 81, 86, 399–400, 404, 407
Committee on Medical Aspects of Food Policy (COMA)   271, 277
communication
  disorders   217
  family   351
  health promotion   515
  mass, *see* media
  pre-verbal   336
  see also information; speech and language
community issues   8–9, 16–18, 542, **550–69**
  accidents   184–90, 559, 565
  adolescent risk-taking   247–8
  child abuse   326–7, 466, 559, 560, 565
  diagnosis   376, 475, 545, **550–69**
  disasters   437
  ethnic minorities   429
  health promotion   513–14, 517–20
  health services   463–4, **465–6**, 469, **470**, 471–6, **550–67**

community issues (*cont.*)
  immunization 498–9, 505, 507–8
  nutrition 284, 290, 560, 565
  pollution management 171
  poverty 376, 553, 566
  war and children 117
  see also intersectoral issues
computerization 508, 509
conception 156, 164, 259–61
  see also fertility and infertility
condoms 241–2, 246, 248, 516–17
  see also birth control
conduct, *see* behavioural factors
conflict, armed 43, 109–27, 285
congenital problems
  child health services 463
  community diagnosis 559
  ethnic minorities 423–4
  infant mortality 98, 385
  in vitro fertilization 260
  outcome measures 485, 492–4
  pollution 163–7
  rubella 58, 422, 499–500, 502, **503**
  SIDS 301
  special needs 334
  substance abuse 321
  syphilis 498
  see also fetus
consanguinity 424
consensual unions 75, 81, 86, 399–400, 404, 407
contraception, *see* birth control
coping strategies 118, 442, 520, 544
  see also resilience
cot deaths 98, 140, **297–309**, 385, 488
counselling
  accident prevention 187, 189
  adolescents 247
  breast-feeding 273
  child abuse 326
  family 409
  genetic 389, 423, 425, 490
  HIV 133, 139, 141
  SIDS 304, 305
  special needs 337
crack cocaine 142, 240–1
cultural issues
  accidents 185
  child abuse 310, 314, 322–3
  childhood 196–8, 200, 201
  community participation 552
  family breakdown 406
  growth and development 213, 215
  health promotion 513, 515
  low birth-weight 380, 386
  nutrition 276, 280, 282, 284–5, 289–91
  quality of life 572, 575–6, 579, 581
  special needs 332, 341, 343
  see also ethnic minorities

cystic fibrosis 346, 349, 485, 584
cytomegalovirus 136, 143, 300

Darwin, C. 210
data collection, *see* information
death, *see* bereavement; mortality
demographic issues 69–108
  child health services 460–3
  developing countries 45–8, 59–60
  ethnic minorities in UK 415–17
  illegitimacy 77–8, 81–2, 86, 369–70
  low birth-weight 380
  migration 86, 89, 90–2, 397, 510, 578
  special needs 95, 333–5, 341–4
  see also age factors; birth rates; cultural
    issues; education; epidemiology;
    families; fertility and infertility;
    gender issues; genetic factors;
    information; life expectancy;
    marriage; migration; morbidity;
    mortality; population issues; racial
    factors; religious belief;
    social/socioeconomic issues
dental caries 103, 245, 484
depression
  adolescents 227, 238, 346, 347
  child abuse 315, 317, 321
  ethnic minorities 418–19, 421, 429
  growth and development 215, 219
  risk/resilience 435–8, 444, 446–8
  war and children 113–15, 117, 118, 121
deprivation, maternal 214, 262
deprivation, social
  health care 25
  health promotion 475
  HIV infection 142–3
  immunization 505
  parent partnership 545
  sensory 266–7
  SIDS 297, 298
  see also cities; poverty
developing countries 45–67
  accidents/injuries 57, 176–7, 183, 185, 187
  child abuse 322
  community participation 551, 554
  environmental issues **46**, 48, **59–60**, **64–5**, 374
  immunization 50–1, 53, 56, **58–9**, 62–4, 498
  infant mortality 50–3, 58–9, 61, 275, 285
  nutrition 45, 48, 50–4, **55–7**, 61–2, 275, 285, 291
  parent partnership 541–2, 545–6
  poverty 45, **48**, 59, 65, 361, 368, 374, 376
  quality of life 59, 573
  special needs 48, 50, 52, 341–3, 353
development, *see* growth and development
diabetes 50, 95, 104

Subject index

adolescents 344, 351, 352
   outcome/performance measures 485, 493
diagnosis and detection 459, 463, 541
   child abuse 311, 314–17 **323–5**, 326–7
   community 376, 475, 545, **550–69**
   developmental progress 222
   pollution-related disease 166
   special needs 331, 332, **336**, 388
   see also screening
diarrhoea, *see* gastroenteritis/diarrhoea
Dickens, C. 202
diet, *see* nutrition/nutritional disorders
diphtheria 498, 500, **502**, 505, 509
   developing countries 53, 58, 62
   SIDS 301
disability 347, 386–90
   see also special needs
discipline, *see* punishment
discrimination 38, **39**, 361, 429–30, 517
disease, *see* morbidity
divorce and family breakdown 397–411
   adolescent risk-taking 236, 403
   child abuse 319
   child health services 460
   demographic trends 75, 78, 79, 81–5
   growth and development 216, 403
   HIV infection 139
   outcome/performance measures 486
   poverty 367
   quality of life 582, 584
   risk/resilience 402, 409, 437, 439
drowning accidents 100, 177, 181–3, 187, **230–1**, 234
drug abuse
   adolescents 225–7, **233–4**, 235–44, **245**, 246–8
   child abuse 313–14, 321
   child health services 460
   community diagnosis 560
   HIV infection 130, 134–5, 140–3
   intersectoral approaches 472
   outcome/performance measures 479, 486
   SIDS 299
   UN Convention 43
   'unfit' mothers 203
dust pollution 159, 161, 171

'Earth Summit', Rio de Janeiro (1992) 151, 169
eating, *see* nutrition/nutritional disorders
ecological issues, *see* environmental issues
economic issues, *see* social/socioeconomic issues
eczema 104
education
   accident prevention 183, 186, 189
   adolescents 226–7, **236–7**, 242, **244**, 246–8, 345

child abuse 316, **318**, 320, 321, 325–6
   in child care 290
   developing countries 50, 51, 60–1
   environmental 170
   ethnic minorities 421–2
   growth and development 214–16, 222–3
   of health professionals 18, 508, 544, 548, **567–8**
   and health promotion/services 460, **461**, 463–5, 514, 516, 519–20
   historical perspectives 197, 202–4, 206–7
   HIV infection 143
   immunization 505, 508
   intersectoral approaches 473, 475
   literacy 50, 59, **60–1**, 96, 183, 573, 582
   low birth-weight 386, 388
   maternal 50–1, 61, 78
   and nutrition 283
   outcome/performance measures 478, 484, 485
   parental participation 544
   peace education 122
   in personal relationships 407
   and quality of life 577, 578, 583–4
   right to 43–4
   in social paediatrics 10, 18–20, **24–6**, 29–30
   special (needs) 202, 331–4, **335–8**, 343, 386
   truancy 113, 244, 316, 318, 421
   war shortages 111–12, 122
   see also cognitive factors; health education; school-age children
emotional development 211, 218
emotional problems, *see* psychological issues
employment, *see* child labour; social/socioeconomic issues
encephalopathy 136, 137
energy
   developing countries 48, 64–5
   International Atomic Energy Commission 169
   nuclear power 155, 156, 165, 168
   nutritional 274–8, 285–8
enuresis 113, 117, 213, 316, 421, 484
environmental issues 151–91
   adolescent risk-taking 226, 239
   child abuse 317, 327
   community participation 560
   desertification 46
   developing countries 48, **59–60**, **64–5**, 374
   European morbidity trends 103–4
   growth and development 216–17, 221–2
   health promotion 512, 513, 518, 520
   hospitals 525–39
   immigrants 420
   intersectoral approaches 473–5
   obesity 286

environmental issues (*cont.*)
  outcome/performance measures 478, 485–7, 490, 495
  quality of life 576, **577–8**, 579, **580**
  reproductive technologies 266
  risk/resilience 433–4, **435**, 437–44, 449
  SIDS 299
  special needs 332, 333
  see also accidents; cities; food; global issues; housing; pollution; poverty; public health; social/socioeconomic issues
epidemiology
  accidents 176, 183, 189
  child abuse 311–14
  community participation 555, 558–60, 564–8
  divorce 398–402
  outcome/performance measures 480, 488, 494–5
  pollution 167–8, 170
  refugees 416–19
  SIDS 298–9, 302
  see also demographic issues; information; population issues
epilepsy 262, 343, 385
EPI programme 58, 498
ESSOP 21–2, 26, 30, 32, 363, 377
ethical issues 10, 143, 259–60, **263–4**, 65, 568
ethnic minorities 412–32
  adolescents 235, 421, **422**, 426
  Afro-Caribbeans 289, 420–2, 424–6, 429
  child abuse 314
  Chinese 289–90
  in developing countries 45, 61–3
  language problems 213
  low birth-weight 383, 424–5
  nutrition 276, 279–82, 286, **289–91**, 412, 421, **426**
  poverty 367–8
  special needs 332, 429
  Vietnamese 289–90, 322, 414
  see also Asians; cultural issues; racial factors; refugees
European Community 63, 64, 274–5, 290
European Development Fund 63
European Society for Social Paediatrics (ESSOP) 21–2, 26, 30, 32, 363, 377
European Society for the Study and Prevention of Infant Death 306
European Standards Centre 169
evacuees 116
  see also refugees
evaluation issues
  community participation 552–3, 556–7
  health service planning 462, 464, 467
  immunization coverage 504–5
  outcome/performance measures 477–97

parent partnership 546–7
quality of life 570–85
technology 264
exercise 88, 518, 560
Expanded Programme on Immunization (EPI) 58, 498
exploitation 38, **43**, 319, 323

Faculty of Community Medicine 363
failure to thrive 136, **217–18**, **316–17**, 320, 421
falls 99, 176–7, 180–1, 187, 234
families
  accident prevention 189, 190
  and adolescents 227, **236**, 346, 349, 353–4
  binuclear 404
  breakdown of, *see* divorce and family breakdown
  child growth and development 211, **215–16**, 217–8, 222–3, 403
  demographic trends 78, 81–94
  ethnic minorities 421–2, 426, 428–9
  extended 81, 86, 319, 460, 579
  family health 8, 556, 566
  health promotion/services 397–8, 405, **406–10**, 464–5, 514, 520
  historical perspectives 197–202, 207
  HIV infection 139, 142–3
  hospital neonatal care 528, 531, **532**, **535–6**
  intersectoral approaches 469–76
  lone-parent, *see* single-parent families
  nuclear, *see* nuclear families
  nutrition 286–91
  one-parent, *see* single-parent families
  outcome/performance measures 478, 485–6, 495
  poor, *see* poverty
  public health 17
  quality of life 573, 577–84
  rights lobby 546
  risk/resilience 402, 409, 433–7, 439–43, 447–50
  SIDS 299, 304–6
  size 78, 82–6, 89, 197, 372, 577, 579
  special needs **336–7**, 346, 349, **350–2**, 353–4, 388–90, 463
  structure 75, 83, 89, 200, 397–8, 460, 579
  violence, *see* child abuse
  in wartime 111, 113–17
  see also parents
family planning, *see* birth control
family practitioners 24, 189, 507, 556, 559–61, 565
  see also primary health care
fathers
  adolescent 242

child abuse 313
  European family life 82
  family breakdown 409
  growth and development 216
  war and children 117
  see also parents
fear
  child abuse 320, 321
  health promotion 516–17
  pollution 165
  premature babies 527
  war and children 113, 117–18, 120
fertility and infertility
  adolescents 245
  conception 156, 164, 259–61
  demographic trends **75–9**, 81–2, 84, 86, **89**, 90–2
  pollution 164–5
  regulation, see birth control
  technologies 259–63, **264–8**, 381, 390, 527, 531
  voluntary childlessness 77, 82
  see also birth rates; sexual behaviour
fetus 259–60
  damage to 156, 159, 162–4, 167, 321, 389, 427
  diagnosis 490–1
  fetal alcohol syndrome 245
  gestational age 380–2
  HIV transmission 50, 129–134, 138, 140, 143, 203
  maturation of 75, 156, 259–60, 267–8, 389
  protection of 83, 87, 202, 260, 459
  rights 259
  stillbirths 134, 481
  see also congenital problems; pregnancy
firearm accidents 100, 231
fires 100, 181, 187, 234
  see also burns
fluoridization 103
food
  consumption 65
  hospital 428
  intolerance 103
  poisoning 103
  policies 271, 277, 286, 291
  pollution 154–8, **159**, 160–2, 169–70
  solid 275–6, 282, 286, 288, 289
  wholefoods 287
  see also nutrition/nutritional disorders
Food and Agriculture Organization 169, 274
formaldehyde 159, 160, 163
formula feeding 272, **273–5**, 276–7, 280–3, 286, 290
  see also bottle feeding
fostered children 25, 143, 261, 319
Foucault, M. 203–5, 207
Freud, S. 202, 210, 581

G–6–PD deficiency 425–6
gamete intrafallopian transfer 390
gastroenteritis/diarrhoea
  breast-feeding 138
  child abuse 316, 317
  developing countries 50–4, 56–8, 62
  ethnic minorities 62, 426, 429
  HIV infection 136, 143
  nutrition 275
  oral rehydration 51, 53, 64
  water pollution 165
gender issues
  accidents 184, 229, 230
  adolescent risk-taking 226, 229–33, **234–5**, 238–40, 244
  child abuse 312–13, 323
  child rearing 207
  communication disorders 217
  divorce sequelae 402–3
  family functions 401–2
  HIV infection 128, 141, 142, 243–4
  morbidity/mortality 97, 99–100, 462
  nutrition 277
  poverty 372
  quality of life 576, 581
  risk/resilience 433, 439–40, 442
  SIDS 298, 299
  special needs 334–5, 342–4, 346
  toxic effects 162
  war 113, 120–1
  see also women
general practice/practitioners 24, 189, 507, 556, 559–61, 565
  see also primary health care
genetic factors 464–6, 513
  adolescent risk-taking 226–7, 238–9
  counselling 389, 423, 425, 490
  ethnic minorities 412, 425–6
  in vitro fertilization 261
  low birth-weight/prematurity 385, 386, 389
  obesity 286
  quality of life 577, 579
  SIDS 299
  special needs 333–5
  see also gender issues
Gesell, A. 210
gestational age 380–2
GIFT 390
girls, see circumcision, female; gender issues; rubella
global issues 3, 8, 10
  accidents 184, 185, 186
  community participation 550
  divorce 401
  immunization 498
  pollution 154, 155, 157
  quality of life 570–1, 577

global issues (*cont.*)
  war 43, 109–27, 285
  see also environmental issues; Health for All by the Year 2000; HIV infection; poverty
glucose–6–phosphate dehydrogenase (G–6–PD) deficiency 162, 425–6
gonorrhoea 240, 243, 316
'greenhouse effect' 154, 155
grief 305
growth and development 101–2, 210–24
  accidents/injuries 180–1, 188
  adolescents 214–15, 219, **227–9**, 249, 279
  child abuse 211, 214, 316, 320–2, 325–7, 433
  community diagnosis 560
  developing countries 56, 64
  divorce sequelae 216, 403
  ethnic minorities 421
  failure to thrive 136, **217–18**, **316–17**, 320, 421
  fetal 75, 156, 259–60, 267–8, 389
  health care 464–5
  historical perspectives 205
  HIV infection 141
  hormone treatment 221
  information on 461
  intersectoral approaches 215, 470
  low birth-weight/prematurity 218, 386, 389, 527, 532
  nutrition 101, 212, 218, 278–9, 283–4, **285–6**, 287–90
  outcome/performance measures 222, 487, 493–5
  parental diagnosis of problems 542
  pollution 156, 164
  poverty 363, 371
  puberty 215, **344–5**, 346–7, 353, 495
    see also adolescents
  quality of life 219, 574–7, 579, **580**
  risk/resilience 433, 434, 442–4, 447–8
  social paediatrics research 27
  special needs 222–3, 332–6, 347–9
  war 112
  see also cognitive ability; height; motor skills; sexual behaviour; weight
gypsies 299, 413, 499

haemoglobinopathies 425, 427
haemophilia 130, 140–1
handicap 347, 386–90
  see also mental handicap; special needs
headache 113, 346, 372
health
  definitions of 12, 59, 513, 570–2
  determinants of, *see* environmental issues; genetic factors; psychological issues;social/socioeconomic issues

  family 8, 556, 566
  global 3, 8, 10
    see also Health for All by the Year 2000
  v. illness 21, 518, 525, 570–1
  inequalities **174–91**, 361–3, 368, 371–5, **376–7**, 475, 513
  MCH programmes 7, 551–3
  mental, *see* psychiatric problems; psychological issues
  and nutrition in childhood 290
  public, *see* public health
  right to 186
  status 101, 475, **477–97**, 527, 555, 578
  surveillance 20, 25, 463–4, 487, 494, 508
  UNICEF programme 183–4
health care/services
  access to 142, 485
  accidents 174, 189–90
  antenatal **132–3**, 138, 242, 389, **422–6**, 490–1, 535
  community participation 463–4, **465–6**, 469, **470**, 471–6, **550–67**
  coordination, *see* intersectoral issues
  cost/effectiveness 477–80, 487–91, 510–12, 571
  curative v–vi, 21, 25, 96, 140, 459–60, 463–5, 489, 571
  developing countries 45, 48, 51–3, 63
  ethnic minorities 427–30
  evaluation, *see* evaluation issues
  goals of 477–9
  HIV infection 140–3, 463
  holistic 465, 513
  immunization 459, 506–9
  neglect of 318
  neonatal intensive 73, 262, 265, 381, **384–5**, 388–9, **527–39**
  planning **457–68**, 530, 545–7, 550–6, 567
  poverty 363, 376
  preventive, *see* prevention
  quality of 489, 512–13
  rehabilitative 459, **463**, 465
    see also special needs
  special needs 353, 459, 461, 463, 466
  war shortages 111–12
  see also health professionals; health promotion; hospital care; primary health care; public health; social paediatrics; voluntary sector
health education 517–19
  accident prevention 188
  community participation 551, 562–4
  ethnic minorities 425, 427–8
  family demographics 89, 91
  and health promotion 514, 518
  immunization 507
  nutrition 273, 280–1, 287, 291, 541
  pollution management 170–1
  public health 15

Subject index

risk/resilience 445
SIDS 302, 304
see also health promotion; information
Health for All by the Year 2000 (WHO) v, vi, 12, **16–20**, 513, 517
 accident prevention 184, 186
 family environment 397, 475, 477
 immunization 498
 parent partnership 542
 poverty **362–3**, 372, 376 542
 quality of life 570–1, 574, 577
health professionals
 accident prevention 188, 189
 adolescent risks 247
 breast-feeding 272–3
 child abuse 310–11, 315
 community participation 553–68
 conflicting advice 291, 506, 515
 coordination, *see* intersectoral issues
 dietary practices 286, 288–91
 ethnic minorities 428
 family breakdown 404, 409
 general practitioners 24, 189, 507, 556, 559–61, 565
 health promotion 512
 HIV infection 143
 hospital neonatal care 529, **530**, 535–6, **537**
 immunization uptake 502–9
 nurses 24, 215, 306, 536–8
 outcome/performance measures 477–80, 487, 490, 495
 paediatricians 24, 29, 482
 and parents 540–9, 562
 pollution management 171
 poverty 376–7
 SIDS 304–6
 in social paediatrics 23–5
 teamwork, *see* multidisciplinary approaches
 training 18, 508, 544, 548, **567–8**
health promotion 13–16, 25, 27, 463–5, **512–23**
 family breakdown 397–8, 405–10
 immunization 507
 intersectoral 469–76, 517–18
 nutrition 281, 512, 515, 518
 and pollution 169
 and poverty 376
 see also prevention
health services, *see* health care/services
healthy cities projects 16, 363, 469, **474–6**, **519**
hearing
 growth and development 210
 iodine deficiency 284
 parental diagnosis 542
 pollution 154, 165
 premature babies 267, 386
 quality of life 580

height
 adolescents 345
 child abuse 320–1
 growth and development 101–2, 217, 219, 221
 nutrition 278, 284, 285, 288
 outcome/performance measures 495
 poverty 371, 373
 quality of life 576
hepatitis
 adolescents 142
 child health services 463
 community participation 566
 developing countries 55, 58
 ethnic minorities 423, 426
 immunization/prevention of 131, 510
hereditary factors, *see* genetic factors
heroin 142, 234
herpes 141, 243, 316
heterosexual activity 128, 142, **231–2**, 515, 517
 see also sexual behaviour
historical aspects 193–209
 accident mortality 174
 child abuse 198–9, 208, 310, 319, 322
 child protection 207, 260
 demographic trends 82
 health promotion/services 457–60, 464, 512–13
 MCH programmes 552
 mortality 174, 200, 298, 572
 parent partnership 540–3
 poverty 368
 public health 13
 quality of life 572
 social paediatrics 3–7
 special needs education 335
 UN Convention 36–8
HIV infection 128–49, 510, 514–17
 adolescents 140, **141–2**, 225, 240–8
 developing countries 50, 55, 63
 health promotion/services 140–3, 463, 517
homelessness 246, 323
homicide 100, 177, 231, 240
homosexuality 128, 142, 517, 232
hospital care 459, 465
 accidents 177
 child abuse teams 327
 developing countries 63
 ethnic minorities 428
 immunization/infectious diseases 502, 508
 outcome/performance measures 494
 premature babies 262–3, 525–39
 preparing children for 449
 social paediatrics 9, 24–5
housing
 community participation 559
 ethnic minorities 429
 homelessness 246, 323

housing (*cont.*)
  and hospital admission   262–3
  intersectoral approaches   475
  outcome/performance measures   485
  pollution   168
  poverty   363, 368, 373, 374, 376
  quality of life   577, 578, 580–1, 584
human papilloma virus   243
hydrocarbons   157, 164
hydrocephalus   262
hygiene   48, 512
  see also public health
hyperactivity   320, 321
hypoxia   300

iatrogenesis   257–69, 527, 541
illegitimacy   77–8, 81–2, 86, 369–70
illiteracy   50, 59, 60–1, 96, 183, 573, 582
illness, *see* morbidity
immigrants, *see* ethnic minorities
immunization   498–511
  child abuse and neglect   318
  child health services   459, 506–9
  developing countries   50–2, 53, 56, **58–9**, 62–4, 498
  ethnic minorities   62, 422–3
  and HIV infection   137–8
  influenza   58, 500, 510
  outcome/performance measures   492–4
  SIDS   301
  social paediatrics   25
  wartime   123
impairment   386, 388
  see also special needs
imprisonment   43
incest   313, 315, 321, 323, 324
income levels, *see* social/ socioeconomic issues
incubators   265–7, 384, 527, 530–5
infant feeding
  bottle feeding   138, **273–5**, 298, 426
  child health services   459
  COMA reports   271
  education in schools   290
  ethnic minorities   289, 421, 426
  formula feeding   272, **273–5**, 276–7, 280–3, 286, 290
  health education leaflets   541
  iodine deficiency   284
  and obesity   286
  premature babies 280, 283, 380, 532–3
  SIDS   298
  vegan diets   287
  vitamins   280
  weaning   56, 275–7, 280, 282–3, 288–9
  see also breast-feeding; nutrition/nutritional disorders
infanticide   297–8, 310, 323

infant mortality   **69–80**, 88, 90–1, **95–9**
  accidents   183
  child abuse   319, 322
  developing countries   50–3, 58–9, 61, 275, 285
  ethnic minorities   423–5
  European Society for the Study and Prevention of Infant Death   306
  family size   197
  health service planning   462
  HIV infection   134, 136–40
  intersectoral approaches   472, 473
  in vitro fertilization   260
  low birth-weight/prematurity   262, 368–70, 381–5, 389–90
  neonatal, *see* neonatal mortality
  nutritional problems   275, 285
  outcome measures   481–3, 492
  perinatal, *see* perinatal mortality
  poverty   368–70
  quality of life index   573, 582
  socioeconomic factors   97, 368–70
  stillbirths   134, 481
  sudden unexpected   98, 140, **297–309**, 385, 488
infants
  accidents   180, 188
  of adolescent parents   241–2
  birth, *see* childbirth
  bonding   135, 213–14, 325, 384
  crying   559
  death, *see* infant mortality
  drug–affected   203, 314, 318
  ethnic minorities   289, 421–6, 429
  growth and development   213, 215, 217
  HIV infection   134–5, 138, 141, 143
  immunization   58, 502–3
  low birth-weight, *see* low birth-weight
  nutrition, *see* infant feeding
  obese   286
  pollution   155, 156, 159, 163, 167
  premature, *see* prematurity
  quality of life   580–1
  risk/resilience   440–1
infectious diseases   96, 257, 499–505
  adolescents   245
  candida   136, 137, 141
  child abuse   316
  child health services   459, 463
  chlamydial   243, 316
  community participation   565
  cytomegalovirus   136, 143, 300
  developing countries   45, 48–52, **53–5**, 57, 62, 64
  herpes   141, 243, 316
  human papilloma virus   243
  malaria   50–2, **54–5**, 62, 426, 498
  meningitis   58, 372
  nutritional deficiency   283, 285

Subject index

opportunistic 136, 137, 143
pollution 154, 158, 161
premature babies 532
refugees 62
SIDS 299–302
wartime 112, 123
see also gastroenteritis/diarrhoea; hepatitis; HIV infection; immunization; parasitic infections; respiratory problems; sexually transmitted diseases; tuberculosis
infertility, *see* fertility and infertility
infibulation 427
influenza vaccine 58, 500, 510
information 19–20
   accidents 176, 185, 186, 188
   child abuse 325
   community participation 552, 554, 556, **557–9**, 562
   ethnic minorities 427
   family breakdown/demographics 91–2, 406
   growth and development 461
   health promotion 514–15, 518
   immunization 504–5, 508
   low birth-weight/prematurity 390, 527, 529–30, 535
   nutrition 270, 278, 284
   outcome/performance measures 492, 494
   parent partnership 540, 543, 545
   pollution management 168–70
   poverty 364, 371, 377
   records 291, 504, 508, 542, **546**, 547
   special needs 337, 348
   see also epidemiology; health education
injuries, definition of 174–5
   see also accidents
intelligence
   child rearing 207
   family breakdown 406
   outcome/performance measures 495
   pollutants 164–6
   see also cognitive factors
intensive care, neonatal 73, 262, 265, 381, **384–5**, 388–9, **527–39**
interdisciplinarity, *see* multidisciplinary approaches
International Atomic Energy Commission 169
International Classification of Diseases 175
International Labour Office 169
International Society for the Prevention of Child Abuse and Neglect 310
interpersonal relationships
   child abuse 313, 321, 437
   community participation 554, 559, 567
   family breakdown 397–9, 401
   health promotion 515, 517
   historical perspectives 196, 198, 199, 202

   HIV infection 141
   hospital neonatal care 533
   maternal bonding 135, 213–14, 325, 384
   quality of life 572, 574, 578–80
   risk/resilience 437–8, 441, 443, 448
   special needs 332
   wartime 113, 114
   see also families; peer groups; sexual behaviour; support networks
intersectoral issues 17, **25–6**, 30, **469–76**
   accidents 176, 184–8
   community participation 556, 558
   growth and development 215, 470
   health promotion/services 462, 465–6, **469–76**, 517–18
   hospital neonatal care 538
   poverty 376–7, 473
   see also community issues; multidisciplinary approaches
interventions
   accident prevention 187–8
   adolescents 247–8, 349, 353
   community participation 559–60
   effectiveness of, *see* evaluation issues
   family breakdown 404, 407, 409
   growth and development 219, 221–3
   nutrition 284, 290–1
   pollution emergencies 170
   v. prevention 488
   quality of life 571
   SIDS 302–3
   special needs 333–4, 335–8, 349, 353
   see also health education; health promotion; legislation; policy issues; prevention
in vitro fertilization 260–1, 390
invulnerability, *see* resilience
iodine 56, 156, 162, 274, **284**
iron deficiency 56, 160, 274–9, **281–4**, 288–90, 426

Japanese encephalitis 58
juvenile delinquency 119, 242, 244, 320
   see also behavioural factors

'kangaroo method' 58, 264, 266
kwashiorkor 50, 56, 318

language, *see* speech and language
lead pollution 153–70
learning, *see* cognitive ability; education
legislation
   adolescent risk-taking 249
   child abuse 311, 326
   child protection 459
   family breakdown 407
   fertility 82–3, 87, 202–3, 264, 459
   health promotion 469, 519–20

legislation (*cont.*)
  immunization 505
  pollution 169
  quality of life 576, 582
leukaemias 165, 321
life-events 405–6, 435–7, 444–6, 579, 583–4
life expectancy/survival 45, 48, **69–72**, 95
  accident prevention 183
  historical perspectives 200
  HIV infection 137
  low birth-weight/prematurity 268, 385, **386–8**, 488, 529
  outcome/performance measures 479, 488
  physical contact with infants 322
  quality of life 571–3, 577, 582
  reproductive technology 259, 262
  see also mortality
lifestyle factors 59, 88–9
  AIDS 514–17
  community participation 551, 560
  health promotion/services 460–1, 513, 518, 520
  and low birth-weight 380, 388, 389
  poverty 361, 372, 376
  see also alcohol; drug abuse; environmental issues; families; sexual behaviour; smoking; social/socioeconomic issues
literacy 50, 59, **60–1**, 96, 183, 573, 582
loss experiences 438, 440
low birth-weight 380–96
  adolescent parents 241, 245
  cerebral palsy 262, 386, 388, 389
  developing countries 48, 50–1, 58
  ethnic minorities 383, 424–5
  European trends 69–80, 98
  growth and development 218, 386, 389, 527, 532
  HIV infection 134, 140
  hospital care 527–39
  infant mortality 262, 368–70, 381–5, 389–90
  in vitro fertilization 260
  nutrition 280, 283
  outcome/performance measures 488, 495
  pollution 165
  poverty 370, 371, 373
  SIDS 298, 299, 385
  wartime 112
  see also prematurity
lymphadenopathy 136, 137

malaria 50–2, **54–5**, 62, 426, 498
malformations, *see* congenital problems
malnutrition, *see* nutrition/nutritional disorders
marijuana 233–45, 321
marriage
  arranged 422

  breakdown, *see* divorce and family breakdown
  cohabitation 75, 81, 86, 399–400, 404, 407
  consanguineous 424
  demographic trends **75–9**, 81–5, 89–91
mass media, *see* media
maternal age 75, 78, 82
  adolescents 241–2
  low birth-weight 380, 389, 390
  SIDS 298
maternal and child health programmes 7, 551–3
maternal bonding 135, 213–14, 325, 384
maternal deprivation 214, 262
maternal mortality 51, 89, 139, 183
maternity leave 409
MCH programmes, *see* maternal and child health programmes
measles 498–500, **502–3**, 504–5, 509
  developing countries 52–3, 58–9, 62
  outcome/performance measures 492
  poverty 371
measurement issues, *see* evaluation issues; information
media
  accident prevention 186, 188
  adolescent risk-taking 248
  divorce 407, 582
  health promotion 475, 514, 517, 520
  immunization 505–7
  nutritional deficiency 288
  and war 121
medical care, *see* health care/ services
medical profession, *see* health professionals
medicine 19, 512
  community 363, 567–8
  traditional 427, 541
  see also health care/services
Mediterranean Action Plan 169
men, *see* gender issues
meningitis 58, 372
mental handicap/retardation 42, 222–3, 332
  adolescents 343, 345
  child abuse 317, 320, 321, 324
  developing countries 50
  iodine deficiency 284
  prematurity 262, 386
  quality of life 573
  toxic pollutants 163
  see also special needs
mental health, *see* psychiatric problems; psychological issues
mercury 153, 155–8, 161–3, 165
migration 86, 89, 90–2, 397, 510, 578
milk
  breast, *see* breast-feeding
  cow's 275–7, 280–4, 286, 289, 426
  school 278

MMR vaccination 500, 502, 503
morbidity 95–108
  adolescent risk-taking 245, 247
  child abuse 316, 317, 324
  chronic, *see* special needs
  clinical paediatrics 21
  communicable/notifiable 103, 504, 509–10
    see also infectious diseases
  community participation 555, 560–1
  developing countries 48, 52–3, 56
  divorce 402
  ethnic minorities 412, 422–7
  health promotion/services 461–2, **463**, 512–13, 516, 518
  International Classification of Diseases 175
  in vitro fertilization 260
  'new' 103, 257–357
  nutritional, *see* nutrition/nutritional disorders
  outcome/performance measures 478–80, 484–7, 488–9
  pollution 166
  poverty 371–2
  premature babies 386–7, 389
  prevention of, *see* prevention
  quality of life 525, 573, 578
  severity of 488
  SIDS 301, 304
  see also diagnosis and detection; health; names of individual conditions
mortality 88, 95–108
  child abuse 311–12, 317, 319, 320, 322
  community issues 555, 560
  developing countries 45, **48–51**, 52–62, 275, 285
  divorce 400, 402
  ethnic minorities 423–5
  health promotion/services 461–2, 512
  historical perspectives 174, 200, 572
  HIV 134, 139–41
  homicide 100, 177, 231, 240
  infanticide 297–8, 310, 323
  infectious diseases 498, 502
  in vitro fertilization 260
  maternal 51, 89, 139, 183,
  nutrition 270, 275, 278, 285
  outcome measures 478–80, **481–3**, 484–5, 488, 492
  poverty 368–70, 373
  refugees 62
  substance abuse 234, 245
  war 111
  see also accidents; infant mortality; life expectancy/survival; suicide
mothers
  age, *see* maternal age
  bonding 135, 213–14, 325, 384

child abuse 314, 317, 324
community participation 565
conflicting advice 541
drug-addicted 203, 314
education of 50–1, 61, 78
ethnic minorities 427–8
health promotion 514
health status 56, 75, 116–17, 134, 380
HIV infection 50, 129–134, 138, 140, 143, 203
hospital neonatal care 527–39
infants deprived of 214, 262
in vitro fertilization 261
MCH programmes 7, 551–3
mortality 51, 89, 139, 183
nutrition 56, 286
parity of 75, 78, 298
quality of life 578–80
risk/resilience 445
single, *see* single-parent families
smoking 299
special needs children 337
in wartime 116–17
working 81
see also breast-feeding; childbirth; parents; pregnancy
motor accidents, *see* traffic accidents
motor skills
  child abuse 316
  growth and development 210, 222
  nutrition 284, 288
  premature babies 262, 265–8
  quality of life 576
  special needs 336, 338, 342
multidisciplinary approaches 7–8, 17–21, 30
  adolescent risk-taking 247–8
  child protection teams 327
  community participation 557, 560, 562
  growth and development 211
  health service planning 465–6
  HIV infection 143
  hospital neonatal care 537
  nutritional problems 284, 290
  quality of life 571, 575–6, 585
  special needs 332, 335–7
  see also intersectoral issues
multiple sclerosis 343
mumps 58, 136, 492, 500
Munchausen's syndrome by proxy 314, 317

nature–nurture debate 332, 487
needs 183
  child abuse 320, 324
  community assessment 550, 553–8, 565
  health promotion/services 464–7, 469, 476, 519
  historical perspectives 197, 200, 207
  outcome/performance measures 479–80

needs (*cont.*)
  and parents 528, 531, 542
  quality of life 572–3, 576
  and technology 260, 264–6, 268
  UN Convention 38
  see also special needs
neonatal intensive care 73, 262, 265, 381, **384–5**, 388–9, **527–39**
neonatal mortality 382
  accidents 183
  child health services 462
  developing countries 50, 51, 53
  European demographic trends 73, 97
  HIV infection 134
  outcome measures 481, 492
  poverty 368–9
  prematurity 384, 385, 389
  see also infant mortality
neurological problems
  adolescents 343, 344
  HIV infection 136
  in vitro fertilization 260
  nutritional deficiency 284, 288
  pollution 156, 162, 163
  prematurity 263, 385, 386, 388
  risk/resilience 434
noise pollution 154
nomads 62
non-organic failure to thrive 136, **217–18**, **316–17**, 320, 421
nuclear families
  child abuse 319
  demographic trends 81, 83, 86
  family breakdown 404, 407
  health promotion 514
  historical perspectives 195, 198, 205
  quality of life 580, 582, 583
nuclear power 155, 156, 165, 168
nuclear war 112, 120–1
nurses 24, 215, 306, 536–8
  see also health professionals
nutrition/nutritional disorders 270–96
  adolescents 242, **279**, 280, 283–6, 344
  calcium 160, 274, 277–8, 287–8, 290
  calorie intake 50, 56, 62, 460, 486
  cereals 275–6, 282, 290, 460
  child abuse 316, 320–1, 323
  community participation 284, 290, 560, 566
  cult/inappropriate diets 271, 287–8, 318
  developing countries 45, 48, 50–4, **55–7**, 61–2, 275, 285, 291
  dietary reference values 271
  eating disorders 315–16, 351, 421
  ethnic minorities 276, 279–82, 286, **289**, 412, 421, **426**
  European demographic trends 96
  G-6-PD deficiency 162, 425–6
  growth and development 101, 212, 218, 278–9, 283–4, **285–6**, 287–90
  health promotion/services 281, 459, 460, 463, 512, 515, 518
  iodine 56, 156, 162, 274, **284**
  iron deficiency 56, 160, 274–9, **281–4**, 288–90, 426
  outcome/performance measures 485, 486
  poverty 282, 285, 289–90, 363, 374–6
  quality of life 579
  recommended daily amounts 271, 277
  refugees 62
  rickets 275, **279–81**, 288–90, 421–2, 426
  social paediatrics research 27
  trace elements 158, 274–5
  vegetarian diets 280, 282, 287, 288, 426
  vitamins 56, 275–83, 287–9, 426
  wartime 112, 113
  see also food; infant feeding; protein/protein deficiency

obesity 100, 104, **218–21**, 275, 278, **286–7**
  see also weight
oral rehydration 51, 53, 64
orphans 25, 55, 139–40, 198, 319, 323
otitis media 484
outcome measures, *see* evaluation issues
ozone 154, 157, 160, 163, 169

paediatricians 24, 29, 482
paediatrics
  clinical v–vi, 21, 29, 459–60, 463, 465
  community 568
  developmental 8
  preventive, *see* prevention
  social, *see* social paediatrics
parasitic infections
  developing countries 45, 48, 50, 52, 53, **55**
  ethnic minorities 421, 426
  pollution 154
parents 540–9
  abusive, *see* child abuse
  adolescents 226–7, 236, 239–42, 249
  attitudes/expectations 211, 322, 372, **421**, 461, 544
  community participation 559–62, 565–6
  ethnic minorities 421, 428
  immunization decisions 502, 505–9
  lone, *see* single-parent families
  pollution 156, 166
  poverty 372, 376
  premature babies 268, 388, 389, **527–39**
  rights and responsibilities 39–40, 264, 337, 540–3, 546
  separation from, *see* family breakdown; orphans

single, *see* single-parent families
   special needs **336–7**, 338, 351, 541, **544–5**
   see also families; fathers; mothers
parotitis 58, 136, 492, 500
paternity leave 409
peer group relationships
   adolescents 226–9, **236**, 238–9, 345–8, 353
   child abuse 326
   health promotion 514
   quality of life 579, 581
   risk/resilience 435, 448
   war and children 113
performance measures, *see* evaluation issues
perinatal mortality
   accidents 183
   child health services 462
   developing countries 50
   ethnic minorities 423–5
   in vitro fertilization 260
   outcome measures 481–2
   poverty 368–70
   premature babies 262
   quality of life index 582
   see also infant mortality
personality factors
   adolescents 226, 349, 351
   child abuse 317, 319
   child rearing 206
   family breakdown 403, 406
   growth and development 218
   quality of life 577, 579–80
   risk/resilience 226, 440–2, 449–50
pertussis 498, 500, **502**, 504–6, 509
   developing countries 53, 58, 62
   poverty 371
   SIDS 301
Pestalozzi, J.H. 210
pesticides 163, 164
Piaget, J. 205
play, *see* recreation
pneumonia 54, 58, 372
poisoning
   food 103
   health promotion 515
   mortality 99, 177–83, 370
   pollution 153–62, 166, 168, 169
   pregnancy 260
policy issues
   accidents/safety 174, 180, 183–90
   adolescent risk-taking 248
   aid programmes 63–4, 551
   child abuse 326
   community participation 556, 563–4
   ethnic minorities 429–30
   health promotion 469, 474, 512–14, 520
   historical perspectives 198
   immunization 499, 505, 508

nutrition 271, 277, 286, 291
parent partnership 544
pollution 171
poverty 363, 376, 377
quality of life 570–1, 573, 576
special needs 338, 353
see also priority setting
poliomyelitis 498–9, **500**, 501, 504–5, 509
   developing countries 53, 58, 62
   and HIV infection 138
   parental diagnosis 542
political issues
   accidents 185
   child abuse 319
   developing countries 59, 65
   family breakdown 407
   family demographics 81, 86
   health promotion/services 465, 474, 476, 513, 518–19
   MCH programmes 552
   poverty 373, 377
   priority setting 488–9
   public health 17, 20
   quality of life 571, 582
   reproductive technologies 264
   special needs 341
   war and children 118
pollution **103–4**, **151–73**, 374, 566, 577–8
   see also air pollution
population issues 81, 84, 89–91
   growth patterns 290
   health promotion 512, 518
   immunization 510
   quality of life 571, 574
   and social paediatrics 3
   see also community issues; demographic issues; epidemiology; information
pornography 43
post-traumatic stress disorder 114–15, 117, 321
poverty 359–79
   adolescent parents 242
   child abuse 316–19, 323, 324
   community participation 376, 553, 566
   developing countries 45, 48, 59, 65, 361, 368, 374, 376
   European demographic trends 96
   intersectoral approaches 376–7, 473
   malnutrition 282, 285, 289–90, 363, 374–6
   outcome/performance measures 485, 486
   pollution 159, 168
   pregnancy 373, 545
   quality of life 577, 579
   special needs 332, 343, 372
   and war 122
   see also deprivation, social; social/socioeconomic issues

power
  exercise of 203–7
  nuclear 155, 156, 165, 168
pregnancy 69–80
  antenatal care 132–3, 138, 242, 389, **422–6**, 490–1, 535
  developing countries 51, 52–3, 56, 64
  ectopic 134, 243, 260
  health promotion 516
  HIV infection 131–4
  hospital care 529
  pollution 162, 164, 165, 167
  poverty 373, 545
  protection 83, 87, 202, 260, 459
  rubella 503
  SIDS 299, 300, 305–6
  teenage, *see* adolescents
  teratogenesis 164, 321
  termination of, *see* abortion
  unplanned 87, 225, 235, 240, **241–2**, 246, 248, 460
  vitamin D deficiency 280, 426
  see also fetus
prematurity 262–8, 381–5
  child abuse 312, 324, 325
  developing countries 48, 50–1, 58
  HIV infection 134, 140
  hospital care 262–3, 527–39
  in vitro fertilization 260
  rickets 280
  special needs 262–3, 384, 386, 388, 390, 488
  see also low birth-weight
prenatal care **132–3**, 138, 242, 389, **422–6**, 490–1, 535
pre-school children
  child abuse 312, 318
  child health services/education 461
  community participation 559
  ethnic minorities 420, 421, 426
  growth and development 216
  low birth-weight 386, 388
  morbidity in Europe 100, 371, 505
  mortality in developing countries 50
  nutrition 277–8, 283
  parent partnership 542, 544
  special needs 335
prevention 459–60, 462, 465
  accidents 27, 174–6, 179–80, 183, **184**, 185–90
  adolescents 246–9, 471
  child abuse 310–11, 325–7
  community participation 551–2
  developing countries 57–9
  European demographic trends 96
  health inequalities 373, 376
  hepatitis 131, 510
  HIV 140, 144, 515, 517

infant mortality 306
  v. intervention 488
  low birth-weight/prematurity 381, 388–90
  nutrition 278, 280–1, 283–4, 286
  pollution 168, 170, 171
  quality of life 571
  social paediatrics 9–10, 27
  see also health promotion; immunization
primary health care 463–5
  community participation 551, 553, 556, 562, 564, 566
  GPs 24, 189, 507, 556, 559–61, 565
  health promotion 513
  parent participation 541
  pollution management 171
  poverty 376
  see also immunization
priority setting
  accident prevention 180
  community participation 554–7, 563–4
  nutrition 291
  outcome/performance measures 477, 480, **488–9**, 491
  see also policy issues
prostitution 43, 130, 142, 246, 316, 321
protection
  children, *see* child protection
  fetus/pregnancy 83, 87, 202, 260, 459
  health 13–16
  see also legislation; prevention; resilience; safety
protein/protein deficiency 274, 277–8, **285–6**, 287–8
  child health services 460
  developing countries 50, 56, 62
  outcome/performance measures 486
psychiatric problems
  adolescents 227, 238, 246, 343–7
  child abuse 311, 317, 324
  child health services 461
  divorce 402
  outcome/performance measures 484
  quality of life 570, 574–9
  refugees 418
  risk/resilience 433, 435, **436–7**, 438, 441, 444–7
  screening programmes 516
  war 114–18, 121
  see also anxiety; depression; fear; mental handicap
psychoanalysis 202, 205
psychological issues
  adolescent risk-taking 226–7, 237–8
  alienation 103, 143, 288
  child abuse 317–18, 320–1
  child health promotion 512–13
  ethnic minorities 421–2
  newborn children 580

non-organic failure to thrive   136, **217–18**, **316–17**, 320, 421
pollution   165, 170
public health   13
refugees   418, 420
risk/resilience   433, 435, 438–40, **441–2**, 447
schoolchildren   100
SIDS   305
special needs   332–4, 336, 346, 349–51
war   112–15, 120
see also attitudes;
    behavioural factors; intelligence;
        interpersonal relationships;
        personality factors; quality of life;
        resilience; self-esteem; stress
psychotic illness, *see* psychiatric problems
puberty   215, **344–5**, 346–7, 353, 495
see also adolescents
public health   3, 12–21, 541
    accidents   185, 188
    community participation   568
    developing countries   48
    infectious diseases   498
    intersectoral approaches   475
    'new'   257, 513
    pollution   154, 157, 170, 171
    quality of life   570
    and social paediatrics   8
    special needs   344
    see also environmental issues
public opinion, *see* attitudes
punishment
    child abuse   310, 324, 326
    ethnic minorities   422
    health promotion   519
    historical perspectives   203–5, 207
    UN Convention   43, 44

quality of care   489, 512–13
see also evaluation issues
quality of life/well-being   12, 525, 570–85
    accidents   183, 573, 578, 582
    developing countries   59, 573
    ethnic minorities   420–7
    growth and development   219, 574–7, 579, **580**
    health promotion/services   459, 514, 516
    historical perspectives   198
    pollution   153
questionnaires
    community participation   563
    hospital neonatal care   528
    quality of life   576, 583
    social paediatrics in Europe   22–3, 26, 32–5
see also evaluation issues

racial factors
    asthma   372
    discrimination/harassment   429–30
    low birth-weight   383, 424–5
    quality of life   576
    rickets   280, 421–2, 426
    risk/risk-taking   225–6, 231–3, 241
    see also ethnic minorities
radiation/radioactivity   154–7, 161–9
radon   154, 159
records, patient   291, 504, 508, 542, **546**, 547
recreation
    accidents   175, 180–1, 184
    community health promotion   472
    hospital care   527
    outcome/performance measures   485, 486
    pollution   154, 158, 159, 161, 169
    quality of life   581
    rights to   43–4
refugees   412–20, 426–7
    developing countries   61–3
    family breakdown   397
    pollution   154
    UN Convention   43
    war and children   116
rehabilitation   459, 463, 465
    see also special needs
religious belief
    adolescent risk-taking   226, 237, 239
    childhood   201
    developing countries   59
    divorce   398, 402
    European demographic trends   82
    growth and development   215
    nutrition   287–8, 289
    war and children   119
renal problems   156, 164, 349
reproduction, *see* fertility and infertility
research issues
    accidents   177, 186
    breast-feeding   273
    family breakdown/formation   397
    growth and development   210, 221, 222
    nutrition   290
    parent partnership   546–7
    pollution   170
    quality of life   571, 573, 575
    reproductive technologies   261, 265
    risk/resilience   433, 440, 444
    SIDS   299, 306
    social paediatrics   9, 18–23, **26–9**, 30–5
    special needs   332, 349, 350
    war and children   115, 117, 121
    see also evaluation issues; information; questionnaires
resilience (protective factors)   442–55
    adolescents   225–56, 433–55, 519
    child abuse   321

resilience (*cont.*)
    cognitive factors   433–4, 449, 579
    coping strategies   118, 442, 520, 544
    families   402, 409, 433–7, 439–43, 447–50
    outcome/performance measures   486–7
    personality factors   226, 440–2, 449–50
    public health   14
    quality of life   579
    special needs   351, 354
    war and children   112–13
    see also psychological issues
resources
    accident prevention   179, 185
    allocation/implications   42, 478–80, 484, 488–90
    community participation   552–3, 556–9
    developing countries   48, 52, 55, **64–5**
    family breakdown   406
    growth and development   215
    health promotion   469, 512
    poverty   372, 377
    quality of life   570–4, 577
    see also environmental issues
respiratory problems   100, 103
    adolescents   245, 343
    community participation   559
    developing countries   50, **54**, 62, 64
    ethnic minorities   429
    pneumonia   54, 58, 372
    pollution   163–7
    poverty   372
    premature babies   380, 386, 389
    SIDS   298–300
    see also asthma; tuberculosis
rickets   275, **279–81**, 288–90, 421–2, 426
rights   36–44
    community participation   551
    ethnic minorities   415, 418
    family rights lobby   546
    fetal   259
    to immunization   507
    to know origins   261
    v. needs   260
    newborn babies   533–5
    parents   39–40, 264, 337, 540–3, 546
    safety   184, 186
    social paediatrics research   29
    special needs   331, 337, 338
    see also UN Convention on the Rights of the Child (1989)
risk factors/risk-taking   433–55
    accidents   185–9, 436
    adolescents   225–56, 433–55, 519
    AIDS   141, 514–17
    child abuse   304, 312, 324–6
    divorce   402–3, 409, 437, 439
    immunization   499
    in vitro fertilization   260

low birth-weight   380
obesity   219
poverty   367–8, 377
public health   14, 15
quality of life   572, 577, 579
SIDS   302–4
war and children   113, 121–2
see also resilience
ritual abuse   318
road accidents, *see* traffic accidents
Roman Catholic Church   83, 86, 87, 260
Rousseau, J–J.   203
rubella   58, 422, 499–500, 502, **503**

safety
    accidents   100, 174, 179–81, **183–90**
    adolescent   249
    belts   247
    health promotion   515
    outcome/performance measures   486
    pollution   155, 169–70
    public health   14
    'safe sex'   515
    of vaccines   502
    see also protection; risk factors/risk-taking
salutogenesis   405–10, 570, 579
satisfaction   105–6, 486–7, 491–5, 547, 572, 583–4
    see also quality of life
school-age children
    low birth-weight   386, 388
    morbidity   100, 105
    nutrition   271, 278, 279, 290
    obesity   221
    quality of life   581
    risk/resilience   435–40, 444–7
    rubella immunization   503
    special needs   333, 335
    see also adolescents
schools/schooling, *see* education
screening
    accident hazards   188
    antenatal   **132–3**, 138, 242, 389, **422–6**, 490–1, 535
    ethnic minorities   423, 425–6
    growth and development   222
    health promotion   516
    health surveillance   20, 25, 463–4, 487, 494, 508
    HIV   130, 131, **132–3**, 134, 138–9, 143
    iron deficiency   283
    outcome/performance measures   478, 490, 494
    see also diagnosis
self-esteem
    adolescents   227, 237–8, 345–7, 349
    child abuse   317, 321, 323, 326

Subject index

health promotion 515–16
  quality of life 574, 579–84
  risk/resilience 442–3, 447–51
self-help 541, 544
sewage 154, 155, 156, 158
sexual abuse 312–16, 318, 321–4
  adolescents 246
  ethnic minorities 422
  historical perspectives 199, 208
  morbidity trends 105
  outcome/performance measures 479
  risk/resilience 437
  UN Convention 43
sexual behaviour
  adolescents 141–2, 225–7, **231–3**, 235–48, 345, **347–8**, 581
  after child abuse 321
  childhood 202
  cultural differences 323
  demographic trends 81, 82, 86
  and disability 347
  family breakdown 401
  growth and development 211, 214
  health promotion/services 461, 515–18
  heterosexual 128, 142, **231–2**, 515, 517
  HIV infection 141–2
  homosexuality 128, 142, 517, **232**
  prostitution 43, 130, 142, 246, 316, 321
  see also fertility and infertility
sexually transmitted diseases
  adolescents 142, 225, 235, 240–1, **242–4**, 246, 248
  child abuse 316
  congenital syphilis 498
  developing countries 54
  see also HIV infection
sickle-cell disease 349, 422–3, 425
SIDS 98, 140, **297–309**, 385, 488
single-parent families
  adolescent risk-taking 227, 236
  birth-weight 78
  European family trends 82, 83, 89
  growth and development 216
  health promotion/services 460, 514
  obesity 286
  outcome/performance measures 486
  poverty 367, 369, 370
  quality of life 579
skin problems 100
  child abuse 314
  pollution 154, **161**, 162, **164**, 166
  premature babies 268, 534–5
sleep problems
  apnoea 299, 300, 306, 317
  child abuse 315, 321
  community participation 559
  ethnic minorities 421
  premature babies 532–4

SIDS 300–2
war and children 113, 114
smoking
  adolescents 227, **233–4**, 235–40, **245**, 249
  community participation 560
  health promotion/services 460, 516, 519
  mortality in Europe 88
  outcome/performance measures 486, 494, 496
  parental 372–4, 389
  pollution 157, 162–5, 167
  SIDS 299
socialization of children 200–3, 206, 332–4, 401, 514, 581
social/socioeconomic issues
  accidents 177, 183–5, 370
  adolescent risk-taking 226–7, 231, 233, **235**
  birthweight 373, 380, 383, 386–9
  child abuse 313–16, **319–20**, 323–4, 326
  childhood 196, 199, 200, 207
  community participation 552, 558–60
  dental health 103
  developing countries 48, 51–2, 59, 63–5
  divorce/family breakdown 397–8, 400, 409
  ethnic minorities 412, 415
  European demographics 69–108
  growth and development 75, 102, 211–12, **214–15**, 216–21, 371, 464
  health promotion/services 459, **460–1**, 462–6, 513, 516, 518
  HIV infection 142–3
  immunization 506
  infant mortality 97, 368–70
  nutrition 270–8, 282, 285–91
  outcome/performance measures 478–9, 485, 489, 495
  public health 13, 17, 18, 20
  quality of life 570–84
  refugees 414
  risk/resilience 433, 447–8
  schoolchildren 100
  SIDS 298–9
  social paediatrics research 9, 29
  social services 463, 465, 475, 491
  special needs 332–3, 336, 341, 344, 347, 352
  unemployment 323, 363, 367–9, 460, 475, 566
  see also community issues; cultural issues; demographic issues; deprivation, social; education; environmental issues; families; historical perspectives; housing; interpersonal relationships; legislation; lifestyle factors; needs; policy issues;

social/socioeconomic issues (*cont.*)
political issues; poverty; psychological issues; resources; support networks; technology in society; violence
social paediatrics 22–35
associations 29
concepts/definitions **3–10**, 17–21, 23, 30
ESSOP 21–2, 26, 30, 32, 363, 377
practice/practitioners 19–20, 23, **24–6, 525–39**
research 9, 18–20, 22–3, **26–9**, 30–5
special needs 25, 29, 335, 463
teaching/training 10, 18–20, **24–6**, 29–30
social services 463, 465, 475, 491
soil pollution 153, 156, **158**, 159, 161, 170
soldiers, child 43, 112, **120**, 123
special needs (chronic illness and disability) 331–57
adolescents 334, 341–57
child abuse 318, 320, 324
community participation 560–1, 564
developing countries **48**, 50, 52, 341–3, 353
education 202, 331–4, **335–8**, 343, 386
ethnic minorities 332, 429
European demographic trends 95, 333–5, 341–4
growth and development 222–3, 332–6, 347–9
health promotion/services 353, 459, 461, **463**, 466
outcome/performance measures 479
parent partnership **336–7**, 338, 351, 541, **544–5**
poverty 332, 343, 372
premature babies 262–3, 384, 386, 388, 390, 488
quality of life 571, 573, 584
social paediatrics 25, 29, 335, 463
UN Convention 42
in war 122
see also mental handicap/retardation
speech and language
child abuse 320
child development 210, 213, **216–17**, 218, 222
ethnic minorities 419–20, 427
nutritional deficiency 288
prematurity 388
special needs 332, 333, 336
spina bifida 345, 347
sports injuries 175
staffing issues, *see* health professionals
starvation, *see* nutrition/nutritional disorders
stature, *see* height
stereotyping 347, 412, 420, 430, 517
stillbirths 134, 481

see also neonatal mortality
stress
child abuse 323–6
divorce 402
growth and development 218, 221
mortality in Europe 88
pollution 154, 165
post-traumatic stress disorder 114–15, 117, 321
pregnancy 516, 545
premature babies 527, 533–4
quality of life 572
resilience 442
at school 461
SIDS 302
special needs 349, 350–1
wartime 114, 115
substance abuse, *see* alcohol; drug abuse; smoking
sudden infant death syndrome (SIDS) 98, 140, **297–309**, 385, 488
suicide
adolescents 100, 231, 240
child abuse 321
quality of life index 582
refugees 418
unemployment 460
sunlight 154, 164, 279–80, 426
support networks
child abuse 326
community participation 564
family breakdown 398, 402–3, 406, 409
HIV infection 142–3
intersectoral approaches 469
low birth-weight babies 388–90
parent partnership 544–6
quality of life 576–84
risk/resilience 442, 449–50
see also interpersonal relationships
survival, *see* life-expectancy/survival
syphilis 142, 240, 316, 498

targets
child health services 495–6
healthy city 363
WHO, *see* Health for All by the Year 2000
teaching, *see* education
technology in society 515
developing countries 51, 59
diagnostic 512
infant mortality 98
pollution 154
reproductive 259–63, **264–8**, 381, 390, 527, 531
special needs 344, 353
teenagers, *see* adolescents
teeth 103, 245, 484
temperament, *see* personality factors

Subject index

temperature
  extemes of 154
  premature babies 380
  SIDS 301–2
teratogenesis 164, 321
terrorism 437
tetanus 498, 500–2, 509
  developing countries 53, 58, 62
  SIDS 301
thalassaemia 422–3, 425, 490–1
tobacco 245
  see also smoking
toddlers, see infants; pre-school children
torture 43, **114**, 310, 318
toxicity, see poisoning
toys, see recreation
trace elements 158, 274–5
traditional medicine 427, 541
traffic accidents 175–7, 180–4, 188–9
  adolescents **229–30**, 234, 240, 249
  developing countries 57
  outcome/performance measures 485
  poverty 370
  quality of life 578, 582
training, see education
truancy 113, 244, 316, 318, 421
tuberculosis
  BCG vaccination 54, 58, 138, 500
  developing countries 53, 54, 58
  ethnic minorities 421, 426
  and HIV infection 136, 138, 142–3, 510

ultrasound testing 381, 423
ultraviolet light 154, 164, 279–80, 426
UN Conference on Environment and
    Development (1992) 151, 169
UN Convention on the Rights of the Child
    (1989) v, vi, 36–44
  accidents/safety 183
  family breakdown 406, 407
  nutrition 270
  parent partnership 542
  poverty 362–3
  quality of life 577, 582
  reproductive technologies 259–61, 264
  war and children 43, 122–3
unemployment 323, 363, 367–9, 460, 475, 566
UN Environmental Programme 169
UNESCO 60–1
UNICEF 6, 56, 58, 122, **183–4**, 577
urban areas, see cities
urinary problems 164, 300, 316

vaccination, see immunization
varicella vaccine 510
vegetarian diets 280, 282, 287, 288, 426

verbal skills, see speech and language
Vietnamese 289–90, 322, 414
violence
  accidents 183
  adolescents 246, 462
  family 199, 211
  institutionalized 202
  military/war 111–23
  punishment 204, 422
  torture 43, **114**, 310, 318
vision 100
  growth and development 210, 213
  prematurity 262, 267, 386
  quality of life 580
  special needs 342, 345
vitamins 56, 275–83, 287–9, 426
voluntary sector
  accident prevention 186, 187, 190
  community participation 563
  health promotion 472–3, 475
  HIV infection 143
  special needs 337
vulnerability, see risk factors/risk-taking

war 43, 109–27, 285
water pollution 153–6, **158**, 159–62, 165, 169–70, 374, 566
weaning 56, 275–7, 280, 282–3, 288–9
weight
  child abuse 316–17, 320
  nutrition 278–9, 285, 288
  outcome/performance measures 495
  quality of life 576
  special needs 332, 345
  see also low birth-weight; growth and development; obesity
welfare/well-being, see psychological issues; quality of life
WHO 7
  accident prevention 185, 186
  breast milk substitutes 272–4
  child survival and development 56
  EPI 58, 498
  health definition 12, 513, 572
  health promotion 513
  healthy cities programme 363
  HIV and immunizations 138
  pollution management 169
  special needs definitions 386–8
  targets, see Health for All by the Year 2000
whooping cough, see pertussis
women
  HIV 128, 132, 139, 142–3, 517
  immunization 502
  smoking 516
  see also gender issues; mothers

World Health Organization, *see* WHO

yellow fever vaccination 58
young adults
  developing countries 54
  growth and development 215
  health promotion 514–19
  health target 16–20
  quality of life 579
  risk-taking 225, 245–6
  sexuality 54, 515–17
  special needs 334, 341–57
  unemployment 460
  and war 111, 119, 120, 121
  see also adolescents